Meeting Children's Psychosocial Needs Across the Health-Care Continuum

Meeting Children's Psychosocial Needs Across the Health-Care Continuum

Judy A. Rollins, PhD, RN
Rosemary Bolig, PhD
and
Carmel C. Mahan, MSEd, CCLS

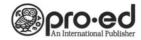
pro·ed
An International Publisher

8700 Shoal Creek Boulevard
Austin, Texas 78757-6897
800/897-3202   Fax 800/397-7633
www.proedinc.com

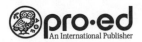
An International Publisher

© 2005 by PRO-ED, Inc.
8700 Shoal Creek Boulevard
Austin, Texas 78757-6897
800/897-3202   Fax 800/397-7633
www.proedinc.com

Library of Congress Cataloging-in-Publication Data

Rollins, Judy.
    Meeting children's psychosocial needs across the health-care continuum / by Judy A. Rollins,
Rosemary Bolig, and Carmel C. Mahan.
        p. cm.
    Includes bibliographical references and index.
    ISBN 0-89079-992-X (alk. paper)
    1. Pediatrics—Psychological aspects.   2. Pediatrics—Social aspects.   3. Children—Hospital
care—Psychological aspects.   4. Children—Hospital care—Social aspects.   5. Children—Diseases—
Psychological aspects.   6. Children—Diseases—Social aspects.   7. Sick children—Psychology.
8. Child health services.   9. Physician and patient.   I. Bolig, Rosemary.   II. Mahan, Carmel C.
III. Title.

RJ47.5.R656 2005
618.92—dc22

2004052942

Art Director: Jason Crosier
Designer: Nancy McKinney-Point
This book is designed in Janson Text, Triplex, Gill Sans, Helvetica, and OPTISchneidler.

Printed in the United States of America

1 2 3 4 5 6 7 8 9 10   08 07 06 05 04

Contents

3   Play in Children's Health-Care Settings   77
Rosemary Bolig

4   The Arts in Children's Health-Care Settings   119
Judy A. Rollins

5   The Child with Special Health-Care Needs   175
Elizabeth Ahmann and Judy A. Rollins

9 Spiritual Issues in Children's Health-Care Settings   351
Lynn B. Clutter

10 Cultural Influences in Children's Health Care   421
Lacretia Johnson

11 Ethical, Moral, and Legal Issues in Children's Health Care   455
Teresa A. Savage

Illustrations

FIGURES

TABLES

CASE STUDIES

Preface

Throughout history, families and concerned professionals have overcome many challenges in their efforts to humanize health-care encounters for children. Many programs aimed at educating health-care professionals now include content about meeting the psychosocial needs of children and their families. Today's financially driven health-care climate, with its emphasis on managed care, threatens to undermine these accomplishments and curtail the development of new approaches.

Significant changes have occurred in health-care services for children, and the system itself remains in transition. Federal legislation, financial considerations, and societal expectations of the role of families often shift, depending on where the services take place and who provides them. In addition, not since the turn of the 20th century has the United States experienced more cultural diversity than in the last two decades, a factor that creates a whole new dynamic in children's health care. A renewed interest in "healing" health care to complement "curing" health care has sparked attention to alternative and complementary medicine practices as well.

It is time to revisit these critical issues in children's health care. *Meeting Children's Psychosocial Needs Across the Health-Care Continuum* integrates current research and theory within the framework of the new and transitioning health-care environment. Despite the changes we experience now and in the future, children in health-care settings—in the home, child care center, school, community agency, ambulatory setting, or hospital—continue to need what they have always needed: the basics, such as nurturing, predictability, adequate stimulation, interaction, a sense of control, and mastery of their environments.

The brisk pace of medical discoveries enables more children to be saved through science and technology today than ever in the past. Accompanying each new discovery, treatment, or protocol are implications for psychosocial and developmental concerns. We hope that this book will foster a commitment in the reader to keep pace with new discoveries and to consider the impact they may have, not only on children's bodies but also on their young minds and spirits.

Judy A. Rollins
Rosemary Bolig
Carmel C. Mahan

Authors and Contributors

Judy A. Rollins, PhD, RN
Rollins & Associates, Inc.
1406 28th Street NW
Washington, DC 20007
   and
Georgetown University School of Medicine
Department of Family Medicine
Washington, DC 20007

Rosemary Bolig, PhD
University of the District of Columbia
Faculty of Early Childhood Education
   and
Child Associates
3839C Rodman Street, NW
Washington, DC 20016

Carmel C. Mahan, MSEd, CCLS
Baltimore County Public Schools
Southeast Infants and Toddlers Program
7801 E. Collingham Dr., Room 109
Baltimore, MD 21222

Elizabeth Ahmann, ScD, RN
3307 Belleview Avenue
Cheverly, MD 20785

Lynn B. Clutter, MSN, RN, BC, CNS
Langstrom University, Tulsa
School of Nursing & Health Professions
700 N. Greenwood, North Hall, Room 360
Tulsa, OK 74106-0700

Lacretia Johnson, MA
University of Vermont
Community Service Department of
   Student Life
48 University Place
Burlington, VT 05405

David A. Julian, PhD
The John Glenn Institute for Public
   Service and Public Policy
Center for Learning Excellence
807 Kinnear Road
Columbus, OH 43212-1421

Teresa W. Julian, PhD, RN, CFNP
Columbus Children's Research Institute
Columbus Children's Hospital, Inc.
700 Children's Drive
Columbus, OH 43205

Lois J. Pearson, MEd, CCLS
Children's Hospital of Wisconsin
PO Box 1997
Milwaukee, WI 53021

Teresa A. Savage, PhD, RN
University of Illinois at Chicago
College of Nursing
845 S. Damen, Room 846
Chicago, IL 60612

Mardelle McCuskey Shepley, DArch
Texas A&M University
College of Architecture
College Station, TX 77843-3137

Introduction

The past century has produced tremendous changes in the way health-care professionals view the needs of children and families. In the first half of the century, it was common practice for children to be admitted to hospitals for lengthy stays with only limited family contact. Staff observed that children cried when their parents left, and because it was so time-consuming to console them, they concluded that parental visits were "disruptive" to the children. At about this time, researchers began to look at the impact of increasing parental presence on parents' satisfaction with their child's hospitalization. When staff observed that parental presence changed children's behavior, the research expanded to include children's reactions, preparation, length of stay, pain management, and other issues.

During this time, children were commonly "seen and not heard," and their feelings and needs were rarely discussed when family decisions were made, including decisions that involved their health care. Health-care professionals, in fear of upsetting the child, frequently counseled parents to avoid telling their child that he or she was going to the hospital. Naturally, the child was most upset when suddenly separated from the parents without explanation, changed into unfamiliar clothes, put into a strange bed, and subjected to painful and frightening tests, procedures, and surgeries.

Since the mid-1930s (Beverly, 1936), research on children's reactions to hospitalization, surgery, or other health-care encounters has demonstrated that children are vulnerable to and have adverse emotional reactions to these events that may persist over time. Findings from early studies—Edelston (1943), Levy (1945), Prugh, Staub, Sands, Kirschbaum, and Lenihan (1953), Skipper and Leonard (1968), Vaughn (1957), Vernon, Schulman, and Foley (1966), and others—consistently demonstrated such effects.

Today, lengthy hospitalizations are rare, with the average pediatric stay at 3½ days (Owens, Thompson, Elixhauser, & Ryan, 2003). Children undergo surgery in the out-patient setting in the morning and are home by afternoon. Advances in technology, such as monitors and other medical equipment designed for home use, have led to sophisticated home treatments that previously were delivered to children only in hospital intensive care units. At the same time, illness and injury prevention and health promotion have brought primary care to the forefront in health care for both adults and children. In an environment of multiple health-care settings and levels of care, professionals and families concerned with humanistic health care have focused attention on smooth and seamless transitions for children as they move throughout the health-care system.

The Continuum of Care

Most children in today's health-care system experience several phases of care. These various phases are often referred to as the *continuum of care:* the progression through and between the various phases of care (Olson, 1999), which varies from child to child, depending upon diagnosis and individual needs. Although every experience is unique, each of the 10 phases has inherent psychosocial stressors for the child and family. Considering the circumstances children and families experience at each phase is helpful because circumstances, in part, dictate differences in stressors and therefore help predict their responses (see Table I.1).

Another way to view health-care services is to look at levels of care. There are three levels: primary, secondary, and tertiary. For definitions of these levels and the services provided, see Table I.2.

A child's continuum of care need not include all of the phases or levels of care, and circumstances determine where the child enters the continuum. For example, a child injured playing football may enter the continuum through emergent care, receive treatment, and be sent home to recover. Another child may be diagnosed with leukemia as part of a routine health examination at the primary care provider. He or she may be sent to an outpatient specialist—a pediatric oncologist—for a complete diagnostic workup, moved to intermediate care within a hospital for initial chemotherapy, sent home with instructions to return to the oncologist at scheduled times, moved back to the hospital with fever and neutropenia, and sent home when the crisis has passed. Later, the child may again return to the hospital for intermediate care or be transferred to an intensive care setting for a bone marrow transplant.

Managed Care

Movement along the continuum of care requires coordination. Perhaps the most significant health-care trend in the 1990s was the proliferation of managed care. In 1992, more than half of the U.S. workforce was covered by a traditional indemnity plan provided by an employer; by 1998, an estimated 85% of Americans with employer-based coverage were enrolled in managed care plans (The Robert Wood Johnson Foundation, 1998).

Managed care is differentiated in several respects from the traditional academic medicine model in which physicians are trained. Managed care's

Table I.1

xxiii

Phases of Care and Selected Considerations

Phase	Selected Considerations
1. Identification of illness or injury	Sudden or prolonged Part of routine health examination or traumatic Requires immediate attention or a slower pace
2. Urgent care	Familiar care provider in familiar surroundings or unfamiliar care provider in strange surroundings
3. Emergent care	Transported in familiar mode (family car) by family member or unfamiliar mode (ambulance, helicopter) by unfamiliar health-care providers Family available or unavailable Retained at original facility or transferred to another facility with required specialty or pediatric expertise
4. Acute care setting within a hospital	Emergent or planned admission Pediatric or adult hospital Placed with age-mates or by diagnosis Family members accommodated (e.g., cot for parent at bedside) or not
5. Intensive care	Transfer planned or unplanned Familiar primary care provider's continued involvement or total transfer to pediatric specialty Family members welcomed or not
6. Intermediate care	Transferred from higher level of care (intensive care, with family accustomed to close monitoring of child) or from lower level of care (outpatient facility) Transfer decision considered family's readiness or transfer dictated by the facility
7. Rehabilitation	Transferred to unit within present facility or transferred to a different facility Rehabilitation included in medical insurance benefits or not included
8. Outpatient specialty care	Occurred as part of diagnostic workup or as part of recovery and follow-up care Involved surgical/invasive procedures or uninvasive monitoring Involved preparation at home before arrival or no preparation Involved follow-up instructions for home care or no follow-up home care
9. Home care	Initiated with previous hospitalization or without previous hospitalization Included multiple care providers or a limited number of familiar care providers
10. Transition from acute to chronic illness	Expected or unexpected (e.g., occurred over time due to recurrence of health problem or natural course of disease, or as a complication of illness or injury) Response of child and family to diagnosis and treatment focus similar from response to acute illness, or different

Note. Adapted from "Acute Illness: The Continuum of Care," by C. Olson, 1999, in M. Broome & J. Rollins (Eds.), *Core Curriculum for Nursing Care of Children and Their Families* (pp. 215–221). Pitman, NJ: Jannetti. Copyright 1999 by Jannetti. Adapted with permission.

Table I.2

Levels of Care

Level	Definition	Services
Primary	Basic health services for medical monitoring, care of routine health problems, immunizations, and anticipatory guidance in the clinic or office setting	Health promotion and prevention Routine acute illnesses and injuries Ongoing management/monitoring of nonroutine problems Child and family education and counseling Family support and networking services Case management
Secondary	Direct services by members of an interdisciplinary team of specialized consultants, as needed, for complex and unusual health problems in a community hospital setting	Complex and specialized interdisciplinary services Child and family education and counseling Education and training for primary health-care providers Development of a service and education plan for community
Tertiary	Direct services by highly specialized members of an interdisciplinary team and specialized consultants, as needed, for complex and unusual health problems in a medical center or university health science center setting	Highly complex and specialized services by interdisciplinary team Child and family education counseling Education and training for primary health-care providers and other professionals Development of individualized hospital discharge plans Development of collaborative community service projects Research

Note. Adapted from "Chronic Conditions: The Continuum of Care," by W. Nehring, 1999, in M. Broome & J. Rollins (Eds.), *Core Curriculum for the Nursing Care of Children and Their Families* (pp. 331–341). Pitman, NJ: Jannetti. Copyright 1999 by Jannetti. Adapted with permission.

foundation is population-based medicine, which is essentially prevention. This means pooling resources to achieve a maximally fair distribution of resources. The ethic in managed care is to do what works and only what works. A different set of values guide the academic medical model: Everything that can possibly be done is done for the individual patient and continues to be done even when a situation looks futile. Another key difference involves decision making. In a managed care medical model, the physician uses a set of regulations and guidelines to decide on a course of action, and must present strong justification for doing otherwise. The academic model promotes autonomous decision making that results in huge variations in the quality of care and little in the way of effective standardized treatment, which is sometimes called "evidence-based medicine." Recognizing these and other significant differences in models, innovative training programs aimed at preparing physicians to work effectively in managed care settings are being implemented (see box).

Children's Voices

Today, we recognize that children have strong feelings about, reactions to, and the right to full participation in events in their lives, or the lives of their family members, friends, and classmates. According to the United Nations Convention on the Rights of the Child, child participation entails the act of encouraging and enabling children to make their views known on the issues that affect them (Bellamy, 2003). In *The State of the World's Children 2003*, Bellamy disputes some of the common myths about child participation (see Table I.3).

Along the continuum of care, ethicists and other concerned professionals and parents have advocated for policies that give children a greater voice in matters that affect them. Researchers, rather than asking only parents or health-care professionals about children's experiences, now also are more likely to ask the children themselves. Research methods such as drawing, which allow children to use more developmentally appropriate "languages," are on the rise. We have learned that children, given the proper forum, have little difficulty in expressing their points of view.

Psychosocial Care Across the Health-Care Continuum

There are now almost 80 years of increasingly sophisticated research on the effects of hospitalization and other health-care experiences on children and their families. With a rapidly changing health-care environment, the health-care system for children both looks and serves children differently than it did in the recent past.

A major question, however, still remains: Are children different? Are their needs and capacities to cope with the demands of illness, treatments, and health-care environments different than those of children during the previous periods of health care? Although home care may alleviate separation, are there other new risks in treating children? Do children require less continuity of care and support from those closest to them during periods of most demand? Do children acquire or express knowledge in new ways? Are they

<table>
<tr><td>

Preparing Physicians To Work in Managed Care Settings

</td><td>

Employers, government agencies, medical students, and graduates have demanded curricular revision in medicine and training in managed health-care environments to prepare physicians for practice in managed care settings. Through the work of the Council on Graduate Medical Education (COGME), educators, clinicians, and government officials have defined core competencies that are requisite to the education and preparation of future physicians. For a discussion of these core competencies and suggested strategies for implementation, see MacKinnon (2000).

</td></tr>
</table>

Table I.3

Child Participation: Myth and Reality

Myth	Reality
Child participation means choosing one child to represent children's perspectives and opinions in an adult forum.	Children are *not* a homogeneous group, and no one child can be expected to represent the interests of his or her peers of different ages, races, ethnicities, and gender. Children need forums of their own in which they can build skills, identify their priorities, communicate in their own way, and learn from their peers. In this way, children are better able to make their own choices as to who should represent their interests and in which ways they would like their viewpoints represented.
Child participation involves adults handing over all their power to children who are not ready to handle it.	Participation does *not* mean that adults simply surrender all decision-making power to children. The Convention on the Rights of the Child (CRC) is clear that children should be given more responsibility—according to their "evolving capacities" as they develop. In many cases, adults continue to make the final decision, based on the best interests of the child—but with the CRC in mind, it should be a decision informed by the views of the child. As children grow older, parents are encouraged to allow them more responsibility in making decisions that affect them—even those that may be controversial, such as custody matters following a divorce.
Children should be children, and not be forced to take on responsibilities that should be given to adults.	Children should certainly be allowed to be children, and to receive all the protection necessary to safeguard their healthy development. And no children should be forced to take on responsibilities for which they are not ready. But children's healthy development also depends upon being allowed to engage with the world, making more independent decisions, and assuming more responsibility as they become more capable. Children who encounter barriers to their participation may become frustrated or even apathetic; 18-year-olds without the experience of participation will be poorly equipped to deal with the responsibilities of democratic citizenship.

(continues)

In 1996, the Pew Charitable Trusts launched a network of pilot residency programs called Partnerships for Quality Education (Boodman, 1999). Designed to improve the training of young doctors, these partnerships train primary care residents to practice high-quality medicine in managed care settings by pairing academic institutions with managed care companies. Participants include Georgetown University Medical Center and Kaiser Permanente, Harvard Medical School and Harvard Pilgrim Health Care, and Cornell University Medical College and Empire Blue Cross Blue Shield.

Table I.3 *Continued.*

Child Participation: Myth and Reality

Myth	Reality
Child participation is merely a sham. A few children, usually from an elite group, are selected to speak to powerful adults who then proceed to ignore what the children have said while claiming credit for "listening" to kids.	Child participation, in many instances, has proven to be very effective. Rather than setting up an ineffectual system, it is up to all of us to devise meaningful forms of participation that benefit children and, in turn, society as a whole.
Child participation actually only involves adolescents, who are on the verge of adulthood anyway.	The public, political face of child participation is more likely to be that of an adolescent than of a 6-year-old, but it is essential to consult children of all ages about the issues that affect them. This means participation within schools and families when decisions about matters there are being discussed. At every age, children are capable of more than they are routinely given credit for—and they will usually rise to the challenges set before them if adults support their efforts.
No country in the world consults children on all the issues that affect them, and no country is likely to do so soon.	That is partly true. However, all countries that have ratified the Convention on the Rights of the Child have committed themselves to ensuring participation rights for children (e.g., the rights to freely express their views on matters that affect them and the freedom of thought, conscience, religion, association, and peaceful assembly). And almost every country can now show significant advances in setting systems and policies in place to allow children to exercise these rights.
Children may be consulted as a matter of form but their views never change anything.	Where children's views are sensitively solicited and sincerely understood, they often create a great deal of change: they may reveal things that adults would never have grasped independently, they can profoundly change policies or programs and, in some cases, they can protect children from future harm. The consultation of even very young children can produce remarkable results. The problem is that such careful consultation of children remains rare.

(continues)

Table I.3 *Continued.*

Child Participation: Myth and Reality

Myth	Reality
Children's refusal to participate negates their rights.	Actually, resistance itself can be an important part of participation. Whether in the give and take of the home, in the refusal to accept punishment at school, or in one's attitude towards civic engagement in the community, resistance can signal a child's or adolescent's opinion about an issue or feeling about the terms of his or her involvement. Adults should recognize resistance as a form of communication and respond to it through understanding, dialogue, and negotiation, rather than by trying to prevent it through force or persuasion. In no situation should children be forced to participate.

Note. From "The State of the World's Children," by C. Bellamy, 2003, New York: UNICEF.

more adaptive than we previously believed? Do the programs and policies instituted to respond to the earlier identified causes of children's upset completely mitigate the stresses faced in today's hospital, home care, and associative settings? Or are there new demands, new risks, new challenges for children and families?

Meeting Children's Psychosocial Needs Across the Health-Care Continuum reopens the dialogue as we look at children's health care in today's environment.

Chapter 1: Children's Hospitalization and Other Health-Care Encounters highlights the impact of a developmental approach to pediatric and family-centered care, and explores interventions that may make a difference in the reactions of children, siblings, and other family members to hospitalization and other encounters with the health-care system.

Chapter 2: Preparing Children for Health-Care Encounters explores stress and coping as well as the history and theories behind various methods of preparing children for health-care encounters.

Chapter 3: Play in Children's Health-Care Settings describes play, its functions and forms, the present state of theory and research on play, and the current thinking of play researchers in health care and other contexts.

Chapter 4: The Arts in Children's Health-Care Settings discusses ways that children use the arts as tools for coping with illness and health-care experiences, describes related research findings and applications, and concludes with recommendations for individuals wishing to use the arts with children or to establish arts programming in children's health-care settings.

Chapter 5: The Child with Special Health-Care Needs addresses psychosocial issues for children with special health-care needs in hospitals, the home, and the community.

Chapter 6: The Child Who Is Dying looks at the needs and issues of the child who is dying, the impact of death at home or in the hospital within the context of palliative care, and the unique characteristics of grief for parents, siblings, grandparents, and others.

Chapter 7: Families in Children's Health-Care Settings explores issues that health-care professionals need to consider when working with families along the health-care continuum, with an emphasis on the health-care professional as an agent for change.

Chapter 8: The Health-Care Environment summarizes terms and objectives of psychosocial issues as defined by environmental psychologists, provides examples of alternative design philosophies, offers guidelines for pediatric hospitals and alternative caregiving environments, and describes more controversial dimensions of healing environments.

Chapter 9: Spiritual Issues in Children's Health-Care Settings provides an overview of spirituality, followed by theoretical and developmental aspects of spirituality and a description of spiritual care.

Chapter 10: Cultural Influences in Children's Health Care presents the dimensions of culture, the within-group complexity found among members of any given culture, and information about developing cross-cultural competence.

Chapter 11: Ethical, Moral, and Legal Issues in Children's Health Care reviews familiar ethical, moral, and legal issues; challenges conventional thinking on these issues; and raises new issues to be faced.

Chapter 12: Relationships in Children's Health-Care Settings explores the types of relationships that develop between health-care professionals and the children and families they serve, and the relationships that develop among members of the health-care team.

Meeting Children's Psychosocial Needs Across the Health-Care Continuum concludes with an epilogue that addresses trends in children's health care, providing thought-provoking ideas for new directions in psychosocial care of children and their families across the health-care continuum.

References

Bellamy, C. (2003). *The state of the world's children 2003*. New York: UNICEF.

Beverly, B. (1936). The effects of illness upon emotional development. *Journal of Pediatrics*, *8*, 533–543.

Boodman, S. (1999). The education of Dr. Kulick. *The Washington Post Health*, *15*(5), 12–15, 17.

Edelston, H. (1943). Separation anxiety in young children: Study of hospital cases. *Genetic Psychological Monographs*, *26*, 3–95.

Levy, D. (1945). Psychic trauma of operations in children. *American Journal of Diseases of Children*, *7*, 69–70.

MacKinnon, G. (2000). Preparing medical students for the changing healthcare environment in the United States. *Journal of the American Osteopathic Association*, *100*(9), 560–564.

Nehring, W. (1999). Chronic conditions: The continuum of care. In M. Broome & J. Rollins (Eds.), *Core curriculum for the nursing care of children and their families* (pp. 331–341). Pitman, NJ: Jannetti.

Olson, C. (1999). Acute conditions: The continuum of care. In M. Broome & J. Rollins (Eds.), *Core curriculum for the nursing care of children and their families* (pp. 215–221). Pitman, NJ: Jannetti.

Owens, P., Thompson, J., Elixhauser, A., & Ryan, J. (2003). *Care of children and adolescents in hospitals.* Rockville, MD: Agency for Healthcare Research and Quality.

Prugh, D., Staub, E., Sands, H., Kirschbaum, R., & Lenihan, E. (1953). A study of the emotional reactions of children and families to hospitalization and illness. *American Journal of Orthopsychiatry, 23,* 70–106.

Skipper, J., & Leonard, L. (1968). Children, stress and hospitalization. *Journal of Health and Social Behavior, 9,* 275–287.

The Robert Wood Johnson Foundation. (1998). Does managed care fit for rural America? *Advances, 4,* 1–2.

Vaughn, G. (1957). Children in hospitals. *The Lancet, 272,* 1117–1120.

Vernon, D. T. A., Schulman, J. L., & Foley, J. M. (1966). Changes in children's behavior after hospitalization. *American Journal of Diseases of Children, 111,* 581–593.

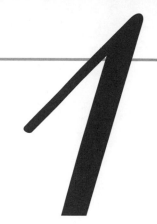

Children's Hospitalization and Other Health-Care Encounters

Lois J. Pearson

Objectives

At the conclusion of this chapter, the reader will be able to:

1. Describe the course of children's development and the potential impact of hospitalization and other health-care encounters at various stages.
2. Indicate the various reasons for children's responses at different stages and the counterinterventions appropriate to each stage.
3. Discuss the social, economic, technological, medical, and knowledge changes that have contributed to changes in child health-care policies and practices.
4. Suggest current and future challenges to children's abilities to cope and adapt in child health-care encounters.

Those of us who have spent many years working in hospitals have come to take much for granted. We know we are kind, benevolent, capable people interested in healing, the alleviation of suffering and the prolongation of life. However, a child coming into the hospital for the first time may see us quite differently. No matter how well we do our job, we are not his parents, the hospital bed is not his own, and the world we provide is an unfamiliar and frightening one. It is a world in which children are hurt. Every body orifice may be entered and when these are exhausted we create new openings by injection, by IV, cut-down or by surgery.

—Robinson, 1972, p. 1

These words, written in 1972 in a paper titled "The Psychological Impact of Illness and Hospitalization Upon the Child—Infancy to Twelve Years" by Mary Robinson, summarized the state of health care for children at the time and challenged pediatric health-care professionals to reform caregiving to better meet the unique psychosocial needs of children and families. The challenge came at a time when current research was documenting the deleterious effects of hospitalization on children of all ages. A review of more than 200 articles in 1965 concluded that emotional distress was common both during the period of hospitalization and after discharge. Between 1963 and 1983 many additional research articles documented the prevalence of psychologic upset following discharge from the hospital, including behavioral changes, increased separation anxiety, increased sleep anxiety, and increased aggression toward authority (Gaynard et al., 1990). In addition, retrospective studies noted that children who were hospitalized as young children demonstrated adjustment difficulties as adolescents, especially children who were hospitalized for longer than 1 week or had multiple admissions before the age of 5 years (Douglas, 1975; Quinton & Rutter, 1976).

Significant changes in pediatric health-care in the last 25 years, especially the institution of principles of family-centered care, have affected both the way that health-care is delivered to children and the psychosocial outcomes. A study in 1984 by Chess and Thomas documented that for school-age children, psychologic development sometimes includes stress, but that within a supportive environment with opportunities for mastery, hospitalization may result in psychologic benefits.

This chapter begins with a description of the characteristics of children in hospitals today. Next, the impact of a developmental approach to pediatric care is highlighted and the particular interventions that may make a difference in children's reactions to hospitalization are explored, along with a brief discussion on vulnerable and resilient children. Parents' and siblings' reactions to a child's hospitalization are explored, followed by a description of the emergency room experience. The chapter concludes with an overview of ambulatory and home health-care for children.

Characteristics of Children Hospitalized Today

According to Owens, Thompson, Elixhauser, and Ryan (2003), nearly two thirds of all childhood hospital stays are for newborns and neonates (babies up to 30 days old); nearly 95% of these stays are for the birth of infants in the hospital. The remaining third of pediatric hospital stays are for pediatric illnesses besides neonatal care and adolescent pregnancy (3%).

Although children younger than 1 year constitute only 1% of the U.S. population, they account for nearly 13% of all hospital stays; children 1 to 17 years account for 5% of all hospital stays (Owens et al., 2003). Excluding neonates and pregnant adolescents, 45% of hospital admissions for pediatric illness are routine, nonemergency admissions, and 44% are emergency department admissions. Children from low-income areas are 25% more likely to enter through the emergency department than children from higher income areas.

Infectious disease is a common reason for hospitalization throughout childhood. Injuries, including leg injuries, medication poisonings, and head injuries, are among the top reasons for hospital stays for 13- to 17-year-olds. However, asthma and pneumonia remain among the top 10 reasons for hospitalizations among all pediatric age groups (Owens et al., 2003).

Length of hospital stay for children varies by diagnosis. However, on average, children's stays in the hospital are 29% shorter than adult stays

(Owens et al., 2003). The following diagnoses are associated with the longest length of stay (p. 33):

- Prematurity, low birth weight, and fetal growth retardation
- Respiratory distress in infancy
- Leukemia
- Respiratory failure
- Pre-adult mental disorders
- Cardiac and circulatory birth defects
- Aspiration pneumonitis
- Anxiety and personality disorders
- Affective disorders (primarily depression)
- Complications of device, implant, or graft

At discharge, children are less likely to receive home health-care services or long-term care than are adults. Thus, because demand for posthospital specialized care can be relatively infrequent for children, high-quality posthospital pediatric care may be limited in many areas.

A Developmental Approach

Children's reactions to hospitalization and other health-care experiences can be best understood through the lens of psychosocial development. Erikson's (1963) theory of personality development is the most widely accepted and used in pediatrics (Wong, Perry, & Hockenberry, 2002). Built on Freudian theory, Erikson's theory emphasizes a healthy personality as opposed to a pathological approach. According to Erikson, specific changes are assumed to take place during eight predictable age-related stages. Individuals face a unique conflict at each stage, which has two aspects: favorable and unfavorable (Erikson, 1959):

- Trust versus mistrust (birth to 1 year)
- Autonomy versus shame and doubt (1 to 3 years)
- Initiative versus guilt (3 to 6 years)
- Industry versus inferiority (6 to 12 years)
- Identity versus role confusion (12 to 18 years)
- Intimacy and solidarity versus isolation (the 20s)
- Generativity versus self-absorption (late 20s to 50s)
- Integrity versus despair (50s and beyond)

No core conflict is ever mastered completely. However, the individual must adequately resolve each conflict before progressing to the next stage.

Children's reactions to hospitalization at every developmental age are precipitated by the presence of stressful events. These may include separation, loss of control, bodily injury, and pain (Wong et al., 2002). In addition, the unfamiliarity of the hospital setting and reduced opportunities for developmentally appropriate activities contribute to the level of experienced stress (Johnson, Jeppson, & Redburn, 1992). How children respond to these stressors will be influenced not only by developmental age, but also by previous experience with illness, separation or hospitalization, innate or acquired coping skills, seriousness of the diagnosis, and available support systems (Wong et al., 2002).

The traditional belief is that children cared for on intensive care units will have more troublesome responses than will children cared for in general pediatric wards. However, recent research indicates this may not be the case. Rennick, Johnston, Dougherty, Platt, and Ritchie (2002) compared the psychologic responses of children hospitalized in a pediatric intensive care unit (PICU) with those hospitalized on a general ward to identify clinically relevant factors that might be associated with psychologic outcome. The researchers followed 120 children for 6 months after PICU and ward discharge, comparing groups of children based on their sense of control over their health, medical fears, posttraumatic stress, and changes in behavior, and examining relationships between children's responses and their age, the invasive procedures to which they were exposed, severity of illness, and length of hospital stay. As anticipated, children in the PICU spent more time in the hospital. However, because children admitted to hospital wards today are much sicker than those who were hospitalized a decade ago, Rennick et al. found that the children on the general wards received just as many invasive procedures as did the children on the PICU. The primary difference was that the children on the PICU received more pain medication and sedation than did the children in the general wards. They concluded that, although no significant group differences were found, children who were younger, more severely ill, and who endured more invasive procedures had significantly more medical fears, a lower sense of control over their health, and ongoing posttraumatic stress responses 6 months post discharge.

Although other factors affect the child's response to hospitalization, as mentioned above, a developmental approach is the most commonly used method for addressing psychosocial needs. The following sections describe concerns, responses, and interventions for children—infants through adolescents—who are hospitalized.

Infants: Newborn to 6 Months

I was wheeled over to Julia, and got my first good look at her. I felt like I'd been drenched in ice water. She had on only the little hat and a tiny diaper. She had tubes up her nose, in her arms, and in her feet. She had electrodes on her chest, back, and sides. Her eyes were covered to protect them from the lights, which shone around the clock. She looked so frail, helpless, and so small. I started to cry and didn't stop until long after I was

*in my new bed. J couldn't do anything to help her, and J was
so afraid that she would die. (Rapacki, 1991, p. 15)*

The hospitalization of a newborn creates a myriad of stresses for new parents. The presence of complex medical equipment in a strange and unfamiliar environment, and the reality of a very ill baby, challenge the basic parenting skills that usually focus on becoming acquainted with, feeding, and comforting a new little person. Frequently exhausted by the emotional and physical demands of labor and delivery, the process of integrating medical information comes at a time when parents are least able to do so.

Care in the neonatal intensive care unit (NICU) is required to be family-centered as much as "infant-centered" (Thurman, 1990). Numerous studies have demonstrated that supporting parents in the NICU helps reduce stresses and positively affects the parent–infant relationship over time. A study by Lally and Phelps (1994) documents the importance of security, protection, and intimacy for a level of trust to develop between infant and family. When these needs are not met, infants may become depressed, develop failure to thrive, or show signs of hospitalism. (The term *hospitalism* was first used by Spitz [1945] to describe the inability of infants to survive in institutional settings.)

Family-centered care principles within the neonatal intensive care unit recognize that, over time, the family has the greatest impact on a baby's health and well-being. Dr. Gretchen Lawhon states, "When two critically ill infants have the same clinical diagnosis, the one who has family present, pulling for him or her and actively participating in care, will almost always do better" (Johnson, 1995, p. 11). In addition to open and 24-hour visiting, family-centered care includes family advocacy, family-to-family support, and a view of parents as participants in care—not visitors to the NICU (Johnson, 1995). (For more details on family-centered care, see Chapter 5: The Child with Special Health-Care Needs.) Innovative programs to support these practices include the following:

- Parent advisory councils to address parent concerns
- Weekly parent support group meetings
- Parent representation with staff on hospital family-centered care committees to plan environmental modifications to improve family comfort
- Improved communication between professionals and parents, such as orientation videos for parents and parent communication books

The Newborn Individualized Developmental Care and Assessment Program (NIDCAP) was developed as a foundation for the provision of developmentally supportive care in the neonatal intensive care unit (Als & Gilkerson, 1995). The plan begins with detailed observations of infant behavior and builds on the infant's unique strategies in creating a plan of care, including the infant's autonomic, motor, and state systems. These observations help both professionals and parents to respond to the infant's many cues in providing supportive care.

The NIDCAP framework also describes a developmental care environment that includes

- *Consistency of care giving*—Each infant is assigned a primary multidisciplinary care team that includes the family to create an individualized care plan;
- *Structuring the infant's 24-hour day*—Cares should be clustered to respect the infant's sleep–wake cycles and to promote growth;
- *Pacing of care giving*—The family is an integral part of care giving as the infant begins to recognize parents' voice, touch, and feel and receives comfort and more stable physiological measures with family presence and participation;
- *Supports during transitions*—Infants often need increased support between care giving activities and between sleep and wakeful periods;
- *Appropriate positioning*—Placing the infant in special positions for cares and rest enhances the infant's ability to seek comfort and encourages stability;
- *Individualized feeding support*—Both method and schedule of feeding need to be based on each infant's individual needs and competencies, so that feeding is perceived as pleasurable;
- *Opportunities for skin-to-skin holding*—Kangaroo Care (see Figure 1.1) encourages respiratory stability and more restful sleep for infants, while helping parents to feel less anxious and more fulfilled;
- *Collaborative care*—All exams, procedures, and tests should be planned with the infant's primary care giver and parents present to provide comfort and lessen stress;
- *Quiet, soothing environment*—Measures like rocking chairs or recliners at the bedside for parents, homelike family spaces, and the ability to personalize the infant's bedside with family photos, soft music, clothing, and blankets help decrease family stress. Subtle lighting to reflect day/night sequencing and reduction of noise levels in special care nurseries are also important to reduce potentially harmful stimuli; and
- *Developmental support*—The caregiving team should include developmental care specialists as well as other disciplines to provide psychosocial care including social work, pastoral care, and child life. (Als & Gilkerson, 1995, pp. 5–6)

Research documenting the importance of developmental care principles for newborn intensive care units has demonstrated that high-risk infants (e.g., very low birth weight, ventilated patients) have improved medical outcomes, including decreased intercranial hemorrhages, reduced severity of chronic lung disease, improved growth, and earlier discharge. Similar results

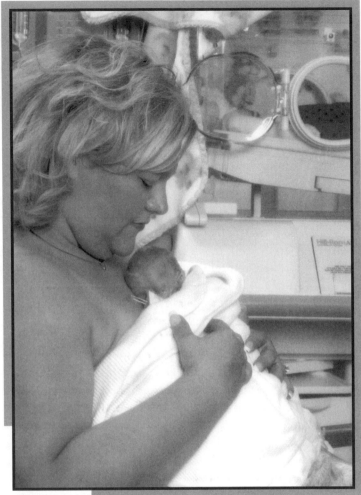

Figure 1.1.
Kangaroo Care offers the opportunity for skin-to-skin holding.
Note. Photograph used with permission of Children's Hospital of
Wisconsin.

are seen in healthy preterm infants, indicating that supporting and protecting the infant's developing nervous system improves brain functioning (Als
et al., 1994).

Older Infants: 6 Months to 1 Year

*Many years later a mother recalls her child's first hospital ad-
mission, "I stood outside the door of the treatment room for what
seemed like hours while they drew blood and started an IV. She
never stopped screaming but no one would let me come in to
comfort her."*

The developmental needs of older infants continue to be based on the ability of the infant to develop trust. Consistent, nurturing, and loving caregivers help the older infant become trusting. While the primary threat to this age group is separation anxiety (see next section), older infants are rapidly developing their own unique and engaging personalities. They control their environments and get their needs met by emotional expressions such as crying and smiling. When these cues are missed and the infant is unable to elicit nurturing responses, a feeling of distress and decreased sense of control may increase the infant's stress levels. Additional distresses result from restriction of movement (e.g., arm or leg restraints, IVs, lab draws) and changes in rituals and routines. Maximizing parental presence and participation in cares provides the greatest protection for the older infant's successful developmental growth and minimizes the disruptive effects of hospitalization. Creating a homelike environment that includes family photos, comfort objects such as familiar blankets and stuffed animals, favorite quieting music, and opportunities for exploration and movement beyond that possible within the crib, helps to ensure ongoing learning for the older infant.

Separation Anxiety

The primary source of stress for middle infancy through preschool-age children (ages 6 months through 3 years) is separation anxiety. Classic studies by Robertson (1958) and Bowlby (1960) describe a series of three stages in a young child's response to separation. The initial stage, *protest*, is an active and aggressive response to the absence of the parent, and is characterized by crying, screaming, or kicking while constantly watching for signs of the parent's return. The child refuses the attention of anyone else, and seems inconsolable. The protest stage may last from several hours to as long as a week. In the next stage, *despair*, the child stops crying and appears depressed. Bowlby describes this stage as one of increasing hopelessness. The child may continue to cry intermittently, but more often appears withdrawn and quiet. This behavior originally formed the basis for parent visiting policies in the 1950s and 1960s when the return of the parent caused the child to once again cry vigorously. The child's ability to bring his or her feelings of acute distress back to the surface was misinterpreted as "re-upsetting" the calm and complacent child who, in reality, had been in despair. The final stage, *detachment*, appears after a long period of parental absence and is characterized by the child's reinvestment in his or her surroundings and normal activity. The child copes with the pain of the parent's absence by forming superficial attachments to others, becoming increasingly self-centered, and becoming more interested in material objects (Bowlby, 1960). While the child appears to be recovering, the return of the parents is met with apathy and the child's inability to reattach. Detachment is the most serious stage, in that the adverse effects are less likely to be reversed. One of the positive outcomes of improvements in pediatric policies and increased family involvement in care is that the stage of detachment is seldom observed within the hospital setting. However, the first two stages—protest and despair—are more frequently observed, even with brief separations from either parent.

Toddlers: 1 to 3 Years

The parent of a 22-month-old child recalls, "The part that frightened me most was when he came back from a procedure completely sedated, and a staff member commented on how 'peaceful' he looked lying there. That immediately made me think of a comment often heard at funerals. It was the defining moment of feeling so helpless when prior to that I had always been able to make things better for him. All I wanted was for him to wake up and say 'Momma.' I didn't appreciate the peacefulness of that moment. Toddlers aren't supposed to be peaceful!"

As infants grow into toddlers, hospitalization creates new challenges as developmental norms focus on increasing autonomy and goal-directed behaviors. While parental presence is still the greatest need, toddlers learn by moving, exploring, playing, and engaging in socializing activities. With limited verbal skills, egocentric toddlers make their needs known in demonstrative ways, often reacting with frustration to restrictions of movement or changes in routine. They may perceive the hospital as punishment and if they experience pain for the first time, they may feel more confused when the parent does not rescue them from painful procedures. For this age group, the need to master experiences and gain autonomy is met through play. The presence of child life programming and opportunities to play at the bedside or in a playroom are crucial for the toddler, to ensure ongoing development (see Chapter 3: Play in Children's Health-Care Settings). While engaged in developmentally appropriate play activities, the toddler begins to master the new experience.

Because the hospital environment differs so drastically from the home environment, toddlers require the greatest attention to minimizing these differences as much as possible. Activities of daily living, home routines of bathing, eating, and playing should be respected as much as possible within the requirements of medical treatment. When toddlers experience severe restrictions and changes of routine, feelings of unpredictability and loss of control may cause them to regress to earlier and more secure developmental levels. While this regression may appear to provide comfort to the toddler, giving up newly acquired skills is difficult and may make toddlers more susceptible to negative responses to hospitalization (Wong et al., 2002).

It is important to remember that because toddlers have not yet developed a sense of body image or boundaries, intrusive procedures may be highly stressful regardless of whether pain is actual or perceived. This age group is able to remember painful procedures and may respond to similar tests and routines with physical resistance and uncooperativeness. Toddlers are often able to understand far more than they are able to express in words, and subsequently they benefit from preparation for procedures (see Chapter 2: Preparing Children for Health-Care Encounters). Parental participation in toddler interventions is important, both to provide security for the toddler during new experiences, but also to lessen a parent's anxiety by allowing the parent to engage in anticipatory coping. The presence of a prepared and less anxious parent will most often be evident in a more cooperative and less frightened toddler.

Preschoolers: 4 to 5 Years

A four-year-old bargains with the nurse, "Please don't give me a shot. I'll be good!"

Preschoolers are more secure than toddlers if they have had opportunities to develop trusting relationships through life experiences. Yet they are still very vulnerable to the stresses of hospitalization and medical care. In fact, Stanford and Thompson (1981) identify children ages 9 months through 4 years to be the most vulnerable to the negative effects of hospitalization. More independent than toddlers, preschoolers also suffer most from physical restrictions and loss of control. They may continue to view the hospital as punishment but now also engage in magical thinking: They believe that they have the ability to wish things to happen. For preschoolers, the reason for hospitalization, tests, and treatments must be concrete and hands-on. Using real equipment for preparation helps preschoolers understand and communicate. Again, play is the critical determinant for coping (see Chapter 3). Opportunities for medical play, preparation, and expressive play help the preschooler to understand, as well as help adults detect a child's fears, concerns, or misconceptions. Perhaps the egocentric nature of the preschooler is most obvious when a medical person appears at the playroom door and every preschooler in the playroom responds with the certainty that the person is there for them!

Preschoolers are particularly vulnerable to threats of bodily injury, as their concept of body integrity is not yet fully developed. Fears of mutilation are common and their inability to understand body functioning limits their ability to understand the need to "fix" a body part through surgery. In addition, a preschooler's concept of the cause of illness is complicated by their inability to separate themselves from the external world. Therefore, they perceive that you get a cold if you go out in the cold. This understanding includes a sense of blame or responsibility, reinforcing the preschooler's feelings of having done something wrong to be deserving of punishment. Addressing these preschool misconceptions in play and preparation provides the child with increased coping skills and lessened anxiety, while enabling the child to gain support through distraction (see Chapter 2).

Finally, in addressing the needs of the older infant, toddler, and preschool-age child, it is important to clearly establish *safe* places for children. Because the child's bed should be the ultimate "safe place," all invasive procedures should be done in a treatment room away from the child's bedside (Anderson, Zeltzer, & Fanurik, 1993). Without attention to this need for safety, a young child may not be able to sleep soundly, fearing that he or she will be approached at any moment for a painful procedure.

However, results of a more recent study (Fanurik et al., 2000) suggest that better guidelines for decisions related to the use of bedside versus treatment room need to take into account child-specific, procedural, and situational factors. Nurses surveyed in this study responded to a series of vignettes for children ages 3 years, 9 years, and 14 years who were scheduled for an intravenous insertion and a lumbar puncture, as to where they would want to perform each procedure. Nursing decisions considered the child's age, level of invasiveness of the procedure, child's coping skills, health condition, type of hospital room, developmental status, and parent's ability to assist their child. While decision making in some situations focused on medical issues, such as the stability of the patient to be moved, availability of equipment, and urgency of the procedure, others did consider psychosocial factors such as whether moving the patient to an unfamiliar space might heighten the child's anxiety level. The study did not consider levels of perceived or actual pain for the child, nor did the study attempt to define "invasiveness" of procedures. Implications for this research indicate that parents and children need education about the advantages and disadvantages of each setting and should be active participants in making the choice for bedside or treatment room use (Fanurik et al., 2000). It also prompts a greater awareness that what healthcare professionals view as invasive or noninvasive may not be similarly defined by the child. When a decision is made to use a treatment room, it should be designed to obscure the view of endless shelves of medical equipment and enhance coping through changes in lighting, music, or visual aids. The room should be large enough to accommodate not only the required medical staff performing the procedure, but also the child's identified support person, whether that be a child life specialist or family member, or both.

The other truly safe place should be the playroom where children may safely engage in play activities without the fear of intrusive examinations or procedural tasks being completed (see Chapter 3). Considerations of "psychosocial safety" for the child need to be continually emphasized as each new group of students, residents, and staff persons enters the pediatric environment.

The School-Age Child: 6 to 12 Years

They looked into my mouth and into my ears, they looked into my eyes and they touched my tummy. But they never looked at me.
                    —7-year-old hospitalized patient
(Association for the Care of Children's Health, 1990, p. 19)

School-age children are less vulnerable to the anxieties of hospitalization due to a number of developmental achievements. They are more social, able to be separated from parents for longer periods of time, and capable of cognitive reasoning. In addition, they are able to form trusting relationships with other adults and peers (Stanford & Thompson, 1981). As concrete operational thinkers, they are able to process information and understand relationships between events and experiences.

Earlier research on school-age children's ability to tolerate parental separation was based primarily on adult recollections. Yet in a more recent study, hospitalized children ages 8 through 11 years rated "being away from my family" higher than any other fears associated with hospitalization (Hart & Bossert, 1994). This is attributed to the psychosocial challenge of hospitalization and a tendency to regression, both of which increase the child's need to be with his or her family. Interventions to support family contact are important, including easy access to phone or email, unlimited family visiting, and supportive services for families while at the hospital.

Other significant fears identified in this study included "having to stay a long time, getting a shot, having my finger stuck, and the doctor or nurse telling me something is wrong with me" (Hart & Bossert, 1994, p. 87). Anticipated responses that were *not* supported by research or identified by the children as stressful were concerns about missing school or fears that they might die. These results also support Erikson's stage of industry versus inferiority, and the importance of school-age children performing the normal routines and tasks of their age group. It becomes important for school-age children to know the implications of disease or treatment and hospitalization for the present and also the future, as they are able to reason and cognitively process events and consequences.

The abilities identified above help to clearly define interventions to benefit the school-age child in the hospital. Activities of industry such as arts and crafts, creative writing or journaling, playing games, role-playing, socializing with other patients, and computer programming such as STARBRIGHT World (see box), help children express feelings, master experiences by learning new skills, and cope with required procedures and treatments. Involvement in child life programming and hospital school programs are critical for a child of this age to normalize the medical setting, provide structure and routine, as well as offer opportunities for peer group interaction. Because changes in appearance and body function are also important to this age group, the hospital serves as a safe and sheltered place where children can practice new skills and gain competence and confidence with physical changes that may result from illness or injury.

A final implication of the unique research of Hart and Bossert (1994) demonstrated no significant differences in the identified fears of chronically ill or acutely ill children, suggesting that prior experience or familiarity with the health-care system does not lessen children's fears. The authors attribute this finding to the fact that unknown fears are replaced by known fears. The need for preparation and supportive interventions seems to be just as great for chronically ill children who have been hospitalized before as for acutely ill children (Hart & Bossert, 1994).

Bossert (1994) also asked school-age children what stressful things happened to them in the hospital. From all of the children's responses, interviewers

STARBRIGHT
World

In November of 1995 an interactive computer network was launched specifically for children with serious medical conditions in hospitals. STARBRIGHT World is an integrated program based upon five methods of intervention: interpersonal communication, peer support, self-expression, knowledge and information, and distraction/affective elevation. Developed by the STARBRIGHT Foundation, the network links hospitalized children with serious illnesses to their homes all over the country. It offers children a virtual playground: an information center, games, text chat spaces, bulletin boards, e-mail, video conferencing, and a search engine to find others based on criteria such as medical condition, age, or interests. It reduces isolation and loneliness by connecting children in any part of the country who are facing similar chal-

identified six categories of events and examples of each as stated by the children. Table 1.1 lists the categories in descending order of frequency.

Adolescents

If you get sick and are suddenly thrown into a situation where strange people are poking at you, asking personal questions, sticking needles into your arms, and telling you why they want to put a plastic tube into your chest, it's really overwhelming.
—Elizabeth Bonwich, age 16
(Krementz, 1989, p. 68)

Erikson's developmental stage of adolescence is "Identity versus Identity Confusion" and therein lies the key to working with the hospitalized adolescent. Naturally seeking to separate from parents and family, teenagers develop a heightened dependence on peers and social groups. The hospital experience becomes threatening as it separates the teen from normal group activities, disrupts future plans, and increases insecurities about appearance and self-worth. The period of mid-adolescence, ages 14 to 18 years, is described as the most difficult time for an adolescent to be hospitalized. It is during this time when the peer group is especially important to developing self-image and independence, and doubts about sexual functioning are of greatest concern.

In addition to loss of social supports, hospitalization and illness frequently result in loss of independence and control, and adolescents may respond with feelings of anger and frustration. In general, younger adolescents are less vulnerable to these inherent risks because they have yet to develop strong emancipatory drives and more easily handle the increased dependency precipitated by the hospital experience (Stanford & Thompson, 1981). Simi-

lenges because of their condition or illness. Research demonstrates that children engaged in the distractive STARBRIGHT World activities experience less pain and anxiety and are more willing to return for treatment. The network is monitored and children may access other prescreened and approved Internet sites. The STARBRIGHT Foundation has recently begun a scholarship program that provides home computers to seriously ill children who otherwise do not have access to a computer at home so they can stay connected with supportive friends and resources. STARBRIGHT also develops educational CD-ROMs and videos with information and activities to assist children in coping with specific medical conditions.

Note. Adapted from STARBRIGHT World. Available at www.starbright.org/projects/sbworld/KCWK.html Adapted with permission.

larly, older adolescents, having attained a confident level of independence, develop improved parent relationships and may approach the stresses of hospitalization with adult-like coping skills (Hoffman, Becker, & Gabriel, 1976).

Interventions for adolescents should focus on peer group support. An adolescent unit that features an environment and policies specifically designed for adolescents will increase both coping and cooperation. Access to appropriate activities, video games, movies, cooking, a pool table, and music and computer access should all be featured in a teen room with programming designed exclusively for teens. As caring for children and their families is the sole mission of children's hospitals, claiming space for such a room or even a separate ward for adolescents typically is not an issue. However, for pediatric units in a general hospital, designating a separate room for this purpose may be challenging and perhaps not a priority for hospital decision makers. Nevertheless, with an awareness of the importance of such space for meeting the psychosocial needs of teenagers, health-care professionals have been very creative in capturing bits of space, for example, claiming a small seating area at the end of a corridor for teens to gather. Others have designated an area of the hospital playroom for teens only, and refer to the playroom as an "activity" room to label the space as appropriate for all ages.

Liberal visiting policies and opportunities for peer socialization require guidelines that are different from other areas of the hospital. Staff who understand and enjoy adolescents and who possess appropriate communication skills also have a positive effect on the coping of an adolescent. Information and preparation will lessen teen fears and anxiety while enhancing anticipatory coping. The ability to listen to adolescent concerns, answer questions, and enhance decision making should be an integral part of developmentally appropriate care.

Being in isolation is difficult for a child of any age, but it becomes especially difficult during adolescence, when peer relationships are often a central focus of everyday life and activity. When medical treatment will require isolation for a period of weeks, such as that required for a bone marrow

Table 1.1

Stressful Events School-Age Children Experience When Hospitalized, in Descending Order of Frequency

Category	Operational Definition	Examples
Intrusive events	Any event involving entry into the body through the skin or a natural body orifice	Injections, blood work, intravenous insertion, surgery, pills, nasogastric tubes, suppositories
Physical symptoms	Any physical symptom or sensation relating to the illness or treatment	Pain, nausea, side effects of medications such as blurry vision, dizziness, burning of intravenous medication
Therapeutic intervention	Any activity relating to treating or assessing the physical status of the child	Physical exam by doctor, palpation of abdomen, waking after surgery, being woken up at night, dressing change, removal of stitches
Restricted activity	Limitation of normal or desired activity due to illness or hospital rules	Bed rest, holding still during X rays, not allowed to leave unit, can't go outside
Separation	Any expression of concern due to separation from family, friends, or pets due to hospitalization	Parents' leaving, missing friends or pets
Environment	Any physical or interpersonal aspect of the child's environment	Cords and wires on walls that look like monsters at night, changing rooms, unpleasant or noisy roommates, impatient or "mad" doctors and nurses

Note. Adapted from "Stress Appraisals of Hospitalized School-Age Children," by E. Bossert, 1994, *Children's Health Care, 23*(1), pp. 33–49. Copyright 1994 by Erlbaum. Adapted with permission.

Theme Rooms

The child life specialist on an oncology unit helps teenagers prepare for isolation required for bone marrow transplants by creating a "theme room." After touring the unit and talking about the adolescent's likes and dislikes, favorite activities, and usual routines, the new patient and staff design the room around a theme. It might be a place that the teen hopes to visit, or perhaps a fantasy place from his or her own imagination. Seventeen-year-old Cheri chose "Cheri's Cabana" as her theme. With the participation of staff, Cheri transformed her room into a tropical island. Posters of sunny beaches adorned the walls, and palm trees and fish were crafted out of paper. Butterflies and tropical birds hung from the ceiling. When visitors were allowed into her room, they were often given a Hawaiian lei to wear with their required hospital isolation gown. A bright orange stuffed monkey sat near

transplant, anticipatory coping may include a unique kind of environmental planning (see box).

Attention to privacy and confidentiality is also essential for adolescents to feel trusting and able to participate in their own treatment planning. Respecting wishes and honoring confidences are essential principles to build trust and acceptance. Assuring a teen's privacy during personal cares and treatments is often an ongoing struggle within a large teaching hospital. Members of the psychosocial team may need to intervene to help adolescents feel assured that their needs will be met. Because of an adolescent's preoccupation with appearances, interpreting the value of personal care needs to medical personnel may also be necessary. One adolescent girl remembers little about her critical illness and ICU stay except for the day when she was helped to have her hair washed! Simple touches like replacing the blankets to cover a teen after an examination may make a significant difference to an adolescent.

An interesting research study documented the memories of adolescent patients 4 years after their discharge from the hospital (Denholm, 1990). In the original study, five basic adolescent needs were identified: privacy, peer visitation and contact, mobility, independence, and educational continuity (Denholm & Ferguson, 1987). Using telephone interviews and written approaches, the researchers contacted 22 adolescents from the original study of post-hospitalization reactions and asked them to share their recollections of care and to offer suggestions for changes in hospital environments. The majority of positive memories concerned relationships with nursing staff, other patients, family members, and visitors. The next largest category of positive memories focused on the availability of activities, especially television, VCRs, and the activities room. Fewer negative memories were identified in this follow-up study and focused on nursing care and lack of preparation for procedures, as well as inconveniences of cares, such as being awakened during the night. Suggestions for improved care identified more privacy, appropriate gowns, better explanations of procedures, more family rooms, and

Cheri's bed and filled the room with monkey noises when squeezed. The bathroom door had a sign reading "Spa," and favorite staff people often were given "fantasy" titles in keeping with her theme. Like any adolescent, Cheri looked forward to turning 18 and so painted an island lounge and cocktail bar in a mural along one wall, complete with other tourists sitting at the bar sipping umbrella-topped fruit drinks. "You don't feel like you're in the hospital," said Cheri. "You feel like you're in a make-believe land."

Note. Courtesy of Cynthia and Damien Amore.

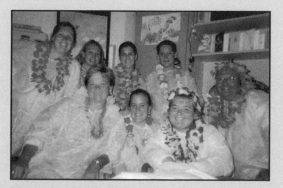

Hospital staff members join in a celebration of a teenager's "island" theme room.

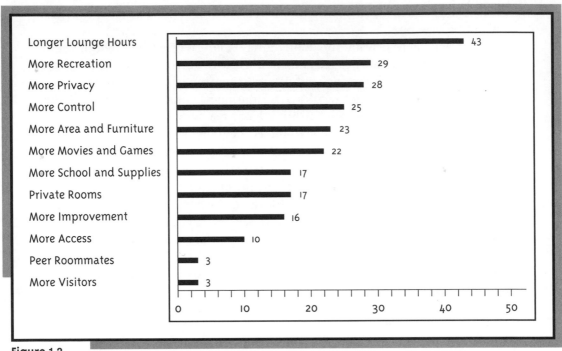

Figure 1.2.

Percentage of adolescents suggesting changes in each of 12 areas. *Note.* From "The Experience of Hospital-ized Adolescents: How Well Do We Meet Their Developmental Needs?" by J. L. Gusella, A. Ward, and G. S. Butler, 1998, *Children's Health Care,* 27(2), pp. 138–140. Copyright 1998 by Lawrence Erlbaum. Reprinted with permission.

more time to be alone. Conclusions of this study indicate that the study group expressed little evidence of long-term emotional upset. Additionally, the adolescents identified feelings of positive self-worth, increased coping abilities, and a greater appreciation of life. It is noteworthy that these adolescents were cared for in a hospital that had a designated ward for adolescents.

A study of Canadian adolescents demonstrated that 90% felt satisfied overall with their hospital experience (as measured by a computerized questionnaire), but 91% of these adolescents also were able to make suggestions for improvements (Gusella, Ward, & Butler, 1998). The results of this study are summarized in Figures 1.2, 1.3, and 1.4.

Vulnerable Children

Some children, regardless of age or developmental level, have been described as psychologically vulnerable (Petrillo & Azarnoff, 1997). Despite the advances in meeting the unique needs of children through child life, play preparation, and family presence, these vulnerable children need individualized

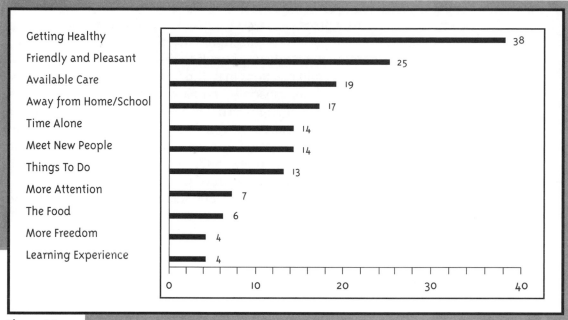

Figure 1.3.

Percentage of adolescents listing advantages to being in the hospital, by category. *Note.* From "The Experience of Hospitalized Adolescents: How Well Do We Meet Their Developmental Needs?" By J. L. Gusella, A. Ward, and G. S. Butler, 1998, *Children's Health Care*, 27(2), pp. 138–140. Copyright 1998 by Lawrence Erlbaum. Reprinted with permission.

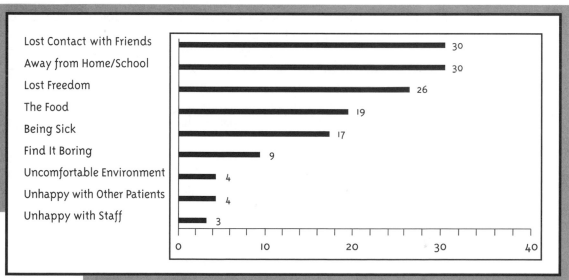

Figure 1.4.

Percentage of adolescents listing disadvantages to being in the hospital, by category. *Note.* From "The Experience of Hospitalized Adolescents: How Well Do We Meet Their Developmental Needs?" By J. L. Gusella, A. Ward, and G. S. Butler, 1998, *Children's Health Care*, 27(2), pp. 138–140. Copyright 1998 by Lawrence Erlbaum. Reprinted with permission.

approaches to meet their needs. This group may include young children and previously hospitalized children who may have misconceptions or over-whelming fears about past hospitalizations and treatments. Another group, children with emotional disturbances, tends to distort perceptions about illness or injury. Parent–child reactions may also have a role in the maladaptive behaviors of some children, especially if a parent exhibits extreme anxiety requiring the intervention of an impartial professional to correct misinformation and reduce levels of fear. Another group of especially vulnerable children includes those who are sensory impaired, neurologically compromised, or developmentally delayed. For these children, the usual methods of preparation and coping through play or expressive arts may not be as effective, and a more individualized approach must be adapted to each child's abilities (Petrillo & Azarnoff, 1997).

Resilient Children

Despite the many risks posed by health-care experiences for many children, it is possible, as stated earlier, for some children to adapt to the experience without negative sequelae. These children may be labeled as *resilient*. Resiliency is defined as the ability to return rapidly to a previous psychologic or physiologic state (Rutter, 1987). Children who are described as resilient tend to respond more quickly and appropriately to major life events such as divorce or hospitalization or to adapt more positively to chronic and ongoing stresses. They may cope better with the isolation and immobility required during treatment for limited periods of time if they are able to rely on their strengths and ability to develop supportive relationships.

Protective factors that encourage resiliency in children focus on involvement in action and the ability to give directions. A resilient school-age boy who was hospitalized for many months with severe burns coped by insisting not only on removing his own dressings before each whirlpool treatment, but also on doing it at his own pace. This method seemed agonizingly slow and frustrated all of the therapists who wished to accomplish the undesirable task as quickly as possible. Yet, for the patient, it was critical to his ability to adapt to the experience and maintain some measure of control. Bolig and Weddle (1988) identified the following additional psychosocial principles that support resiliency:

1. Relating a child's actions to reactions or outcomes (e.g., "When you relax your arm, your IV runs smoothly").
2. Providing social reinforcement upon the performance of a task, rather than before.
3. Rewarding degrees of effort (e.g., how hard a child works rather than how successful he or she may be at that work, such as holding still for an IV start).

4. Encouraging extraordinary effort and tasks even under stress.
5. Modeling both expression of feelings and self-talk.
6. Training new skills and practicing old behaviors.

Children may become more resilient if they are helped to perceive experiences constructively, are supported with policies that lessen separation from family members, and are encouraged to express their feelings (Bolig & Weddle, 1988). A summary of issues for all ages and developmental stages with suggested interventions to help in coping is found in Table 1.2.

Family Reactions

The hospitalization of a child creates stress for the entire family. How a family handles the stress varies greatly depending on a family's coping abilities, past experience with an ill child and circumstances of the hospitalization caused by the illness or injury, and acute or chronic illness. Bossert and Hart (1999) list the sources of stress for parents during a child's acute illness:

- Child's illness
  - Diagnosis
  - Decisions about management of illness including consents for painful treatment for procedures
  - Perceived severity of the illness
- Hospital environment
  - Unfamiliar equipment, routines, policies
  - Uncertainty about parental roles and participation in cares
  - Unknown expectations of parents by staff
  - Personnel roles, number of caregivers
- Type of admission
  - Expected—with time for planning
  - Unexpected—from clinic with need to change family routines quickly
  - Emergency—most stressful due to suddenness of illness or injury
- Length of stay
- Changes in child's behavior
  - Loss of developmental milestones
  - Changes in child's emotional responses
  - Physical changes due to illness or injury including pain, altered appearance, ability to communicate, loss of mobility or strength
- Changes in routines of daily family life especially rooming in, child care arrangements, and work responsibilities (pp. 157–158)

(*text continues on p. 24*)

Table 1.2

Understanding Children Who Are Hospitalized: A Developmental Perspective

Age Group	Erikson	Piaget
Infant (0–1 years)	Trust vs. Mistrust • To get • To give in return	Sensorimotor • Exploration of physical self and environment • Object constancy • Cause and effect
Toddler (1–3 years)	Autonomy vs. Shame and Doubt • To hold on • To let go	Sensorimotor Preoperational (preconceptual phase) • Can hold and recall images • Increasing use of symbolization • Highly egocentric perception of world
Preschooler (3–6 years)	Initiative vs. Guilt • To make (going after) • To "make like" (playing)	Preoperational (preconceptual phase) Preoperational (intuitive phase) • Transition period between— depending solely on perception, and depending on truly logical thinking • Better able to see more than one factor at a time that influences an event
School-ager (6–12 years)	Industry vs. Inferiority • To make things (completing) • To make things together	Concrete operations • Increasing ability to think logically in the physically concrete realm • Understands the meaning of series of actions, of order and sequencing

Table 1.2 *Continued.*

23

Understanding Children Who Are Hospitalized: A Developmental Perspective

Hospitalization Issues	Possible Troublesome Responses	Interventions
Separation Lack of stimulation Pain	Failure to bond Distrust Anxiety Delayed skills development	Maximize parental involvement Maximize parental information Provide stimulation • Visual • Auditory • Tactile • Kinesthetic • Vestibular
Separation Fear of bodily injury and pain Frightening fantasies Immobility or restriction Forced regression Loss of routine and rituals	Regression (including loss of newly learned skills) Uncooperativeness Protest (verbal and physical) Despair Negativism Temper tantrums Resistance	Maximize parental involvement Maximize parental information Facilitate medical play Promote therapeutic play • Environmental exploration • Freedom within limits • Routine and ritual • Self-expression • Movement activities • Sensory stimulation games
Separation Fear of loss of control, sense of own power Fear of bodily mutilation or penetration by surgery or injections, castration	Regression Anger toward primary caregiver Acting out Protest (less aggressive than toddler) Despair and detachment Physical and verbal aggression Dependency Withdrawal	Maximize parental involvement Maximize parental information Facilitate medical play Promote therapeutic play • Environmental exploration • Freedom within limits • Routine and ritual • Self-expression • Movement activities • Sensory stimulation games
Separation Fear of loss of control Fear of loss of mastery Fear of bodily mutilation Fear of bodily injury and pain, especially intrusive procedures in genital area Fear of illness itself, disability, and death	Regression Inability to complete some tasks Uncooperativeness Withdrawal Depression Displaced anger and hostility Frustration	Maximize parental involvement Maximize parental information Encourage education and teacher involvement Facilitate medical play and information Promote therapeutic play • Skill building • Meaningful projects • Group activities • Peer support • Freedom within limits • Self-expression

(continues)

Table 1.2 *Continued.*

Understanding Children Who Are Hospitalized:
A Developmental Perspective

Age Group	Erikson	Piaget
Adolescent (12–18 years)	Identity and Repudiation vs. Identity Diffusion • To be oneself (or not to be) • To share being oneself	Formal operations • Deductive and abstract reasoning • Can imagine the conditions of a problem—past, present, and future—and develop hypotheses about what might logically occur under different combinations of factors

Parents may have feelings of guilt about their role in the need for hospitalization, perhaps questioning their timeliness in seeking medical care. They worry and fear the outcome, and may feel anger about the circumstances or generalized burden of the hospitalization and its impact on the whole family. If a child has been very ill at home, a parent may also feel some measure of relief that the child will now be hospitalized. Nearly all parents share a generalized feeling of anxiety.

Bossert and Hart (1999) identified a series of priorities that families use to cope with the disruption in family routine caused by hospitalization. These priorities, in order of importance, are as follows:

1. *Needs of the hospitalized child.* Most parents believe that they should be with the child as much as possible, and mothers generally spend more time in hospital than fathers. As the child's condition improves, less time may be spent at the bedside.

2. *Needs of the siblings.* Caring for the siblings at home is an area that most parents will accept outside help to manage.

3. *Work responsibilities.* Again, mothers usually take more time off from work than fathers do, and her work seems to take a lower priority than his.

4. *Home responsibilities.* Other caretakers or older siblings may help with essential tasks like preparing meals, while other home tasks may be ignored. Whether a parent rooms-in or visits, a parent's personal needs for exercise, socialization, and time with spouse may all be difficult. (p. 159)

Table 1.2 *Continued.*

25

Understanding Children Who Are Hospitalized:
A Developmental Perspective

Hospitalization Issues	Possible Troublesome Responses	Interventions
Dependence on adults	Uncooperativeness	Encourage peer group activities
Separation from family and peers	Withdrawal	Provide privacy
	Anxiety	Respect independence (choices)
Fear of bodily injury and pain	Depression	Encourage self-expression
Fear of loss of identity		Address body image, sexual image, and future concerns
Body image and sexuality		Facilitate medical preparation
Concern about peer group status after hospitalization		Encourage education and teacher involvement
		Facilitate visits with peers

Note. From *From Artist to Artist-in-Residence: Preparing Artists to Work in Pediatric Healthcare Settings* (p. 24), by J. Rollins and C. Mahan, 1996, Washington, DC: Rollins & Associates. Copyright 1996 by Rollins & Associates. Reprinted with permission.

Special attention must be given to the availability of personal comforts for parents, such as showers, computers for e-mailing family or friends, meal trays, laundry facilities, and areas for relaxation away from the bedside.

The use of parent pagers is an innovative program that has helped parents take time for personal, family, and business needs. Parents often feel pressured by the child not to leave the bedside for a shower or a telephone call for fear that a procedure or test will be done in their absence. Parents often are reluctant to leave the bedside, fearing that they might miss a physician's visit and the opportunity to discuss medical information; however, parents must be able to leave the bedside to share information with family members or make care decisions. The provision of a pager for parent use enables them to be readily available as needed at the bedside, helps them to feel a measure of control, and enhances their participation in their child's care (Ashenberg, Lambert, Maier, & McAliley, 1996).

A new understanding of the needs of the hospitalized child has resulted in a change of expectations for parents. Whereas previously parents relinquished most measures of control of their child, now they are expected to remain with their child and participate in cares (Darbyshire, 1994). Parental presence has altered the perceived and identified needs of parents when a child is hospitalized. Parents overwhelmingly identify the need for information as critical to their coping. Not only do parents need information, but also they need to receive it in understandable language with the opportunity to ask questions for clarification. Filling this need for information helps a parent to feel in control of what is happening in the hospital (Hallstrom, Runesson, & Elander, 2002). Parents also report that contributing their input makes them feel recognized as competent partners in the care of their child. At the same time, parents also feel vulnerable to the moods and temperament of the medical staff, and may be reluctant to express frustration or criticism, fearing that it might affect their child's care.

Bossert and Hart (1999) also describe phases in a parent's coping. In the initial phase of illness, parents may be passive and acquiesce to recommendations of professionals. Next, parents may enter a phase of information seeking wherein they gather information from many different professionals, analyze literature, and develop a personal understanding of the diagnosis and management. As parents become more comfortable with the environment and information, they often become strong advocates for their child's treatment, reaffirming their roles as parents who best know their child's needs and responses.

Phases of Parent's coping →

In a study of stress appraisal and coping in 35 mothers of NICU infants, Reichman, Miller, Gordon, and Hendricks-Munoz (2000) found that 60% of the participants presented with clinically significant levels of distress, and that 58% of the variance in distress could be explained by four variables. Increased distress was associated with the appraisal of uncontrollability, confrontive coping, and escape-avoidant coping. Decreased distress was associated with the coping strategy of accepting responsibility. They found that mothers who had greater satisfaction with their child's physician claimed to feel greater control over the situation and to function better. The authors conclude that it would be helpful if basic cognitive–behavioral strategies for anxiety reduction were taught to staff, family, and friends, and that a supportive NICU environment is essential.

One further need identified in research by Ward (2001) was the need for parental assurance that their child was receiving the best possible care. This study of parents during their first week in the NICU acknowledged that parents frequently identified feelings of shock, anticipation, and uncertainty about the outcome for their infant. An interesting finding of the study was that fathers and mothers differed significantly in the ranking of needs. Fathers ranked assurance and information as less important than did mothers. During the first week of hospitalization, both fathers and mothers placed support needs as least important. (The author did note that the research was conducted in a setting where parent support groups were not available.)

The 10 most important needs identified by parents in this study were:

- To know exactly what is being done for my infant
- To see that the NICU staff provide comfort to my infant, such as giving my infant a pacifier, using blankets to support my infant's body, and talking softly to my infant
- To know how my infant is being treated medically
- To have questions about my infant answered honestly
- To be able to visit at any time
- To be assured that the best care possible is being given to my infant
- To know the expected outcome for my infant
- To feel that the hospital personnel care about my infant

- To know that my infant is being handled gently by health care providers
- To know specific facts concerning my infant's progress

The 10 least important needs identified by parents were:

- To have someone be concerned about my health
- To have a bathroom near the waiting room
- To have a pastor, clergy, or other person from my church visit
- To have someone help with transportation
- To be allowed to have my infant's siblings visit
- To receive help in responding to the reactions of my infant's siblings
- To have another person with me when visiting the NICU
- To have comfortable furniture in the waiting room
- To be able to talk to other parents whose infant is in the NICU or has a similar situation
- To have a support group of other families available (Ward, 2001, p. 284)

Findings related to least important needs may be significant in light of the attention presently being given to parents' comfort within the critical care setting and the perceived need to create more homelike environments for parents. However, this study may also be unique in that the infants whose parents participated in the research had a length of stay no longer than 30 days. It may be that once the needs of greatest importance have been addressed and the parents are assured that the care their infant is receiving is knowledgeable and nurturing (presumably demonstrated within the first month of hospitalization), they may then turn their attention to other parental needs, such as comfortable surroundings and convenient services.

Sibling Reactions

While much attention is focused on the child who is the patient and on the needs of parents, siblings are also affected by the experience. Brothers and sisters may experience a wide range of feelings and concerns, and may be forced to identify and deal with these concerns in the absence of the parent who is either physically separated or emotionally unavailable to the well siblings. How they adapt and cope is dependent on a number of important variables that include the following:

- Sibling age and developmental level
- Acuity, nature and knowledge of the illness or injury
- Changes in parent interactions
- Changed routines and substitute care arrangements
- Socioeconomic status of family
- Past experiences

Parents may underestimate the stress that is felt by siblings until behavioral or physiologic symptoms are noted. These may include changes in eating or sleeping patterns; inability to concentrate in school; acting nervous, withdrawn, or angry; physically acting out with siblings or friends; and being reluctant to be away from parents. Craft (1993) identified the child's age and developmental level, the nature of the threat, the sibling–ill child relationship, the nature of the changes, and the family's socioeconomic status as factors influencing sibling responses to hospitalization.

Child's Age and Developmental Level

The ability of a sibling to understand and cognitively perceive events may cause children under the age of 7 years to be the most vulnerable (Craft, 1993). In a study by Knafl and Dixon (1983), the most negative reactions of siblings occurred between the ages of 4 and 11 years. The nature of the illness itself is concerning to siblings who may worry about the outcome, fearing that their brother or sister might die. Young siblings may experience guilt, imagining that they caused the illness or injury. They may also worry about developing the same illness or injury. In one research study (Craft, 1986), 50% of siblings were fearful of getting the same illness as the hospitalized child. In addition, younger children are more vulnerable to separation from parents because of their poorly developed concept of time. Older siblings may feel guilty if a contagious illness or intentional injury is the reason for hospitalization, and they may have a perceived or actual belief that their actions had a role in the cause of the illness or injury. Older siblings also may experience more feelings of anxiety as they become increasingly able to conceptualize the impact of future outcomes. They may feel anger toward the ill sibling, or toward parents for placing more responsibilities on the older sibling at home, either in caring for other siblings or performing household tasks (Bossert & Hart, 1999).

Nature of the Threat

A sudden acute and life-threatening illness or injury creates more stress for siblings. Time elapsed since diagnosis is also a factor, as stress levels for siblings are higher with a new diagnosis of progressive illness as opposed to a previously diagnosed condition (Craft, 1993).

Sibling–Ill Child Relationship

Siblings who have a close relationship with the hospitalized child report greater stress than those whose sibling relationships are not perceived as close. A sibling's perception of the relationship with an ill or injured brother or sister may also affect the associated feelings of guilt, anger, or anxiety. These feelings are common when a new baby is born and requires hospitalization, changing the family structure and function and the role of other children in the family.

Nature of the Changes

Physical separation from parents and the ill sibling is a major source of stress for well siblings. They may feel physically or emotionally abandoned, interpreting these events as a loss of love, or they may feel they are being punished. The effects of separation, especially in younger children, may be similar to the separation anxiety as described earlier in reference to the hospitalized child. In addition, changes in caregivers and routines may be difficult for well children, especially if they are cared for outside the security of their own home. Often substitute caregivers may have different parenting styles and expectations for siblings.

Family Socioeconomic Status

Family income generally has an impact on the availability of resources and supports, an important variable for siblings. The negative effects of parental separation may be lessened if both parents are available to share the responsibilities for the ill child as well as the healthy siblings. The level of a mother's education and occupation also has been demonstrated to lessen siblings' anxiety (Craft, 1993). It is speculated that with more education may come an increased sensitivity to the effects of hospitalization on siblings and a greater sense of responsibility to provide support and information.

Assistance and Support

Many studies have documented the importance of including siblings in the experience of hospitalization. Siblings who are supported with developmentally appropriate explanations of the causes of illness or injury, participate by being present with the ill brother or sister, and are provided with opportunities to express their feelings demonstrate fewer adverse responses. The responsibility for supporting siblings during the hospital experience should be shared by parents and the health-care team. Perhaps the professional with the greatest ability to support siblings is the child life specialist who possesses not only the knowledge and ability to explain causative factors in developmentally appropriate language to children, but also has a wealth of resources to engage siblings in expressing feelings and concerns. The ability to visit is critical, especially for younger children who have not yet reached the developmental stage of being able to think abstractly or process information cognitively (see Figure 1.5). Any time children visit the hospital, especially within critical care settings, developmentally appropriate

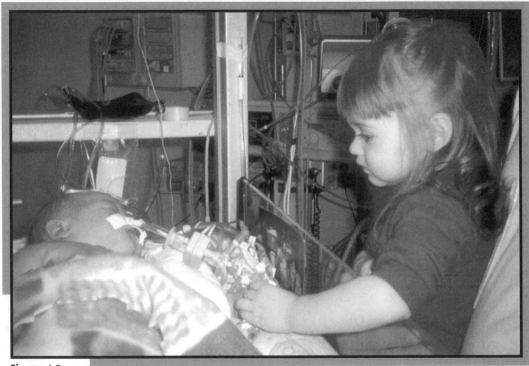

Figure 1.5.
The ability to visit is especially important for young children. *Note.* Photograph used with permission of Children's Hospital of Wisconsin.

preparation is essential. The use of dolls, puppets, and photographs, as well as inclusion in preadmission programming, all provide important support for siblings (see Chapter 2). If siblings are unable to visit due to distance from the hospital, similar illnesses, or other reasons, parents may be encouraged to communicate through telephone calls, letters, or audio or videotapes. While siblings gain a sense of inclusion by participating in creating these resources at home to send to the ill child (see Figure 1.6), parents may send similar resources back home to help the well siblings cope with the separation and alternative care arrangements.

The Emergency Room Experience

The reactions of children to health-care experiences and the effects of hospitalization may be exaggerated in the emergency room. The physical environment is overwhelmingly frightening as evidenced by the presence of complex medical equipment and supplies for emergency care, from simple suturing of lacerations to the treatment of life-threatening traumatic injuries. The surrounding activity is usually busy and sometimes chaotic, with ob-

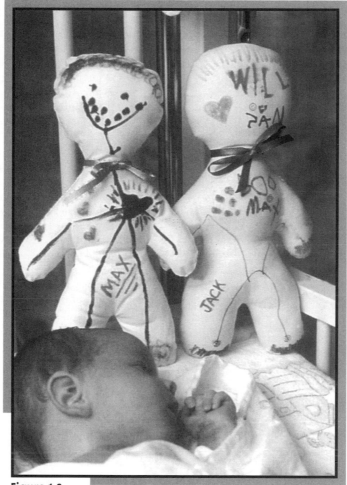

Figure 1.6.

Creating a special drawing or doll for a brother or sister who is hospitalized helps siblings feel included. *Note.* Photograph used with permission of Children's Hospital of Wisconsin.

servable and heightened anxiety levels of staff, parents, and other children. The presence of police, emergency transport personnel, and other strangers not usually associated with the hospital may add to a child's sense of fear. Crowded waiting areas and the sights of other sick and injured children awaiting care may cause more anxiety for the child about to encounter his or her own medical experience, perhaps for the very first time.

Although the emergency room visit is one of the most common experiences a child and family will have with a hospital, its psychology is among the least studied and understood. Yet understanding and responding to the psychosocial aspects of an emergency are essential elements of effective care. In Table 1.3, Brunnquell and Kohen (1991) have listed children's typical reactions by age and interventions that may support children in the emergency room.

Table 1.3

Developmental Issues in Emergency Settings

Developmental Phase	Stressors to the Child	Intervention Strategy
Infancy (0–12 months)	Separation from parent	Enable parent to remain with child to provide emotional support Minimize number of caregivers
	Impaired basic trust	Minimize intrusive procedures Do not involve parents as actors in intrusive procedures; rather, enable their presence to comfort child
Toddler (12–30 months)	Separation from parent	Involve parent in noninvasive cares Enable parent to remain with child to provide emotional support Provide choices in age-appropriate activities Minimize number of caregivers
	Loss of autonomy	Actively involve child in treatment, when possible Prepare child for procedures, including play and medical equipment
	Restriction of movement	Provide age-appropriate activities while waiting Minimize use of excessive restraint
Preschool (30 months– 5 years)	Separation from parent	Encourage parental involvement in noninvasive cares Enable parent to remain with child to provide emotional support
	Fear of mutilation Magical thinking	Provide accurate preparatory information Offer psychological preparation prior to and following procedures Ask questions and model honest communication
	Loss of competence and initiative	Teach planned coping strategies Provide age-appropriate activities and play
School age (6–12 years)	Loss of bodily control	Ensure preparation for and involvement in procedures Encourage choices among options if possible (e.g., IV in right or left hand)
	Enforced dependence	Involve patient in care Teach planned coping strategies that encourage mastery
	Loss of competence	Provide age-appropriate activities Help children recognize aspects of their effective coping
Adolescence	Lack of trust Enforced dependence Threat to bodily competence	Communicate honestly Involve patient in care and decisions Discuss potential psychological changes and physical responses Address long-term issues in follow-up
	Threat to future competence	Provide opportunity for follow-up discussion and guidance as needed

Note. From "Emotions in Pediatric Emergencies: What We Know, What We Can Do," by D. Brunnquell and D. Kohen, 1991, *Children's Health Care, 20*(4), p. 243. Copyright 1991 by Erlbaum. Reprinted with permission.

Brunnquell and Kohen (1991) also developed a series of steps to assist families in coping with emergency treatment while reducing the threatening aspects of the experience.

1. Avoid matching the emotional level of the patient and family if they are upset. Instead, respond with empathy and calmness to help the family reach a calmer level of emotional arousal.
2. Assure that someone is specifically attending to emotional care, especially if the primary medical caregiver does not have time to do so, and explicitly tell the patient, family, and designated person this task is being assigned.
3. Meet the intense information needs of patients and families. Recognize that feelings of loss of control are exacerbated by incomplete, conflicting, or delayed information.
4. Prepare patients and family members present for specific procedures as clearly as possible. Also prepare them for emergencies such as seeing their child in distress, where he or she will be going next, and how best they can support their child.
5. Take specific actions to control pain. If using anesthetics, allow sufficient time for them to take effect; many children report they begin to feel numb after a procedure is carried out. Also, use alternative interventions, such as relaxation/mental imagery techniques in the emergency situation. Recognize that anxiety increases pain. (p. 246)

In a growing number of settings, the presence of a child life specialist in the emergency room has demonstrated the effectiveness of preparation and psychosocial support for emergency room treatment while lessening the anxiety for the child and family (Alcock et al., 1985; Christian & Thomas, 1998; Krebel, Clayton, & Graham, 1996). In addition, the presence of parents during procedures is also helpful for both patient and staff, provided that the parent knows what to expect and how to be supportive to increase their child's coping. There is a growing movement in emergency medicine and critical care areas to permit parents to be present during resuscitation when accompanied by a staff person whose only role is to support and give information to the parent (McGahey, 2002).

Ambulatory Care

The challenges of meeting the psychosocial needs of children have increased as more and more children and adolescents are treated in outpatient rather than inpatient settings. The systems for providing such care have seen a greatly increased volume of patients as well as the necessity to meet more complex medical needs of patients and families (Johnson et al., 1992). Pediatric ambulatory care must be provided in ways that

- enhance the strengths of families,
- support the child's development,
- promote multidisciplinary communication and cooperation, and
- build partnerships with community-based health, early intervention, education, social service, and other human service organizations and agencies. (Johnson et al., 1992, p. 424)

Facilities providing ambulatory care should be designed to meet the varied needs of families, including accessibility to public transportation, qualified staff including interpreters for non–English-speaking families, and attention to a family's entrance into the clinic. Also necessary are comfortable waiting and well-equipped play areas for families who often spend many hours in outpatient settings. Research has documented that families of children who are engaged in meaningful activities express greater satisfaction with care, even in settings where lengthy waits are the norm (Ipsa, Barrett, & Kim, 1988). Educational efforts in the waiting area may be more subtle, where the availability of children's books provides children with activities while waiting, but also encourages interaction between parents and children. One pediatric hospital formed a liaison with a local used bookstore chain to place book carts in every clinic waiting area. Books on these carts are intended for children and families to take home when they leave the clinic, with the hope that parents will continue to encourage reading together as a family experience.

When setting up a new office, physicians are advised to consider pediatric needs, including not only child-size exam tables and exam room equipment, but also toys, magazines, music, educational videos, and aquariums to engage pediatric patients while waiting (Nazarian, 1999). Adolescents require space that is comfortable and not located in the same waiting area as younger children.

The ability to provide ambulatory care is also challenged by societal issues of poverty, drug and alcohol abuse, homelessness, and violence. An educational component of care should be provided with resources and information readily available to families. Education for parents regarding normal growth and development must be supplemented with resources to address risk areas for each developmental stage. In addition, medical care services may be located in community areas, such as school-based clinics and early intervention programs where children are already receiving other services. These resources should be designed to meet the needs of working families or those with limited transportation, making more services available during evenings and weekends.

Preparing children for outpatient treatment may be more challenging because professional resources to address psychosocial needs are often focused on inpatient settings (Johnson et al., 1992). Parents may have difficulty in establishing a trusting relationship with a primary physician due to changes required by insurance providers and the consolidation of physician services into larger and larger practices as the economic demands of health care are continually being challenged. Although the issues of health-care economics will not be easily solved, parents should be encouraged to use clinics and physician groups that attempt to meet children's unique psychosocial needs as well as their medical needs. The child who feels comfortable and safe in a waiting area designed especially for children may more easily adapt to being treated by more than one familiar and trusted physician. Encouraging simple medical play at home as part of usual play activities with attention to the positive aspects of medical care also may prepare children for future health-care experiences in inpatient or outpatient settings.

Home Health Care

As the health-care environment changes, children with complex medical needs are frequently returning home to be cared for by in-home nursing staff with increasing parental responsibility for care. This trend is often welcomed by families who hope to return to some measure of normalcy after weeks or months in the hospital. Yet it is not a trend without risks, as factors that affect both parents and siblings within the hospital may be exacerbated in the home environment. The ongoing responsibility of understanding the operation and functions of medical equipment without the backup of readily available professionals creates additional stress. Siblings may feel less recognized or supported due to additional time devoted to the care of the ill child at home. They may also feel more conspicuous or different in the community and may be reluctant to have their peers visit.

For all of these reasons, planning for the transition from hospital to home is essential for every member of the family. While parents learn the responsibilities of home health care, attention needs to be given to sibling involvement and adjustment. The opportunity to anticipate changes and develop positive coping styles may be facilitated by child life or other members of the health-care team. Ongoing opportunities to express feelings and concerns through creative activities, journaling, art, and music should be provided. Specific interventions may include a school visit by a health-care professional or peer preparation for the return of a child with complex medical needs. Creating a role for siblings in these specific interventions may be helpful, both in assessing siblings' understanding of the situation and in helping them master a challenging experience. As in most other aspects of the health-care experience, the inclusion of siblings as active participants rather than observers will facilitate positive coping. Special attention may be required over time as the developmental needs and concerns of both the ill child and his or her healthy siblings may change significantly through each new developmental stage. Additional support for well siblings of a chronically ill child may include professional counseling and support group involvement with peers in similar situations.

Recent programming developed for children with complex medical needs includes medical day care settings where children's medical needs, therapies, and socialization are provided in a group setting. Staffed by a variety of health-care professionals, including developmental teachers; speech, physical, and occupational therapists; and child life specialists, these centers fill a unique role in allowing parents to work and maintain activities of daily living. Centers provide the children with an environment that emphasizes individual growth and development within an appropriate social setting rather than in the isolated environment of home. Outdoor play, field trips, and special events are possible with a staff of trained health-care professionals. Many children make extraordinary psychosocial and physical progress within this developmentally appropriate and engaging day care setting. Because these facilities are most often located within or near hospitals, the challenges of frequent hospitalizations for these children may be more easily managed due to familiar staff and smoother transitions from one setting to another.

Conclusion

> *I'm the same person I was before I got sick. I can't run or play as much as before, but I can read and sleep and do work and think—most things that everybody else does.*
> —Adam Rojo, 7 years old
> (Krementz, 1989, p. 25)

Children in hospitals today are different than in years past. Infants are surviving earlier and longer with medical conditions that for many years had few treatment options and little hope of survival. Children of all ages are living with chronic illnesses that once were referred to as terminal. They may be hospitalized more often for new treatments and procedures but stay for shorter periods of time and return home with medical needs previously only managed in the inpatient setting.

In addition, injuries are now an increasing threat to children and adolescents, resulting in more hospital admissions. The result is that hospital pediatric units are now occupied by infants, children, and adolescents who are more critically ill than in the past. The one variable that has not changed is that these patients are children with emotional, developmental, educational, and socialization needs that must be met (Johnson et al., 1992). The commitment to meet these unique psychosocial needs, in addition to the increasingly complex medical needs, requires attention to all aspects of family-centered care. It also requires health-care professionals to provide not only a physical environment that is designed specifically for children and families, but also a caring and nurturing environment that welcomes every child as part of a family.

Study Guide

1. Describe the conditions for children in hospitals 25 years ago, and discuss why and how changes occurred.

2. What is the *developmental* approach to pediatric care?

3. Beyond age or developmental level, what factors influence children's responses to health-care experiences?

4. Discuss how the recent research is refuting some long-held beliefs about children's responses to health-care encounters.

5. Using the developmental approach, describe a typical response by children in one age range to the inpatient health-care experience, and draw implications for practice.

6. How does an *individualized care plan* assist staff, children, and families in coping with health-care experiences?

7. Explain the concept of resiliency and how it can influence children's health-care encounters. Describe methods of supporting resiliency.

8. Recent research has identified various parental needs. Describe changes in facilities, practices, and policies that could assist parents in their children's health-care experiences.

9. With increased ambulatory and home health-care, there are new issues and challenges for children and families. Cite several of these and discuss implications for health-care systems and practitioners.

10. Considering the trends in child health, disabilities, and chronic illnesses; technological and medical advances; and socio-economic factors, describe children's hospitalization and other health-care encounters 25 years from now.

References

Alcock, D., Goodman, J., Feldman, W., McGrath, P., Park, M., & Cappelli, M. (1985). Evaluation of child life intervention in emergency department suturing. *Pediatric Emergency Care, 1*(3), 111–115.

Als, H., & Gilkerson, L. (1995). Developmentally supportive care in the neonatal intensive care unit. *Zero to Three, 15*(6), 2–10.

Als, H., Lawhon, G., Duffy, F. H., McAnulty, G. C., Gibes-Grossman, R., & Blickman, J. G. (1994). Individualized developmental care for the very low birth weight preterm infant: Medical and neurofunctional effects. *Journal of American Medical Association, 272,* 853–858.

Anderson, C. T. M., Zeltzer, L. K., & Fanurik, D. (1993). Procedural pain. In N. L. Schechter, C. B. Berde, & M. D. Yaster (Eds.), *Pain in infants, children, and adolescents* (pp. 435–458). Baltimore: Williams & Wilkins.

Ashenberg, M. D., Lambert, S. A., Maier, N. P., & McAliley, L. G. (1996). Easing the wait: Development of a pager program for families. *Pediatric Nursing, 22*(2), 103–107.

Association for the Care of Children's Health. (1990). *Shaping the future of children's health care*. Washington, DC: Author.

Baygirl 163. (2003). Kids connecting with kids. STARBRIGHT World. Retrieved on March 1, 2003, from http://starbright.org/projects/sbworld/baygirl.html

Bolig, R., & Weddle, K. D. (1988). Resiliency and hospitalization of children. *Children's Health Care, 16*(4), 255–260.

Bossert, E. (1994). Stress appraisals of hospitalized school age children. *Children's Health Care, 23*(1), 33–49.

Bossert, E. A., & Hart, D. E. (1999). Acute illness: Effects on the child's family. In M. Broome & J. Rollins (Eds.), *Core curriculum for the nursing care of children and their families* (pp. 155–164). Pitman, NJ: Jannetti.

Bowlby, J. (1960). Separation anxiety. *International Journal of Psychoanalysis, 41,* 89–113.

Brunnquell, D., & Kohen, D. P. (1991). Emotions in pediatric emergencies: What we know, what we can do. *Children's Health Care, 20*(4), 240–247.

Chess, S., & Thomas, A. (1984). *Origins and evolution of behavior disorders*. New York: Guilford Press.

Christian, B., & Thomas, D. (1998). A child life program in one pediatric emergency department. *Journal of Emergency Nursing, 24,* 359–361.

Craft, M. J. (1986). Validation of responses reported by school-aged siblings of hospitalized children. *Children's Health Care, 15*(1), 6–13.

Craft, M. J. (1993). Siblings of hospitalized children: Assessment and intervention. *Journal of Pediatric Nursing, 8*(5), 289–297.

Darbyshire, P. (1994). *Living with a sick child in hospital*. London: Chapman & Hall.

Denholm, C. (1990). Memories of adolescent hospitalization: Results from a four year follow-up study. *Children's Health Care, 19*(2), 101–105.

Denholm, C. J., & Ferguson, R. F. (1987). Reactions of adolescents following hospitalization for acute conditions. *Children's Health Care, 15*(3), 183–187.

Douglas, J. W. B. (1975). Early hospital admissions and later disturbances in behavior and learning. *Developmental Medicine and Child Neurology, 17,* 456–480.

Erikson, E. (1959). Identity and the life cycle. *Psychological Issues Monograph*. New York: International Universities Press.

Erikson, E. (1963). *Childhood and society* (2nd ed.). New York: Norton.

Fanurik, D., Schmitz, M. L., Martin, G. A., Koh, J. L., Wood, M., Sturgeon, L., & Long, N. (2000). Hospital room or treatment room: Where should inpatient pediatric procedures be performed? *Children's Health Care, 29*(2), 103–111.

Gaynard, L., Wolfer, J., Goldberger, J., Thompson, R., Redburn, L., & Laidley, L. (1990). *Psychosocial care of children in hospitals: A clinical practice manual.* Bethesda, MD: Association for the Care of Children's Health.

Gusella, J. L., Ward, A., & Butler, G. S. (1998). The experience of hospitalized adolescents: How well do we meet their needs? *Children's Health Care, 27*(2), 131–145.

Hallstrom, I., Runesson, I., & Elander, G. (2002). Observed parental needs during their child's hospitalization. *Journal of Pediatric Nursing, 17*(2), 140–148.

Hart, D., & Bossert, E. (1994). Self-reported fears of hospitalized school age children. *Journal of Pediatric Nursing, 9*(2), 83–90.

Hoffman, A. D., Becker, R. D., & Gabriel, H. P. (1976). *The hospitalized adolescent.* New York: The Free Press.

Ipsa, J., Barrett, B., & Kim, Y. (1988). Effects of supervised play in a hospital waiting room. *Children's Health Care, 16*(3), 195–200.

Johnson, B. H. (1995). Newborn intensive care units pioneer family-centered change in hospitals across the country. *Zero to Three, 15*(6), 11–17.

Johnson, B. H., Jeppson, E. S., & Redburn, L. (1992). *Caring for children and families: Guidelines for hospitals.* Bethesda, MD: Association for the Care of Children's Health.

Knafl, K. A., & Dixon, D. M. (1983). The role of siblings during hospitalization. *Issues in Comprehensive Pediatric Nursing, 6,* 13–22.

Krebel, M., Clayton, C., & Graham, C. (1996). Child life programs in the pediatric emergency department. *Pediatric Emergency Care, 12*(1), 13–15.

Krementz, J. (1989). *How it feels to fight for your life.* Boston: Little, Brown.

Lally, R., & Phelps, P. (1994). Caring for infants and toddlers in groups: Necessary considerations for emotional, social, and cognitive development. *Zero to Three, 14*(5), 1–6.

McGahey, P. R. (2002). Family presence during resuscitation: A focus on staff. *Critical Care Nurse, 22*(6), 29–34.

Nazarian, L. F. (1999). The well-equipped office. In M. Green, R. J. Haggerty, & M. Weitzman (Eds.), *Ambulatory pediatrics* (pp. 530–539). Philadelphia: Saunders.

Owens, P., Thompson, J., Elixhauser, A., & Ryan, K. (2003). *Care of children and adolescents in U.S. hospitals.* Rockville, MD: Agency for Healthcare Research and Quality.

Petrillo, M., & Azarnoff, P. (1997). Preparation programs and new strategies. In P. Azarnoff & P. Lindquist (Eds.), *Psychological abuse of children in health care: The issues* (pp. 59–79). Tarzana, CA: Pediatric Projects.

Piaget, J. (1960). *The child's concept of the world.* Patterson, NJ: Littlefield, Adams.

Quinton, D., & Rutter, M. (1976). Early hospital admissions and later disturbances of behavior: An attempted replication of Douglas' findings. *Developmental Medicine and Child Neurology, 18,* 447–459.

Reichman, S., Miller, A., Gordon, R., & Hendricks-Munoz, K. (2000). Stress appraisal and coping in mothers of NICU infants. *Children's Health Care, 29*(4), 279–293.

Rapacki, J. D. (1991). The neonatal intensive care experience. *Children's Health Care, 20*(1), 15–18.

Rennick, J., Johnston, C., Dougherty, G., Platt, R., & Ritchie, J. (2002). Children's psychological responses after critical illness and exposure to invasive technology. *Journal of Developmental Behavioral Pediatrics, 23*(3), 133–144.

Robbins, W. (2001, January 25). No stopping her now: Teen is breaking new ground in fighting leukemia. *Kenosha News,* p. D1.

Robertson, J. (1958). *Young children in hospitals.* New York: Basic Books.

Robinson, M. (1972, May). *The psychological impact of illness and hospitalization upon the child—Infancy to twelve years.* Paper presented to the Metropolitan Washington, DC, Association for the Care of Hospitalized Children, Washington, DC.

Rollins, J., & Mahan, C. (1996). *From artist to artist-in-residence: Preparing artists to work in pediatric healthcare settings.* Washington, DC: Rollins & Associates.

Rutter, M. (1987). Psychosocial resilience and protective mechanisms. *American Journal of Orthopsychiatry, 57,* 316–331.

Spitz, R. (1945). Hospitalism: An inquiry into the genesis of psychiatric conditions in early childhood. *Psychoanalytical Study of the Child, 1,* 53–74.

Stanford, G., & Thompson, R. H. (1981). *Child life in hospitals: Theory and practice.* Springfield, IL: Thomas.

Thurman, S. K. (1990). Parameters for establishing family centered neonatal intensive care services. *Children's Health Care, 20*(1), 34–39.

Ward, K. (2001). Perceived needs of parents of critically ill infants in a neonatal intensive care unit. *Pediatric Nursing, 27*(3), 281–286.

Wong, D. L., Perry, S. E., & Hockenberry, M. J. (Eds.). (2002). *Maternal child nursing care.* St Louis, MO: Mosby.

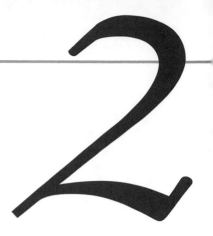

Preparing Children for Health-Care Encounters

Carmel C. Mahan

Objectives

At the conclusion of this chapter, the reader will be able to:

1. Discuss the purposes of *preparation* and the various theories underlying its use with children.
2. Determine strategies for preparation derived from theories.
3. Describe the evolution of preparation strategies and the knowledge and attitudes that influenced these changes.
4. Delineate the value of a research base to practice and policy for preparation.
5. Analyze the current use of computer technology, and project future demands for preparation strategies.

$\mathcal{I}$ n Chapter 1: Children's Hospitalization and Other Health-Care Encounters, a discussion of the reactions of children to health-care encounters revealed that hospitalization, doctor and clinic visits, ambulatory care and emergency room visits, and home health-care encounters prove stressful for children and their families. Much of the literature used to support that theory also supports the use of preparation as a means to reduce stress and to promote more effective coping. In fact, particularly in the early literature, it is sometimes difficult to separate the effects of the health-care environment itself from the effects of treatments and procedures on children and their families.

This chapter explores stress and coping and the history and theories behind various methods of preparing children for health-care encounters. The importance of timing, the child's stage of development, learning styles, culture, family support, the nature of the procedure, and the health-care setting are addressed with respect to planning appropriate methods of preparing children and adolescents for health-care encounters.

Stress and Coping

The literature reveals two categories of stressors in children: normative and nonnormative (Berk, 1997). Normative stressors are the common, developmental stressors of daily life (e.g., being left out of the group, having parents who fight, getting bad grades), while nonnormative stressors arise from unusual or traumatic experiences (e.g., serious illness of the child or parent, child abuse, community disasters).

What a child finds stressful is closely related to his or her age, gender, and developmental level. Growth, maturation, and expansion of environmental influences that occur with increasing age also change the nature of stressful experiences (Berk, 1997). For example, troubled peer relationships with same-sex friends are very stressful for school-age children, while troubled peer relationships with the opposite sex would likely be more stressful for teenagers.

Three classic definitional orientations have been used to describe stress: stimulus definitions, response definitions, and relational definitions. Until the 1960s, the major stress theorists were concerned with what constituted a stressful situation (the stressor) and the physiologic and psychologic reactions of the individual to the stress (the stress response; Janis, 1958; Selye, 1974). Lazarus's work (1966) began to shift the emphasis of study from a stimulus–response perspective to a process orientation of psychologically coping with stress. The most commonly used definition of stress, stressors, or stressful situations today considers both external and internal factors and includes the additional feature of appraisal. Stressors are "external and/or internal demands that are appraised as taxing or exceeding the resources of the person" (Lazarus & Folkman, 1984, p. 141).

The concept of stress, according to Lazarus (1966), is not a variable but a rubric consisting of many variables and processes. However, some researchers and writers have been troubled about the tendency to expand the concept of stress to include all the activities normally considered under the rubric of adaptation. Much of what people do to adapt occurs routinely and automatically through cognitive processes, specific actions, and styles of living that do not necessarily involve stress. However, if stress is regarded as a generic concept, its sphere of meaning must be delimited; otherwise, stress will come to represent anything and everything that is included in the concept of adaptation (Lazarus & Folkman, 1984).

Stressors may be social, cultural, psychologic, physiologic, or a combination of stimuli impinging on the individual (Lazarus & Folkman, 1984). Cognitive appraisal is the mental judgment about a stressor. It is an evaluative process that determines why and to what extent a particular transaction or series of transactions between the person and environment is stressful. These mental processes intervene between the encounter with the stressor and the resulting reaction. Not a static event, coping is the process through which the individual manages the demands of the person–environment relationship that are appraised as stressful and the emotions they generate. The process of coping does not imply success, only effort (Walker, Wells, Heiney, & Hymovich, 2002).

No specific models or theories currently exist to explain the entire process of children's stress and coping; however, Lazarus and Folkman's (1984) transactional model developed for adults is the model most commonly applied to children. According to their model, after judging the stimulus as stressful, the individual performs a secondary appraisal to determine what can or might be done to address it. After appraisal, the individual uses some form of cognitive or behavioral coping effort (Lazarus & Folkman, 1984). The individual's personal resources and constraints affect the choice of coping efforts. Constraints for children may include developmental age or limited life experiences. Efforts to cope may be problem focused, emotion focused, or a combination of the two.

The outcome or results of these coping efforts are either adaptive or maladaptive. Lazarus (1981) cautions about judging whether a given coping effort is adaptive or maladaptive. Value systems can impinge on this determination; for example, an individual's value system may judge denial as maladaptive, yet denial may be an appropriate response for a certain individual or in a particular situation. Coping effort is also related to time; for example, denial may be adaptive from a short-term perspective but maladaptive in the long term. Cultural factors, as well as the perspective of the individual and the function the effort serves (short- or long-term), must all be considered when interpreting the benefits or limitations of a coping effort.

Theoretical Framework for Preparation

In response to the information gained from the studies of children's reactions to health-care experiences cited in Chapter 1, pediatric health-care professionals began to develop preparation programs for children and families to help reduce anxiety and promote effective coping with health-care encounters. During the mid-1970s, studies demonstrating the positive effect of preparation programs on children's responses to hospitalization and surgery came to the attention of health-care professionals. Several of the most widely known studies, such as Wolfer and Visintainer (1975), Melamed and Siegel (1975), and Petrillo (1972), identified the following key elements of effective programs (Stanford & Thompson, 1981):

- Conveying information to the child in a developmentally appropriate manner
- Encouraging the expression of feelings about the information or event
- Including the participation of parents or other significant family members
- Establishing a trusting therapeutic relationship with staff members

In one of the early studies, Vaughn (1957) described an experimental condition in which two groups of children were admitted to the hospital for strabismus repair. A control group received no intervention, while the experimental group met for 15 to 25 minutes with a psychiatrist who reassured and supported each child and provided a brief, developmentally appropriate explanation of the surgery planned for the following day. Results indicated that the control group demonstrated more severe and persistent emotional disturbance than did the experimental group, during hospitalization and at 3 and 6 months following discharge. The intervention proved more effective in children 4 years old and older. All of the children under age 4 still had some behavioral disturbances at the 6-month follow-up.

One possible explanation for the continued upset of younger children in this study is that parents had limited contact with their children. Skipper and Leonard (1968) demonstrated that an intervention with mothers that involved both preparation and support reduced parental anxiety, as expected. It also demonstrated that their children scored lower on both physiologic and psychologic measures of distress, even though no intervention was directed at the children. In light of this, many subsequent studies included the factor of either liberalized parent visiting or rooming in, as well as other social supports in addition to a preparation program. This may confound the preparation data per se, but it has led to more comprehensive support for pediatric patients and their families as health-care workers noted the benefits to children, families, and staff when such support is offered.

In another classic study, Wolfer and Visintainer (1975) added "stress-point supportive care" to a preparation program that included role rehearsal, and reported that the experimental group demonstrated less upset on both psychologic and physiologic measures. Participants in the experimental group also had better post-hospital adjustment scores than those in the control group. Once again, this effect was observed to be greater in children age 6 years and older. Further, the authors noted that

> the exact causal sequence of this involved process is complex and unknown … The net effect of the preparation and supportive care can be described as stress reducing. However, the precise nature of this dynamic cognitive and affective process remains to be determined. (Wolfer & Visintainer, 1975, p. 254)

More recently, Zahr (1998) evaluated therapeutic play as a surgical preparation method for preschoolers in Lebanon. An intervention group of 50 children received an interactive puppet show 1 day before surgery; a control group of 50 children received routine care without the puppet show. Children in the intervention group demonstrated significantly less anxiety and more cooperation than the control group. They also had lower mean blood pressure and pulse rates during a preoperative injection. Following discharge, the intervention group had lower scores on the Post Hospital Behavior Questionnaire. The author concludes that therapeutic play is an effective way to reduce stress responses among preschoolers in Lebanon.

The complex, multivariate interactions among children, families, staff, and environment continue to be the focus of research in the area of preparation. More recent research focuses on methods of preparation and differences in coping styles, variables that were not considered in earlier research. Zeitlin and Williamson (1994) define *coping efforts* or *strategies* as the specific cognitive or behavioral actions taken to manage tension-generating events. *Coping style*, on the other hand, refers to the way an individual routinely uses certain types of strategies, rather than others, to manage his or her world. While portraying a characteristic way of behaving (i.e., typical behavioral patterns), coping style does not describe the specific actions an individual will use in a particular situation. Children learn coping strategies from infancy onward, and many strategies learned in childhood continue into adulthood. Although patterns develop, children learn additional coping modes from parents, peers, teachers, and relatives. Further, children seldom use only one strategy at a time.

An example from the adult literature evaluates hypnosis as a preparation method, and concludes that its effectiveness relates not only to hypnotic ability, but to other individual differences such as coping style, differences in coping demands, and past medical and surgical experiences (Kessler & Dane, 1996). The article cites one study in which clients receiving cognitive behavioral hypnotherapy exhibited at least 70% greater improvement than those receiving cognitive behavioral therapy without hypnosis. The authors conclude that an intervention tailored to the individual needs of the client and presented in a hypnotic context would be beneficial to the majority of clients (Kessler & Dane, 1996).

Other studies examined the use of pamphlets (Stone & Glasper, 1997), books (Felder-Puig et al., 2003), or videotapes (Moix, Bassets, & Caelles, 1998) to prepare children and families for surgery. These methods were found to be effective and to result in an increase in parental satisfaction with the surgical experience. With the increase in day surgery in many acute settings (Murphy-Taylor, 1999), these methods may increase the availability of preparation materials to families who live too far away to come in for a preparation program. Some hospitals now offer "virtual tours" and interactive children's programs on their Web sites.

Two meta-analyses addressed some of the limitations of the preparation research. Kleiber and Harper (1999) analyzed 26 studies dealing with the effects of distraction on children's pain and distress during medical procedures: 16 studies on distress behavior, and 10 on children's pain. Combining the studies gave sample sizes of 491 and 535, respectively, to address the limitation of small sample size in each of the original studies. They concluded that distraction had a positive effect on distress behaviors across the populations represented, and that the effects of distraction on children's pain (self-reported) were influenced by moderator variables.

O'Connor-Von (2000) reviewed 400 articles on preparing children for surgery. Twenty-two met both exclusion and inclusion criteria, yielding a sample size of 1,263. This analysis found that "further research is needed to examine the efficacy of preparation strategies, address diverse populations, and include patient and parent involvement in the preparation process" (O'Connor-Von, 2000).

Each year in the United States approximately 3 million children undergo anesthesia and surgery; 40% to 60% of these children develop significant behavioral stress prior to surgery (Kain, Caldwell-Andrews, & Wang, 2002). A study at a university children's hospital in the northeastern United States demonstrated that perioperative distress can result in negative behavioral changes, including bad dreams, crying, temper tantrums, and fear of doctors and hospitals for up to 2 weeks following surgery (Kain, Mayes, O'Connor, & Cicchetti, 1996). In a later study (Kain, Mayes, Wang, & Hofstadter, 1999), children undergoing anesthesia and surgery were given either sedation with acetaminophen (paracetamol) or acetaminophen alone prior to induction of general anesthesia. The sedated children demonstrated fewer negative behaviors during the first postoperative week than those not sedated.

A study in Sweden evaluated an anesthetic sedation-free method of transurethral catheterization in children through the use of written and oral child-adapted information and practical instructions to prepare children and their families (Gladh, 2003). A simple questionnaire was given to 115 consecutive children undergoing transurethral catheterization. Of the 99 children who returned the questionnaire, 95 found the preparation "good" or "very good" and tolerated the catheterization procedure well. Gladh concluded that careful preparation of children and their parents can allow the majority of diagnostic studies that require urethral catheterization to be accomplished without anesthesia.

The literature available on preparing children for medical procedures identifies a small study (Blount, Powers, Cotter, Swan, & Free, 1994) that showed that teaching children distraction as a coping strategy, with parents as coaches, resulted in increased coping and decreased distress after one treatment session. In two of the three children ages 4 to 7 years, this change persisted over the course of treatment. Additional research is needed to clearly demonstrate the effectiveness of various types of preparation on the dimensions of children's and parents' behavior such as anxiety, coping, and resilience.

In a survey of pediatric oncology centers, McCarthy, Cool, Petersen, and Bruene (1996) asked staff about the use and effectiveness of cognitive behavioral interventions to help children and their families cope with pain and anxiety during lumbar punctures and bone marrow aspirations. The survey revealed that the majority of centers use various cognitive behavioral interventions, and that these were most often provided by nurses. Interventions that require more time and training on the part of the staff were less frequently used. A variety of support services were available by consultation, but not on an ongoing basis. The authors concluded that nurses should continue to study ways to incorporate the use of effective cognitive behavioral interventions into the routine care of children with cancer. Liossi and Hatira (1999) conducted a study involving pediatric cancer patients and found that patients receiving either hypnosis or cognitive behavioral training to relieve pain and distress during bone marrow aspiration reported less pain and anxiety than a control group, and than their own baseline. The two strategies were similar in their effectiveness at pain relief, but children in the cognitive behavioral group reported more anxiety and demonstrated more behavioral distress than did the hypnosis group. These authors maintain that it is the ability to *cope* well with a stressor that demonstrates a positive effect, even—or perhaps especially—in the face of evidence that the event *is* inherently stressful.

Becoming increasingly popular in pediatric oncology settings, art therapy is being used to help prepare children with cancer for the many procedures inherent in their treatment to prevent anxiety, fear, and prolonged emotional distress. Favara-Scacco, Smirne, Schiliro, and Di Cataldo (2001) studied the use of art therapy with 32 children ages 2 to 14 years before, during, and after lumbar punctures using the following modes: (a) clinical dialogue to calm children and help them cope with painful procedures; (b) visual imagination to activate alternative thought processes, decrease the attention toward overwhelming reality, and raise the peripheral sensitivity gate; (c) medical play to clarify illness, eliminate doubts, and offer control over threatening reality; (d) structured drawing to contain anxiety by offering a structured, predictable reality (the drawing) that was controllable by children; (e) free drawing to allow children to externalize confusion and fears; and (f) dramatization to help children accept and reconcile themselves to body changes. The responses of children hospitalized before art therapy was initiated at the hospital in 1997 were compared to those of children hospitalized after. Favara-Scacco and colleagues reported that children hospitalized before the program began exhibited resistance and anxiety during and after painful procedures, while children provided with art therapy from the first hospitalization exhibited collaborative behavior.

Melnyk, Small, and Carno (2004) described an innovative program that engages parents in preparation activities for their children. The program, called Creating Opportunities for Parent Empowerment (COPE), consisted of educational information, delivered in audiotaped and written form, that included child behavioral information about children's typical responses to critical illness and parental role information that provided mothers' suggestions about how they could facilitate their children's adjustment. Mothers also received a parent–child activity workbook with three activities to perform with their children: (a) puppet play, (b) a "Jenny's Wish" book, and (c) therapeutic medical play. A comparison group was given audiotaped information about the hospital's services and policies and comparison activities including coloring, reading a book, and playing with clay. Melnyk et al. reported that mothers in the COPE program (a) reported less negative mood state and less parental stress; (b) provided more support to their children during intrusive procedures; (c) provided more overall emotional support to their children, as rated by primary nurses blind to study group; and (d) reported less posttraumatic stress symptoms following hospitalization.

Studies on preparation can be found in journals from the fields of medicine, nursing, psychology, rehabilitation, hospital administration, patient education, art therapy, and others. What is clear is that this body of work has informed and changed many past practices in children's health care. It needs to continue so that our practice can continue to reflect the changing needs of children and families in an evolving health-care system. This is borne out in the work of O'Byrne, Petersen, and Saldana (1997), who surveyed the preparation programs of pediatric hospitals for evidence of the impact of health psychology research on practice. Results indicated that while there had been a dramatic increase in the use of techniques validated by the research literature (75% of hospitals had greatly increased the use of effective preparation strategies such as filmed modeling and coping skills training), many programs still used methods that were not supported by research. For example, 87% of child surgery patients receive tours, despite a lack of empirical evidence of their effectiveness. The authors call for a greater dissemination of the available research regarding the effectiveness of preparation programs for children.

Developmental Perspective

Children are dynamic beings, constantly growing and changing. Their cognitive, physical, emotional, and social skills emerge at varying rates based on individual and environmental factors. Consequently, it is important to tailor any preparation to each child according to his or her developmental level. This may or may not correspond to chronologic age. Still, there are guidelines that can help to generally shape the preparation experience to meet the needs of each child. In Chapter 1, Table 1.2. Understanding Children Who Are Hospitalized: A Developmental Perspective offers some general guidance based on children's cognitive and emotional development, and the types of reactions to health-care encounters one might expect at each developmental stage.

It is interesting to note that the literature fails to consistently demonstrate any benefit to preschool children participating in preparation programs (Kain, Mayes, & Caramico, 1996; Vaughn, 1957). Despite this, in clinical practice, preschoolers are the age group most likely to have elective surgery, and also are generally considered to be the most at risk for negative emotional reactions to surgery (Mahan & Mahan, 1987). Consequently, they are the target age group for many preparation programs.

Many of these studies concerning preschool children measure anxiety, a variable that is used to draw the conclusion that preparation does not help (Kain, Mayes, & Caramico, 1996; Melamed & Siegel, 1975). However, a more recent study to determine if a preparation program that included role play could reduce anxiety prior to ENT surgery noted a positive effect of the preparation program *especially* among children under 5 years of age (Hatava, Olsson, & Lagerkranser, 2000). Other studies confirm the finding that preparation is not helpful for younger children, but also measure effectiveness of coping strategies employed by the children. Pediatric research on the effects of individual differences on the response to preparation include Petersen and Toler (1986), who concluded that an information-seeking disposition predicted question asking during anesthesia induction, as well as observed distress following surgery. Age, however, had an even more decided effect, influencing the majority of stress variables measured (Petersen & Toler, 1986). This study also found that information seeking increased with age. Corbo-Richert (1994) observed the coping behaviors of children undergoing chest tube insertion in a pediatric intensive care unit (PICU). The predominant coping behaviors were self-protective, followed by reaching out and controlling behaviors, and information-seeking behaviors. Weisz, McCabe, and Dennig (1994) classified coping strategies as primary control (attempts to alter conditions), secondary control (attempts to adjust to conditions), or relinquished control (no attempt to cope). Secondary control coping was positively associated with general behavioral adjustment and illness-specific adjustment.

Kain, Mayes, and Caramico (1996) conducted a perioperative anxiety study with children ages 2 to 10 years who were scheduled for outpatient surgery and general anesthesia, and their parents. The authors measured temperament and anxiety using an observer, self-report, and parent report scale at two stress points: (a) while waiting in the holding area and (b) on separation from parents at the operating room. Parent anxiety levels also were measured both by self-report and observer scales. Parents completed a post-hospital behavior rating scale 2 weeks later. The results of this study were that children between 2 and 3 years of age and children with a history of previous hospitalizations were more anxious if they had participated in the preparation program than those who had not participated. Children older than 6 years were least anxious if prepared 5 to 7 days in advance of the surgery, and most anxious if prepared only 1 day before surgery. The authors conclude that:

> the application of behavioral preparation is best undertaken with knowledge of the child's age, and his or her past medical experiences. Specifically, children who are at least 6 years old should receive the preparation at least one week prior to surgery ... The program had a negative effect on children age 3 years and younger and on children with a history of previous surgery or hospitalization, and these populations should not be offered preoperative preparation programs. (Kain, Mayes, & Caramico, 1996, p. 513)

To date, these findings have not been widely applied to clinical practice. Many settings routinely prepare children 2 to 3 years of age, and also children with previous medical or surgical experience. It would be interesting to revisit this study and add a component dealing with coping strategies. Anecdotal reports suggest that children who remain anxious still cope more effectively when prepared for surgery.

Some approaches, however, have universal appeal with children (and adults) regardless of age. In an ethological study of 18 children ages 3 through 6 years who were hospitalized in a PICU, Snyder (2004) found one intervention successful in gaining children's cooperation with all of the study participants: offering a choice or control over what was happening, such as offering to postpone the procedure, asking what limb or bodily location they preferred for device application or insertion, or negotiating how the procedure should be performed. "When nurses did offer a choice, the children exhibited better cooperation regardless of their age" (Snyder, 2004, p. 39).

Language

When preparing children, language is one aspect of development that must be considered. Child life specialists and nurses generally begin offering preparation programs to children between 2½ and 3 years of age. At this age, many children are able to ask questions and participate verbally in the program, although most will learn more by manipulating and exploring objects, and by visual demonstrations. As children mature, they are increasingly able to process verbal information and ask appropriate questions about it. Table 2.1 outlines some general expectations concerning language development in young children. For specific information about communicating effectively with children, see Table 2.2, box, and Figure 2.1.

Table 2.1

53

Sequence of Language Acquisition

Age	Characteristics
Newborn	Cries as first means of oral communication
4–6 weeks	Coos
5 months	Makes monosyllabic sounds (e.g., "ba," "ga")
6–8 months	Babbles ("mamamama") Attends to own name
10 months	Uses first specific words with appropriate reference (e.g., "mama," "dada") Should comprehend word "no"
12 months	Uses 1–2 words other than "mama/dada" Increases vocabulary at an average of one word per week Comprehends simple commands
18–20 months	Uses an average of 20 words
24 months	Has a vocabulary of around 50 words Acquires one or more words per day Uses two-word sentences ("want up") Should be able to follow simple two-step commands (e.g., "sit down and drink your juice")
24–30 months	Uses telegraphic speech as 3–5 word sentences with subject, object, and verb (e.g., "me want juice")
36 months	Has receptive language of about 800 words Understands simple prepositions (e.g., "put the ball under the table")
4 years	Uses intelligible speech most of the time

Note. From "Cognitive and Psychosocial Development," by M. Baroni, 1999, in *Core Curriculum for the Nursing Care of Children and Their Families* (p. 39), by M. Broome and J. Rollins (Eds.), 1999, Pitman, NJ: Jannetti. Copyright 1999 by Jannetti. Reprinted with permission.

Another language issue related to preparation is the use of medical terminology with children. Many of these words are unfamiliar and ambiguous, even to parents. Using them may contribute to fantasies or misunderstandings on the part of children about what will occur. When medical terminology should be used because the child will hear it, or because it is the correct name for a body part, the words should be explained to children in language they will understand, and opportunities for questions or clarification should be offered. Words or phrases that are helpful to one child may be threatening to another. Health-care providers must listen carefully and be sensitive to the child's use of and response to language. For example, children may interpret "shot" as "with a gun" or "PICU" as "pick you." For an excellent commentary on choosing language, see Gaynard et al. (1990).

Table 2.2

Age-Specific Considerations

Age Group	Considerations
Infants	Consider body language, such as gestures and posture, as well as pitch, intonation, and intensity of voice.
	Nonverbal behaviors work especially well for infants, with cuddling, patting, or some other form of gentle physical contact often quieting them.
	Maintain a calm voice and avoid sudden, loud noises. The actual words spoken are not as important as the way they are spoken.
	Because infants can begin fearing strangers as early as 6 months, holding out the hands and asking the older infant to "come over" is seldom successful. If handling is necessary, the best approach is to pick up the infant firmly without using gestures.
	Infants are usually more at ease when upright, and in visual contact with and close proximity to their parents.
Preschool and young school-age children	Avoid quick approaches. Let the child make the first move whenever possible.
	Broad smiles and other facial contortions may appear threatening.
	Avoid extended eye contact until after the child is comfortable.
	Position yourself at the child's eye level. You will appear less threatening to the child and the child's smallness will be de-emphasized.
	Children may be more responsive when remaining close to the parent, such as sitting on the parent's lap.
	Be direct and concrete with young children because they are unable to deal with the abstract or separate fact from fantasy. For example, young children attach literal meanings to common phrases such as "a frog in the throat" or "hold your horses."
Older school-age children	Continue using relatively simple explanations to facilitate understanding as children get older.
	Children this age want concrete explanations and reasons for everything, for they rely more on what they know than what they see when faced with new problems. They use knowledge seeking as a coping strategy. Learning new things about how their bodies work offers children this age an opportunity to master some aspects of the hospital experience.
Adolescents	Be prepared to deal with a wide range of emotions and behaviors. Give concrete explanations that focus on the adolescent's concerns, even though the capacity to think in abstract terms increases with age.
	It is unnecessary to be fluent in teen jargon, but ask for clarification when needed.
	To enhance communication, exchange information without using coercive questions. Initially confine discussions to less threatening topics to allow time for trust to develop.
	Ask broad, open-ended questions before specific questions, such as "How's school?" before asking, "What is the best or worst thing about school?"

Note. Adapted from "Communicating Effectively with Young Children," by L. Clutter, C. Hess, K. Nix, J. Rollins, D. Smith, N. Stevens, and D. Wong, 1987, *Children's Nurse, 5*(4), pp. 1–3; and "Communicating Effectively with Older Children and Adolescents," by L. Clutter, C. Hess, K. Nix, J. Rollins, D. Smith, N. Stevens, and D. Wong, 1988, *Children's Nurse, 6*(1), pp. 4, 6, 8.

Communication Techniques

1. *Give children an opportunity to express their thoughts, concerns, and feelings.* Listen and respond to underlying messages rather than just verbal content. Be attentive, try not to interrupt, and avoid comments that convey disapproval or surprise.

2. *Acknowledge and validate the child's feelings.* Instead of denying them with a statement such as, "Don't be angry," say, "You sound really mad." This permits the child to accept the emotion and begin to deal with it.

3. *Avoid negative "you-messages," that often start with "you" followed by something that tends to blame, accuse, or attack the person to whom the message is directed.* Use alternatives such as:

   • *Describe the child's situation or problem without mentioning the child.* For example, instead of saying, "You took off your bandage," say, "The bandage is off; it needs to be on."

   • *Send "I-messages" to communicate thoughts, feelings, expectations, or beliefs without imposing blame or criticism.* For example, say, "I feel frustrated when I cannot hear what Johnny is trying to tell me because of all the noise in here."

   • *Provide descriptive praise to point out the child's attributes or to identify your feelings about the child.* For example, after obtaining a blood sample, saying, "You sat very still and told me it hurt instead of moving your arm," is more helpful than making an evaluative statement such as, "You're a great patient," which may cause the child to feel doubt, denial, or fear of not measuring up at a later time. In summary, comment on the behavior, not the person.

   • *Use the third person technique by expressing a feeling in terms of "he," "she," or "they."* This gives the child an opportunity to agree or disagree without being defensive. For example, say, "Sometimes children who are sick tell me they feel angry or sad because they cannot do what others can do." Then wait silently for a response or encourage one by saying, "I wonder if you have ever felt that way."

Figure 2.1.

Communication techniques. *Note.* Adapted from "Communicating Effectively with Young Children," by L. Clutter, C. Hess, K. Nix, J. Rollins, D. Smith, N. Stevens, and D. Wong, 1987, *Children's Nurse*, 5(4), pp. 1–3; and "Communicating Effectively with Older Children and Adolescents," by L. Clutter, C. Hess, K. Nix, J. Rollins, D. Smith, N. Stevens, and D. Wong, 1998, *Children's Nurse*, 6(1), pp. 4, 6, 8.

Preparation Techniques

Preparing children for surgery and procedures requires some knowledge of and sensitivity to the emotional and cognitive abilities of children at different ages and stages of development. An entire profession, the field of child life, has grown up around our increasing understanding of the psychosocial needs of children and families in health-care settings, including the need for preparation. Now an integral part of many interdisciplinary teams in children's health care, child life specialists are trained to assess the developmental needs of children and to plan appropriate interventions, including preparation, within the context of the children's abilities, family relationships, and medical conditions (see Figure 2.2).

Other individuals who may contribute to or assume the preparation role in a given setting include nurses, therapists, physicians, social workers, and parents. Pediatrician Morris Wessel, MD, offers this account of his routine for preparing his young patients for surgery:

> Early in my practice in 1953, I visited a child (age 8) preoperatively and took her for a walk down to the surgical suite. I stopped at the door, and she asked, "Why can't we go in? Isn't this where I will be going tomorrow?" I had no ready answer so I pushed the door open. It was in the evening and the nurses were very gracious when I said, "This is Suzy. She is going to have surgery tomorrow and I thought it would be nice if she could see where she was going and meet you." … This became a regular routine in my practice the night before elective surgery. Many surgeons approved and appreciated this role. However, over the years the anesthesiologists took offense, saying that the preoperative preparation of the child was their responsibility. They seemed be unaware that, as good as they were, they were newcomers to the child and family, where, as a primary pediatrician, I already had a relationship with them. I kept this up throughout my practice…. I cannot measure the success of my intervention, but it was satisfying to me. And when I retired, this intervention was mentioned by many children and parents. (Wessel, as cited in Stein, Rothstein, & Kennell, 2001, p. 428)

General Strategies for Communicating Effectively with Children

1. Use a calm, unhurried, and confident voice.
2. Speak clearly, be specific, and use as few words as possible. As a general guide, use sentences with a sum of words that is equal to the child's age in years plus one.
3. Use play as a strategy for getting to know the child. For example, if the child has a doll or stuffed animal, you can begin by speaking to the toy, then initiate conversation with the child by asking simple questions about the toy.
4. Listen to and observe the child at play. Often, children will express important information such as complicated or difficult feelings through this familiar medium.
5. Look for opportunities to offer the child choices, but offer them only when they exist. For example, when a child must change into a gown, a statement such as, "I need your dress off so I can listen to your chest. Shall I help you take it off?" gives the child an explanation, a choice, and some measure of control.

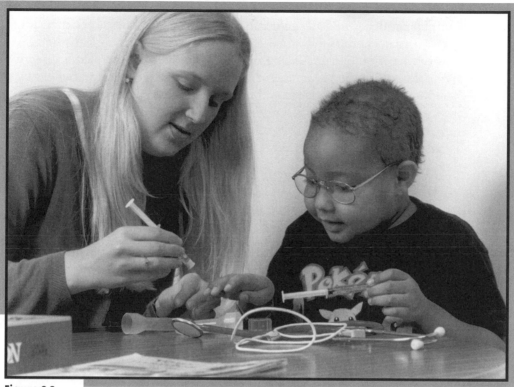

Figure 2.2.
Child life specialists are trained to assess the developmental needs of children and to plan appropriate interventions, including preparation. *Note.* Photograph used with permission of Children's Hospital of Wisconsin.

6. Be honest. It is best to describe how something might feel than to simply say, "It will hurt."

7. Avoid phrases that might be misinterpreted. For example, the statement, "Let's see how warm your body is," is preferred to, "Let's take your temperature." The child may wonder what you are going to do with his or her temperature and if you are planning to give it back. Words such as "shot" can be frightening if a child envisions a shot from a gun. Instead substitute with the phrase, "Putting some medicine under the skin."

8. Avoid expressions with dual meanings, such as "put to sleep."

9. Substitute words that may be interpreted as threatening with words that are less emotionally charged, such as replacing "stick" with "gently slide."

10. State directions and suggestions in a positive way. For example, say, "You need to stay very still" rather than, "Don't move."

11. Avoid prying, asking embarrassing questions, and lecturing when giving advice.

Note. Adapted from "Communicating Effectively with Young Children," by L. Clutter, C. Hess, K. Nix, J. Rollins, D. Smith, N. Stevens, and D. Wong, 1987, *Children's Nurse,* 5(4), pp. 1–3; and "Communicating Effectively with Older Children and Adolescents," by L. Clutter, C. Hess, K. Nix, J. Rollins, D. Smith, N. Stevens, and D. Wong, 1998, *Children's Nurse,* 6(1), pp. 4, 6, 8.

Very young children may need only basic information, but the opportunity to explore the equipment and environment with a supportive adult is reassuring to them (see Figure 2.3). As children grow and learn, mastering new information becomes more important to their ability to cope effectively with a stressful experience. Preschool and school-age children benefit by rehearsing expected behaviors and participating in choices about which coping strategies are most useful to them. Adolescents need even more complex information about what to expect before, during, and after the procedure. In addition, they can sometimes gain support by talking to another teen who has coped effectively with a similar situation.

Infants and Toddlers: Birth to 2.5 Years

In some settings, infants and toddlers under age 2 years are offered preparation, despite a lack of any empirical evidence of benefit (Kain, Mayes, Caramico, 1996; Vaughn, 1957). In anecdotal reports, however, children as young as 9 months of age can attempt to use medical equipment appropriately and may benefit from familiarizing themselves with the equipment (Gaynard et al., 1990). Sensory exploration is the primary way that infants and toddlers learn about their world (Allen & Marotz, 1989). These children generally enjoy and may benefit from an opportunity to explore materials that will be used in their care. This exploration may lead even the youngest child to an increased sense of mastery over objects and events that take place in health-care settings. Demonstrating the use of medical equipment may stimulate older infants and toddlers to imitate the behavior. Because such young children have a limited concept of time, these interventions may take place immediately or shortly prior to an examination or treatment. It is not until nearly age 4 that a child can usually understand a sequence of daily events, and even later that a child learns to tell time (Allen & Marotz, 1989).

For children so young, perhaps the most effective intervention of all is the presence of social support—a parent or other caring adult who can comfort the child during periods of stress (Clutter et al., 1987). In fact, according to Skipper and Leonard (1968), preparing the parents of very young children for what to expect from the procedure, and how they can help care for their child may lead to lower stress levels for both parent and child. Beginning a preparation session with some humor for anxious parents (e.g., "Do you know the definition of minor surgery? It's when it's happening to someone else's child.") can be an effective way to break the ice.

The following are some guidelines for preparing infants, toddlers, and their parents for health-care encounters. An example of preparing an infant is found in Case Study 2.1.

■ **Introductions.** Introduce yourself to the parents. Attempt to engage the infant with a game of "peek-a-boo" or another game without touching or getting too close to the infant.

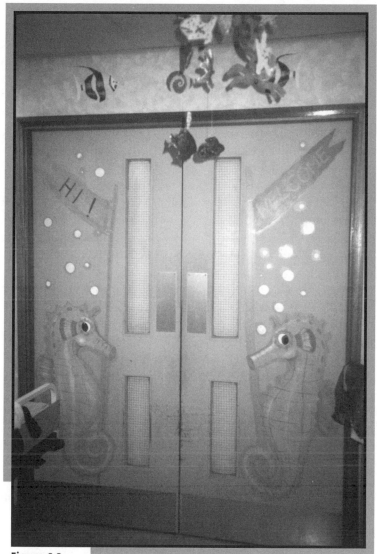

Figure 2.3.
Visiting surgical and recovery areas ahead of time can be an important part of preparation. *Note.* Photograph of Leicester Royal Infirmary.

Case Study 2.1
Preparing an Infant for Craniofacial Surgery

Eleven-month-old Kevin was scheduled for craniofacial surgery. He arrived at the surgery center the week before surgery for a "preoperative tour" with his parents, who were very anxious. The referring physician and nurse believe that the tour is primarily to benefit the parent, but often the parents expect their child to gain from the experience as well.

The child life specialist encouraged Kevin to explore the toys in the playroom and the medical equipment in the preoperative area (e.g., stethoscopes, thermometers, bandages). This was followed by a demonstration of the use of the inhalation mask, and Kevin was asked to imitate. The mask was sent home with the family so that they could rehearse that behavior for the day of surgery.

The family was then taken to the Pediatric Intensive Care Unit, where Kevin would wake up. The child life specialist demonstrated the room and bed controls, and introduced the family to some of the staff who would be caring for Kevin. She explained policies for the various areas where Kevin would be during and after surgery and gave them a handbook with additional policies and resources for families.

As she escorted the family out, the child life specialist offered Kevin the opportunity to turn off lights, push the elevator buttons, and open the automatic doors. This provided Kevin with a sense of mastery over these experiences. Kevin's parents reported that they felt very reassured by the visit. The child life specialist asked them to call her if they had any additional questions or concerns.

- **Exploration.** While explaining procedures to the parents, offer the child an opportunity to explore the various medical equipment that will be used during his or her surgical experience.
- **Demonstration.** Show the baby or toddler an anesthesia mask. Demonstrate its use on yourself, then parents. Ask the child to imitate this behavior. Send home the mask, along with a pre-made surgical doll with all tubes and bandages the child will have. Tell the child he or she will have what the doll has when he or she comes to the hospital. Instruct parents to reinforce the teaching at home using these materials.
- **Mastery.** Show parents and the child around the environment, introduce them to the staff. Allow the child to work the television controls, light switches, and automatic doors, with assistance, if necessary.

Preschoolers: 2.5 to 5 Years

Reports from perioperative nurses and parents in the author's acute care setting suggest that the combination of preparation and social support results in lower anxiety for parents and children, even in the preschool age group. This preparation is given 5 to 7 days in advance, and includes sensory information, role rehearsal, demonstration of medical equipment, and reassurance for child and parents. The following are some techniques found to be useful with this age group. An example of preparing a preschooler is found in Case Study 2.2.

- **Introductions.** State your name and your role on the staff (e.g., "Hi, my name is Kim. My job is to talk with children about what will happen when they come to the hospital."). Then, clearly state

Case Study 2.2
Preparing a Preschooler for Surgery

Four-year-old Alex was scheduled for a tonsillectomy, adenoidectomy, and myringotomy with tubes. His mother, a single parent, had asked for books to read with him that might help them through this experience. One week before surgery, Alex came to the surgery center with his mother for preparation. He appeared shy and clung to her during introductions. The first stop was the playroom in the waiting area. Alex explored the toys, and did not want to leave to proceed with the preparation. He was given a choice to drive the toy car or ride in the wagon to the next room, and he chose the car. In the pre-operative area, Alex tried out the scale and the blood pressure cuff, but declined to try the thermometer. His mother tried to cajole him, but was told: "Today Alex can choose not to try the thermometer. But next week, the nurse will need to measure his temperature."

The next stop was the pre-op playroom, where Alex and a child life specialist rehearsed what would happen to Alex, using a doll as the patient. Alex named the doll, chose a "flavor" for his anesthesia mask, and helped hold the mask to the doll's face while it fell asleep. Alex became anxious when offered an opportunity to start the doll's IV, as did his mother. After a reminder that he would be asleep, and would neither feel nor remember getting the IV, Alex decided to help. He and his mother were surprised and relieved to learn that a needle would not stay in his arm, just a tiny, flexible tube. Then Alex learned that while the medicine made him stay asleep, his doctor would take out his tonsils and adenoids so he would not get so many sore throats, and put tubes in his ears so he would get fewer earaches.

Alex saw a picture of the recovery, or "Wake-Up," room. He was told that when he got to the second wake-up room his mother would be there, and that his jobs would be to drink juice and eat popsicles, and to tell his mother or a nurse if he was hurting. He was told how he would get medicine to help stop the hurting, and things he could do to help himself (e.g., watch a movie, take deep breaths, drink something cold). Lastly, he was told that when his IV was removed, he could get dressed, choose a sticker, and go home with his mother. He agreed to practice choosing a sticker the day of his preparation, which he took home along with his doll "patient." The child life specialist told him that if there was anyone at home who had not come to the preparation, Alex could use the doll to show them what he learned. She mentioned to his mother that hearing this would be a way to assess how much Alex learned, and if she needed to correct any misinformation or confusion, she could do so at home or call the child life specialist for help.

what will and will not occur on this occasion (e.g., "Today we will look around the hospital, talk about your surgery, and play with doctor toys. You will come back on another day for your surgery. Nothing we talk about will happen to you today."). This clarification allows the child to attend to the session without fearing what will happen next.

- **Exploration.** Next, show the child and parents where they will be on the day of surgery. Point out facilities and resources, and provide an opportunity for the child to explore the toys in the play area.
- **Explanation.** Show the preoperative area where the child will get ready for surgery, and emphasize that the parents will be with the child during this time. Describe admission procedures, who the child will meet, and what will happen up until the time of surgery. Then, using dolls and medical equipment, demonstrate anesthesia induction (see Figure 2.4). Explain how the IV works, and allow the child to insert the IV in the doll. Briefly explain what the doctor will

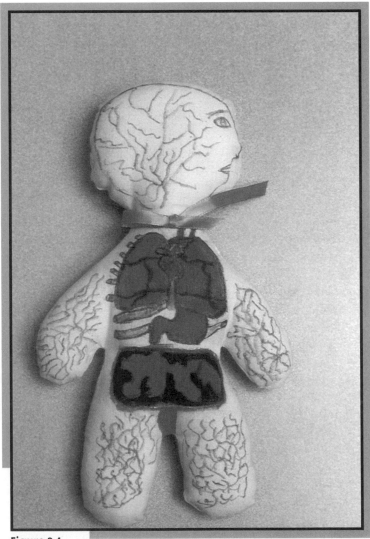

Figure 2.4.
Simple dolls can play an important role in preparation for a wide age range of children. *Note.* Photograph used with permission of Children's Hospital of Wisconsin.

do and how it will help child's health. Then, discuss waking in the recovery room and tell the child when he or she will be reunited with parents.

- **Appropriate Choices.** Offer the child appropriate choices at every juncture. Children feel more confident when they are in control of some aspects of the procedure. For that reason, many settings use a "flavored anesthesia" program as one way of offering choice. Other choices may include who—the child's mother or father—goes to the operating room with the child, what toys to bring to the hospital, and which movie to watch in recovery. Letting the child know in advance the available choices will give him or her positive issues to focus on when talking with parents between the preparation and the time of surgery. Do *not* offer a choice that the child does not have. This often leads to a lack of trust and diminished cooperation.

- **The Child's Role.** Inform the child of the "jobs" he or she needs to do related to the procedure. For example: "You will need to drink juice and eat popsicles when you come back from your surgery." Or, "You will need to remember not to touch your IV. Only the nurse or doctor may do that." This is another means of enlisting cooperation—helping children feel they are important in the process.

- **Coping Strategies.** Teach the child coping strategies such as deep breathing, singing, playing, or other forms of distraction or active coping. Enlist parents as coaches, which gives them a positive role and may reduce their anxiety as well. Inform children that they may use these strategies to relieve pain or anxiety, either before or after surgery.

- **Cues.** Children may remain fearful unless they know when a task is complete. As you explain, tell the child how to know when each step is finished (e.g., "When the IV is out, the nurse will put on a bandage. That is when it will be time for you to put on your clothes and go home with your parents.").

- **Questions.** Ask if the child or parent has any questions. Both parents and children need to feel that their questions have been answered during the preparation session. Many preschoolers are reluctant to speak to the child life specialist, nurse, or other staff member who is conducting the session. Offer the child the chance to whisper a question to the parent, who then asks the staff member. Always offer one or more ways the parent or child may contact the staff if further questions arise.

- **Positive Ending.** Offer stickers or other rewards to help the child have a concrete, positive representation of the preparation session. In the author's setting, the child is allowed to keep the preparation doll, and is encouraged to use it to explain his or her procedure to family members or classmates. While escorting the child out at the conclusion of the session, a demonstration on how to work the automatic doors of the surgery area is given and the child is offered the opportunity to open each one on the way to the exit. Opening the doors is usually the first thing the child wants to do upon entering the hospital on the day of the surgery.

School-Age Children: 6 to 11 Years

The school-age years are characterized by an increasing ability to understand rules, a concept of fairness, and cooperation with others. Children in this age group gain mastery and a sense of competence by demonstrating knowledge and skills. Preparation for children in this age group can include the techniques listed above, and those listed below. For an example of preparing a school-age child, see Case Study 2.3.

- ■ **More Information.** Children ages 6 years and older are increasingly curious about how body systems work. Include an explanation of the affected organ system and how the procedure will improve the condition. Use graphics or dolls with organ systems the child can visualize or manipulate (e.g., "The tube that brings urine from your kidneys to your bladder (indicate on doll) needs to be moved so that you won't get so many kidney infections." See Figure 2.5). Answer any follow-up questions, or refer the child to his or her surgeon if you do not know the answer to a specific situation.

Case Study 2.3
Preparing a School-Age Child for Surgery

Kenisha is an 8-year-old girl scheduled for bilateral ureteral reimplants. During her preparation, she tours the surgery center and has her anesthesia and surgery explained, as did Alex in Case Study 2.2. At this age, children begin to fear that they will not wake up from surgery, or that they will wake up during surgery and experience pain. To counter this, the child life specialist explains: "The medicine makes you stay asleep so you won't feel or remember anything about your surgery. When the surgery is done, the doctor stops giving you the medicine, and that lets you wake up."

The child life specialist uses a life-size doll that opens to reveal kidneys, ureters, and bladder; the workings of the urinary tract are briefly explained. The doll is used to explain how the surgery will fix the problem, and to show Kenisha how her urinary catheter will work after the surgery. Kenisha manipulates the doll's internal organs, and asks questions about their function and about what will happen during surgery. She also manipulates the Foley catheter in the doll, and asks why it is necessary and if it will hurt. She is reassured that it will be placed while she is asleep, but is also told that she may feel some "stinging" or pain when it is removed and during her first few voids. She elects to practice relaxation breathing to help with that part of her recovery.

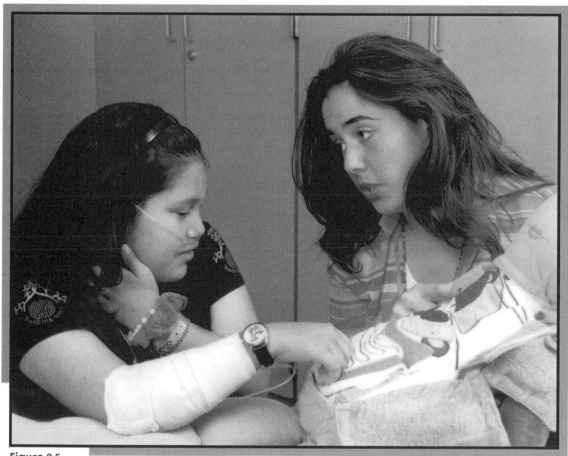

Figure 2.5.
Dolls with organ systems are excellent tools for preparation. *Note.* Photograph used with permission of Children's Hospital of Wisconsin.

- **More Complex Coping Strategies.** School-age children may wish to use creative visualization, listen to favorite music or inspirational tapes, choose whether to watch and participate in appropriate aspects of care, or identify other ways to help them feel more control in the situation. Help them choose from among several options (e.g., "Some children like to pretend they are in a favorite place while this is happening. We can practice what that would be like. Others bring music to listen to, or hold someone's hand during the difficult parts. What do you think would help you the most?"). These are only a few of the many choices you may offer a child.
- **More Opportunities To Participate in Care.** Indicate those areas in which the child might like to participate during the procedure (e.g., "You may help the nurse remove the old bandage," or "You can hold the thermometer in your mouth while we measure your temperature."). Older children may be more cooperative if they feel their choices are being respected as often as possible.

- **Timing.** Tell older children about events at least a week in advance to allow them to acclimate to the information and to plan and rehearse their preferred coping strategies. If treatment will involve more than one intervention, provide a schedule, along with what kinds of issues might cause a change in the schedule. Encourage the child and parents to inform you of any special events that conflict with the treatment schedule. Let them know that, although the child's health comes first, some changes might be possible to coordinate with very important events. Frequently review the long-range plan with the child and family, as children and parents under stress may lose sight of the long-range plan when dealing with day-to-day crises.

Adolescents: 12 to 18+ Years

Adolescents face a number of physical, emotional, social, and cognitive changes. The physical growth spurts of puberty are accompanied by an increase in hormonal activity that causes the body to become more sexually and physically mature. Along with these changes come strong emotions about fitting in socially with peers, feeling attractive to potential partners, and developing close friendships. In addition, teens feel that they are maturing intellectually and should participate more in their own decision making.

A health-care encounter that involves medical tests, procedures, or surgery is perceived as a threat to many of the developmental milestones of adolescence. Like younger children, teens may regress (act younger) when faced with a threat. However, they may simultaneously feel shame about their regression, and a need to act "tough" and "grown up" in the face of such encounters. It is not unusual for patients in this age group to act immature and frightened one minute, and cool and indifferent the next. It is sometimes difficult for parents to help because the teen may ask for help one minute and push them away the next. "Trying on" adult roles is a natural part of adolescent development.

Many of the strategies for younger children will work with teens, with some modifications and the following additions. See Case Study 2.4 for an example of preparation techniques with a teenager.

- **Question List.** Encourage teens to come to the session with a list of questions they would like to ask. Let them know that adults do this, as it is easy to forget what they planned to ask once they are distracted by the medical setting.
- **More Adult Teaching Tools.** Use photographs of the procedure instead of, or in addition to, dolls and drawings, according to the teen's cognitive and emotional abilities.
- **Coping Strategies.** Focus on coping strategies at every step of the process. Ask: "What do you think will help you with the IV? Do you usually look or turn away? Does counting, or humming, or relaxation breathing help? Let's practice it now."

Case Study 2.4
Preparing a Teenager for Procedures

Danita is a 14-year-old girl who visits the hospital repeatedly for tests, procedures, and IV medications. She prepares for the outpatient days by baking cookies for the staff and patients, and visiting with people she knows while waiting to be called for her procedure. Afterwards, she leaves as quickly as possible.

If her treatment requires an inpatient stay, she brings her own sheets, pillow, blanket, and seasonal decorations for her room. She chooses to make the environment as much her own as she possibly can. She also brings music, videos, and the book of all her friends' e-mail addresses so that she can communicate with them on the computer. She surrounds herself with friends and family, and makes an effort to learn the names of the doctors, nurses, and staff members taking care of her.

When it is time for a procedure, she turns on her compact disc player, tunes out everything else, and copes very effectively with the experience. Her family supports her through these times, calming her with their presence and providing distracting activities to help pass the time. She has put together a very comprehensive plan for dealing with the stressors of multiple health-care encounters using a variety of coping strategies.

- **Privacy Issues.** Be especially mindful of privacy issues. Let teens know who will need to examine them and why. Make suggestions about how they can protect their own privacy (e.g., "If the nurse forgets to close the curtain around your bed, ask her to do so," or "Even though they want you to use the urinal, you can still go to the bathroom and close the door for more privacy."). Ask about any specific privacy concerns the teen may have.
- **Unexpected Menstruation.** The stress of having a procedure or surgery may bring on menstruation unexpectedly. Assure teens that this is normal, and suggest that they may want to bring some of their own supplies for comfort. Also let them know that the hospital will have what is needed in case they forget.
- **Active Participation in Care.** Encourage teens to actively participate in their care. Teens can choose their menus, ask what their vital signs are, help to take them, and ask to see their plan of care and talk with doctors, nurses, and parents about how they can take charge of some of the issues. This will help them to feel empowered and offer a sense of mastery, instead of encouraging a feeling of dependence.
- **Peer Group Contact.** Encourage teens to keep in touch with their peer group. In this age group, peer relationships are more important than ever before, and visits from friends and classmates with shared interests will go a long way toward facilitating a quick

recovery. Feeling accepted by peers in the face of a threatening event is a major concern for adolescents, and no reassurance by adults can take the place of the experience of visiting with friends and being treated as one of the group.

Emergency Admissions or Procedures

If the preparation is for an emergency hospital admission or a procedure that was not anticipated, there might not be the luxury of time for the child and parent to acclimate to the information presented. In such instances, it is still important to focus on active coping, locus of control, support from parents, and on what to expect from staff.

The following strategies can be used for emergency procedures. See Case Study 2.5 for an example of helping a child cope with an emergency procedure.

Case Study 2.5
Helping a Child Cope with Emergency Procedures

Nine-year-old Georgia was admitted from the Emergency Department with suspected aseptic meningitis. She needed an IV and a lumbar puncture (LP) to rule out that diagnosis and begin proper treatment. When the child life specialist met her, Georgia had been in the treatment room for 45 minutes or more, and had been through two failed IV insertion attempts. Georgia stated she was afraid of getting stuck with the needle, that it would hurt, and that she "wasn't ready."

EMLA Cream* had been applied, and the child life specialist explained that it took time to work, and that while they were waiting, they would do some doctor play to learn about getting an IV. She stated to Georgia, "When we're finished playing, the cream will be working, and it will be time to get your IV." They proceeded to do therapeutic medical play with a cloth doll and IV equipment. Georgia chose not to participate very actively, especially at first, but she watched everything intently. For her, the best part was seeing that what would stay in her arm was not a needle, but a soft, flexible catheter that she was allowed to touch so that she would know how it felt. She learned that she could do "the pinch test" to see if the EMLA was working, so she would not have to rely on information from anyone else, but could decide for herself how it would feel. She discussed ways she had coped in the past with unpleasant things, and chose two strategies. She would count until the needle was out, and she would use her imagination to pretend to be in her own room (i.e., creative visualization).

When the time came for the IV start, Georgia decided that her mother would hold one hand, a medical student would help her hold her arm still, and the child life specialist would help coach her counting and imagery. She was quite anxious, and did a lot of screeching, but she held still and counted, even though more than one IV attempt had to be made and one of them was without EMLA. She was praised by everyone in the room for doing such a great job holding still, counting, and doing her imagery, and she seemed very proud of herself. Now that the IV was in place, it was used as a vehicle for sedation for the LP.

As discussed earlier, therapeutic medical play, as well as rehearsing coping strategies for possible future procedures, can be helpful for children traumatized by difficult procedures. The focus should be on the child's ability to use the chosen strategies successfully. Children will often perform to our expectations, and if we indicate we expect them to succeed, they are much more likely to do so.

*EMLA Cream is a thick, white cream that contains two commonly used anesthetic agents, lidocaine and prilocaine. Normally these agents need to be injected to numb the skin; however, EMLA Cream is formulated to carry the agents through the skin surface to directly numb the area.

- **Behavioral Limits.** Offer the child some behavioral limits as well as choices (e.g., "You may yell as loudly as you like when you get your blood test, and I really need you to hold your arm still during the test. If it is too hard to do by yourself, we can have someone hold it to help you remember."). A similar explanation can be used if restraints are needed (e.g., "The medicine makes you too sleepy to remember not to pull out the tube in your mouth. These bracelets are here to help you remember. When someone is here to hold your hand, we can take them off for awhile."). Children do need limits as well as choices, and they expect adults to supply them.
- **Negotiations.** Once it is time for the procedure, begin on time and do not allow "negotiations" for changes in rules to be used as a delaying tactic. In a child- and family-centered setting, any accommodations have presumably been made, and the only result of further delays is a power struggle that no one can win.
- **Skilled Professionals.** Whenever possible, ensure that a child life specialist or another pediatric health-care professional skilled in preparation and coaching is present to assist with the procedure. It is much more effective to be proactive than to try the procedure and then ask for help once the child and parents are upset and traumatized.
- **Honesty.** Remember the Golden Rule: BE HONEST! It actually reads: "Do unto others as you would have others do unto you," but the results are much the same. Any adult would feel betrayed and insulted if the professionals in a given situation said one thing and did another. Children deserve no less respect in this regard. We cannot reasonably ask them to cooperate with painful or invasive procedures if we are not honest about how it will feel, how long it will take, and how they will know when it is over. It is uncomfortable to say to a child, "Yes, this will hurt." Naturally, no one wants

a child to experience pain, so we do not want them to have to anticipate it. However, as part of a comprehensive plan to help children
and families cope more effectively with health-care encounters,
honesty is paramount. Nothing else will succeed without it.

When There Is No Time for Preparation

In emergency situations, sometimes preparation simply is not possible. At
those times, coaching a child through the procedure and offering ideas for
coping strategies is the next best thing. You might say, "Some children tell
me it helps if they blow bubbles" (or listen to music, sing, or employ whatever distractions are available). "What do you think will help you?" Positioning can also help. Sitting a child in a parent's lap with the arm that needs
an IV extended flat on a table in front of them is a much less threatening position than is being held down lying supine. Stephens, Barkey, and Hall
(1999) present a comprehensive model for assisting children with invasive
procedures. It includes preparation, parent participation, use of the treatment
room, and positioning for comfort. Also stressed is the need to maintain a
positive and calming atmosphere throughout the procedure.

Postvention

In the worst-case scenario, a child arrives at the hospital or other health-
care setting having had a traumatic emergency admission with no preparation, no coaching, and no support. Now what? One goal of this book is to
prevent that from ever happening. But when it does, staff members can offer
support, encouragement, and opportunities for the child and parents to develop trust in the health-care professionals now caring for them.

A helpful strategy is therapeutic medical play:

1. Offer the child a doll or stuffed animal as the "patient," and medical
   supplies such as needles, syringes, tubing, stethoscopes, Band-Aids,
   and casting materials, and allow the child to manipulate the materials
   while caring for the "patient."
2. Use open-ended questions to encourage verbalizations about the
   play (e.g., "Why does your doll need a needle in the face?").
3. Correct any medical misconceptions the child either verbalizes or
   expresses through play.

Medical play also offers children an opportunity to experience some
mastery over things that have been used on them in the medical setting. This
process can be very empowering. For more information on medical play, see
Chapter 3: Play in Children's Health-Care Settings.

If the examples of preparation or helping children cope with procedures
in Case Studies 2.1 through 2.4 were "how to" in nature, the example in Case

Study 2.5 definitely falls into the "what not to do" category. There were so many opportunities that were not taken to make the experience less frightening for this child that by the time there was an intervention, she was almost beyond her ability to take advantage of it. This is exactly the type of scenario we hope to eliminate by disseminating the information in books such as this.

Conclusion

To calm a child during a procedure, he or she can be given a sedative, permitted to have a parent present, or be prepared psychologically. Current practice is often determined by the child's health-care system. Consider, for example, a child scheduled for surgery. Although sedation and parental presence are common in the United Kingdom, in the United States most children are taken into the operating room awake and alone (Larkin, 1997).

However, pre-medication for surgery and other procedures is becoming increasingly more common in the United States. Yet some argue that in busy operating rooms, schedule delays that are secondary to sedation administration may not be tolerated. Fortunately, recent research has focused on seeking out evidence that medications such as midazolam can be administered 10 minutes before a surgical procedure and produce significant anterograde amnesia (Kain et al., 2000).

Short-acting general anesthetic agents such as propofol are becoming increasingly common for outpatient nonsurgical procedures that children formerly were expected to tolerate without anesthesia, and sometimes even without sedation. Endoscopies, bone marrow aspirations and lumbar punctures are among the procedures for which these agents are used. As a result, the children need preparation mainly for the IV start, and do not need to be supported through the procedure because they are not conscious. This is changing the practice of child life specialists and other professionals who have prepared and supported children through such procedures in the past. As new research and technology advances the science, health-care practice will continue to shift to meet the changing needs of children and families in all types of health-care settings.

Children and families can learn to cope effectively with many major stressors, including those associated with illness, surgery, and medical procedures. Our task as health-care professionals is to offer them the tools that will increase their skills in this area. Yet researchers must continue to explore all resources, including medications, that may serve to reduce both the number and intensity of stressors children experience in health-care settings. Also, research is needed to determine whether children's hospitalizations are shorter and pain medication needs are lower when children are pre-medicated. Such evidence could influence hospitals and third-party payers to change current practice and focus on humane strategies that are in everyone's best interest.

Study Guide

1. What is *preparation*?

2. When was preparation for hospitalization and procedures first recognized as important to young children and their families? Why?

3. What were the results of the early (1950s–1980s) studies in preparation?

4. What were the characteristics of preparation in the 1970s and 1980s?

5. How did preparation change by the 1990s? What knowledge, research, and attitudes influenced these changes?

6. Explain the advantages and disadvantages of repression or expression of feelings at the time of events for children at various stages of development.

7. Define the concept of "stress" and its use to both explain and predict children's responses to health-care encounters.

8. How does the "stress reduction" approach to preparation affect children's responses?

9. Define "coping styles," and discuss the ways in which coping styles interact with health-care events.

10. Discuss the pros and cons of various methods of preparation.

11. Discuss the findings of recent meta-analyses of preparation studies and list 3 to 5 studies or strategies essential to strengthening this body of research.

References

Allen, K. E., & Marotz, L. (1989). *Developmental profiles, birth to six*. Albany, NY: Delmar.

Baroni, M. (1999). Cognitive and psychosocial development. In M. Broome & J. Rollins (Eds.), *Core curriculum for the nursing care of children and their families* (pp. 33–44). Pitman, NJ: Jannetti.

Berk, L. (1997). *Child development* (4th ed.). Boston: Allyn & Bacon.

Blount, R. L., Powers, S. W., Cotter, M. W., Swan, S., & Free, K. (1994). Making the system work. Training pediatric oncology patients to cope and their parents to coach them during BMA/LP procedures. *Behavior Modification, 18*(1), 6–31.

Corbo-Richert, B. H. (1994). Coping behaviors of young children during a chest tube procedure in the pediatric intensive care unit. *Maternal Child Nursing Journal, 22*(4), 134–146.

Clutter, L. B., Hess, C., Nix, K. S., Ogle, M. B., Rollins, J., Smith, D., Stevens, N., & Wong, D. (1988). Communicating effectively with older children and adolescents. *Children's Nurse, 6*(1), 4, 6, 8.

Clutter, L., Hess, C., Nix, K., Rollins, J., Smith, D., Stevens, N., & Wong, D. (1987). Communicating effectively with young children. *Children's Nurse, 5*(4), 1–3.

Favara-Scacco, C., Smirne, G., Schiliro, G., & Di Cataldo, A. (2001). Art therapy as support for children with leukemia during painful procedures. *Medical and Pediatric Oncology, 36*(4), 474–480.

Felder-Puig, R., Maksys, A., Noestlinger, C., Gadner, H., Stark, H., Pfluegler, A., & Topf, R. (2003). Using a children's book to prepare children and parents for elective ENT surgery: Results of a randomized clinical trial. *International Journal of Pediatric Otorhinolaryngology, 67*(1), 35–41.

Gaynard, L., Wolfer, J., Goldberger, J., Thompson, R., Redburn, L., & Laidley, L. (1990). *Psychosocial care of children in hospitals: A clinical practice manual*. Bethesda, MD: Association for the Care of Children's Health.

Gladh, G. (2003). Effect of thoughtful preparation on the catheterization of children undergoing investigative studies. *Neurourology and Urodynamics, 22*(1), 58–61.

Hatava, P., Olsson, G., & Lagerkranser, M. (2000). Preoperative psychological preparation for children undergoing ENT operations: A comparison of two methods. *Paediatric Anaesthesia, 10*(5), 477–486.

Janis, I. (1958). *Psychologic stress: Psychoanalytic and behavioral studies of surgical patients*. New York: Wiley.

Kain, Z. N., Caldwell-Andrews, A., & Wang, S. (2002). Psychological preparation of the parent and pediatric surgical patient. *Anesthesiology Clinics of North America, 20*(1), 29–44.

Kain, Z. N., Hofstadter, M. B., Mayes, L. C., Krivutza, D. M., Alexander, G., Wang, S. M., & Reznick, J. S. (2000). Midazolam: Effects on amnesia and anxiety in children. *Anesthesiology, 93*(3), 676–684.

Kain, Z. N., Mayes, L. C., & Caramico, L. A. (1996). Preoperative preparation in children: A cross-sectional study. *Journal of Clinical Anesthesia, 8*(9), 508–514.

Kain, Z. N., Mayes, L. C., O'Connor, T. Z., & Cicchetti, D. V. (1996). Preoperative anxiety in children. Predictors and outcomes. *Archives of Pediatric and Adolescent Medicine, 150*(12), 1238–1245.

Kain, Z. N., Mayes, L., Wang, S., & Hofstadter, M. B. (1999). Postoperative behavioral outcomes in children: Effects of sedative premedication. *Anesthesiology, 90*(3), 758–765.

Kessler, R., & Dane, J. (1996). Psychological and hypnotic preparation for anesthesia and surgery: An individual differences perspective. *The International Journal of Clinical and Experimental Hypnosis, XLIV*(3), 189–207.

Kleiber, C., & Harper, D. C. (1999). Effects of distraction on children's pain and distress during medical procedures: A meta-analysis. *Nursing Research, 48*(1), 44–49.

Larkin, M. (1997). Calming children preoperatively curbs anxiety. *The Lancet, 350*(9086), 1228.

Lazarus, R. (1966). *Psychological stress and the coping process.* New York: McGraw-Hill.

Lazarus, R. (1981). The costs and benefits of denial. In J. Spinetta & P. Deasy-Spitta (Eds.), *Living with childhood cancer* (pp. 50–67). St. Louis, MO: Mosby.

Lazarus, R., & Folkman, S. (1984). *Stress, appraisal, and coping.* New York: Springer.

Liossi, C., & Hatira, P. (1999). Clinical hypnosis versus cognitive behavioral training for pain management with pediatric cancer patients undergoing bone marrow aspirations. *International Journal of Clinical and Experimental Hypnosis, 47*(2), 104–116.

Mahan, C., & Mahan, K. (1987). Patient preparation in pediatric surgery. *Clinics in Podiatric Medicine and Surgery, 4*(1), 1–9.

McCarthy, A. M., Cool, V. A., Petersen, M., & Bruene, D. A. (1996). Cognitive behavioral pain and anxiety interventions in pediatric oncology centers and bone marrow transplant units. *Journal of Pediatric Oncology Nursing, 13*(1), 3–12.

Melamed, B. G., & Siegel, L. J. (1975). Reduction of anxiety in children facing hospitalization by use of filmed modeling. *Journal of Consulting and Clinical Psychology, 43,* 511–521.

Melnyk, B., Small, L., & Carno, M. (2004). The effectiveness of parent-focused interventions in improving coping/mental health outcomes of critically ill children and their parents: An evidence base to guide clinical practice. *Pediatric Nursing, 30,* 143–148.

Moix, J., Bassets, J., & Caelles, R. M. (1998). Effectiveness of audiovisual materials as preparation for surgery in pediatric patients. *Cirugia Pediatrica, 11*(1), 25–29.

Murphy-Taylor, C. (1999). The benefits of preparing children and parents for day surgery. *British Journal of Nursing, 8*(12), 801–804.

O'Byrne, K., Petersen, L., & Saldana, L. (1997). Survey of pediatric hospitals' preparation programs: Evidence of the impact of health psychology research. *Health Psychology, 16*(2), 147–154.

O'Connor-Von, S. (2000). Preparing children for surgery—an integrative research review. *Association of Operating Room Nurses Journal, 71*(2), 334–343.

Petersen, L., & Toler, S. (1986). An information seeking disposition in child surgery patients. *Health Psychology, 5*(4), 343–358.

Petrillo, M. (1972). Preparing children and parents for hospitalization and treatment. *Pediatric Annals, 1*(3), 24–41.

Rollins, J., & Mahan, C. (1996). *From artist to artist-in-residence: Preparing artists to work in pediatric healthcare settings.* Washington, DC: Rollins & Associates.

Selye, H. (1974). *Stress without distress.* New York: The New American Library.

Skipper, J. K., & Leonard, R. C. (1968). Children, stress and hospitalization: A field experiment. *Journal of Health and Social Behavior, 9,* 275–287.

Snyder, B. (2004). Preventing treatment interference: Nurses' and parents' intervention strategies. *Pediatric Nursing, 30*(1), 31–40.

Stanford, G., & Thompson, R. (1981). *Child life in hospitals: Theory and practice.* Springfield, IL: Thomas.

Stein, M., Rothstein, P., & Kennell, J. (2001). Preparing a 3 year old and his parents for an elective surgery. *Journal of Developmental and Behavioral Pediatrics, 22*(6), 425–429.

Stephens, B. K., Barkey, M. E., & Hall, H. R. (1999). Techniques to comfort children during stressful procedures. *Accident and Emergency Nursing, 7*(4), 226–236.

Stone, K. J., & Glasper, E. A. (1997). Can leaflets assist parents in preparing children for hospital? *British Journal of Nursing, 6*(18), 1054–1058.

Vaughn, G. F. (1957). Children in hospital. *The Lancet, 272*(2), 1117–1120.

Walker, C., Wells, L., Heiney, S., & Hymovich, D. (2002). Family-centered psychological care. In C. Baggott, K. Kelly, G. Foley, & D. Fotchman (Eds.), *Nursing care of children and adolescents with cancer* (pp. 365–390). Philadelphia: Saunders.

Weisz, J., McCabe, M., & Dennig, M. (1994). Primary and secondary control among children undergoing medical procedures: Adjustment as a function of coping style. *Journal of Consulting and Clinical Psychology, 62*(2), 324–332.

Wolfer, J. A., & Visintainer, M. A. (1975). Pediatric surgical patients' and parents' stress responses and adjustment. *Nursing Research, 24*(4), 244–255.

Zahr, L. K. (1998). Therapeutic play for hospitalized preschoolers in Lebanon. *Pediatric Nursing, 24*(5), 449–454.

Zeitlin, S., & Williamson, G. (1994). *Coping in young children: Early intervention practices to enhance adaptive behavior and resilience.* Baltimore: Brookes.

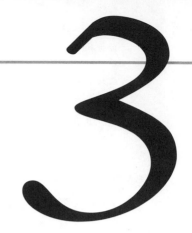

Play in Children's Health-Care Settings

Rosemary Bolig

Objectives

At the conclusion of this chapter, the reader will be able to:

1. Discuss the importance of play to development and coping and the implications of its absence.
2. Indicate the values of play in health-care settings for children at various stages of development and in different stages of illness.
3. Describe the factors that have influenced the amount of and type of play provided in health-care settings.
4. Illustrate current and future challenges to play and play facilitation in child health-care settings.

Since the earliest recognition of the negative impact of institutionalization and hospitalization on young children, play and the relationships that ensue have been among the primary prescribed antidotes (Richards & Wolff, 1940):

> Through play a child grows, develops, expresses his emotions, and adjusts to his environment. Play becomes a safety valve for his hidden wishes and fears and a balance for the tensions that are a part of every growing child's life. Ill or well, the child needs play. (p. 229)

The dosage of play and the processes and procedures for assuring its quality frequently have been in debate. However, those who advocate for or provide psychosocial care agree that play is critical for children's expression, mastery, and learning about their experiences—whether in nursing or occupational therapy contexts, or in specialized play, activities, or education programs.

Health care and health-care settings have changed dramatically over the past 10 years, however, and so have perceptions of and provisions for play in such experiences and environments. Especially in its normative forms, play appears to be less prevalent and perhaps less valued than it was a few years ago. Play in health-care professional journals is also a topic receiving less attention today. Little research on play in health care has been conducted since the late 1980s, as is true of basic and quantitative research on play in other contexts.

Change, of course, is inevitable, and the failure of systems and organisms to adapt results in decline if not extinction. Health-care systems and specific programs and disciplines supporting play have changed with the demands of the times (Kleinberg, 1987; Wilson & Chambers, 1996). But just as health-care professionals serving children must continue to acknowledge that children are unique and different than adults, they cannot forget that play is a primary means for children to develop and to cope with life's demands. Pioneers in changing health-care practices for children and their families—researchers such as Robertson (1958) and practitioners such as Plank (1962)—fought against prevailing beliefs about children and systems of care. With over 60 years of experience and research, and with the expanding body of knowledge about mind–body interactions and the recognition of the bio-psychosocial model of health care (Engel, 1980), positions about the uniqueness of children in general, as well as children in health-care settings—and hence play—may need to be re-articulated.

Children *are* different and childhood is very brief. Experiences that *do not* occur within specific time ranges may have as much impact on the course of development as those that do occur; the manner in which experiences happen also may have short- as well as long-term effects. However, in many instances, the impact of an experience is not determined for months, if not years. What may appear as a short-term gain, may instead cause long-term pain. Children may be more resilient than once believed, but they also may be more vulnerable in ways that are only beginning to be understood. For example, recent brain research on children suggests that there are a finite number of years in which neurons must be used or connected to one another, and that stress and constant threats can re-wire emotion circuits: The more this aberrant pathway is used, the easier it is to trigger (Begley, 1996). A continual high alert state affects cortex development and thus children have trouble assimilating complex information such as language. Quinton and Rutter (1976), for example, found that among children with repetitive hospitalizations there were significant reading problems, which may be explained by this recent research on brain functioning.

Children are bringing to health care, as they are to other settings, their unique experiences and family situations—and, new risks and opportunities. Nevertheless, and most important, they are *children* who need nurturing, support, and protection from overwhelming anxiety and stimulation. They are neither more adaptive than previous generations, just because they seemingly had more to adapt to, nor are they simply "information processors" that future views of them may attempt to argue. They are children who, like Kasey, so poignantly described by child life specialist Debbie Kossoff (1996) in a tribute in *The Advocate*, need the reassurance and safety that play environments and facilitators provide:

> When I would appear she would always ask to go to the playroom in her wagon … and at the end of her life, once we were all in the playroom, Kasey expressed an interest in creating a card using the materials I had prepared earlier for Secretary Day. Kasey always enjoyed participating in planned art projects during her hospital visits, but on this day she did not make a card for a secretary. Instead, she asked me to fill the card with love messages for her mommy, auntie, sister, uncle, daddy, and teacher and others important to her. Kasey's younger sister helped with the finishing touches by putting stickers on the card for decoration. When the cards were completed, we moved Kasey and her wagon into the middle of the room, and sat around her in a circle of love, comfort, and support and waited for the inevitable to occur. (p. 29)

Play, for Kasey, even in the last moments of her life, provided the means for solace, communicating, interpreting, and perhaps regulating events around her.

In this chapter, what play is and is not, its functions and forms, the present state of theory and research on play, and the current thinking of play researchers in health care and other contexts will be presented, as will methods and contexts for facilitating play. We will explore multiple, interacting factors that have very little to do with the nature of children or their needs but that influence the perceived importance of play. We will describe the increased research on play and play-based programs, especially in health-care settings, which is vital for its revival and perhaps its survival (Power, 2000; Thompson, 1995). Beyond this imperative for data-based information on play, especially in health care, there are other systems, beliefs, and attitudes toward children that need to be considered in response to new challenges and demands in health care, technology, family life, and society in general to encourage the conditions that are supportive of children's play.

Play in Psychology, Education, and Anthropology

Play is one of, if not *the*, quintessential behaviors of childhood. It has been of significant research interest since the 1930s and has been the subject of much debate throughout the years (Power, 2000). Power (2000) reports that the research interest in play was at its height in the 1970s, with interest waning ever since. There have been various "waves" of research, according to Fein (1997), that include determining ways to investigate play, training studies, correlational investigations of categories of play and, most recently, qualitative studies. Over the past 10 years, however, there has been less interest in the quantitative study of children at play and variable support for play in early childhood settings. With the changing of nature research on play (Fein, 1997), recent qualitative work may have expanded and deepened the understanding of its complexity. Qualitative research, however, often takes longer to conduct and has been less likely to be published, although an increasing number of journals are devoted to or include this work.

Play Perspectives

First and foremost, play is fun. Play—to be playful—is within the control and imagination of children. With these characteristics, it is not surprising that throughout recorded history play often has been a metaphor for *freedom* and even for *power* (Sutton-Smith, 1995). Play frightens some and appears frivolous to others. Particularly in the United States' culture, play often is seen as diverting, interfering, or subverting more purposeful activity.

Sometimes play is thought to decrease motivation. Play appears to be too random, too pleasurable, too self-serving to serve any important function. Play also gives control to children, making some adults feel out of control. When lives and times of adults are chaotic, structure is often imposed on children, with play often being one of the first behaviors to suffer.

With the changes that have occurred either through demographics, immigration or migration, world wars, and technology in the United States, and the concurrent feelings of both optimism and lack of control, it is not surprising that, at various times, the belief in the importance of play has retreated in lieu of more direct means of socializing, educating, and effecting the growth and development of children. In the early part of the 20th century, for example, members of the Child Study Movement fought back against the establishment of the highly structured Froebelian kindergarten and Montessori programs. Despite their contrast to prevailing teaching practices in their countries of origin, these methods were not child-centered or truly play-oriented. In the rapidly changing 1960s, an out-of-control period in the opinions of some, and with the rapid increase in demand for child care, the Montessori approach was accepted, albeit adapted for this country. Behavioral theories with token economies and reinforcement schedules in education also were widely accepted in the 1960s and 1970s. Public education systems are constantly being buffeted by these changes in perspective on how children develop and learn (Glickman, 1988).

Even the development of theory and research is not immune from these forces. Products of their times, theories reflect the prevailing viewpoints, values, and expectations as well as "knowledge" and, in turn, affect their times. Various views or paradigms have influenced not only the development of theories about human (and non-human) growth and development, but—because play has long been recognized as a behavior of children—play theory as well. Early theories or classical theories included explanations of play as means for discharging natural energy (Spencer, 1873/1951); renewing energy (Patrick, 1916); reliving periods of history of the human species (Hall, 1904); and practicing for adulthood (Groos, 1901). With the exception of recapitulating evolution, all these theories have had some impact on current theories about play. By the 1930s, psychoanalytic theory began to dominate views of human development, with Freud's (1952) psychosexual theory and Erikson's (1950/1963, 1972) psychosocial theory predominant in the understanding of the critical importance of play.

Current perspectives on play include competence motivation and arousal-seeking. Competence motivation theory posits that children receive satisfaction in developing competency via play, regardless of whether there are any external rewards (Spodek & Saracho, 1988). "Play enables children to act on their environment, becoming more effective and thus receiving personal satisfaction" (Spodek & Saracho, 1988, p. 15). Arousal-seeking theory states that children need to be continually involved in information processing, but that play is the way children mediate the amount of stimulation to achieve an optimal level of arousal.

Play has thus been viewed through various lenses with resultant perspectives, which have affected the nature of scholarly inquiry as well as practice. According to Sutton-Smith (1995, pp. 279–291), these perspectives revolve around five themes:

- *Play as Progress*—Among scholars in the 20th century, there was an obsession to demonstrate that children learn something useful from their play; although this continues today, the specific focus has shifted from physical skills, to emotional, to cognitive, depending upon prevalent theories.
- *Play as Adaptation*—A curvilinear relationship has been found between play participation and general adaptation. Those children who do not get to play with others because they are too withdrawn or aggressive generally also perform badly at school.
- *Play as Power*—Although this conceptualization of play often has been more common among historians, sociologists, and anthropologists—and has to do with concepts of contest, conflict, group identity, and traditions—psychologists often deal with this in terms of intrinsic motivation, autotelia, stimulus arousal, and free choice or free will.
- *Play as Fantasy*—Play as imagination, creativity, and flexibility has been a relatively recent area of inquiry, and one that focuses on the importance of the individual. Often, imaginative play is seen as "higher order" and has been found to be related to reading and other academic areas of ability.
- *The Play of Self*—Play is increasingly cited as an optimal experience or peak experience. Csikszentmihalyi (1990) describes play as the subjective experience that integrates all of learning and capacities of the individual, in much the same way that the state of "flow" does for adults.

Rethinking Children's Play

By Diane E. Levin, PhD

Has something changed in society and childhood in recent years that is affecting play? Is there really cause for concern and, if so, what can the adults who care for children do about it? Why is play important? Play is vital to most aspects of children's social, emotional, and intellectual development and academic learning. It is one of the most powerful vehicles children have for trying out and mastering new skills, concepts, and experiences. Play can help children develop the knowledge they need to connect in meaningful ways to the challenges they encounter in school—for instance, learning literacy, math, and science, as well as how to interact positively with others. Play

Functions of Play

Play has been viewed as serving multiple, often overlapping functions, dependent upon theoretical perspective or discipline (see boxes). Among educators, for example, play is thought to have the functions of understanding the world and providing experiences with symbolic possibilities. According to Mallory and New (1994), play provides:

> a context for children to practice newly acquired skills and also to function on the edge of their developing capacities to take on new social roles, attempt novel or challenging tasks, and solve complex problems that they would not (or could not) otherwise do. (p. 328)

A more comprehensive list includes social, cultural, and emotional functions as well. Play provides a means to do the following:

- express and represent concepts and feelings
- integrate and deal with emotions
- resolve conflicts in a microsphere
- expand imagination and fantasy
- express in fantasy what is unacceptable in reality
- ingest experiences through repetition and transformation
- become empowered
- build competence
- encourage novel and challenging responses
- self regulate stimuli
- promote positive effect and relaxation
- practice and prepare for a variety of roles
- communicate
- behave with flexibility
- express cultural values and beliefs symbolically

also contributes to how children view themselves as learners. As they play, they resolve confusing and disturbing social, emotional, and intellectual issues. They come up with new solutions and ideas and experience the sense of power that comes from being in control and figuring things out on their own (something children often do not get to do in real life). This helps develop a positive attitude toward learning—about how to find interesting problems to work on and how to solve them in creative ways. Play is a dynamic and endlessly diverse process.

Note. From "Rethinking Children's Play," by Diane E. Levin, October 2004, in *Our Children, 25*, 8–11. Retrieved May 14, 2004, from www.pta.org//parentinvolvement/adcouncil/oc_rethinking.asp

White Paper #6: *The State of Children's Play*

Play, in particular, is the special manifestation of freedom in childhood. It is quite common in modern societies to regard the existence of play in childhood as an indication that childhood is proceeding naturally and that, indeed, a child is even working on growing up as he or she plays the roles of parent, teacher, banker or any of the other manifestations of older and more powerful beings. If this isn't happening, or if it is happening in ways that seem different from those of our own childhoods, we may be alarmed.

Research on play has established that it has benefits for cognitive, social, and emotional development. Children who are allowed to play with certain materials show evidence of higher creativity and problem solving ability on related tasks; children allowed to play frequently with others show higher levels of social competence; and giving children an opportunity to play symbolically with upsetting situations enables them to cope more ef-

- experience peer culture and cohesion
- experience pleasure and fun

Defining Play

Although opinions differ among child practitioners as to what behaviors are play, increasingly most play researchers agree that some of the following criteria must be met. Play must be

- voluntary
- internally motivated
- pleasurable, relaxed
- "as if" or pretense present
- organism rather than object dominated
- unique, unpredictable
- active, both motorically and cognitively

"True" play, or acts and behaviors meeting all these criteria might indeed be very rare. Reviewing all the literature on play, Rubin, Fein, and Vandenberg (1983) found six recurring criteria cited: (a) intrinsic motivation; (b) orientation toward means rather than ends; (c) internal rather than external locus of control; (d) noninstrumental rather than instrumental actions; (e) freedom from externally imposed rules and expectations; and (f) active engagement. However, Smith and Vollstedt (1985) found that trained observers characterize an activity as play when there is a combination of non-literality, positive effect, and flexibility.

Alternatively, although many child practitioners often label the majority of children's behaviors as "play," *not play* is literal, with intense, neutral (or intense) effect, inflexible or predictable. Studies of what children define

fectively. Sociologist Janet Lever of Northwestern University found more complexity in the games of boys than girls in later childhood and saw that as advantageous to their development of social and organizational skills. University of Illinois play specialist Lynn Barnett found that preschool children anxious about the start of school who were allowed a period of free play showed decreases in distress while those who listened to stories did not.

The value of play has not been lost on educators. Some have attempted to incorporate play into the curriculum, and through "play training" have even shown the ability to increase a child's creativity and problem solving ability. But one can rightly question the remaining character of play in such situations, when adults have most of the control over the situation. Promoting the values of play without killing the essence of play brings us back to the question of structure....

Note. From "White Paper #6: The State of Children's Play." Retrieved May 14, 2004, from www.academyofleisure sciences.org/alswp6.html Copyright by Academy of Leisure Sciences. Reprinted with permission.

as play, however, have found that it is the context in which the activity occurs. The single most important factor for kindergartners in one study was whether the activity was "voluntary" or who decided on the activity and its goals (King, 1979). Among younger children (3- and 4-year-olds), play was found to be viewed as a personal, ongoing activity (*I Play*), distinct from functional activities such as eating and napping.

To illustrate play and not play, consider the differences between the *exploration* and *play* of young children. When presented with an unknown object, toddlers will hold it, look at it intensely, and manipulate it in a way similar to most other toddlers. However, once explored, the object then takes on the variations characteristic of the individual child: to be tossed, batted, sat on—and usually with smiles and giggles—or to become a plane or sun. Likewise, consider the concentration of an 8-year-old reading the directions for putting together a model airplane, as opposed to use of the object after it is finished. In the first instance, it is prescribed and predictable; after completion and exploration, it is less so. Exploration of the ball and the construction of the plane are purposeful and goal-oriented. Play, then, is idiosyncratic and process-dominated; one's own ideas are imposed on the object or situation.

Categories of Play

Piaget's (1962) and Smilansky's (1968) classifications of play types have been most influential, especially in studying play. Piaget (1962) distinguished between practice play, symbolic play, and games with rules. Smilansky (1968) elaborated by renaming practice play as "functional play," adding constructive play, naming symbolic play "dramatic," and retaining the category games with rules. There is current controversy as to whether constructive play is indeed play because it appears to be goal-oriented or product-focused. Adults, however, are especially likely to view this form of activity as "play." The other types of play, according to Rubin et al. (1983), are as follows:

- *Functional play*—simple, repetitive muscle movements with or without objects
- *Dramatic play*—substitution of an imaginary situation to satisfy child's personal needs and wishes
- *Games with rules*—acceptance of prearranged rules and adjustments to these rules

Smilansky's (1968) categories of play frequently are nested with Parten's (1932) categories of social participation (e.g., unoccupied, solitary, parallel, associative, cooperative), so that play is described as "functional–parallel," for example. Smilansky (1968) and Parten (1932) assumed a developmental, hierarchical sequence to their types of play. However, more recent studies have not found this; for example, constructive play remains steady throughout childhood, as does solitary play. In addition, language play and rough-and-tumble play were not considered by these theorists and were largely ignored until recently.

Content, Types, and Forms of Play

Content of play is largely the result of a transaction between children (e.g., their ages, personalities, gender, relationships among playmates, psychologic states) and the environment (e.g., people in it, space, equipment, time). *Theme* is another term used to describe play content. There are gender differences, as well as age differences, in the themes in which children most frequently engage. Boys are more likely to engage in themes and roles more distant from the house/home roles of girls, for example.

Type and forms of play are a result of context and content. A variety of typologies, continuums, or polarities are used to conceptualize and juxtaposition various forms of play; for example, an unstructured–structured play polarity (Delpo & Frick, 1988) and a freeplay-to-work continuum (Bergen, 1988). Each of these approaches attempts to distinguish forms of play on a number of criteria, including the degree of adult involvement, choice of objects, nature of intent of play (from adult perspectives), and type of objects, among others.

Research on the Effects of Play

Although specific knowledge about the short-term effects of play exists, there is not an impressive amount of research on its effect on development (Power, 2000). Questions continue about whether play is a result of development or if it influences development, although many believe play both reflects and affects development. There are many explanations for the difficulties in discerning the effects of play—not least of which is that play may be related to *all* aspects of development, and that play may interact differently for individuals. Indirect or even sleeper effects of play's quantity and quality, and its relationship to cognitive, social, emotional, and physical development may be much more difficult to discern. The lack of specifications for minimal amount or type of play required for normal development, or the amount required for optimal development is also an issue, as is definition and measurement (Power, 2000). What is known, however, is what happens if there is *no* play. Children who do not play often are under extreme emotional or physical distress or have cognitive or emotional limitations. This is so even in cultures or families who do not facilitate or value play. Play has been found to be related to creativity, reading ability, and a host of other specific skills. Play seems to cause, at least in the short term, other effects, such as (a) even more play, (b) problem solving, and (c) decreased anxiety (Power, 2000).

The following characteristics, however, consistently have been found in qualitative and descriptive studies (Hughes, 1995; Johnson et al., 1999; Roopnarine, Johnson, & Hooper, 1994):

- Children play in every human culture, past and present.
- There are vast differences in the amount and types of play, cross-culturally and within cultures.
- Children from less technologically advanced cultures and from lower socioeconomic backgrounds engage in less complex, less frequent, and less sophisticated make-believe play.
- There are distinct differences in the play of children related to gender.
- Play frequency, complexity, and category changes with age and experiences.
- Play is related to cognitive, emotional, social, and physical factors.
- Play development is predictable and orderly, yet unique to the situation and to the individual.
- Physical and psychologic safety is essential for play to occur.

While the 1970s and 1980s were times of research inquiry into the influences of play in cognitive development, today there is a renewed interest in the social and emotional impact of play. New, more valid and reliable measures appropriate for young children may yield more information about these relationships. Further, play research, like research on love, has received little widespread funding support; play researchers have had difficulty in obtaining consistent funding. Thus, there have been waves of research rather than consistent lines of inquiry into the etiology and effects of this "natural" behavior of children in health care, childcare, early education, child development, or child psychology.

Today some researchers are beginning to view play as an integrative process, the "glue" holding together aspects of being. Others are beginning to study play's neuro-physiologic impact and sources. For example, evidence indicates that when children are playing their heart rates are lower and more variable (as opposed to exploration when they are higher and less variable). The earlier models of play and brain development (Tipps, 1981), and of symbolic play and interhemispheric functioning (Weininger & Fitzgerald,

1988), are receiving support through recent imaging studies of the brains of children. Increasing evidence indicates that larger and longer term dosages of play, in play-based early childhood education curricula, for example, have long-term positive and more enduring effects on children's self-esteem, interpersonal relationship skills, academic skills, and achievement than do directive or eclectic approaches (Power, 2000).

Play in Health Care

Play—which includes initiation of actions by children and the responsiveness to children by others—is one of the most powerful processes by which children regulate their experiences and environments. In health-care contexts, although play is regarded as important for children to express their feelings and regain feelings of control and competency, it is less likely to occur or be encouraged than in years past because of changing environments and expectations. Less time in acute settings and more intense illnesses and treatments have made it appear that more direct instruction is essential. There is especially less emphasis on play as a normalizing experience—that is, that play is a comforting, familiar activity involving symbols and signs not related to the illness or hospitalization experience—or on its value for relationship-building. Play has an important role in *prevention*, providing for integrating experience, emotion, and cognition as experiences are occurring, so that *intervention* is less necessary. This role is less frequently cited in the professional literature, even as conceptual or theoretical articles, than in the past. As is true for play in education, therapy, and cultural contexts, there have been diverse studies on play in health care, with most quantitative investigations occurring in the 1970s and 1980s.

Advocates and facilitators for children's psychosocial needs in health-care settings, representing different health-care disciplines, different theoretical perspectives, and at different times, have argued cogently and emotionally for the importance of play or play opportunities for children in health-care settings. They worked diligently to create affective and physical environments necessary for play to occur in health-care settings—time, space, equipment, as well as supportive and, if possible, nonthreatening relationships with adults. Education of staff on the needs of children and families, including the values of play and play as a diagnostic tool, was also instituted (Green, 1974; Po, 1992). Rather than being concerned merely for "user-friendly" environments or services, many administrators also began to see the vital aspects of providing play and play-focused programs. These efforts flourished during the 1970s and 1980s, particularly in large teaching or children's hospitals. This period also was a time of rapid medical and surgical advances, when many life-threatening diseases became less so. Hospitals were transformed by changes in visiting policies and parent participation, increased ambulatory care, and new technologies.

By the 1990s, however, expansion and growth of organized play programs slowed in the United States (Bolig, 1990). In child life and nursing services, play—especially in its unstructured forms—began to be challenged by the assertion that structured play and other interventions were more effective. Spiraling health-care costs, increased reliance on technology, as well as a lack of a research base for play or play program practice, all interacted in undermining the support for play and organized play-based programs in health-care settings. Managed health care and ever-expanding services in same-day surgery and outpatient care greatly influenced the length of hospitalizations, thus affecting the nature of inpatient care and those using it. Care shifted to ambulatory and home care settings. Programs and services to families in these contexts generally have not included play.

Today play is often viewed as less efficient, if not less effective, than other, more direct means of informing children about impending procedures and events, or in reducing anxiety, despite the fact that little research supports or refutes either position. Some psychosocial advocates and facilitators contend that because children in hospitals are admitted for shorter periods, are sicker, and are subjected to more intense intrusive procedures than their counterparts of just a few years ago, there is not time for children to become sufficiently acclimated to the environment, or to develop relationships with staff or other children to play, especially spontaneously. Even playing with adult modeling, interaction, or permission-giving is difficult given the constraints cited. Further, children in inpatient environments are sometimes viewed as too ill to play. Yet, length of hospitalization has been found to have little to do with post-hospitalization upset. Quinton and Rutter (1976) found that multiple, short hospitalizations have a negative effect on children. Fahrenfort (1993) found that it was lack of parental presence (play was not measured) rather than shortness of stay that most affected outcomes.

Therefore, without conditions occurring to foster spontaneous play, facilitators often rely on more direct means of bringing children into contact with the symbols, signs, concepts, and knowledge related to their illness and procedures. Medical play, particularly that which is more structured, appears more direct and therefore is often more valued in acute care milieus (Bolig, Yolton, & Nissen, 1991; McCue, 1988). More specific and tailored to the individual, medical play may have greater acceptance in health-care settings because it looks like a "treatment." Ambulatory settings lack trained volunteers or professionals or consistent efforts at providing these play opportunities; even fewer exist for home care.

Perspectives on Play in Health-Care Settings

Until the 1970s and 1980s, psychoanalytic theories were used to support and explain the value and functions of play in health-care settings. These theories posit that play reduces anxiety by giving children a sense of control over the world and an acceptable way to express forbidden impulses. As in other environments, by the 1980s the cognitive-developmental theories, which view play as a means to facilitate the general cognitive development and to consolidate previous learning while allowing for the possibility of new learning in a relaxed atmosphere, gained acceptance (Hughes, 1995). More recent theories, such as arousal modulation and neuro-psychologic, have had a less direct influence on explanations of the value of play or into specific practices in health-care settings despite what would appear to be an obvious appeal to those with a physiologic aspect to their practice. Perhaps because the interest in play and play research has waned, less incentive exists to frame play within the context of recent theories and research.

Functions of Play

Perspectives by various child health-care practitioners on the functions of play—that is, what play does for children—are highly variable, ranging from diversion and stimulus-reduction to mastery and internalization of control. These differing perspectives, as in other contexts, are largely a result of training in various disciplines, the timing of training, and the types of roles engaged in "playing" with children.

Over time, however, two theories of play have dominated the thinking of a number of health-care disciplines. Psychoanalytic theory, for example, was originally the most widely held belief about play for hospitalized children, and has persisted in influencing beliefs that play is *cathartic* (allowing children to express what they can not handle rationally), and that through play children can come to *master* situations or come to grips with pain in reality. But Piaget's (1962) cognitive theory began to add another dimension in understanding functions of play. According to Piaget (1962), play is the way younger children abstract or assimilate experiences into their existing schema or internal cognitive structures.

The American Academy of Pediatrics Committee on Hospital Care (2000), in its Child Life Policy Statement, focused on the importance of play:

> Engaging in developmentally appropriate play and reading activities moderates children's anxiety and minimizes the possibility that health care encounters will disrupt normal development. Child-directed play and guided (or issue-specific) play experiences allow children to be active and exert control over their endeavors. Observation of play offers insight into the patient's concerns and level of understanding of the health care events and, thus, affords the opportunity to correct misconceptions. These observations are shared with the rest of the health care team so that all are better prepared to respond appropriately to the individual patient. To help cope with painful treatments and instrusive procedures, a child life specialist often uses "medical play," involving nondirective exploration of medical equipment, dramatic themes in which situations encountered by the child are reenacted, use of games or puzzles depicting medical themes, or the creation of art work using health care materials (e.g., bandage strips, tongue depressors, syringes). Such activities allow a child to approach the threatening situation with greater familiarity and a sense of mastery. (p. 1156)

Therapeutic play, a term associated with play in health-care settings, is play that is used to prevent psychologic injury (Matthews, 1991), and aims to

- meet children's ongoing developmental needs;
- help children cope with the unfamilar hospital environment;
- increase children's understanding of their hospitalization and treatment;
- promote a sense of control, mastery, and positive self-concept;
- facilitate self-expression; and
- meet children's need to cope with separation and deprivation.

The National Association for Hospital Play Staff (NAHPS) in England further elaborated on the functions of play in hospital (www.nahps.org.uk). According to NAHPS (2000), play

- creates an environment where stress and anxiety are reduced;
- helps the child regain confidence and self-esteem;
- provides an outlet for feelings of anger and frustration;
- helps the child understand treatment and illness. Through play, children are able to effectively learn the sensory and concrete information they need to prepare for hospital procedures and treatment;
- aids in assessment and diagnosis; and
- speeds recovery and rehabilitation.

Play as therapy, that is, play to assist with alleviating psychosocial injury, according to the Association for Play Therapy, Inc. (2000), is used as a

mechanism for developing problem-solving and competence skills; as a process that allows children to mentally digest experiences and situations; as an emotional lavoratory in which the child learns to cope with his/her environment; as a way of talking, in which toys are the child's words; and as a way of dealing with behaviors and concerns through playing it out.... And play is a natural medium for self expression, facilitates child's communication, is conducive to cathartic release of feelings, and can be renewing and constructive. (p. 4)

The primary purposes of play in health-care settings are prevention, restoration, and cure. Details regarding these purposes are found in Table 3.1.

Definitions, Types, Content, and Forms of Play

In the professional health-care literature, play has been described in various ways—from all activities in which children engage to those that have the characteristics cited earlier. Although perhaps causing few problems in practice, this lack of consensus causes a major difficulty in research design, with play defined variously and sometimes not even measured. But a consistent definition or description, with subtypes, would be very helpful not only for researchers but also for practitioners; defining play as one process to

Table 3.1

Primary Purposes for Play in Health-Care Settings

	Prevention	**Restoration**	**Cure**
Goals	To prevent deterioration, diffusion, regression To maintain internal sense of control/efficacy	To restore after situational distress/imbalance To assess rapidity of return to previous state	To cure imbalance as a result of a situation and temperament or personality problems
Population	All children Groups	All children Small groups Individuals	Children who do not respond to restorative play or identified as having emotional problems
Forms of Play	Nondirective Unstructured	Structured Guided	Structured Directive
Functions of Play	To maintain a sense of control To encourage interaction with peers in a familiar setting with objects and materials for age range and individual interests	To express feelings To obtain mastery through play with objects and roles associated with health-care encounters	To express fantasies, anxieties, and defenses through repetition and by developing a relationship with therapist through situation/objects specific to the individual

evaluate when considering outcomes such as length of stay, type or intensity of pain medications, and other similar measures would be beneficial.

Types of play in health-care settings include those cited in the previous section on types, although again this schema for the description of play has rarely been systematically employed. Descriptions of forms of play have, however, included normative, educative, and therapeutic play (Bolig, 1984). McCue (1988) also discussed various forms and types in health-care settings, specifically medical play.

Research on Play in Health-Care Settings

Little research was conducted on the play of hospitalized or ill children, or in health-care settings in the 1990s. Most of the research interest, like that on play in general, was in the late 1960s, 1970s, and early 1980s. Few Master's and PhD students in nursing, occupational therapy, child development, or related areas of study are conducting research on play of children in today's health-care settings, and few conceptual or theory articles have been published. Instead, recent research on children's responses to health-care encounters has focused on individual variation in responses to specific illnesses or disabilities. Some articles have focused on the play issues of specific groups of children, such as those receiving bone marrow transplantation

(Kuntz et al., 1996). Parental responses to home care have also been a focus of research, rather than the reactions or behaviors of children.

A primary method of achieving the goals of health-care play and activities programs is termed *child life* in the United States (Child Life Council, 2000). However, play has rarely been studied in child life contexts or used as either a dependent or independent variable. Instead, researchers have studied play in its directive or nondirective forms within nursing care or specific therapeutic contexts as a mediating variable. Play also is viewed as a primary method of determining children's psychosocial state, especially among nursing staff (Po, 1992). The general goals of these play studies have been that of imparting knowledge about impending procedures and reducing anxiety (e.g., therapeutic play, or play therapy). Findings indicate that short-term (e.g., one-shot, 30-minute) forms of play in nursing care contexts generally have been significant in reducing anxiety, although methodology and interpretation of some of the results have been a concern (Phillips, 1988). No studies, however, have determined whether play behaviors or anxiety reduction via play—either in play and activities programs, nursing care contexts, or occupational therapy—are related to post-hospital or treatment behaviors or later adjustment (Thompson, 1985, 1995). A few studies have examined play in child life outpatient play and activities programs. Perhaps because outpatient settings are less complex and the children focused on more limited activities for shorter periods of time, serious empirical inquiry is viewed as less complex for these settings. Inpatient play and activities programs widely vary in objectives and methods or "curricula." Programs vary from those that are diversionary to those that are therapeutic (Bolig, 1984, 1988). Further, programs also vary in the extent to which playrooms are the focus for activities, play, and relationships, the consistency with which staff are available, the educational backgrounds of staff, and in the ratio of staff to children, making comparative studies particularly difficult to conduct. Additional factors affecting complexity of description and comparison of programs are (a) age ranges of children served, (b) variations in types of illness represented, and (c) the equipment and play materials available. All of these variables have been found to be important predictors of variations in programs and of program outcomes in other settings involving children (Pellegrini & Perlmutter, 1989).

Research on play in the hospital has focused on the disruption of play in hospitalized children (Cataldo, Bessman, Parker, Pearson, & Rogers, 1979; Tisza, Hurwitz, & Angoff, 1970) aggression in play (Vredevoe, Kim, Dambacher, & Call, 1969), and the choice of play materials used by hospitalized children in relation to their anxiety levels (Gilmore, 1966; Tarnow & Gutstein, 1983). A few studies have focused on play interventions and their relationship to children's play behaviors in outpatient settings (Cataldo et al., 1979; Ispa, Barrett, & Kim, 1988; Pearson, Cataldo, Turemen, Bessman, & Rogers, 1980; Williams & Powell, 1980), while others have investigated the effect of play therapy or information and educative play on children's anxiety. No studies of children's play in extended care or home settings have been published.

Data on the disruption of play indicate that the hospital environment, at least temporarily, alters the patterns of play of hospitalized youngsters.

Data from a study on aggression in play indicate no increase in aggressive play behaviors with either hospitalization in general, or with surgery (Vredevoe et al., 1969). Gilmore (1966) studied the selection of play materials of children suffering from anxiety related to hospitalization. On the whole, research indicates that children who are neither highly anxious nor highly defensive often will select toys that are relevant to their particular situation. Children presented with choices will select hospital play materials if they are not too frightened; the most highly anxious children are least likely to select such toys if they are in a freeplay situation. But the presence of an adult can modify this response and help children feel more comfortable with anxiety-producing materials (Bolig, 1992).

Studies focusing on play interventions have found that short, supervised play sessions with materials related or unrelated to the medical setting may help children to cope more effectively with hospitalization (e.g., Clatworthy, 1981; Lockwood, 1970; Schwartz, Albino, & Tedesco, 1983). One experimental study, using a control group, examined a nurse's use of medical play with a doll and hospital equipment; results indicated that although the doll play did not reduce children's stress scores, anxiety-defense scores of the experimental group were found to be significantly lower after engaging in the play session (Lockwood, 1970). Clatworthy's (1981) experimental study also investigated the effect of play interventions on anxiety levels. The control group children were found to be more anxious at the final evaluation than were children in the experimental group. However, play intervention did not serve to decrease the anxiety levels of children over the course of hospitalization. Instead, the control group children evidenced increased anxiety levels over the course of hospitalization, whereas the experimental groups' anxiety levels held constant. Rae, Worchel, Upchurch, Sanner, and Daniel (1989) found that short sessions of therapeutic play (i.e., nondirective but reflective and interpretative with symbolic objects) were significantly more effective in reducing self-reported fears of 5- through 12-year-olds than diversionary play, verbal support, or no treatment. In a study of latency-age youngsters hospitalized for a minimum of 10 days, Fosson, Martin, and Haley (1990) presented them with a single 30-minute session with medical play or a control of television viewing with the investigator. Findings included a decline in anxiety in both groups, from admission to discharge; although not significant, a greater decline occurred among those children in the medical play group.

Schwartz et al. (1983) found in an experimental study that an opportunity to play under the supervision of a supportive adult—whether the play materials were related to the source of stress or not—was somewhat effective in altering children's manifestation of anxiety. A control group received no preoperative preparation from an adult, whereas one experimental group was allowed to play with toys unrelated to their upcoming medical procedure in the presence of the child life specialist. A third experimental group was given information by the child life specialist about the upcoming procedure through the use of medical play techniques. Findings indicated that both of the groups of children who participated in an adult supervised play session were consistently more cooperative and less upset than were the control group children. The children in the two play groups (related to and unrelated to upcoming surgery or procedures) varied significantly in anxiety at only one point—during induction of anesthesia. During this procedure, those children who had been in the play group related to the surgical procedure fared better than did those in the unrelated play group.

The investigation of programs and play and activities rarely has been studied. In a quasi-experimental study, Clegg (1972) attempted to assess the effectiveness of a comprehensive child life program and reported significant reduction in anxiety levels of children who had participated in child life programs. However, no control groups were used for comparison. Bolig (1980) found that children participating in an activities-based child life program increased in (internal) locus of control, although the level of anxiety was not affected. Wolfer, Gaynard, Goldberger, Laidley, and Thompson (1988), in a quasi-experimental study of a model child life program with a preparation rather than a play focus, found positive effects on a variety of outcome measures such as coping, adjustment, and recovery variable. Pass and Bolig (1993), in a naturalistic study of children's play in two forms of child life programming foci (i.e., playroom/group versus nonplayroom/individual), found no differences in the frequency and complexity of play, although there was a trend toward significance for therapeutic and educative play occurring more in the playroom-focused setting.

In a field experiment with play type as an outcome variable, Bolig (1992) varied the amount of time a child life-supervised playroom was available and the type of equipment, and found that young children played the majority of the time under any condition. Most of children's play was functional, constructive, and normative, and by or with a parent, child life specialist, or volunteer. Play type and form was, however, influenced by the addition of symbolic objects and the presence of adults, in interaction with amount of time in the playroom. Both functional and dramatic forms increased with added symbolic material, with significantly more dramatic group play in the 2-hour condition. Child life specialists and volunteers were more likely to maintain play at higher levels (i.e., dramatic play, games with rules) than were parents.

It seems that supervised play sessions with materials, whether related or unrelated to the hospital setting, may prove helpful in reducing children's anxiety or behavior distress during hospitalization (Thompson, 1985). Type of organized program also appears to affect children differently, although, in the few studies conducted thus far, the outcome variables have differed. Amount of time in the inpatient setting and amount of time in a supervised playroom also influence the amount and types of children's play. Lastly, there is some initial evidence that parents and professionals encourage different levels of play. Whether short periods of no play, maintenance of children's pre-hospitalization play level, or enhancement of play have any long-term sequalae have yet to be studied.

Variables Affecting Hospitalized Children and Their Play

Many variables have been found to affect the psychosocial and behavioral responses of hospitalized children (Thompson, 1985), and may have an impact on their play behaviors, including play environment, parent contact, age, length of hospitalization, type of illness, and gender. Each of these variables will be explored and discussed below.

The Play Environment. For many years researchers and practitioners in child development and early childhood education (e.g., Bruner, Jolly, & Silva, 1976; Frost & Klein, 1979; Piaget, 1962; Shure, 1963; Smith & Connolly, 1981) have recognized that the immediate physical and affective environments affect behavior. Through the presence and permission of adults, young children in particular gain assurance and encouragement to interact with objects and people. Through the stimulation of various concrete, symbolic objects, children first explore and then express uniquely. Some researchers indicate that knowledge of a particular environment is a more reliable predictor of a peoples' behaviors than knowledge of demographic variables or individual behavior tendencies (Barker, 1968).

Examinations of the relationship between preschool environments and children's behaviors have shown that the various interest areas or learning centers in preschools appear to have a powerful influence on the types of behavior displayed in each area. In a survey of day care environments in which the focus was to determine indicators of quality programs, the quality of physical space was positively correlated with the teachers warmth and the children's interest and involvement in activities (Kritchevsky, Prescott, & Walling, 1977). Nash (1981), in a 3-year period of observation of children in planned and unplanned environments, concluded that children's creative, cognitive, and language development was enhanced in planned environments. In most recent research focused on the effect of selected environmental variables upon the behavior of preschool children, desirable behaviors were more likely to be found in higher quality environments than in those of lower quality (Smith & Connolly, 1981).

However, limited investigation of play environmental factors in hospital settings has taken place. Tisza et al. (1970) found that amount of time in the hospital was related to exhibition of play behaviors. Three days were necessary for the young children studied to begin to play. Harvey and Hales-Tooke (1970) noted that the presence of a play leader was necessary for children to engage in "settled play." Likewise, in outpatient settings, the presence of a play facilitator was found to be related to more play and less anxious behaviors (e.g., Williams & Powell, 1980). Type of play materials was found to be related to children's anxiety and defensiveness. Gilmore (1966) found the presence of anxiety to be an important influence on the choice of toys; either a marked increase or decrease in interest was noted. Burstein and Meichenbaum (1979) also found that level of anxiety influenced selection of play materials. Children low in defensiveness prior to hospitalization actively played with relevant materials in the pre-hospital period and displayed minimal anxiety following discharge. Children high in defensiveness avoided one pre-hospital play with hospital-relevant toys, and had higher anxiety following hospitalization. But type of equipment or toys, room arrangement, and space relationship to child behaviors, including play, has not been studied in hospital programs, with one exception. Eisert, Kulka, and Moore (1988) reported that a play structure, developed to facilitate symbolic play of children with disabilities, significantly increased amount of time in partial play, symbolic play, and total play (Eisert et al., 1988). Bolig (1992) found that the longer children were in a (supervised) playroom, the more likely they were to engage in higher levels of play. Also, the presence of symbolic and thematic materials enhanced plays, as did the presence of the parent and child life specialist.

Parent Contact. Lehman (1975) and Brain and Maclay (1968) reported that "rooming in" (i.e., parents' staying through the hospitalization) has a positive effect on children's responses to hospitalization. Brain and Maclay (1968) studied two groups of preschool subjects—one that had mothers rooming in, and one that did not. Ward personnel and an anesthesiologist recorded observations of the children during induction of anesthesia. The researchers noted significantly more favorable adjustments for those children who had mothers rooming in with them during their hospital stay for tonsillectomy or adenoidectomy. Lehman (1975) conducted an *ex post facto* study of preschool-age children—half of the group's mothers had roomed in with their children during hospitalization and half had not. The mother and nurse of each child completed a questionnaire describing the child's behaviors. The children whose mothers roomed in displayed more aggressive behaviors than did those whose mothers did not room in. Lehman (1975) interpreted this finding as evidence that those children whose mothers did room in felt comfortable enough to express their real feelings regarding hospitalization. Cormier (1979) found that children who exhibited behaviors indicating the probability of depression were those who had little to no parent contact while hospitalized. With the exception of two field studies, the relationship of parent involvement during hospitalization of their children to play behaviors, either in playrooms or other contexts, has not been studied (Thompson, 1985). Hall (1977) noted increased parental play with children after the introduction of a supervised play room; Bolig (1992) found that parental presence was related to increased play, but not as complex forms of play as would occur with a child life specialist.

Age. The majority of research studies indicate that children between the ages of 6 months and 3 to 4 years are the most vulnerable age group for upset, although a few more recent studies suggest that age may be less of a predictor of upset than did studies in the past (Thompson, 1985). Children in the infant to preschool stages frequently show more upset both during and following hospitalization. Children who are older tend to exhibit fewer overt signs of psychologic disturbances; however, adolescents have been studied infrequently. The preschool years are included in the age range most likely to suffer disturbances as a result of hospitalization. The majority of disruption and play intervention studies have been conducted with this age group. As would be anticipated, it is for this developmental stage that play, and especially normative play, may serve the most critical preventative, curative, and equilibration functions. However, for older children, play may also be critical, although different forms may be more effective. Related expressive and efficacy activities, such as art and bibliotherapy, drama, and even humor, need investigation (see Chapter 5).

Length of Hospitalization. Tisza et al. (1970) found evidence that preschool-age children show a disruption in play behavior during the first day of hospitalization. The disruption gradually diminished over the 3-day observation period. Burstein and Meichenbaum (1979) also noted disturbances of play in a study of the relationships among play, anxiety, and defensiveness. They recorded the amount of time each child spent playing with materials for each play session, and found that the children spent significantly less time playing with toys during hospitalization than they did either prior to or after release from the hospital. Burstein and Meichenbaum (1979) attributed the disturbance in play behavior to a "disposition not to play" rather than to the distractions of the novel stimuli in the hospital setting. Pass and Bolig (1993) found that the longer children were hospitalized the more they engaged in educative and rough-and-tumble play and the less they engaged in exploratory behavior.

Type of Illness. Few significant findings have been reported concerning the relationship between the type of illness or subsequent treatment mode and the amount of psychologic upset that hospitalized children experience (Thompson, 1985). However, there is some indication that children who are admitted to the hospital under emergency conditions are more likely to suffer upset upon discharge than are other children (Shade-Zeldow, 1976). It would be anticipated that the more acute illnesses would limit play behaviors, as would restrictions (e.g., IVs, isolation). Pass and Bolig (1993) found that children admitted for surgical procedures engaged in less play, and more unoccupied behavior and reading, than children who were admitted for other medical reasons.

Gender. Gender differences in regard to children's responses to hospitalization have rarely been noted (Thompson, 1985), although differences have been found in other stress studies (Rutter, 1981). The few studies reporting differences have contradicted each other, or have had an intervening variable that may have been the actual cause of the results. For example, in a study of upset during an injection, Torrance (1968) found girls to have a higher level of upset than boys. However, the mean age for girls was lower than that of boys in the study. In self-reported studies of relative upset about hospitalization, Campbell (1978) found boys to be less disturbed; however, Dearden's (1970) similar study found girls to be less disturbed. Pass and Bolig (1987) found that boys engaged in more constructive play than girls in two different child life settings; girls had more onlooker behavior than boys. But, the variety of children's play in nonmedical contexts has been found to be influenced by gender, with girls engaging in less rough-and-tumble and aggressive play and showing interest in a wider variety of toys and play materials than boys (Johnson, Christie, & Yawkey, 1999). It is likely that gender differences in play among hospitalized children may be found when other factors are controlled.

Research Questions for Play in Health-Care Settings

Virtually all basic and applied questions about play of ill or hospitalized children, and in the variety of health-care settings, remain unanswered or even yet to be asked. The few studies that have been conducted have failed to use similar instruments, populations, methodologies, or comparison groups. Replication is necessary, as is improved methodology, because the methodology or analyses in some previous studies may be questionable (Phillips, 1988). More recent theoretical formulations have not generated congruent research questions. Thus, the following are essential basic questions in a systematic inquiry into play in health-care settings:

1. Do children play in the hospital? How much time do children spend at play, as opposed to other activities? Where do they play? With whom do they play? When do children play? In what types and forms of play do children engage? What types of materials do they choose?
2. Does where, and with whom, and with what children play affect the quantity and quality of their play?
3. Are quantity and quality of children's play (e.g., in different settings, with different individuals, in total) related to coping skills, state and trait anxiety, self-esteem, locus of control, cognitive level? What physiologic stress indicators (e.g., heart rate, sweat, urine output) can be used to study the effects of play?
4. Are quantity and quality of children's play (e.g., in different settings, with different individuals, in total) related to nature of illness, number of intrusive procedures, length of hospitalization, whether a parent rooms in, types of medication, or amount of involvement in play activities program?
5. Are quantity and quality of children's play in the hospital setting better predicted by (pre-hospital) personality variables or by hospitalization variables?
6. Are quantity and quality of children's play during hospitalization related to physical recovery variables such as length of hospitalization, number of infections, or amount of pain medication?
7. Are quantity and quality of children's play during hospitalization related to psychosocial and behavioral post-hospital or post-treatment adjustment?

In sum, the major issues are as follows: (a) whether play occurs during health-care encounters and in health-care contexts, and under what conditions; (b) whether play is a valid measure of children's psychologic state during hospitalization or other health-care experiences; (c) what factors contribute to variation in children's play during health-care encounters; and (d) whether children's play during hospitalization, ambulatory care, or even home care contributes to variation in physiologic and psychologic recovery. Further, questions about the types of organized programs (e.g., philosophies, curricula, interactional patterns), variations in facilitative relationships (e.g., professional training, type of relationship, amount of time in relationship), and play physical environment (e.g., where, type of equipment) also need to be addressed.

Facilitating Play in Health-Care Settings

Roles of the adult in children's play are especially critical during health-care encounters. Without sensitivity to the responses of children, adults can turn "play" into "not play" or fail to assist "not play" into "play." This constant adaptation of roles or behaviors of adults in children's play may be indeed one of the most sensitive and nonmedical functions in which health-care practitioners engage. The facilitation of different *types* and *forms* of play may have various effects on children during hospitalization, and are likely to be related to differing post-hospital adjustment patterns (Rae et al., 1989). The inclusion or exclusion of various types or forms of play may favor one aspect of functioning over another (e.g., cognitive over affective). And, typically, adults engaging in play with children favor cognitive functioning, asking questions rather than reflecting children's feelings or intents, for example. Thus, if play provision is to continue to be an integral aspect of today's health care for children, it must be recognized that not all activities in which children engage are play, and the types, forms, and extent to which play occurs are likely to be related to different hospital and post-hospital adjustments of children.

Each of the theories of play has implications for psychosocial and psychoeducational prevention and intervention strategies. As examples, the psychoanalytic theories support the contentions that children need to "express" feelings through play to master events and to avoid repression or fixation, and cognitive theories (e.g., Piaget, 1962) postulate that children acquire "knowledge" through play. The "expression of feelings" and "acquisition of knowledge" perspectives on play have been the predominant positions on the functions of play, with several subtypes. There are underlying theoretical principles, particularly related to which environmental aspects are needed to sustain play, and these may be competing. Unstructured play, for example, congruent with nondirective forms of play therapy and characteristic of psychoanalytic theory, requires different responses from the environment than does guided or co-play, which is characteristic of cognitive theories. Cognitive theories presume a greater transaction between children and their environments—a more or less co-equal interaction/impetus by adult and child. However, the psychoanalytic view requires an initial, supportive relationship with adults for children to feel secure enough to explore and ultimately play with their environment. Thus, a cognitive perspective implies a more active role on the part of the adult in children's play. More active or directive roles have certain dangers; that is, there is a subtle but critical line beyond which adults can turn children's play into "not play," or overstimulate or overwhelm children's regulatory systems. Furthermore, although limited, there is empirical support from studies of children in other

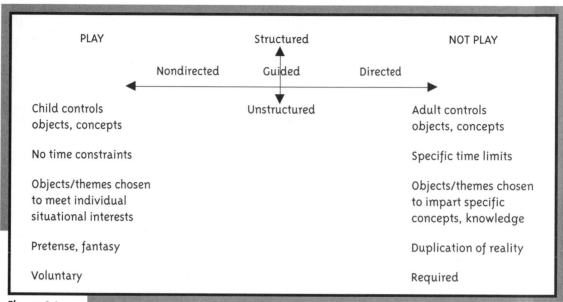

Figure 3.1.

Play to Not Play continuum.

settings that indicate more active play involvement on the part of adults may favor cognitive aspects of development, whereas unstructured and nondirected play might have more social or emotional benefits (Smith, 1995). Alternatively, in health-care settings with little time to develop relationships, the reciprocal play process between adults and children may actually facilitate attachment (Rutter, 1981). This continuum of play to not play is illustrated in Figure 3.1.

Identifying the variety of roles in which adults can engage in children's play, and the resultant differences in quantity and quality of children's play, has precipitated another line of research, particularly in school and childcare settings. Enz and Christie (1997), among other recent descriptive studies, have identified six roles that adults engage in with children's play. Roles can be conceptualized on a continuum that ranges from no involvement to complete control (Johnson et al., 1999). Among children in classroom and childcare settings, the most productive roles are in the middle range of involvement. These middle-range roles (Johnson et al., 1999, pp. 210–213) are as follows:

- *Stage Manager*—While staying on sidelines during play, adult helps children prepare for play and responds to children's requests for assistance with materials and equipment.
- *Co-player*—Adult becomes partner in play, taking on less dominant roles than the children, following the actions and interactions of the children.
- *Play Leader*—Adult extends and expands children's play through suggesting new roles, themes, and elements.

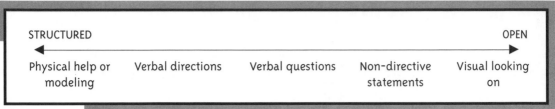

Figure 3.2.
Behavior continuum. *Note.* From "Play Techniques for Preschool Age Children under Stress," by C. H. Wolfgang and R. Bolig, 1979, *Journal of the Association for Care of Children in Hospitals,* 7, p. 7. Copyright 1979 by Erlbaum. Reprinted with permission.

The most effective roles for professionals in health care might be found at the higher end of these middle-range roles, because a greater intensity of interaction might be essential given limited time and other resources. However, greater sensitivity to individual reactions and issues is required at these higher levels of intensity. Specialized training of staff may be required for engagement in more curative forms of play.

Wolfgang and Bolig (1979) identified specific behaviors congruent with these roles through which adults in play encounters with hospitalized children take on more or less "control," as identified in Figure 3.2.

Similarly, the type of materials selected (and who chooses) may also be viewed as contributing to the degree of structure. Items that are structured, such as puzzles, are most likely to be used in the way the item is intended, whereas "open" or fluid materials, such as sand and water, are more likely to be subject to children's feelings or thoughts. Lastly, symbolic objects, including health-care items, are more likely to elicit unique expressions of feeling and experiencing. In this approach outlined by Wolfgang and Bolig (1979), adults interact and transact with children and their play through modifying their own behaviors and materials as children become more or less expressive. The goal is for children to be in control and fully expressive in symbolic forms of play.

Playing into the 21st Century

As we enter the new millennium, there may be a renewed interest in play. Recently a resurgence of interest in animal play has occurred (Bekoff & Byers, 1998). An article in *U.S. News and World Report* (Brownlee, 1997) states that the study of play has gained a badge of respect as biologists have found increasing evidence that, to a variety of species, play is nearly as important as food and sleep. There is increasing evidence that "locomotion play" of young animals forges connections between neurons in the brain, especially in the cerebellum, the region that controls and coordinates movement. Early evidence suggests that play taps into the brain chemicals involved in pleasure.

When rats play, their brains release dopamine, a chemical that in humans induces elation and excitement. Fagen (1995) correlated the current increased interest by scholars in animal play with that of interest in angels:

> Like play, angels have long been a topic of scholarly speculation and popular interest, although scientists seem to disregard them. Indeed the study of angels and the study of play, and the popular ramifications of these enterprises, seem to offer certain similarities. They are based at least in part on speculation, hope, and romanticism. (pp. 26–27)

There is also an increasing consensus that play experiences help to form multiple and hardwired interactions in the brain, and children who do not play may actually have smaller brains (Brown, Sutterby, Therrell, & Thornton, 2002).

And, there is a greater awareness of the importance of research specifically on health services for children:

> The characteristic of childhood as a unique developmental stage of life, the continuity of child health with adult health, and a distinctive child health care system justify a separate focus of health services research on children. Child health services research currently lacks the tools necessary to monitor the impact of the health care system change on children's health and to compare the effectiveness of alternative treatment modalities. (Forrest, Simpson, & Clancy, 1997, p. 1787)

A special commission through the Board on Children, Youth, and Families (1996) has focused discussion on children in the rapidly changing health-care system. Also, play has recently been "discovered" by technocrats and business leaders as a stress reducer and creativity enhancer in the workplace (Gregerman, 2000). Play continues to be a viable aspect of early childhood education and is still the subject of many books in the field despite fewer articles on play as a specific topic in the professional literature. Several organizations are concerned with play, as are a number of professional associations (see Appendix 3.1). The Association for Study of Play (TASP), a multidisciplinary group of professionals committed to play research and its application, continues to support dialog on play research and play theory. The organization recently began publishing a journal, *Play and Culture Series.* The International Play Advocacy (IPA) organization supports dialog on play throughout the world. IPA strongly states its position on the values of play, including that play, "along with the basic needs of nutrition, health, shelter and education, is vital to develop the potential of all children" (International Association for the Child's Right to Play, 2000). Although the Association for the Care of Children's Health has disbanded, the Child Life Council (CLC) continues to uphold play as a primary means "to minimize stress and anxiety for children and to foster continued growth and development and prevent adverse reactions to health care encounters" (Child Life Council, 2000), as does the National Association for Hospital Play Staff (NAHPS) in England. Other groups concerned with play also assure its vitality. These groups include the Association for Play Therapy, Inc. (APT, 2000), which promotes play therapy, conducts and makes available play therapy research, and presents an annual Student Research Award to encourage ongoing play therapy research. The International Council for Children's Play (ICCP) is focused on research on children's play and toys, and through its biannual meetings, it brings together researchers from all over the world. Many countries have play policy statements as well as organizations active in supporting play; the Children's Play Council in the United Kingdom is just one example (www .ncb.org.uk/cpc/). Several organizations provide play training. Additionally, computer technology facilitates individual networking among play professionals and others with an interest in play.

It does appear that the interest in play, from its therapeutic to learning functions, is still significant, and commitment to its implementation is likely to resurge. This renewal may be a response to mechanistic or linear thinking related to computers and computer-learning, overstructuring of children's time, and the increased testing of children. Brain research, too, especially on critical periods and effects of trauma, is likely to provide further evidence of the importance of play—with its relaxation, multiple facets, and internal control aspects.

Play in Health-Care Settings of the Future

Louv (1992) talked about today's children living a childhood of firsts—as each generation does. But children in today's health-care and early childhood settings are different. They are the first childcare generation, the first multicultural generation, the first generation to have single parents, and the first generation to grow up with the computer. In terms of health care, this is the first generation that is likely to spend only 1 day or less in the hospital when born, to be the product of gene therapy, or perhaps, to undergo laser and robotic surgery. They may be informed of impending experiences by a video or CD-ROM or, someday, by virtual reality in a specially equipped fantasy room to guide them through their impending experiences. They can seek out Web sites about their own illness or surgery and can communicate with children all over the world who have a similar disability or disease (Bush,

Play for Peace	**P**lay for Peace: brings children from conflicting cultures together through cooperative play to promote positive relationships among people who have a history of inter-cultural tension. By bring children with unique backgrounds, values, and beliefs together through the seemingly simple act of play, seeds of compassion are sown for a more peaceful today and tomorrow.

Huchital, & Simonian, 2002). In the future, they may have interactive dolls or plush toys to hold on to that interact with them, as does a project prototype at Massachusetts Institute of Technology (Auerbach, 1999, p. 121):

> a fluffy green bug who imitates body movements by picking them up through an antennae-equipped sensor strapped to its back. The toy can sense movements and even the mood of its owner—less of a thing and more of a creature that knows you and your habits.

In the not so distant future, children in health-care settings may have a "nurse" robot that attends to their care and responds to their questions. Undoubtedly, they will spend even less time in acute health-care settings and more in ambulatory and home settings. A computer chip implanted into children with diabetes and asthma may monitor their responses and alert their home health caretakers or parents to an impending crisis. This form of prevention, and more sophisticated knowledge of etiology of illnesses, will lead to fewer diseases affecting children or less acute onset of chronic diseases that are not yet curable by gene therapy.

Less illness and less time in health-care settings may very well enhance quality of life. But as discussed in the beginning of this chapter, children's essential needs for comfort, control, reassurance, information, and human support, will not have changed appreciably, despite all the technologic and medical advances. The challenges in providing play and other child-focused ways of learning and expressing will continue. Sophisticated and costly virtual experiences such as those being supported and investigated by the STARBRIGHT Foundation may influence certain aspects of children's adjustment and coping, but may not be sufficiently different or better than traditional playroom-based experiences and ensuing relationships (Battles & Wiener, 2002) to warrant decrease in support for play.

However, according to Isenberg and Jalongo (1997), the adults who facilitate and advocate for play in this increasingly complex and technological future will, more than ever, need to

- develop a wide range of strategies for a wide range of abilities, situational responses, and physical limits to foster play, creativity and self-expression;

The objectives of Play for Peace are: to promote positive relationships among children from cultures in conflict; to create a nonthreatening environment, free from fear, where children can experience the joy of play; and to influence the behavior of adults through the positive example of children at play.

Note. For more information on Play for Peace, visit the Web site at www.playforpeace.org
Reprinted with permission.

- develop paradigms and approaches to maximize play possibilities in acute care settings;
- expand and refine communication capacities;
- focus on intrapersonal traits and interpersonal skills for developing and maintaining optimal and therapeutic relationships;
- extend knowledge of child and human development with neuro-physiologic theory and research;
- document the impact of their professionals' practices and policies on children's adjustment, recovery, health, and development; and
- assure personal resources and creative energies to face challenges optimistically.

Ultimately play will be revitalized and more clearly understood, for, as Sutton-Smith (1995, p. 290) stated, "What may be adaptive about play may not be the skills that happen to be a part of it, but the willful belief in one's own capacity for a future." And what may be most important about play is our belief in the uniqueness and essential needs of children, as well as what we can learn from children's play (see Play for Peace box).

Conclusion

Life continues to *play* with us all; we are not in full control but use our culture's symbols, relationships, interactions, and resources to *play it (life) back*. Children not only play to gain knowledge but also the time- and culture-bound skills, as well as timeless roles, that enable them to contribute, adapt, heal, and love. In a time of rapidly increasing technology, changing social structures, demands for early achievements, and testing in schools, play may serve a more critical function than in times past when children and adults had more free time to explore, dream, and experiment with ideas, roles, and relationships. Yet at other times, children were at high physical risk, were viewed as "little" adults, or were valued primarily for contributions to the economy of the family; frequently, play might have not been possible. Thus, in these times, it is important to understand that play *plays* within historical, cultural, and economic situations in various ways.

Play will always be a part of childhood in some way in healthy societies and may be a particular hallmark of mental and societal health: Those societies with a high proportion of freedom of expression, choices, and individual control (characteristics of play) may be most productive and interesting, and certainly represent the ideal of democracy. Likewise, play of children in health-care settings and encounters will survive, and must survive: It is both a cause and effect of maintaining a healthy system of care. However, parents and child health-care professionals must continue, as their predecessors, to advocate for play's inclusion and support in the rapidly changing health-care system to assure health for children and health care.

Study Guide

1. Define *play*.

2. Identify the characteristic behaviors of play.

3. Describe the functions of play.

4. Discuss the history of play in health-care settings.

5. Identify the various theories of play in health-care settings.

6. Describe the major research themes on play in health-care settings.

7. Discuss factors leading to more or less emphasis on play in health-care settings.

8. Identify research questions on play in health-care settings that have yet to be addressed.

9. What impact does technology have on play?

10. What will be the future of play in health-care settings?

APPENDIX 3.1
Resources for Play

Play Organizations

The Association for Play Therapy, Inc.
2050 N. Winery Ave., Suite 101
Fresno, CA 93703
USA
Phone: 559/252-2278
Fax: 559/252-2297
E-mail: info@a4pt.org
www.a4pt.org
An international organization dedicated to the advancement of play therapy; conducts and makes available play therapy research.

The Association for Study of Play (TASP)
7507 Clarendon Road
Bethesda, MD 20814
USA
Phone and Fax: 301/656-9479
E-mail: mmfryer@aol.com
www.csuchico.edu/phed/tasp/
A multidisciplinary group of professionals committed to play research and its application.

Alliance for Childhood
PO Box 444
College Park, MD 20741
USA
Phone: 301/513-1777
Fax: 301/513-1777
E-mail: info@allianceforchildhood.net
A partnership of individuals and organizations committed to fostering and respecting each child's inherent right to a healthy, developmentally appropriate childhood.

The Institute for Play
Stuart Brown, Founder
46 W. Garzas Road
Carmel Valley, CA 93924
USA
Phone: 831/659-1740
E-mail: info@instituteforplay.com
www.instituteforplay.com
Provides a mix of information and resources to give a deeper understanding of the nature and importance of play, and connections to helpful people, organizations, and information.

The International Play Advocacy (IPA)
International Membership Secretary
Mr. Gerrit Lekkerkerker, Hoflaan 4
3271 BD Mijnsheerenland
The Netherlands
Phone: 31 10 417 23 58
Fax: 31 10 417 2095
E-mail: scz@bsd.rotterdam.nl
www.ncsu.edu/ipa
Supports dialog on play and advocates for children's right to play throughout the world.

National Lekotek Center
2100 Ridge Avenue
Evanston, IL 60207
USA
Phone: 800/366-7529
TTY: 800/573-4446
Fax: 847/328-5514
E-mail: lekotek@lekotek.org
www.lekotek.org/
Dedicated to promoting access to developmentally appropriate play and learning for children with special needs and their families.

Playing for Keeps (PFK)
Wheelock College
200 The Riverway
Boston, MA 02215
USA
Phone: 617/879-2185
Fax: 617/738-0643
E-mail: playingforkeeps@wheelock.edu
A developing coalition of parents, academics, and toy manufacturers "to foster a climate of constructive play through education, collaboration, and action."

Professional Organizations Supporting Play in Practice

American Occupational Therapy Association (AOTA)
4720 Montgomery Lane
PO Box 31220
Bethesda, MD 20824-1220
USA
Phone: 301/652-2682
TDD: 800/377-8555
Fax: 301/652-7711
E-mail: praota@aota.org
www.aota.org
A professional association of occupational therapists, occupational therapy assistants, and students of occupational therapy dedicated to helping people regain, develop, and build skills that are essential for independent functioning, health, and well-being.

Child Life Council (CLC)
11820 Parklawn Drive, Suite 202
Rockville, MD 20852-2529
USA
Phone: 301/881-7090
Fax: 301/881-7092
E-mail: clcstaff@childlife.org
www.childlife.org
A professional organization composed of child life specialists, educators, students, and others who use play, recreation, education, self-expression, and theories of child development to promote psychological well-being and optimum development of children, adolescents, and their families.

Children's Play Council
8 Wakley Street
London EC1V 7QE
United Kingdom
Phone: 020 7843 6016
Fax: 020 7278 9512
E-mail: cpc@ncb.org.uk
www.ncb.org.uk/cpc/
A campaigning and research organization dedicated to raising people's awareness of the importance of play in children's lives and the need for all children to have access to better play opportunities and services.

National Association for the Education of Young Children (NAEYC)
1509 16th Street, NW
Washington, DC 20036-1426
USA
Phone: 202/232-8777
Toll Free: 800/424-2460
Fax: 202/328-1846
E-mail: naeyc@naeyc.org
www.naeyc.org
An organization of early childhood educators and others dedicated to improving the quality of programs for children from birth through third grade.

National Association for Hospital Play Staff
Chairman of the Trustees
21 Rosefield Road, Staines
Middlesex, TW18 4NB
United Kingdom
E-mail: hospitalplay@msn.com
www.nahps.org.uk
A charity that provides professional support to hospital play staff to promote the physical and mental well-being of children and young people who are patients in hospital or hospice or receiving medical care at home.

Play Training

The Canadian Play Therapy Institute
11E 900 Greenbank Road, Suite 527
Nepean (Ottawa), Ontario, K2J 4PG
Canada
Phone: 613/634-3125
E-mail: cplayti@kos.net
www.playtherapy.org
Serves as one of the world's major resources in play therapy and child psychology. CPTI runs many training programs each year in the field of child psychology and play therapy with a variety of presenters in many regions of the world.

Chesapeake Beach Professional Seminars (CBPS) Play Therapy Training Institute
3555 Ponds Wood Drive
Chesapeake Beach, MD 20732-3916
USA
Phone: 410/535-4942
E-mail: cbps@radix.net
www.radix.net/~cbps/playinst.html
Provides traditional as well as innovative play therapy/child psychotherapy training for mental health professionals and others providing therapy with children.

The National Institute of Relationship Enhancement
4400 East-West Highway, Suite 28
Bethesda, MD 20814
USA
Phone: 301/986-1479
E-mail: info@nire.org
http://www.nire.org
Provides training, supervision, and certification for mental health professionals in The Child-Centered Play Therapy Model, and conducts basic and advanced skills training workshops in play therapy, as well as offering supervision and certification in this effective intervention with children.

The Play Therapy Training Institute, Inc.
PO Box 1435
Hightstown, NJ 08520
USA
Phone: 609/448-2145
E-mail: info@ptti.org
www.ptti.org
Offers a variety of 1- and 2-day Play Therapy Seminars; following a broad-spectrum, eclectic approach to Play Therapy, instruction is available in all the major approaches and techniques.

PLAY-TRAIN
31 Farm Road
Sparkbrook, Birmingham, B11 1LS
United Kingdom
Phone: 440 121 766 8446
E-mail: team@playtrndemon.co.uk
www.playtrn.demon.co.uk
A leading specialist in playwork training in the UK; provides high-quality training and consultancy for organizations working with children; carries out research and development projects, bringing fresh ideas to bear on key issues in work with children.

The Theraplay Institute
3330 Old Glenview Road, Suite 8
Wilmette, IL 60091
USA
Phone: 847/256-7334
E-mail: theraplay@aol.com
www.theraplay.org
Provides training and research in Theraplay, a dynamic and effective short-term approach to treating children's emotional and behavioral problems. Based on the intimacy and physical interplay that characterize healthy relationships between parent and child, Theraplay techniques use structured play to promote the child's self-esteem, competence, and trust in others.

Play Online Discussions

Play-Children
E-mail: play-children-reqest@mailbase.ac.uk
An open list for debate on issues around children's play needs.

Play Therapy E-Mail Discussion Group
Sign-on: http://playtherapy.org/discuss.htm
An e-mail discussion group about play therapy.

References

American Academy of Pediatrics, Committee on Hospital Care. (2000). Policy statement: Child Life programs. *Pediatrics, 106*, 1156–1159.

Association for Play Therapy, Inc. (2000). 2000–01 *Goals and finances.* Available online from www.a4pt.org

Auerbach, S. (1999). *F.A.O. Schwarz: Toys for a lifetime: Enhancing childhood through play.* San Francisco: Universe.

Barker, R. G. (1968). *Ecological psychology: Concepts and methods of studying the environment of human behavior.* Stanford, CA: Stanford University Press.

Battles, H. B., & Wiener, L. S. (2002). STARBRIGHT World: Effects of an electronic network on the social environment of children with life-threatening illnesses. *Children's Health Care, 31*, 47–68.

Begley, S. (1996, February 19). Your child's brain. *Newsweek*, pp. 55–62.

Bekoff, M., & Byers, J. (1998). *Animal play: Evolutionary, comparative, and ecological approaches.* New York: Cambridge University Press.

Bergen, D. (1988). Using schema for play and learning. In D. Bergen (Ed.), *Play as a medium for learning and development: A handbook of theory and practice.* (pp. 169–180). Portsmouth, NH: Heinemann.

Board on Children, Youth, and Families. (1996). *Paying attention to children in a changing health care system.* Washington, DC: National Research Council.

Bolig, R. (1980). The relationship of personality factors to responses to hospitalization in young children admitted for medical procedures. (Doctoral dissertation: Ohio State University, 1981). *Dissertation Abstracts International, 41*, 3732-B.

Bolig, R. (1984). Play in hospital settings. In T. Yawkey & A. Pellegrini (Eds.). *Play: Developmental and applied.* Hillsdale, NJ: Erlbaum.

Bolig, R. (1988). Guest Editorial: The diversity and complexity of play in health care settings. *Children's Health Care, 16*, 132–133.

Bolig, R. (1990). Play in health care settings: Challenges for the 1990s. *Children's Health Care, 19*, 229–233.

Bolig, R. (1992). *Play in child life contexts: A field experience.* Paper presented at the Association for the Care of Children's Health Conference, Atlanta, GA.

Bolig, R., Yolton, K., & Nissen, H. (1991). Medical play: Issues and questions. *Children's Health Care, 20*, 225–229.

Brain, D. J., & Maclay, I. (1968). Controlled study of mothers and children in hospital. *British Medical Journal, 1*, 278–280.

Brown, P., Sutterby, J. A., Therrell, J. A., & Thronton, C. D. (2001). *Play is essential to brain development.* Austin, TX: International Play Equipment Manufacturers Association. Retrieved July 26, 2004, from www.ipema.org/News/default.aspx

Brownlee, S. (1997, February 3). The case for frivolity. *U.S. News and World Report.*

Bruner, J. S., Jolly, A., & Silva, K. (Eds.). (1976). *Play: Its role in development and evolution.* New York: Basic Books.

Burstein, S., & Meichenbaum, D. (1979). The work of worrying in young children undergoing surgery. *Journal of Abnormal Psychology, 7*, 121–132.

Bush, J. P., Huchital, J. R., & Simonian, S. (2002). An introduction to program and research initiatives of the STARBRIGHT Foundation. *Children's Health Care, 31*, 1–10.

Campbell, J. D. (1978). The child in the sick role: Contributions of age, sex, parental status, and parental values. *Journal of Health and Social Behavior, 19*, 33–51.

Cataldo, M. F., Bessman, C. A., Parker, L., Pearson, J. E., & Rogers, M. C. (1979). Behavioral assessment for pediatric intensive care units. *Journal of Applied Behavior. Analysis, 12*, 83–97.

Child Life Council. (2000). *Position statement.* Available online from www.childlife.org

Clatworthy, S. (1981). Therapeutic play: Effects on hospitalized children. *Children's Health Care, 9*, 108–113.

Clegg, R. (1972). Effects of a child life program upon the anxiety levels of children hospitalized for major elective surgery. (Doctoral dissertation, University of Maryland). *Dissertation Abstracts International, 33*, 4882-B.

Cormier, P. P. (1979). Identification of typologies derived from child behaviors in the hospital as predictors of psychological upset. *Journal of Psychiatric Nursing and Mental Health Services, 17*, 28–35.

Csikszentmihalyi, M. (1990). *Flow: The psychology of optimal experience.* New York: Harper-Collins.

Dearden, R. (1970). The psychiatric aspects of the case study sample. In M. Stacey (Ed.), *Hospitals, children and their families: The report of a pilot study.* London: Routledge & Kegan-Paul.

Delpo, E., & Frick, S. (1988). Directed and non-directed play as a therapeutic modality. *Children's Health Care, 16*, 261–267.

Eisert, D., Kulka, L., & Moore, K. (1988). Facilitating play in hospitalized handicapped children: The design of a therapeutic play environment. *Children's Mental Health, 13*, 201–208.

Engel, G. L. (1980). The clinical application of the bio-psychosocial model. *American Journal of Psychiatry, 37*, 535–544.

Enz, B., & Christie, J. (1997). Teacher play interaction styles: Effects of play behavior and relationships with teacher training and experience. *International Journal of Early Childhood Education, 2*, 55–75.

Erikson, E. (1963). *Childhood and society.* New York: Norton. (Original work published 1950)

Erikson, E. (1972). Play and actuality. In M. W. Piers (Ed.), *Play and development.* New York: Norton.

Fagen, R. (1995). Animal play, games of angels, biology, and Brian. In A. D. Pellegrini (Ed.), *The future of play theory: A multidisciplinary inquiry into the contributions of Brian Sutton-Smith.* Albany: State University of New York Press.

Fahrenfort, J. (1993). *Attachment and early hospitalization.* Amsterdam: Thesis.

Fein, G. (1997). *Play and early childhood teacher education: Discussant remarks.* Symposium presented at the annual meeting of The Association for the Study of Play Meetings, Washington, DC.

Forrest, C. B., Simpson, L., & Clancy, C. (1997). Child health services research: Challenges and opportunities. *Journal of the American Medical Association, 277*, 1787–1792.

Fosson, A., Martin, J., & Haley, J. (1990). Anxiety among hospitalized latency-aged children. *Journal of Developmental and Behavioral Pediatrics, 11*, 324–327.

Freud, S. (1952). *Beyond the pleasure principle.* New York: Norton.

Frost, J. L., & Klein, B. L. (1979). *Children's play and playgrounds.* Boston: Allyn & Bacon.

Gilmore, J. (1966). The effect of anxiety and cognitive factors in children's play behavior. *Child Development, 37*, 397.

Glickman, C. (1988). Play in public school settings: A philosophic question. In T. D. Yawkey & A. D. Pellegrini (Eds.), *Child's play: Developmental and applied.* Hillsdale, NJ: Erlbaum.

Green, C. S. (1974). Understanding children's needs through therapeutic play. *Nursing, 4*, p. 31.

Gregerman, A. (2000). *Lessons from the sandbox: Using the 13 gifts of childhood to rediscover the keys to business success.* New York: Contemporary Books.

Groos, K. (1901). *The play of man.* New York: Appleton.

Hall, G. S. (1904). *Adolescence: Its psychology and its relation to physiology, anthropology, sex, crime, religion, and education* (Vol. 1). New York: Appleton.

Harvey, S., & Hales-Tooke, A. (1970). *Play in hospital.* London: Faber & Faber.

Hughes, F. P. (1995). *Children, play and development.* Boston: Allyn & Bacon.

International Association for the Child's Right to Play. (2000). *IPA's declaration of the child's right to play* [Brochure]. Huntington, England: IPA.

International Council for Children's Play. (2000). Mission statement. Ulm, Germany: ICCP.

Isenberg, J. P., & Jalongo, M. R. (1997). *Creative expression and play in early childhood.* Columbus, OH: Merrill.

Ispa, J., Barrett, B., & Kim, Y. (1988). Effects of supervised play in a hospital waiting room. *Children's Health Care, 16,* 195–201.

Johnson, J. F., Christie, J. F., & Yawkey, T. D. (1999). *Play and early childhood development.* New York: Longman.

King, N. R. (1979). Play: The kindergartner's perspective. *Elementary School Journal, 80,* 81–87.

Kleinberg, S. (1987). Child life in the 1990's: Changing roles, changing times. *Children's Health Care, 15,* 240–244.

Kossoff, D. (1996). To die with dignity: In sweet memory of a girl named Kasey. *The Advocate, 2,* pp. 29–30.

Kritchevsky, S., Prescott, E., & Walling, L. (1977). *Planning environments for young children: Physical space.* Washington, DC: NAEYC.

Kuntz, N., Adams, J. A., Zahr, L., Killen, R., Cameron, K., & Wasson, H. (1996). Therapeutic play and bone marrow transplantation. *Journal of Pediatric Nursing, 11,* 359–367.

Lehman, E. J. (1975). The effects of rooming-in on the behavior of preschool children during hospitalization and follow-up. *Dissertation Abstracts International, 36,* 3052-B.

Levin, D. E. (2004, October). Rethinking children's play. *Our Children, 25,* 8–11.

Lockwood, N. L. (1970). The effects of situational doll play upon the preoperative stress reactions of hospitalized children (pp. 133–140). *ANA Clinical Sessions, Miami.* New York: Appleton-Century-Crofts.

Louv, R. (1992). *Childhood's future.* New York: Doubleday.

Mallory, B. L., & New, R. S. (1994). Social constructivist theory and principles of inclusion: Challenges for early childhood special education. *The Journal of Special Education, 28,* 322–337.

Matthews, B. (1991). *A therapeutic play programme for young hospitalized children.* Paper presented at the Early Childhood Convention, Dunedin, New Zealand.

McCue, K. (1988). Medical play: An expanded perspective. *Children's Health Care, 16,* pp. 157–161.

Nash, C. (1981). *The learning environment.* Toronto: Methuen.

National Association for Hospital Play Staff. (2000). *Play in hospital.* NAHPS Web site: www.nahps.org.uk

Parten, M. (1932). Social play among preschool children. *Journal of Abnormal and Social Psychology, 28,* 136–147.

Pass, M., & Bolig, R. (1993). A comparison of play behaviors in two child life program variations. *Child Care, 22,* 5–17.

Patrick, G. T. W. (1916). *The psychology of relaxation.* Boston: Houghton Mifflin.

Pearson, J. E. R., Cataldo, M., Turemen, A., Bessman, C., & Rogers, M. (1980). Pediatric intensive care unit patients: Effects of play intervention on behavior. *Critical Care Medicine, 8,* 64–67.

Pellegrini, A. D., & Perlmutter, J. C. (1989). Classroom contextual effects on children's play. *Developmental Psychology, 25,* 289–296.

Phillips, R. (1988). Play therapy in health care settings: Promises never kept? *Children's Health Care, 16,* 182–187.

Piaget, J. (1962). *Play, dreams, and imitation in childhood.* New York: Norton.

Plank, E. (1962). *Working with children in hospitals.* Cleveland: Western Reserve University.

Po, J. (1992). Nurses, children, play. *Issues in Comparative Pediatric Nursing, 15,* 261–269.

Power, T. G. (2000). *Play and exploration in children and animals.* Mahwah, NJ: Erlbaum.

Quinton, D., & Rutter, M. (1976). Early hospital admissions and later disturbances of behaviour: An attempted replication of Douglas' findings. *Developmental Medicine and Child Neurology, 18,* 447–459.

Rae, W., Worchel, F., Upchurch, J., Sanner, J., & Daniel, C. (1989). The psychosocial impact of play on hospitalized children. *Journal of Pediatric Psychology, 14,* 617–627.

Richards, S. S., & Wolff, E. (1940). The organization and function of play activities in the set-up of a pediatric department. *Mental Hygiene, 24,* 229–237.

Robertson, J. (1958). *Young children in hospitals.* New York: Basic Books.

Roopnarine, J. L., Johnson, J. E., & Hooper, F. H. (1994). *Children's play in diverse cultures.* Albany: State University of New York Press.

Rubin, K., Fein, G., & Vandenberg, B. (1983). Play. In P. H. Mussen & E. M. Hetherington (Eds.), *Handbook of child psychology, 4,* 693–774.

Rutter, M. (1981). Psychosocial resilience and protective mechanisms. *American Journal of Orthopsychiatry, 57,* 316–331.

Schwartz, B. H., Albino, J. E., & Tedesco, L. A. (1983). Effects of psychological preparation on children hospitalized for dental operations. *Journal of Pediatrics, 102,* 634–638.

Shade-Zeldow, T. (1976). Attachment and separation: The effects of hospitalization on pediatric patients. (Doctoral dissertation, Purdue University, 1977). *Dissertation Abstracts International, 37,* 3576-B.

Shure, M. (1963). Psychological ecology of a nursery school. *Child Development, 34,* 979–992.

Smilansky, S. (1968). *The effects of socio-dramatic play on disadvantaged preschool children.* New York: Wiley.

Smith, P. K. (1995). Play, ethology, and education: A personal account. In A. D. Pellegrini (Ed.), *The future of play theory: A multidisciplinary inquiry into the contributions of Brian Sutton-Smith.* Albany: State University of New York Press.

Smith, P. K., & Connolly, K. J. (1981). Social and aggressive behavior in preschool children as a function of crowding. *Social Science Information, 16,* 601–620.

Smith, P., & Vollstedt, R. (1985). On defining play: An empirical study of the relationship between play and various play criteria. *Child Development, 56,* 1042–1050.

Spencer, H. (1870). *Principles of psychology.* New York: Appleton.

Spodek, B., & Saracho, O. N. (1988). The challenge of educational play. In D. Bergen (Ed.), *Play as a medium for learning and development.* Portsmouth, NH: Heinemann.

Sutton-Smith, B. (1995). The pervasive rhetorics of play. In A. D. Pellegrini (Ed.), *The future of play theory: A multidisciplinary inquiry into the contributions of Brian Sutton-Smith.* Albany: State University of New York Press.

Tarnow, J., & Gutstein, S. (1983). Children's prepatory behavior for elective surgery. *Journal of the American Academy of Child Psychiatry, 22,* 365–369.

Thompson, R. H. (1985). *Psychological research on pediatric hospitalization and health care: A review of the literature.* Springfield, IL: Thomas.

Thompson, R. H. (1995). Documenting the value of play for hospitalized children: The challenge of playing the game. In E. Klugman (Ed.), *Play, policy, and practice, 145–158,* St. Paul, MN: Redleaf Press.

Tipps, S. (1981). Play and the brain: Relationships and reciprocity. *Journal of Research and Development in Education, 14,* 19–29.

Tisza, V. B., Hurwitz, I., & Angoff, K. (1970). The use of a play program by hospitalized children. *Journal of the American Academy of Child Psychiatry, 9,* 515–531.

Torrance, J. T. (1968). *Children's reactions to intramuscular injections: A comparative study of needle and jet injections.* Cleveland, OH: Case Western Reserve University.

Vredevoe, D. L., Kim, A. C., Dambacher, B. M., & Call, J. D. (1969). Aggressive postoperative play responses of hospitalized children. *Nursing Research Report, 4,* 4–5.

Weininger, O., & Fitzgerald, D. (1988). Symbolic play and interhemispheric integration: Some thoughts on a neuropsychological model of play. *Journal of Research and Development in Education, 21,* 23–40.

Williams, Y. B., & Powell, M. (1980). Documenting the value of supervised play in a pediatric ambulatory care clinic. *Journal of the Association for the Care of Children's Health, 9,* 15.

Wilson, J. M., & Chambers, E. (1996). Child life can (and must) adapt to the new healthcare environment. *The Advocate, 2,* 36–37. Washington, DC: Association for the Care of Children's Health.

Wolfer, J., Gaynard, L., Goldberger, J., Laidley, L., & Thompson, R. (1988). An experimental evaluation of a model child life program. *Children's Health Care, 16,* 244–254.

Wolfgang, C. H., & Bolig, R. (1979). Play techniques for preschool age children under stress. *Journal of the Association for Care of Children in Hospitals, 7,* 3–10.

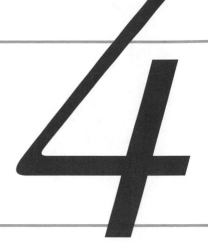

The Arts in Children's Health-Care Settings

Judy A. Rollins

Objectives

At the conclusion of this chapter, the reader will be able to:

1. Discuss the theoretical and cultural explanations for the use of expressive arts for emotional, social, and cognitive adaptation and coping.

2. Review the historical and current thinking about the use of the expressive arts in the healing process with children and youth.

3. Define various forms and relevant functions of expressive arts therapy.

4. Summarize the current body of research about the use of the expressive arts with children in health-care settings and during health-care encounters.

5. Outline resources and supports for the use of the expressive arts in health-care settings.

ealth-care experts agree that hospitalization and other health-care experiences can have serious emotional consequences for children. However, with appropriate support, children can weather, and even grow from, these experiences. The arts can play a significant role in this support.

Although the arts may lack the power to cure, they can promote healing. To more fully understand the use of arts in health-care settings, it is important to understand the distinction between "curing" and "healing." Curing is to bring about recovery from a disease (i.e., to eliminate the disease). Healing is a process of becoming physically and psychologically whole; healing can take place even as the body weakens (Graham, 1993). Some of the most powerful experiences with the arts can occur when cure is no longer an option and impending death is a reality (Rollins, 1994).

The concept of using the arts in health-care settings is not new. The ancient Greeks were greeted by musicians when they entered their temples of healing. But, even before then, art was a healing force. Human beings have always used pictures, stories, dances, and chants as healing rituals (Graham-Pole, 2000). As Western medicine developed with an emphasis on disease processes and cure, the arts were cast aside. Today, however, there is renewed interest in complementary, alternative, or integrative medicine practices, of which the arts often are considered a part. Recognizing the need to investigate and evaluate such practices, the United States Congress mandated the establishment of the Office of Alternative Medicine at the National Institutes of Health (NIH) in 1992 (NIH, Office of Alternative Medicine, 1994), which later became the National Center for Complementary and Alternative Medicine.

Children use the arts in health-care settings much in the same way that they use play (see Chapter 3: Play in Children's Health-Care Settings); however, a distinction can be made. According to Greaves (personal communication, February 1996), "Of course art is play.... It all starts off that way, playing around with ideas. Creativity is play. And children use play as a creative tool. After the play though, the production of the art work then becomes hard work." Offering a combination of creativity and discipline, the arts start from where children are, but make them raise their sights (Rogers, 1995).

This chapter addresses the *therapeutic use of the arts* with children in health-care settings. "Art itself is in many ways therapeutic, for it permits the discharge of tension and the representation of forbidden thoughts and feelings in socially acceptable forms" (Rubin, 1982, p. 57). It is important to distinguish between the therapeutic use of the arts and *expressive* (art, music, dance, poetry, drama) *therapy*. In the first instance, artists and other caring adults facilitate children's engagement in expressive activities that may be therapeutic. For example, children may communicate verbally or nonverbally their thoughts, feelings, and concerns through or while engaging in these expressive activities. *Expressive therapies*, however, are conducted by *expressive therapists* who receive special training to interpret and prescribe specific expressive activities. A certification or licensing process is involved. Individuals without these credentials can do meaningful work with children, but they must be aware of their limitations and not cross the boundary into territory for which they are unprepared.

The term *arts* often first brings to mind the visual arts, yet all forms of the arts (e.g., music, dance, storytelling, poetry, drama, photography) can be used and even mixed when working with children who are ill, disabled, or dying. This chapter begins with a discussion of ways children use the arts as tools for coping with illness and health-care experiences, and describes related research findings and applications. Recommendations for individuals wishing to use the arts with children and to establish arts programming in children's health-care settings follow.

The Arts as Tools for Coping with Illness and Health-Care Experiences

Health-care experiences have long been recognized as stressful for everyone, but research indicates that these experiences can have serious emotional consequences for the developing child (Johnson, Jeppson, & Redburn, 1992; Thompson, 1985). These consequences often are the result of the many stresses inherent in children's health-care experiences. For example, children rarely are permitted to refuse treatments, medications, and procedures. They are constant recipients of "things" being done to them. They may have to "hold still" for a painful procedure, one that they may not understand, and be left feeling powerless and confused. Placed in a passive role with limited opportunities to make meaningful choices, emotions are often intense and confusing.

Creative activities give children an opportunity to express the many emotions associated with illness and health-care experiences. These emotions can include troublesome ones such as fear, confusion, anger, or guilt, as well as happier ones that reflect joy, satisfaction, and personal growth. The creative process is used to transform pain and conflict and foster self-awareness and growth. In the art experience, the person, process, and product are equal.

Participating in the arts can help children deal with several realities of illness and health-care experiences (see Table 4.1). For example, engaging in art experiences can distract children from pain and discomfort. By being positioned in active roles, children are empowered and in control of their world

Table 4.1

Key Concepts: Meeting Psychosocial/Developmental Needs
of Children in Health-Care Settings Through the Arts

In health-care settings, children	The arts provide opportunities for children to
1. May experience pain and discomfort	Develop new coping strategies Distance and distract themselves
2. Have limited opportunities to make decisions	Make choices Be independent
3. Are in passive roles, where they are led, dressed, doctored, and are the constant recipients of things being done to them	Be the active ones Be the ones in charge
4. Experience many emotions, such as fear, confusion, anger, guilt, happiness, joy, and pride	Communicate feelings, both pleasant and unpleasant Safely let go Relive and master traumatic experiences
5. May be physically limited	Draw on their remaining abilities Imagine what they may be unable to do physically
6. Are in a health-care atmosphere with confusing sights, sounds, smells, and strangers	Do something "normal" and familiar Share experiences with others Experience the pleasure and joy of childhood
7. Are in a situation that provides opportunities for learning and growth	Demonstrate understanding of their condition and treatment Experience closure Develop potential for a lifelong interest in the arts and creative expression

Note. Adapted from *Art is the HeART: An Arts-in-Healthcare Program for Children and Families in Home and Hospice Care* (p. 53), by J. Rollins and L. Riccio, 2001, Washington, DC: WVSA Arts Connection. Copyright 2001 by WVSA Arts Connection. Adapted with permission.

as "doers" instead of "receivers." The arts can provide children opportunities to explore safe methods of emotional expression; help them to make the most of their present abilities; engage them in something familiar and enjoyable; and help them to learn, grow, and develop in many significant ways (Rollins, 1995).

Pain and Discomfort

Most children who are ill experience some pain or discomfort. We know that some children engage in play and other expressive activities in an effort to distract themselves from these and other health-care stressors, such as nausea. Although not a substitute for appropriate pharmacologic support, the arts can be integrated into a child's pain management routine. Children often use drawing as a valuable tool to communicate the location and degree of pain, and reports indicate that the arts have been effective to some degree for relief of even severe pain (Rollins, 1995).

The Gate Control Theory can serve as a conceptual framework for the use of the arts in helping people cope with pain (Wall, 1973). This theory proposes that pain impulses are moderated by a gating mechanism that opens to allow nerve impulses to reach the brain or closes to decrease or prevent impulse transmission, depending on the extent to which the gate is open. There is central control, which is the influence that cognitive or higher central nervous system processes have on pain perception via descending fibers to the gating system. Anxiety, anticipation, and excitement may open the gate and thus increase the perception of pain. However, cognitive activities such as distraction, suggestion, relaxation, and imagery tend to close the gate and prevent sensory transmission of pain.

Reduced Opportunities To Make Decisions

Children are rarely permitted to refuse or reschedule treatments, medications, and procedures. The ability to make choices gives children a much-needed sense of control over something in their lives and therefore helps relieve stress. Engaging in the arts, children have endless opportunities to make choices. They can choose colors, what to paint, what musical instrument to play, the ending to a story, poem, or song, and so on (see Figure 4.1). They can even choose not to participate in an activity. This decision, too, has great value; it may be the only real choice the child has had honored that day.

Passive Role

Many of the things that are done to children when they are ill—being poked, prodded, led, doctored, nursed, or dressed—are unpleasant or even painful. Again, they usually have no choice. When children are creating, they are the ones in charge. They can squish lumps of clay and form animals or whatever they wish, pound nails into wood and build airplanes, sing as loud or softly as they like. For that moment, *they* are in control, the captains of their ship, the masters of their universe.

Emotions

Children can experience unpleasant emotions when ill. It is difficult to have to "hold still" for a painful procedure, to be nauseated all the time, to get shots, or to miss school graduation. Health-care experiences are especially confusing for young children. They may wonder why their parents are letting these terrible things happen to them, and be bewildered at their feelings of anger at people as well as at events. They often express anger in misbehavior or refusal to cooperate.

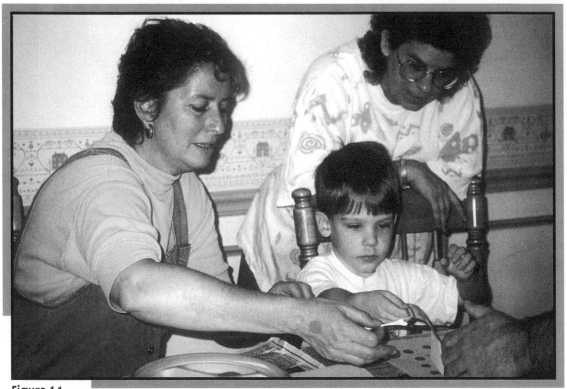

Figure 4.1.

The arts provide numerous opportunities for children to make choices.

Children, particularly young ones, often find it easier to express these feelings and concerns through the arts. Something as simple as the health-care professional or artist saying to a child after a difficult procedure, "Children sometimes tell me that having their blood drawn can be kind of hard. I wonder if you could draw a picture of what it was like for you and we can talk about it," can provide an opportunity for the child to process the experience and the emotions that surround it. Some health-care facilities have very elaborate ways for children to express their emotions. For example, Children's Medical Center in Tulsa, Oklahoma, has a "wet room," a tile room where children are dressed in bathing suits and invited to paint their emotions on the wall. Afterwards, they are encouraged to wash their expressions down the drain, cleansing themselves both literally and symbolically (Express Yourselves, 1997).

In many social settings, such as family or school, children receive the message that expression of strong emotion—anger, fear, grief—will exacerbate interpersonal tensions and hasten rejection. Research indicates, however, that habitual repression of strong emotions can lead to immune deficits that reduce resistance to infection and neoplastic disease (Pert, Dreher, & Ruff, 1998).

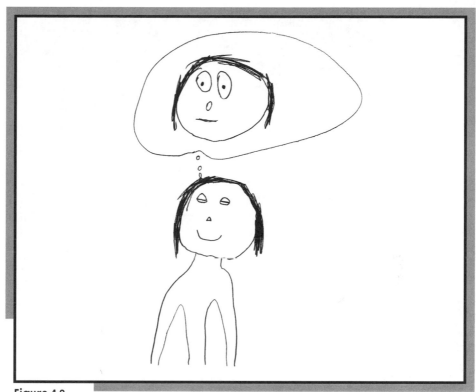

Figure 4.2.
Drawing provided an excellent communication tool for this 7-year-old to express a common presurgery fear: waking up in the middle of the operation.

The creative process facilitates a more honest reflection of what children are thinking and feeling, their hopes, dreams, and fears (see Figure 4.2). Looking at the sequence of cognitive development, children think first in images; as they grow older they learn to translate these images into words. Then they learn to play it safe with words, guarding what they reveal about their thoughts, ideas, or feelings.

Not all of the emotions children experience while ill, hospitalized, or dying are unpleasant. Engaging in the arts can take children, sometimes only for a moment, to a different place—a place of joy and contentment (see Figure 4.3). Children can use the arts to express these good feelings, too.

Physical Limitations

Children may be physically limited, some temporarily (an arm immobilized for an intravenous line), some permanently. Also, certain conditions, such as cystic fibrosis or cancer, can sap a child's energy and therefore limit activity.

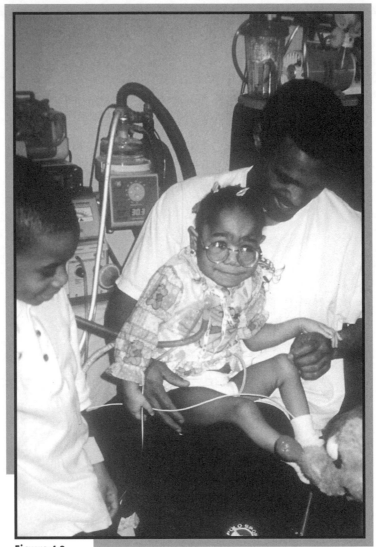

Figure 4.3.
The arts can help children express good feelings, too.

Methods for engaging in an art activity can usually be adapted to meet special needs. For example, children without the use of their arms can learn to hold a paintbrush with their mouths or feet. In other cases, tools can be adapted. For example, foam rubber can be wrapped around crayons or pencils and secured with a rubber band. This shapes the childs hand around the implement, making it harder to drop. Often the children themselves suggest adaptations, recognizing that methods or equipment they use for other activities, for instance, holding a spoon for feeding, can be transferred to arts experiences such as holding a paintbrush.

Redefining the arts experience is another method of adapting. For example, what exactly is "dancing"? We typically think of moving across space on our feet. However, children can dance using only their arms or even simply their eyes. Much of what a child takes away from an arts experience is the good feeling that comes from self-expression, which is acting at whatever level possible in whatever way he or she decides. Even if a child is unable to physically participate in a particular activity, often he or she can still decide the important factors, such as choice of colors for a painting, where a line goes in a drawing, what song to sing, and so on, and direct someone else in the actual execution.

Some children (e.g., children undergoing bone marrow transplants), although physically able to move about, may be physically confined and isolated in a room for infection control or protection. Art experiences can be designed to help these children feel less isolated and part of a "community." For example, in a hospital setting, each child on the unit, including the child in isolation, can be given a blank 35mm slide to decorate with markers, ink, paints, and so on. After the children have completed their work, the slides can be loaded into a slide carousel, put on a slide projector, and taken room to room (or shown on the wall from outside the room) for a "Light Show."

Physical limitations may take on added dimensions for children with special health-care needs. Throughout the course of childhood, most children will miss at least one party or other anticipated event because of illness. For the child with a chronic illness or disability, this may not be a once-in-a-childhood occurrence, but something that happens all the time, something the child comes to expect. These factors all contribute to the enormous sense of isolation many children with special needs and their families experience.

To address this sense of isolation, artist Lacretia Johnson developed the concept of a "Life Necklace," which she uses to create a sense of community and belonging in hospital, community, hospice, and home health-care settings (see Figure 4.4). She asks children and their family members, after making their own beads from polymer clay, if they would like to make a bead for the Life Necklace. Many choose to add their unique beads to the necklace, and the stories of their creative processes are recorded. Through the sharing of the stories of children and their families, the Life Necklace has become a vehicle that fosters a sense of community that extends across generations, ethnicities, cultural and socioeconomic backgrounds, and types of illness and injury (Johnson, 1997).

Health-Care Atmosphere

The health-care atmosphere may mean confusing sights, sounds, smells, and strangers entering the hospital room, treatment room, or even the sanctity of the child's home. This atmosphere does little to foster the normal experiences of childhood. Like play, creating art or engaging in other expressive activities is normal, the essential "work" of childhood. The creative process allows children to escape from their situation and return to the world they know (Greaves, 1996). Children often can share these expressive experiences alongside family members and friends. Parents frequently report that watching their children engaged in normal childhood activities gives them a real sense

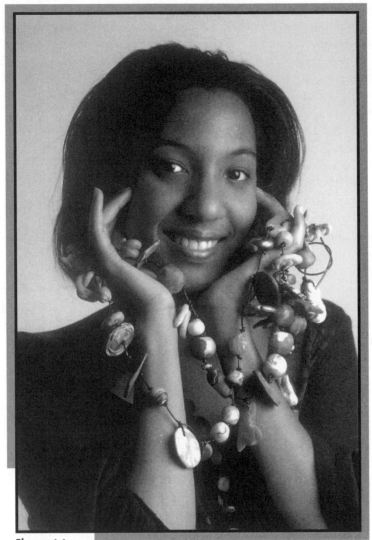

Figure 4.4.
Through the sharing of stories, the Life Necklace fosters a sense of community that extends across generational, cultural, socioeconomic, and illness and injury boundaries. *Note*. Photograph by Siduri. Used with permission.

of hope. In recent years, the potential benefits of hope to the adaptation to varying health states have become a focus of investigation for a growing number of researchers (Hendricks-Ferguson, 1997).

Learning and Growing

Children in health-care settings have the opportunity to learn about physical concerns and about themselves. They can communicate their understanding of their condition and treatment in expressive activities, which gives

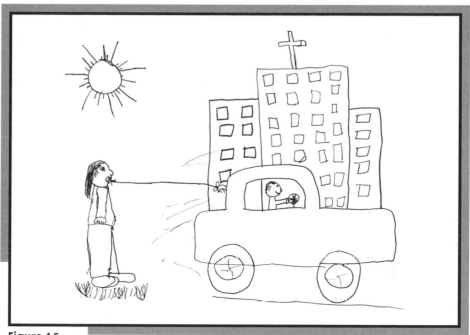

Figure 4.5.

Through her drawing, a 10-year-old girl communicates her knowledge of the reason for her coming to the hospital.

parents and health-care professionals opportunities to discuss a child's understanding and concerns and correct misconceptions. For example, a 10-year-old girl with heart disease was scheduled to have some teeth extracted in preparation for future orthodontic work. Because of her heart condition, the dental surgery was taking place in a hospital to enable appropriate monitoring. She was asked to draw a picture of why she had come to the hospital, which she depicted accurately, if somewhat humorously, in Figure 4.5. Next, she was asked to draw a picture of how she thought the operating room would look. Although she had been hospitalized in the past, she had never been in an operating room. She produced the drawing in Figure 4.6. When she was asked about the obvious hole in the patient's chest, she expressed her concern that because previous hospitalizations were always for her heart condition, the doctor might mistakenly operate on her heart instead of her teeth. This information was passed on to the dental surgeon and the anesthesiologist, both of whom assured her of which parts of her body would be involved and which parts would not. Drawing allowed her to communicate what she had been unable to express in words. Perhaps Bernie Warren, Professor of Dramatic Art at the University of Windsor, Canada, says it best: "Things that are scary are often beyond words" (B. Warren, personal communication, November 2000).

The arts have a unique role for children with chronic conditions who face a lifetime of health-care experiences. Having the opportunity to complete an art activity with a final product allows such children to experience a

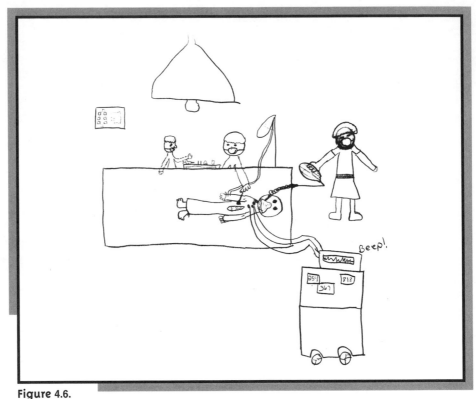

Figure 4.6.
Children often reveal in their drawings fears that they have not been able to put into words.

much-needed sense of closure, plus the personal satisfaction that comes from a job well done. A lifelong interest in the arts may begin in the hospital, clinic, home, or hospice care setting (see Case Study 4.1). For children with chronic or disabling conditions whose occupational choices may be limited, this may be the most important benefit of all.

Although having special meaning for children in health-care settings, creative expression plays a critical role in growth and development for *all* children (Schirrmacher, 1988). Evidence indicates that the arts, particularly music, dance, and the visual arts, develop neural connections and body/brain connections, which further learning in many areas, including math, reading, writing, and general language development (Seidel, 1996). The very nature of creative activities—there is no one right way to express something—promotes success and all of the good feelings that go along with it. Certain experiences also can help the child develop large and small muscle skills. The creative process itself promotes mental or cognitive development, for creating is a series of problem solving and decision making. Creative expression also fosters emotional and social development. Art is a universal language, and children express themselves more naturally and spontaneously through art than through words.

Case Study 4.1
The Long-Term Effect of a Fleeting Contact

Sometimes we are lucky enough to discover that a fleeting contact with a child has a long-term effect. I had been working with a 9-year-old who was recovering from tonsillectomy. My usual procedure is to encourage a child to participate in drawing and painting to pass the time until the parent arrives for discharge. The girl was happily absorbed in the picture making when her mother arrived, and went on to complete the picture. As they were leaving, the mother turned to me and said, "She has always liked art since you gave her some paper and crayons when she was in here six years ago."

Robert Greaves
Monash University
Frankston, Victoria, Australia
1999

Note. Courtesy of R. Greaves, 1999, Monash University, Frankston, Victoria, Australia. Copyright 1999 by Robert Greaves. Reprinted with permission.

Research Findings and Applications

Limited research, particularly quantitative research, has been conducted regarding the use or impact of the arts in health care (Miles, 1997). However, individuals who use the arts with children in health-care settings say that something very special can happen during these experiences; they typically have difficulty identifying and articulating exactly what this "something" is. With exceptions, much of the evidence available to date is anecdotal. In recent years, with increasing interest in complementary, integrative, and mind–body medicine, and greater acceptance of alternative practices, more funding has become available for research in these areas. The development of new quantitative tools and greater acceptance of more sophisticated qualitative measures hold great promise for answers to many of our questions in the near future.

A small but growing body of research indicates that a physiologic process may actually take place through contact with certain images and other forms of the arts. Goldstein (1980) described "thrills"—tingling sensations individuals may experience when exposed to emotionally arousing stimuli. His findings show a relationship between these experiences and the release of endorphins—the body's own pain reliever, relaxer, and mood enhancer. An emerging science that is part of this physiologic research is psychoneuroimmunology (PNI), which is concerned with the correlation between stress and health. Specifically, PNI refers to the study of the relationship between the mind and the brain, nervous system, endocrine system, and the immune system (Linton, 1995). Research findings in this field clearly demonstrate that the mind, brain, and nervous system can be directly influenced, either positively or negatively, by sensual elements in the environment (Gappell, 1995).

Although there is much to learn, the literature on stress provides some rationale for the efficacy of the use of the arts in children's health-care settings. Ryan-Wenger (1992) described 15 categories of strategies children use to cope with stress. Of these, the use of at least five—"behavioral distraction," "cognitive distraction," "emotional expression," "self-controlling activities," and "social support"—can be fostered by an opportunity to engage in the arts. For example, painting, listening to music, or laughing at a funny story can help children set aside the need to deal with stressors for a time.

Humor

Since Norman Cousins wrote about the power of humor to heal and because many forms of the arts are fun and produce laughter, humor has become a popular topic of research in health care. Lambert and Lambert (1995) reported increases in immunoglobulin A (IgA) levels when school-age children participated in a humor program. Included in the list of themes adolescents identified as important for health professionals in caring for adolescents with chronic illness was having a sense of humor (Woodgate, 1998). Researchers have even devised a scale to measure sense of humor. Thorson, Powell, Sarmany-Schuller, and Hampes (1997) found that scores on the Multidimensional Sense of Humor Scale (MSHS) are related positively to a number of factors associated with psychologic health, such as optimism and self-esteem, and related negatively with signs of psychologic distress, such as depression. They conclude that humor is a multidimensional construct that seems to be intimately related to quality of life.

Dowling (2002) provided an extensive account of children's use of humor as a coping strategy, which included the developmental aspects of humor. Piaget's (1962) cognitive stages of development are compared with McGhee's (1979) proposed stages of humor development. For example, children in the concrete operations stage (7–11 years) can (a) understand more abstract and implied incongruities, (b) search for multiple meanings, and (c) explain the reason for their amusement. On the other hand, children in the formal operations stage (11–15 years) have the cognitive ability to appreciate the complex structure of humor and the motivations behind its use. Dowling offers several examples of humor interventions for use with children in health-care settings.

Much overlap exists between the arts, and often more than one modality is used concurrently (e.g., singing and drama as a part of storytelling, dancing to music). However, for organizational purposes, what follows is a selection of research findings categorized loosely by art modality.

Music

Several studies have dealt with the use of music for coping with stress. For example, school-age children with asthma have identified listening to music as one of the four most effective and frequently used strategies for coping with their disease (Ryan-Wenger & Walsh, 1994). Marley (1984) found that music reduced stress-related behaviors in infants and toddlers who were hospitalized. (For a method that puts findings such as this into action, see box). Music also has been useful in producing relaxation during cardiac catheterization (Micci, 1984), and in decreasing preoperative anxiety (Chetta, 1981; Cunningham, Monson, & Bookbinder, 1997; Kain et al., 2004). Molassiotis and Cubbin (2004) reported that music is among the top five complementary and alternative medicine therapies used by pediatric oncology patients. Watkins (1997) reviewed the clinical research literature related to the effect of music; findings that suggest that music may facilitate a reduction in the stress response include decreased anxiety levels, decreased blood pressure and heart rate, and changes in plasma stress hormone levels.

Music has been found effective for increasing pain tolerance to dental procedures (Howitt & Stricker, 1966) and chronic pain (Wolfe, 1978). Studies also reveal music's effectiveness in decreasing pain during intramuscular injection (Fowler-Kerry & Lander, 1987), during bone marrow aspiration (Pfaff, Smith, & Gowan, 1989), after surgery (Dunn, 2004; Steinke, 1991), heel-stick procedures with neonates (Bo & Callaghan, 2000), and with serious illness (Bailey, 1986; Brown, Chen, & Dworkin, 1989; Nolan, 1992).

Music also has proven beneficial in establishing treatment routines as positive experiences for children and their families (Grasso, Button, Allison, & Sawyer, 2000). Routine chest physiotherapy (CPT, an important component of prophylactic therapy for children with cystic fibrosis), requires a significant commitment of time and energy. Grasso and colleagues evaluated the effect of recorded music as an adjunct to CPT, and compared the use of newly composed music, familiar music, and the family's usual routine on children's and parents' enjoyment of CPT. Findings indicate that their enjoyment of CPT significantly increased after the use of specifically composed and recorded music as an adjunct.

The type of music used is an important consideration (see Case Study 4.2). McCraty, Barrios-Choplin, Atkinson, and Tomasino (1998) investigated the impact of different types of music on tension, mood, and mental clarity. Participants completed psychologic profiles before and after listening to 15 minutes of four types of music: grunge rock, classical, New Age, and designer (music designed to have specific effects on the listener). Feeling shifts among participants were observed with all types of music. Of the four types, designer music was most effective in increasing positive feelings and decreasing negative feelings. Findings are summarized in Table 4.2 and suggest that designer music may be useful in the treatment of tension, mental distraction, and negative moods.

(text continues on p. 137)

Baby-Go-To-Sleep

Heartbeat Music Therapy

The Baby-Go-To-Sleep audiotape—which uses real human heartbeat, music, and singing—is being used in a variety of ways with children:

- to help decrease the amount of sedative medications
- to help relax claustrophobic children undergoing magnetic resonance imaging
- to calm babies who are born dependent on cocaine
- to calm fussy, irritable babies
- to help ease premature infants' transition to the home
- to help normal, healthy children who have trouble sleeping

Research findings indicate positive results from the use of the audiotape (Research, n.d.). Nurses in a newborn nursery used the tape with 59 crying babies over a 6-week period in 1985. They found that 94% of the infants stopped crying or went to sleep within 2 minutes when the Heartbeat Musical Therapy recording was played. Researchers in 1999 at The Indiana University School of Nursing found that pain intensity ratings were less for newborns who were played Heartbeat Musical Therapy recordings during and after operations than for babies exposed to no music. Further, the heart rates for babies who had the music intervention remained stable, resulting in higher oxygen saturation rates throughout the procedure.

Case Study 4.2
The Best You Can Be Is You

"Jonathan might enjoy some music," said the Pediatric Intensive Care Unit (PICU) charge nurse that snowy and chilly February evening. Jude and I entered Jonathan's room with guitars and a tattered bag containing our usual supply of small musical instruments. In the darkened room, Jonathan's father stood close to his 5-year-old son's crib. I looked at the frail child, his knee joints so deformed that my first impression was that his legs had been attached to his trunk backwards. The boy's twisted limbs thrashed in constant motion. Much of the motion was spastic, but some seemed directed—at Jonathan's father, who was fending off a seemingly endless barrage of punches and kicks.

"He has been like this all day," his father informed us through a weary smile. I looked at the young father and wondered what I always wonder: "How do parents handle living like this?" I'm certain that if I had asked Jonathan's father this question at this particular moment, he probably would have told me, "You just handle it. What other choice does one have?" I guess the ability of parents such as Jonathan's to continually handle it with such grace is a constant source of amazement for me. The joy children such as Jonathan bring to their parents' lives can sometimes seem quite removed from their present reality. But I guess it is kind of that way with all children, isn't it?

Researchers on the Neonatal Intensive Care Unit at Children's Hospital Medical Center of Akron, in Akron, Ohio, are using the audiotape in their study of the effects of music enhancement and sound reduction on the growth and development of premature babies. Since 1997, the Music Therapy and Sound Reduction/Quiet Time Research Project has been investigating whether changing or reducing the sounds premature babies hear helps them get better faster.

Previous studies on music enhancement and on sound reduction have shown that noise increases a newborn's heart rate and blood pressure, and decreases oxygen saturation levels. Noise also causes babies to spend more time awake or crying. They miss the important sleep time in which they conserve the energy and calories they need for healthy growth.

The study includes NICU babies who are 25 to 30 weeks gestation (born 10 to 15 weeks early), weigh less than 2 lbs. 12 ounces at birth, and are medically stable. Babies are divided into three groups. Group One babies hear the "Baby-Go-To-Sleep" tape, Group Two babies wear foam-plastic earmuffs, and babies in Group Three receive standard NICU care. Participation in the study begins by the time the baby is 7 days old and continues until discharge. Researchers check progress from information gathered during 6-month and 12-month visits to the Neonatal Follow-up Clinic. The 3-year study has recently concluded and findings should be released soon.

The results of this and other studies can have important implications for use of "Heartbeat Music Therapy" in a variety of health-care settings. For more information and a sample of the intervention, contact Terry Woodford at 1-800-537-7748, or write to Healing Light Fund, P.O. Box 550, Colorado Springs, CO 80901.

Note. Used with permission of Audiotherapy Innovations, 2519 W. Pikes Peak Avenue, Colorado Springs, CO 80904.

We introduced ourselves to Jonathan and his father: "I'm Judy and this is my friend, Jude," followed immediately by, "We were wondering if you would like to play some music with us today." This child, like many children who are hospitalized, was conditioned to the notion that strangers entering his room means pain and discomfort. We wanted to make it clear straight away the purpose and nature of our visit.

"What do you think, sport?" his father asked. "Would you like some music?" Perpetual thrashing about was Jonathan's reply.

I wondered if the boy might be in pain. Young children often react to pain with restlessness. His father said that Jonathan had been this way off and on throughout the entire 2 weeks of hospitalization. His theory was that his son was mostly sick and tired of being in the hospital. "He tends to do much better at home, where everything is familiar," he explained.

Jude tuned the guitar and rustled about with other preparations. I searched the bag for materials to make a bell bracelet for Jonathan. I quickly threaded three bells on some pipe cleaners, braided the ends, and connected them to form a bracelet. I handed it to Jonathan's father and said, "He can wear it on his wrist or ankle. If you think he'd like one in both spots, I can easily make more."

After he had attached the bell bracelet to Jonathan's wrist, we asked him to select a percussion or wind instrument from the bag. I believe he chose a maraca, but, because his opportunity to use it was limited, I cannot be certain.

Table 4.2

The Impact of Four Different Types of Music on Tension, Mood, and Mental Clarity

Type of Music	Impact
Grunge rock	Significant increases in hostility, sadness, tension, and fatigue Significant reductions in caring, relaxation, mental clarity, and vigor
Classical	Mixed
New Age	Mixed
Designer	Significant increases in caring, relaxation, mental clarity, and vigor Significant decreases in hostility, fatigue, sadness, and tension

Note. Adapted from "The Effects of Different Types of Music on Mood, Tension, and Mental Clarity," by R. McCraty, B. Barrios-Choplin, M. Atkinson, and D. Tomasino, 1998, *Alternative Therapies in Health and Medicine, 4*(1), pp. 75–84.

Jonathan couldn't talk, so Jude asked Jonathan's father what kind of music Jonathan seemed to enjoy. "Well," he said, "I know that he likes the Barney song, but I think he likes 'You Are My Sunshine' better."

I chose my favorite shaker from the bag, Jude started strumming, and we all began to sing. However, even before beginning the second verse, we realized that this wasn't working. The bells were ringing—Jonathan's contorted arm was flailing about—but something wasn't right. The problem was the song. The lively pace seemed to escalate Jonathan's agitation rather than cheer him up. And the more agitated he became, the more agitated his father became, and their agitation fed into each others' until a circle of swelling agitation filled the room.

We stopped. It was time to reassess the situation. Obviously what the boy liked and what he needed at that moment were quite different. And this likely was also true for his father.

"Let's try the Rory song," I suggested to Jude. Just an hour earlier Jude had introduced me to the children's song writer and singer's music. I had quickly fallen in love with one particular song. Although we had run through it a couple of times, we were still pretty sketchy on the words. But getting part of the way into a song and then not remembering the words was definitely not a new experience for us.

And so we sang Rory's "The Best You Can Be Is You." The words to the song speak of animals that are raised by different kinds of animals, try to be like them, and fail. The message is in the chorus:

Being yourself isn't easy
Still it's the best thing to do
Find your own road
And stick to this code
The best you can be is you (Rory, 1987)

Maybe the magic was the words, the slow soothing melody, or perhaps both, that totally transformed the mood in the room on that cold winter evening. Jonathan's father became very quiet. Instead of using his hands to defend himself from his young son's blows, he began to softly move them over the boy's jittering body, visibly calming him—first his forehead, cheeks, his chest, then radiating out each pitiful limb. It seemed as if he were looking at his son in a new way, perhaps reminding himself of all that his son is, the good and the bad, the sorrows and the joys—his small son simply struggling to be the best he could be. We quietly packed up and left a father and his son to savor a sacred moment together.

Certain types of music are used in palliative care. Therese Schroeder-Sheker (1993), a pioneer in the field of music thanatology, explained that music for the living is meant to engage us, while music for the dying is meant to free us. Although the music is individualized for each patient, chants typically are used because of their tendency to free us:

> The plainchant or Gregorian chant is sung without being attached to rhythm; one cannot count a pulse. There is no rhythmic accent. The body of sung prayer is in neither 4/4 nor 3/4 (three or four beats per measure); therefore, the chants are not stimulating, they are calming. Almost always, symmetrical music in 4/4, regardless of tempo, helps sustain metabolic activity and support the general binding tendency to deepen incarnation and relationship to physical body. (p. 45)

Cultural differences have been reported regarding efficacy and choices of music. For example, results from a study comparing participants from a U.S. study with participants from Taiwan found cultural differences in the both the degree of perceived helpfulness and choices of music. Fewer Taiwanese found the Western music calming, more chose harp music, and fewer chose jazz than U.S. participants. And, not surprisingly when considering how familiarity brings comfort, some Taiwanese participants preferred Buddhist hymns or popular songs heard in Taiwan (Good & Chin, 1998). In another account, Good, Picot, and Salem (2000) reported that Caucasian Americans most often chose orchestral music, piano music, and jazz, while African Americans most often chose jazz and gospel music. However, the investigators caution against stereotyping, urging sensitivity to what may be culturally congruent musical selections for patients. They further note that although soft, instrumental, and melodic music traditionally has been assumed to be soothing, music that is loud, has lyrics, and is strongly percussive or rhythmic should not be ruled out.

O'Callaghan (1996) offered two additional important considerations regarding the use of music. First, not only do people have individual preferences in music, when used inappropriately, music can aggravate pain sensation. The second consideration is a more positive one: Case studies indicate that music is helpful in alleviating the pain experiences of both palliative care patients *and* their significant others.

Ezzone, Baker, Rosselet, and Terepka (1998) tested music as a diversional intervention to see if it would affect participants' perception of nausea and episodes of vomiting. Using 33 adults undergoing bone marrow transplant, they randomly assigned 17 to a control group (that received the usual antiemetic protocol) and 16 to the experimental group (that received the usual antiemetic protocol plus music) during the 48 hours of high-dose cyclophosphamide administered as part of the preparative regimen. They found significant differences between group scores on a visual analog scale for nausea and number of episodes of vomiting, with the experimental group experiencing less nausea and fewer instances of vomiting. Music also has been found effective in reducing nausea after treatments or surgery (Standley, 1992; Steinke, 1991), and after anesthesia or chemotherapy (Keller, 1995).

Music has been the subject of much of the physiologic research in the literature. Listening to music, for example, can increase immune response. Lane (1990) conducted a single live 30-minute music therapy session with children who were hospitalized, and reported a significant increase in salivary IgA, an antibody that provides defense against various infections. The increase was not found in the control group, who did not participate in the music session.

Other studies have investigated the effects of music on infants' oxygen saturation levels, an indicator of respiratory regularity directly affected by the individual's behavioral state and degree of pain. In a study of 17 hospitalized premature infants, Collins and Kuck (1991) reported significant increases in oxygen saturation levels after 10 minutes of music combined with intrauterine sounds played free-field in the isolette. A recent study comparing the oxygen saturation levels of 10 infants who listened to recorded lullabies to those of 10 infants who listened to recordings of their mothers' voices revealed similar yet additional data (Standley & Moore, 1995). On the first day, the infants listening to music had higher oxygen saturation levels than those infants listening to their mothers' voices. However, on the second and third days, the babies hearing music had significantly depressed oxygen saturation levels during the posttest intervals after the music was terminated, while those listening to their mothers' voices did not.

Music, as well as other art modalities, can provide channels through which children can express the fear, anger, sadness, and loneliness of hospitalization. For instance, a sense of isolation may be decreased by asking children to share recollections of home and school experiences through improvised songs (McDonnell, 1983). Audio cassette tapes that feature children talking and singing about their feelings and hospital experiences have helped children who are hospitalized communicate their own thoughts and feelings (Grimm & Pefley, 1990). Hearing about others through story or song helps children realize that they are not alone in a particular situation.

Robb and Ebberts (2003a, 2003b) conducted a small but exciting study examining anxiety and depression levels using a songwriting and digital video production intervention with pediatric patients (9–17 years old) undergoing bone marrow transplantation. Of the 6 study participants, 3 received the music intervention, which consisted of songwriting, digitally recording patients performing their songs, photo and artwork selection, video design, and discussion. The nonmusic group of 3 participants played a board game, a card game, or a video game. Both conditions consisted of six 1-hour sessions over a 3-week period. The investigators reported that 4 participants (3 in the music group and 1 in the nonmusic group) experienced decreased anxiety following a majority of sessions (Robb & Ebberts, 2003a). Further, a patient survey revealed that the participants in the music group rated the music intervention as helping them use their time for something that was fun, to make choices, feel good about themselves, improve their mood, and express feelings (Robb & Ebberts, 2003b). Nonmusic participants indicated that improved mood, using time for something fun, and encouragement to do things normally done outside the hospital were the most beneficial aspects of their sessions. A response to an open-ended survey question is of particular interest to proponents of arts in health care. A member of the nonmusic group said, "Instead of playing games I like to do art" (Robb & Ebberts, 2003b, p. 22).

Visual Arts

Drawing, painting, sculpture, and other visual art modalities offer a means of nonverbal communication. The visual arts can bring out mixed, poorly understood feelings, in an attempt to bring them to order and clarity. Visual art activities provide a vehicle for children to express their anxiety and other feelings related to health-care experiences and illness. While the process of visual expression creates an opportunity for catharsis, at the same time the artwork itself offers a tool to monitor the child's emotional and developmental state and progress. For example, children who are stressed tend to show more emotional indicators in their drawings than do children who are not stressed (Sturner, Rothbaum, Visintainer, & Wolfer, 1980).

Children with cancer have reported engaging in drawing and painting as a means of effectively distracting themselves from even severe pain (Rollins, 1995). In addition to the Gate Control Theory described earlier, brain research over the past 3 decades may offer another explanation for this occurrence. We now know that each hemisphere (left and right) of the brain has its own way of knowing, its own way of perceiving external reality (see Table 4.3; Edwards, 1979).

Drawing is largely a right-brain function. The ability to draw may depend on whether one has access to the capabilities of the right hemisphere (i.e., whether one can "turn off" the dominant verbal left hemisphere and "turn on" the right). And so, while operating in the right hemisphere, the child who is drawing may be aware of pain, but with the left side turned off, he or she does not focus on the words to name, describe, or define it; the focus is on the drawing. The process of creating makes it difficult to think or worry about other things at the same time. Furthermore, with the right hemisphere's sense of timelessness, individuals often emerge from a drawing

Table 4.3

A Comparison of Left-Mode and Right-Mode Characteristics

Left Mode	Right Mode
Verbal—Using words to name, describe, define.	*Nonverbal*—Awareness of things, but minimal connection with words.
Analytic—Figuring things out step-by-step and part-by-part.	*Synthetic*—Putting things together to form wholes.
Symbolic—Using a symbol to stand for something (e.g., the sign "+" stands for the process of addition).	*Concrete*—Relating to things as they are, at the present moment.
Abstract—Taking out a small bit of information and using it to represent the whole thing.	*Analogic*—Seeing likenesses between things; understanding metaphoric relationships.
Temporal—Keeping track of time, sequencing one thing after another. Doing first things first, second things second, and so on.	*Nontemporal*—Without a sense of time.
Rational—Drawing conclusions based on reason and facts.	*Nonrational*—Not requiring a basis of reason or facts; willingness to suspend judgment.
Digital—Using numbers as in counting.	*Spatial*—Seeing where things are in relation to other things, and how parts go together to form a whole.
Logical—Drawing conclusions based on logic: one thing following another in logical order (e.g., a mathematical theorem or a well-stated argument).	*Intuitive*—Making leaps of insight, often based on incomplete patterns, hunches, feelings, or visual images.
Linear—Thinking in terms of linked ideas, one thought directly following another, often leading to a convergent conclusion.	*Holistic*—Seeing whole things all at once; perceiving the overall patterns and structures, often leading to divergent conclusions.

Note. From *Drawing on the Right Side of the Brain* (p. 40), by B. Edwards, 1979, Los Angeles: J. P. Tarcher, Inc. Copyright 1979 by J. P. Tarcher, Inc. Reprinted with permission.

session surprised at the passage of time and how comfortable they were during that period.

Art therapists, play therapists, child life specialists, psychologists, medical social workers, clinical counselors, psychiatric nurses, and other mental health–care professionals have widely used art expression in therapy with children in medical environments, yet until recently very little has been written specifically about "medical art therapy." According to Malchiodi (1993), medical art therapy is the use of art expression and imagery with individuals who are physically ill, experiencing trauma to the body, or undergoing aggressive medical treatment such as surgery or chemotherapy. In the first book devoted to medical art therapy with children (Malchiodi,1999), contributing authors discussed the use of medical art therapy using mandalas (Delue), with children with eating disorders (Cleveland), cancer (Councill), asthma (Gabriels), HIV/AIDS (Piccirillo), burns (Russell), and arthritis (Barton). In a final chapter, Malchiodi discussed somatic and spiritual aspects of children's art expressions.

Rubin (1999, p. 10) pointed out that not only art therapists can make the healing capacity of art available to others: "Many people can—and should—offer children art material in situations of medical stress." Although the use of projective artwork and other art therapy techniques are often best left to certified art therapists, other caring adults can use other techniques, such as the illuminative artwork technique. In this method, the facilitator does not impose his or her analysis of the individual's work, but instead encourages the individual to use the artwork as a communication tool. Spouse (2000) asked individuals to use illuminative artwork in much the same way as metaphors are used to express tacit or preconscious feelings about experiences, and then asked them to explain their significance.

In a study with children with cancer using the illuminative artwork method, Rollins (2003) found that children used this type of drawing in the following ways: (a) as a means of direct expression, and/or (b) as a focal point from which conversation would flow. She calls this second way the "campfire effect," the result of an activity or experience that provides a focal point shared by the individuals involved that serves to increase conversation in both quality and quantity.

A similar method, "draw-and-write," involves inviting children to draw pictures and then write about what is happening in their pictures. Data are richer and more insightful than those obtained through writing alone. This method has proven effective in exploring young children's perceptions about health and illness; it helps the less verbally able to communicate their own health perceptions because the method allows them to draw and then to seek adult help to express their thoughts in writing (Pridmore & Lansdown, 1997).

Rae (1991) used the *ipsative method* for analyzing children's drawings for the purpose of assessment. The ipsative method is a procedure whereby psychosocial adjustment and coping are assessed using the child's own drawings as a standard for comparison. Rather than looking solely at traits, content, or themes in a single drawing, children's psychosocial and emotional progress is evaluated as a function of the changes in their drawings over time. Because children's emotional status can change quickly over time, repeated drawings can offer a more realistic, multidimensional assessment of functioning at a particular time or over a length of time.

Schiller and colleagues (2003) found that drawing could provide an additional dimension of depth and enrichment in the relationship between school-age children with cancer and their nurses. Twenty children, ages 7 to 14 years, were asked to draw self-portraits of how they looked before they became ill and how they looked currently. The children used the process to share their feelings with their nurses, and through their drawings contributed greatly to understanding how the children viewed themselves throughout the various stages of the disease and treatment.

Although children who are ill often communicate thoughts, feelings, fears, or concerns about their illness through their drawings, just as often the content of their drawings may be unrelated to disease. In some cases children use drawing as a way to distract or remove themselves from their current situation. At other times their drawings refer to non–disease-related stressors that are common in the lives of many of today's children—parental divorce and remarriage, geographic mobility, maternal employment and alternative sources of child care, competitive pressures, and various forms of parental insufficiency (Rollins, 1990). Coping with stressors of this nature may be as difficult or even more difficult for the child than coping with disease-related stressors.

Storytelling

Many children find storytelling or reading helpful in coping with stress. Stories can offer a means of dealing with unfaceable fears and untenable realities by doing so indirectly (Freeman, 1991). When a child's unique knowledge and imagination is coupled with an adult's knowledge of child development, fantasy skills can be used as tools for coping, even when the situation is grave. A well-chosen story permits children to discuss their issues and situations if they wish. Other children simply enjoy stories as a fantasy escape that need not be analyzed, and use stories as an opportunity to set things aside for a time (see Case Study 4.3). In other words, children take from a story only what they are ready to find. They may find meaning in their experiences and renewed hope (Heiney, 1995).

Case Study 4.3
Setting Things Aside

When I think about a child setting things aside for a time, 4-year-old Jamal comes to mind. Off and on, Jamal had spent most of the winter in the hospital. An aggressive course of chemotherapy meant that frequently he felt pretty lousy and just stayed in his room. On one good day that had followed a string of very bad ones, Jamal joined us for a story. For a brief time Jamal was not the sickly little boy dealing with nausea and fatigue from the powerful drugs intended to kill the cancer inside him. His single focus was to be the best frog he could possibly be. He puffed out his chest and strutted about the "swamp" with a "gribbitt" that surely would have convinced most any frog that he was kin. Jamal's visit with us was short, but he returned to his room with a sense of pride and renewed vigor, which perhaps empowered him to believe that he could handle more of whatever he must to have that chance of getting well.

Storytelling has been used to help children deal with both mental and physical pain (Heiney, 1995). For example, Kuttner (1988) found that a hypnotic method using the child's favorite story was more effective statistically than behavioral distraction and standard medical practice in alleviating distress, pain, and anxiety during painful bone marrow aspirations.

Indeed, the power of story to distract should not be taken lightly. In 1794, before the use of anesthetics, a young boy had surgery to remove a tumor. He was told such an interesting story during his operation that it absorbed his attention and removed pain from conscious awareness. Eighteen years later, this true believer in the power of story, Jacob Grimm, wrote *Snow White* (Hilgard & LeBaron, 1984).

Storytelling can offer catharsis, which may occur vicariously as feelings of despair, anger, and anxiety are released through the characters in the story (Heiney, 1995). Further, the tone of stories children tell can provide clues to their emotional state. Research indicates that children with higher anxiety levels and poorer adjustment to hospitalization, as measured through observation, tend to tell more negative stories (Hudson, Leeper, Strickland, & Jesse, 1987).

Studies have shown that listening to a humorous story can increase immune response. Relaxation and guided imagery also can affect immune response to disease. Individuals with cancer have been encouraged to imagine "good guys" fighting and overcoming the "bad guy" cancer cells.

Minnesota storyteller and psychologist Elaine Wynne uses storytelling to teach children with asthma ways to manage their disease by exciting their imaginations (E. Wynne, personal communication, March 1999). One tool she helps them learn is relaxation. She tells them, "Pretend you're a rag doll and pretend you're lying in the sun. And the sun is shining on your face and the sun feels very warm on your eyelids, and you feel the warm sun on your arms and hands." Children learn that asthma is not something that just happens. It is something they can control by using relaxation exercises when they begin to have symptoms. Although children who have participated in this program may experience the same number of episodes as other children with asthma, they require fewer physician or emergency room visits. With the current emphasis on controlling health-care costs, programs such as these hold great promise.

The very structure of an individual story—with a beginning, a middle, and an end taking place in a definite timeframe—as well as the structure of a storytelling session itself, can provide a much-needed sense of predictability and closure for children who are ill. This can be especially important for children with chronic conditions who must deal with the ongoing saga of health-care experiences. This same sense of predictability can be enhanced through the telling of familiar stories, old favorites such as "Goldilocks and the Three Bears," "Three Little Pigs," and "Billy Goats Gruff." Hearing something familiar, especially when attempting to cope with an unpredictable illness or the strange surroundings of a hospital, can provide children with a sense of comfort and safety.

Story can do many things. In the words of Susan Gordon, a storyteller in the Studio G artists-in-residence program in pediatrics at Georgetown University Medical Center in Washington, DC:

> I tell stories on pediatric wards because stories entertain; they distract children from their pain and worry. It gives them a chance to play, to create, to imagine, to have sustained human contact, to have choice, to speak, to ask for what they want, to express themselves, to have time enough to say what is really on their minds, to ask questions, to get the story they really need.

Dance and Movement

Before the early 1990s, very little about the significance of dance and movement in pediatrics was reflected in the literature (Goodill & Morningstar, 1993). The goals of dance/movement are, in part, similar to those for other supportive psychosocial services in pediatric health-care settings, and address the whole child rather than focusing on the disease or dysfunction alone.

Dance, described simply, is a statement of emotion expressed through movement. All living organisms, including human beings, at least once in their lives exhibit behaviors that could be referred to as dancing (Warren & Coaten, 1993, p. 58):

> Within all of us there is a dancer. Washing our faces, digging the garden or baking bread can all be viewed as our own personal pieces of choreography, our own special dances.

According to Warren and Coaten (1993), the body is an instrument of expression and in childhood it is through the movement of our bodies that we start to build a picture of our world. We grow and develop and discover what our bodies can do, which ultimately leads to a growing awareness of our body's structure and to the growth of body image. Perhaps of greatest importance is the link between dance/movement and emotion. Our movements—the way we move, the way we stand, our gestures—reflect our inner emotional state. This emotional link is what differentiates dance/movement from the purely mechanical level of physical exercise. At times, intense emotions erupt spontaneously out of a free imaginative movement process; other times, a particular emotion may be deliberately evoked through the music and physical action (Chodorow, 1992).

Dance and movement help the individual (a) gain greater control of isolated body parts, (b) improve body image, (c) achieve controlled emotional release, and (d) become more socially adept (Warren & Coaten, 1993). Hanna (1995) believes that dance may help the healing process as a person gains a sense of control through (a) possession by the spiritual in dance, (b) mastery of movement, (c) escape or diversion from stress and pain through a change in emotion, states of consciousness, and physical capability, and (d) confronting stressors to work through ways of handling their effects.

Although research findings supporting the proposition that dance–movement improves a person's body image have been contradictory, previous work focused on styles such as ballet, jazz, and modern dance. Lewis and Scannell (1995) argued that creative dance–movement, with its less structured approach and absence of predetermined performance standards, has a positive effect on body image. They conducted research with 112 women between the ages of 18 and 69 years who had been actively participating in creative dance–movement courses for periods ranging from 2 weeks to 16.5 years. Participants experienced in creative dance–movement were more satisfied with their appearance, fitness, and body parts than participants with less than 5 years of experience. Given the potential for widespread clinical use of creative dance–movement with children having body-image disturbances, empirical research on the relationship between creative dance–movement and body image is warranted.

Koshland and Curry (1996) described the following four general goals dance/movement can address that can be applied universally to children who are hospitalized:

- *Establishing trust*—Movement, voice tone, sound, gestures, and kinesthetic empathy may be used to tune into the child's non-verbal messages. A peek-a-boo game is a simple way to accomplish this goal with young children.
- *Enhancing body awareness*—Dialogue with the body, dialogue between the child and dance/movement therapist, and movement props such as a feather duster, yarn ball, colorful wand, stretch band, or sounds of bells and music are used.
- *Identifying body sensations*—Although the child has become aware in a general way with what is going on in his or her body, the next step is to learn to identify sensations that may have resulted from the child's illness or injury. A child may learn to regulate breath, physical sensation, or circulation. This goal is facilitated by joining in with the child's movement, or exaggerating the child's movement to intensify and clarify emerging themes and issues.
- *Enabling the expression of feelings*—After a relationship has developed and the child is more aware of and able to identify bodily sensations, he or she is ready to learn how to express feelings. The use of colorful props, stories, and music provide a focus, especially for a child who is frightened, angry, or tired.

Dance–movement has been used successfully with children and adolescents with a variety of acute and chronic diagnoses. For example, Goodill and Morningstar (1993) discussed its use with a 2-year-old boy with cellulitis of the legs to help him express anger and other feelings about his illness; with a 4-year-old who was isolated as a result of exposure to chicken pox and was demonstrating boundary and body-image issues; and with two school-age girls—one with cystic fibrosis and the other with epilepsy—to express hope and to experience exchanging a positive, caregiving activity. Dance/movement has proven effective when used with children and adolescents with cancer, incorporating an array of medical, psychologic, social, and spiritual issues (Cohen & Walco, 1999). Reports indicate that dance and movement also have been integrated successfully into interventions for adolescents with eating disorders (Carraro, Cognolato, & Bernardis, 1998; Laumer, Bauer, Fichter, & Milz, 1997).

Creative Writing

Although a great deal has been said about children's use of nonverbal art forms, many children use creative writing to cope with the stresses of health-care experiences. Children diagnosed with life-threatening diseases often are encouraged to keep a journal to record what is going on in their lives and how they feel about it. Unlined paper also invites drawing to accompany children's words, if they choose. When reviewed at a later date, their journals provide encouraging evidence to children that they are not "in the same place," but have indeed been successful at adapting to some degree to their disease and treatment.

Froehlich (1996) believes that reading literature and writing literature is an inseparable process, just as listening to and experiencing music is linked to creating music: "Experiencing and doing is the ideal synthesis of the creative arts experience. In writing, language is the tool. We choose what we say and how we say it" (p. 202). The link between reading literature and writing it is storytelling. Children too young or otherwise unable to write can dictate a story to an adult to record. Individual books for children featuring their likes and dislikes have become popular over the years in pediatric settings. In a hospital, a group of children can participate in writers' workshops. The goal is to immerse children in a richly literate environment and encourage them to write as real-life authors do (Atwel, 1987; Calkins, 1986).

Writing and reading poetry helps children give voice to situations that touch their hearts (Raingruber, 2004; see Case Study 4.4). Children may be particularly responsive to writing poetry because its nature allows them to express themselves more readily in metaphor. Georgetown's poet-in-residence Adele Steiner works with children individually and in groups to create poetry. She often uses props, such as blowing bubbles, and asks children to tell her what they think of when they see bubbles. One of the children's favorite methods for displaying their poems is through "sky writing" that is placed on the ceiling over their beds (see Figure 4.7). Poetry can be used to address numerous health issues and is appropriate for all health content areas, including palliative care (Robinson, 2004). Massey (1998) described the use of Haiku, a form of Japanese poetry, to promote children's emotional health.

Nurses in the United Kingdom have initiated the "Poem Post" project, which makes a selection of short poems available on postcards in wall mounted

Case Study 4.4
Heartsongs

Mattie Stepanek, who had a rare genetic disease that took his life at the age of 13, began writing poetry at the age of 3 to cope with the death of his brother, who had the same disorder. Many of his poems speak of "heartsongs," which he described as "your inner beauty, the song in your heart that wants you to help make yourself a better person and to help other people do the same. Everybody has one" (*Wisdom Beyond His Years*, 2004, p. 2). During one of his many hospitalizations at Children's National Medical Center in Washington, DC, Mattie's wish to have his poetry published was fulfilled. Within weeks, the book was on the *New York Times* best-seller list. He wrote four additional books of poetry. A peacemaker as well as a poet, Mattie established a close friendship with former President Jimmy Carter, who described Mattie as "the most extraordinary person I ever met" (Wood, 2004, p. 1). Although Mattie used a wheelchair and relied on a feeding tube, a ventilator, and frequent blood transfusions to stay alive, his poetry provided the voice for him to fulfill his life mission to spread peace through the world.

racks within local hospitals. Patients, visitors, and staff contribute poems to the project; feedback has been generally very positive (Macduff & West, 2002).

Another avenue for creative writing is writing music and lyrics. This method may hold special appeal for teenagers. Research findings of North, Hargreaves, and O'Neill (2000) have indicated that music is important to adolescents, and that this is because it allows them to (a) portray an "image" to the outside world and (b) satisfy their emotional needs.

Writing is a wonderful way for children to make sense of their world. Children often are surprised by the insights that emerge as they write. Writing is about discovery. Writing is thinking. Writing is life discovery (Froehlich, 1996).

Drama

Drama, taken from the Greek word meaning simply "doing things" or "action" (Graham-Pole, 2000), has been used successfully with children for health promotion and illness and injury prevention education. For example, drama programs have been designed to increase AIDS awareness (Harvey, Stuart, & Swan, 2000), to communicate HIV/AIDS information (Elliott, Gruer, Farrow, Henderson, & Cowan, 1996; Valente & Bharath, 1999), and to increase knowledge regarding immunization (Gebreel & Butt, 1997). Health education messages in television and radio soap operas and popular serials also have been well-received (Bouman, Maas, & Kok, 1998).

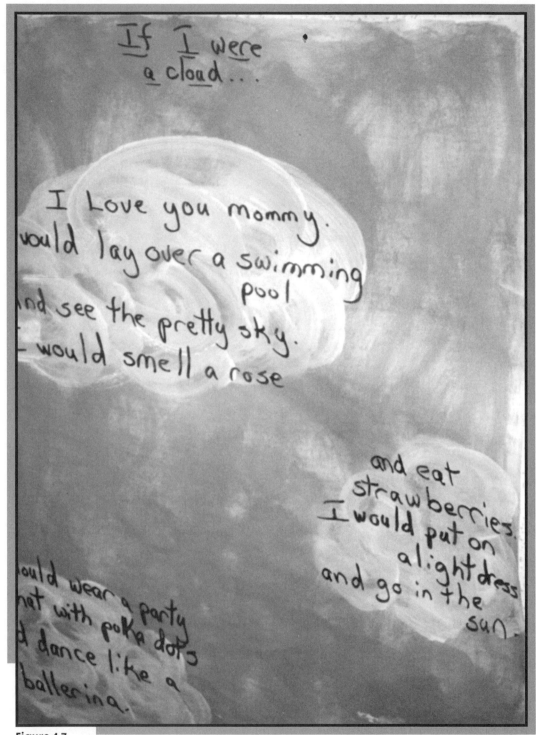

Figure 4.7.
Poetry can be displayed as "sky writing" on the ceiling above the child's bed.

Having children and adolescents participate in role-playing has proven to be an excellent learning tool. For example, Harding and colleagues (1996) used live theater to stimulate thought and discussion among adolescents (Grades 9–12) on topics related to the effects of substance abuse in their lives. A 30-minute professional and contemporary live musical performance was immediately followed by role-playing and discussion. Study findings indicate that live theater is an effective means for stimulating both thought and discussion pertaining to the effects of drugs in the lives of adolescents.

Drama also is an effective intervention for individuals with chronic illness or disability. McKenna and Haste (1999) reported that drama therapy delivered in a one-to-one interaction helped psychologic adjustment to disabilities for individuals recovering from neuro-trauma in four ways. Drama (a) provided them with a sense of personal space in an otherwise institutional setting, (b) allowed escapism and enjoyment, (c) awakened creativity and a sense of potency, and (d) provided a metaphor to explore personal issues. Graham-Pole (2000) described a professor of theater and literature's drama session with depressed teenage diabetics who refused to take their injections. The teens were asked to play parts: "We're going to act—like we're having fun. Fake it till you make it." The professor was after their self-consciousness:

> This is self-awareness of a productive kind. It's getting them to really see themselves right here and now, perhaps for the first time. It's getting them to start taking some real pride in their appearance and their performance. (p. 130)

In time, the previously reluctant and self-pitying teens were trying to outdo each other, expressing themselves, and enjoying the release from their real-life selves.

A discussion of drama and children would be incomplete without a mention of puppetry. Puppets are used in a variety of pediatric health-care settings because they provide safe, vicarious outlets for impulses and fantasies. In working with children and puppetry, it has been observed that the puppet becomes the actual personality of the child. Brounley (1996) explained the significance:

> Since the puppet exhibits no personality conflicts with the child, there is no reason for the child to feel threatened when speaking for the puppet. People speaking through puppets tend to assert themselves more than if they were speaking for themselves. Individuals listening to puppets also tend to accept more from a puppet than they would from another human being, even though they realize that the other human being is speaking. The responses to puppets are possible because they do not threaten. (p. 178)

Puppets are used to educate, to entertain, and to provide opportunities for expressions of emotions, fears, and fantasies. Puppetry is frequently used in preparing children for health-care encounters.

Clowning

Picture a clown at the bedside of a sick child and one imagines the smiling face of a delighted child. However, in past years, some child development specialists have expressed concern about the practice, citing the fact that some children are afraid of clowns, or that some typical clown antics are inappropriate for sick or hospitalized children. Their fears, for the most part, can be put to rest if they use specially trained clowns, such as those in New York's Big Apple Circus Clown Care Unit (CCU), who have been prepared to work with children in hospitals. Founded in 1986, the CCU provides clowns with special training in the needs of children who are ill and hospitalized. The model clown program has been replicated in a dozen countries, including Canada, the United States, France, and Brazil (Oppenheim, Simonds, & Hartmann, 1997).

The clown programs work in close partnership with medical staff at each host hospital, tailoring the program to meet the needs of the facility. The hospital's Chief of Pediatrics reviews the clown program's activities. Clowns visit each hospital 3 to 5 days each week, 50 weeks per year. Clown "doctors," like their medical colleagues, are highly skilled practitioners of their profession. Each member of the clown program is a professional artist—not a volunteer—selected by intensive auditions for high-quality artistry and sensitivity. The clowns work in teams of two or three, with a supervising clown on each team.

Inspired by the Big Apple Circus Clown Care Unit, Caroline Simonds founded Le Rire Medecin (Laughing Doctors) in Paris in 1991. A few years later, Le Rire Medecin decided that, with the emergence of other clown groups, it was important to define the basic principles of their work and to create some rules—a code of ethics—for clowns performing in hospitals. Although the group already had projects for training performers, one of the dilemmas for artists working in a hospital was the question of confidentiality. Simonds (1999, p. 792) explained:

> Is it necessary for a clown to know if a child is in pain, has been molested, or has an incurable illness? Experience has taught us that to remain sensitive to each patient it is important for performers to modify their gestures or physical distance from a patient and even to question the choice of a song.

The performers also felt the need to have the trust of the medical team to work on a long-term basis with their patients. They decided that they needed to define the difference between a "walk around" clown job, family entertainment, and in-depth work interacting with a medical team. The final document consists of 11 basic articles that define standards of professionalism, boundaries of artistic expression, limits of the creative role, responsibility of each artistic act, respect for patients as well as health-care workers, privacy, emotional parameters and distance from patients, basic safety, and even hygiene (Simonds, 1999). To view the code of ethics, see the *British Medical Journal* Web site (http://bmjjournals.com/cgi/content/full/319/7212/792/a/DC1).

Relationship-Centered Care

Intense moments in our lives cry out for human contact. Simply offering a storybook or art supplies to a child who is hospitalized may be helpful and appreciated, but research tells us that people-directed activities are more effective (Banks, Davis, Howard, & McLaughlin, 1993). This makes sense, for a relatively new term, *relationship-centered care*, stresses the concept that interactions among people are the foundation of any therapeutic or healing activity (The Pew-Fetzer Task Force, 1995). In other words, the presence of an artist, musician, storyteller, parent, teacher, child life specialist, nurse, volunteer, or other concerned and caring adult is likely to enhance the child's ability to use the arts in a therapeutic way.

As mentioned earlier, a child's artwork can serve as a communication tool between the child and the caring adult. Through conversation with the adult in an atmosphere of empathy and honest consideration, the child can become more aware of his or her reactions, behavior, intentions, and ambitions. According to Pinchover (1998), the child derives new abilities from these contacts, which moderate anxieties and strengthen healthy energies. Better collaboration and sounder ways of coping with intrusive medical treatment, as well as more trust and hope, seem to emerge from the relationships.

For some activities, such as storytelling, the storyteller's presence is critical. There is a close, caring communication implicit in the storytelling relationship (Freeman, 1991). An analysis of music research in medical treatment determined that the provision of live music was more effective than recorded music when selected and performed by trained music therapists (Bailey, 1983). Although such benefits have not been documented for other types of live music performances in medical settings, it is reasonable to assume that a live musician and recorded music would produce different experiences for children. If the interactions among people are the foundation for a therapeutic or healing activity, then perhaps this difference, too, may be attributed to the interaction between the musician or other artist and the individual.

Olson (1998) believes that bringing live music to the bedside can be a new way of extending the caring tradition of nursing practice, pointing out that bedside musical care is consistent with a holistic nursing philosophy and can be used during pregnancy, childbirth, and in neonatal care. Live music at the bedside can become a part of a treatment plan to foster integrity, well-being, and health.

Greaves (1996) offered an additional benefit of personal interaction between the artist and child. In the health-care environment, children can receive more individual attention in art instruction than would be possible from a teacher in the classroom. Interacting with an artist provides an opportunity for children to develop a potential for artistic interest and expression that can be explored throughout a lifetime (Rollins, 1992).

Professional Artwork

Florence Nightingale (1860) understood the significance of art in health-care settings. She felt strongly that the effect of beautiful objects was not simply on the mind, but also on the body: "Little as we know about the way in which we are affected by form, colour, and light, we do know this: they have an actual physical effect" (p. 59).

Children respond to and often use artwork created by professional artists as tools for coping. Prescott and David (1976) reported that children, who live according to the information provided by their senses, remember places and sensations more than they remember people. Thus, they are likely to be more sensitive to their surroundings than are adults, and may be affected deeply and for a long time by details of which adults are unaware.

Most of the research on the effects of images on people in health-care settings involves adult subjects and focuses on architecture or design issues (see Chapter 8: The Health-Care Environment). For example, Ulrich (1984) found that patients recovering from surgery with views of a small park with trees and flowers had better nurse evaluation, took less medication, and had shorter hospital stays than patients with a view of an adjacent brick wall. Later studies further confirmed that visual exposure to natural environments is more effective in fostering reduction of anxiety and stress than comparable visual exposure to urban environments (e.g., Ulrich et al., 1991). In a later study, Ulrich and colleagues exposed 166 patients in intensive care units to one of six visual stimulation conditions: two nature pictures dominated by water and trees, respectively; two abstract pictures similar in complexity to the nature conditions; and two control conditions (Ulrich, Lunden, & Eltinge, 1993). Patients exposed to the view of water experienced less postoperative anxiety than patients assigned to the other five visual conditions, and required fewer doses of strong pain drugs during the ward phase. Findings suggested that placing photographs of certain natural environments in hospital settings might have positive influences on postoperative recovery.

We know that images can be powerful tools for healing. Simonton, Matthews-Simonton, and Creighton (1981) recommended as an adjunct to standard cancer therapies, a program of relaxation, attitude change, and mental imaging. They suggested that patients form a mental picture of their cancer and of the immune system's victory over the disease. The basis for this technique is an ancient notion that a picture or image held in the mind can effect bodily change (Buttler, 1993):

> Psychologists have long recognized that images are preverbal, deeply linked to our emotions and unconscious mind.… Artists also have recognized that images can communicate feelings in ways our thinking minds cannot understand. Whenever we say that a painting, a photograph, a piece of music, or the smell of a flower moves us in a way we cannot express, we are acknowledging the power of images. (p. 117)

Artist and author Joan Drescher, a specialist in murals for healing environments, uses positive images in paintings she creates for children's health-care settings (see Figure 4.8). Her objective is to use these positive images to support the healing process: kites as symbols of courage and hope, air balloons as symbols of freedom and transcendence, and community-based images and nature images as regenerative symbols (Drescher, 1993).

In 1997, she created the Symbols of Courage Project—a series of seven murals for the Children's Hematology/Oncology Clinic at the Floating Hospital for Children at New England Medical Center in Boston, Massachusetts. In the process of developing the murals, she spent many hours in the clinic talking with the children and their families and sketching her impressions of

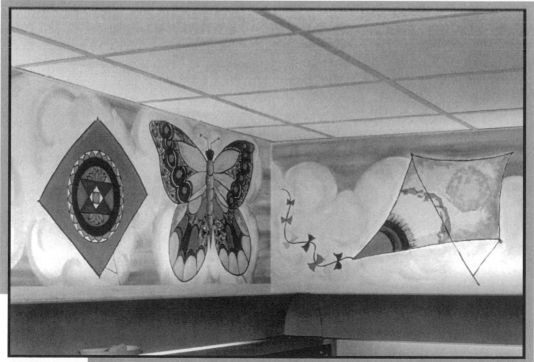

Figure 4.8.

Children at Children's Hospital in Boston, MA, can focus on a "Celebration of Kites" while undergoing radiation treatment. *Note.* Photograph by Joan Drescher. Used with permission.

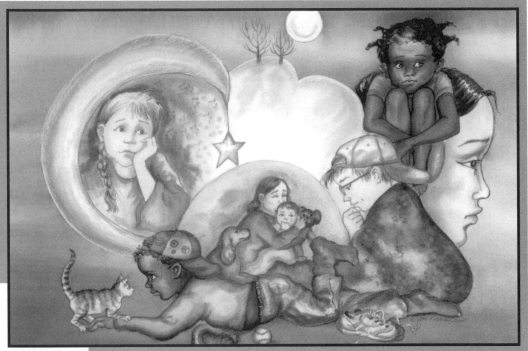

Figure 4.9.
The "Symbols of Courage" murals at the Floating Hospital for Children at New England Medical Center in Boston, MA, empower children with cancer to tell their stories. *Note.* Photograph by Joan Drescher. Used with permission.

the experience. The murals illustrate the journey that children with cancer and their families go through from the first diagnosis through the complete treatment protocol (see Figure 4.9).

Through the use of symbols within the murals, children are empowered to tell their story. In addition to helping children and their families through this difficult journey, the Symbols of Courage Project demonstrates to caregivers and the world what patients and their families go through. According to the clinic's medical director, the murals magnify the ability of all caregivers to understand and even experience the healing process with families, which brings new insight and power to the doctor–patient relationship (L. Wolfe, personal communication, May 1997). This healing art has connected the community and formed a new bridge between the worlds of art and medicine.

Facilitating the Creative Process

Children in health-care settings are, first and above all else, children. Therefore, techniques used to facilitate the creative process in such settings are

Table 4.4

155

Development of Drawing

Approximate Age (years)	Characteristics of Drawing
0–1	The infant has a reflex response to visual stimuli. The crayon is brought to the mouth, but the infant does not draw.
1–2	At approximately 13 months, the first scribble appears: a zig-zag. The infant watches the movement of the crayon leaving its marks on the surface.
2–4	Circles appear and gradually predominate. The circles then become discrete. In a casually drawn circle, the child envisages an object. A first graphic symbol has been made, usually between 3 and 4 years.
4–7	In this stage of intellectual realism, the child draws an internal model, not what is actually seen. The child draws what is known to be there. Transparencies, such as showing people through walls and hulls of ships, are commonly produced. Drawings at this age are expressionistic and subjective.
7–12	During this stage of visual realism, subjectivity diminishes. The child draws what is actually visible. Human figures are more realistic and proportioned. Colors are more conventional. The child distinguishes the right from the left side of the figure drawn.
12+	With the development of the critical faculty, most children lose interest in drawing. The gifted tend to persevere.

Note. Adapted from *Interpreting Children's Drawings* (p. 38), by J. DiLeo, 1983, New York: Brunner/Mazel. Copyright 1983 by Brunner/Mazel. Adapted with permission.

similar to those used with children everywhere. However, children's conditions and the setting itself often require special consideration. For example, as noted in Chapter 1, children often regress when ill or hospitalized. This may be evident in the type of arts experience they are willing to engage in, and often in an art product itself (see Table 4.4 for developmental characteristics of children's drawings). Additionally, pain has been shown to result in regression in children's drawings (Stefanatou & Bowler, 1997).

Children who are ill usually have lower energy levels than their healthy counterparts, and therefore may not appear very enthusiastic about participating in an arts experience. Their responses or affect—the nonverbal expression of their inner state—may be swift, subtle, and therefore difficult to see. Because children's responses usually help artists set the pace for or even decide to abandon a particular project, it is important to become familiar with these subtle and fleeting responses. Also, because we often gauge the success of our work by a child's response, knowing that the child may be having a wonderful time and yet be unable to show it can help us to continue doing this meaningful work without the satisfying feedback that is commonplace with healthy children.

Psychosocial Assessment

Even for artists operating in the role of facilitator and not "therapist," knowledge of various elements of psychosocial assessment can be helpful in planning activities for individual children, monitoring children's responses and progress, and making adaptations and recommendations. Basics of psychosocial assessment include (a) affect, (b) temperament, (c) ability to communicate and interact with peers, adults, and family, (d) personal or family stressors, (e) coping style, (f) amount and type of defense mechanisms used, and (g) self-concept and level of self-esteem (Rollins & Riccio, 2001).

Considering the child's temperament, for example, a visual artist may want to suggest a weaving project for a child who is highly persistent. A child with a low level of persistence might do better with a quick print-making project that allows him or her to see results almost instantly. Considering temperament can help the artist break out of the habit of using the child's age as the sole consideration. For instance, some 6-year-olds have temperaments that welcome very sophisticated, lengthy art projects, while some teenagers would quickly lose interest and prefer creating something that can be completed in one session.

Knowledge of Preceding Events

Children live very much in the here and now. Knowledge of what the child has experienced that day can be an important piece when planning an appropriate arts experience. For example, a child who has just received an injection may be agitated and angry. An activity that allows the child an opportunity to express some of his or her anger, such as pounding on a drum or a lump of clay, may be more appropriate at that moment than attempting to paint with watercolors and a tiny brush.

Basic Concepts

There are several basic guidelines to encourage children's creativity and enjoyment of an arts experience (Rollins & Mahan, 1996, pp. 86–87).[1]

1. *Offer children a wide range of media to explore.* They may never arrive at a finished product, but it's the process that is important.
2. *Erase the line between modalities.* Use music during a visual art activity; sing while dancing; combine singing and chanting with storytelling and drama.

---

[1]*Note.* From *From Artist to Artist-in-Residence: Preparing Artists to Work in Pediatric Healthcare Settings* (pp. 86–87), 1996, Washington, DC: Rollins & Associates. Copyright 1996 by Rollins & Associates. Reprinted with permission.

3. *Encourage children to consider as many details as possible.* Ask questions about their work, such as "Who lives in that tree?"

4. *Provide suggestions for activities.* Provide a list of things the child might wish to draw. Offer ideas for songs, such as making up a singing telegram to be delivered to the child's doctor or nurse.

5. *Respect the importance and uniqueness of a child's emotional life.* Engaging in an expressive activity can bring out all sorts of thoughts, concerns, and feelings, which the child may be reluctant to share, at least at that moment (see box).

6. *Accept the feelings, honest responses, or fantasies that children express symbolically or verbally.* At times a child's response is unexpected, bizarre, regressive, or messy, but as long as there is no realistic harm, the child will get the most benefit from the experience if these responses can be accepted and respected.

7. *Be an extension of and for the child who is physically unable to do all or parts of an activity or project.* The child will still have a sense of empowerment from having the opportunity to problem solve and engage in decision making.

8. *Encourage any special interest or talent in the arts.* Suggest or provide books, tools, or refer the child to a particular artist or artist's work. The curious moment should be captured, for interest is the best motivation for learning.

9. *Help children celebrate their art.* Display their art informally and formally; encourage performances such as mini plays, concerts, or puppet shows; help them create beautiful books for their stories.

Certain children with special needs may need extra help getting started on a project. Once started, they may not work as quickly as other children. It is important to resist interfering with the child's creative process, but to keep alert for signs that the child is struggling and may want help. In such cases it may be best to acknowledge the difficulty of the task and say, for example. "That's a really tough part. Would you like me to help hold the pieces together while you glue them?" Often a simple strategy, such as taping a piece of paper to the table to anchor it for drawing or painting, is all that is needed to adapt an activity for a child's special needs.

Safety Issues

Safety considerations when using the arts with children typically fall under one or more of the following categories: (a) the art materials; (b) the techniques

Respecting the Child's Privacy	**E**ngaging in an expressive activity can bring out all sorts of thoughts, concerns, and feelings. Some children may be reluctant to share them. Children can be given a sketch book and a supply of paper clips. They can express these thoughts and feelings through writing and drawing, then clip

or activities; (c) the child's age and developmental level; and (d) the child's condition (see Table 4.5). Before beginning an activity with a child,

1. *Read the label on art supplies.* Remember that nontoxic refers to acute, short-term health effects.
2. *Use your senses.* Paint, for example, can get moldy, and moldy paint should not be used. When in doubt, throw it out.
3. *Remember that smell is not a good indicator of toxicity.* Some materials, such as markers, can have a strong odor but be nontoxic. Others may have no odor or smell sweet but may be toxic.
4. *Think through each step of an activity.* Consider all equipment needed and techniques to be used.
5. *Consider the child's condition.* Certain odors may bother children who are nauseated. Often children whose immune systems are depressed may not be exposed to certain fresh fruits and vegetables commonly used in children's printmaking activities.
6. *Assess the surroundings.* Some activities require more space than others. Excessively noisy activities may disturb others close by.
7. *Consider supervision requirements.* Some activities require greater supervision than others. When working with a group of children or conducting an activity that requires close supervision, extra help may be needed.

See Appendix 4.1 for resources on safety and the arts.

Home Care Considerations

According to Rollins and Riccio (2001), artists experienced in working with children in hospitals will find that many of their skills transfer quite easily to the home health-care setting. Although similar to working with children in hospitals, working with children in the home is different in several ways (Rollins & Riccio, 2001):

■ *Artists cannot assume that simple supplies will be available, and even if they are, that these supplies are available for the artist's use.* For example,

together the pages they do not want others to see, maybe not now or maybe not ever. Nevertheless, they still have experienced the benefits of expressing them.

Note. Adapted with permission from *From Artist to Artist-in-Residence: Preparing Artists to Work in Pediatric Healthcare Settings* (p. 86), by J. Rollins and C. Mahan, 1996, Washington, DC: Rollins & Associates. Copyright 1996 by Rollins & Associates. Adapted with permission.

Table 4.5

Safety Considerations When Planning Arts Experiences for Children

Variable	Considerations
Materials	Toxic substances can be inhaled, ingested, or absorbed through the skin. Exposure can cause acute or chronic illness, an allergic reaction, or skin damage.
Techniques/Activities	Physical agents such as noise, vibration, repetitive motion, heat, and electrical equipment can cause injury and illness (e.g., loud music may decrease hearing).
Child's age and developmental level	Children under the age of 12 may not understand the need for precautions or carry them out consistently and effectively. Preschool-age children will sometimes deliberately put things into their mouths and swallow them. Habits such as nail biting or thumb sucking increase the risk.
Child's condition	Exposure to art materials or processes, or participation in art activities that exceed an individual child's physical limitations may place the child, especially a child with disabilities, at high risk for further illness or injury. Many of the hazards can be eliminated or reduced with one-to-one supervision or other appropriate measures.

Note. Adapted from *Artist Beware*, by M. McCann, 1992, Guilford, CT: The Lyons Press.

the artist who needs an oven to bake polymer clay beads should bring along a toaster oven. Although most homes have ovens, it could be in use or not available for the artist's use.

■ *Artists need to ask permission before using anything.* This includes something as simple as filling a container of water to rinse a paintbrush.

■ *Paint spills and other accidents may have increased significance in the home.* In the hospital, paint spilling on the bed linen is not a major issue; a quick trip to the linen cart or closet for replacements usually is all that is required. In the home, bed linens may be cherished heirlooms, so bringing along a vinyl tablecloth or other covering is helpful.

■ *To make best use of their time, artists need to be totally prepared for the activity, including being ready to offer alternatives.* Carefully thinking through each step of the planned activity and bringing along whatever may be needed, including something as basic as a container to hold water, will help ensure a good experience for the child, family, and artist.

But perhaps the biggest difference when visiting a child in the home is immediately seeing so many more sides to the child and the family—what they like, how they live, what is important to them—than is seen in the hospital room. In some cases this seems to help establish a bond more quickly, which can contribute significantly in the development of meaningful arts experiences (Rollins & Riccio, 2001).

Starting an Arts Program

Arts programs in pediatric settings come in all shapes and sizes. Learning about existing programs, what they do, and how they got started can be a helpful exercise. There is no one best way to start a program, and, although there often are many similarities, no two programs are ever exactly alike. Some programs pay their artists; others use volunteers. Some programs are hospital-based (e.g., Shands Hospital's Arts in Medicine program in Gainesville, Florida); others are community-based with artists serving children in health-care settings—including the home—through arts organizations (e.g., WVSA arts connection's ART is the heART program in Washington, DC) or museum schools (e.g., Hasbro Children's Hospital's Museum on Rounds in Providence, Rhode Island).

An excellent resource for starting an arts program is available from the Society for the Arts in Healthcare (SAH). With support from the National Endowment for the Arts, SAH has established the Society for the Arts in Healthcare Consulting Service (SAHCS) to provide affordable assistance to organizations wishing to establish or advance the arts in health-care settings (see Appendix 4.2 for contact information for this and other resources).

Selecting Artists

It is critical to spend adequate time selecting appropriate artists to work with children in pediatric health-care settings. Without certain basic characteristics, no amount of preparation and supervision will make a difference. Rollins and Mahan (1996, pp. 1–2) believe that the following are essential characteristics for artists working with children in health-care settings:

1. *A genuine interest in children, a caring attitude, and sensitivity to cultural and ethnic values.* Without an appreciation for the uniqueness of each

child, the trust needed to establish a helpful and enjoyable relationship with children will be absent.

2. *Knowledge and experience in a chosen art form.* If the artists are confident in their ability to do what they do best, they can communicate that to children and help them be successful in what they are trying to accomplish. Although it is desirable for the artist to have knowledge and experience in more than one art form or medium, sometimes it is fun for children and the artist to explore new possibilities together.

3. *A respect for the child's creative process and products.* Respect for the uniqueness of the individual includes respect for each individual's creative process and products of that process. Artists must want to facilitate rather than interfere with that process. In the absence of this quality, disastrous consequences can result.

4. *An appreciation and respect for the power of the arts and an understanding of personal limitations.* Art is a powerful communicator, one that carries both a tremendous potential and an equally great responsibility. An artist who lacks clinical training in art therapy, dance therapy, music therapy, poetry therapy, or any of the other expressive therapies can provide children with genuinely helpful, and in many ways "therapeutic," art experiences. However, Rubin (1984) cautioned those without clinical training about using such experiences to delve deeply into understanding or remediation of internal psychologic problems.

5. *Flexibility.* Artists need to be able to adapt to a variety of children and situations that may change during the course of an activity with an individual child or group of children.

6. *A sense of humor.* Artists who can laugh at themselves and humorous situations convey a sense of warmth that facilitates trusting relationships with children.

7. *The ability to collaborate with others.* Helping children through health-care experiences, illness, dying, and death is a team effort. If artists are to be considered members of the health-care team, they need to be able to work effectively with hospital or health-care agency staff, volunteers, and family members for the most successful outcome.

8. *No health condition that could result in harm to the children or to the artist.* Hospitals and health-care agencies require persons who will have regular contact with children to undergo a limited health screening, which typically includes a PPD test for tuberculosis and proof of either having had or immunization against certain childhood diseases such as measles, mumps, rubella, and chicken pox. On the other hand, artists with certain chronic health conditions need to be aware of the possibility that their health may be compromised by exposure to children with particular diseases or conditions.

Most artists who are interested in working in pediatric health-care settings will bring some experience working with children, but not necessarily. The desire to work with children is probably more important than

A Checklist for Hospital Entertainment Activities

This checklist can be used to ensure that entertainment activities for children in the hospital and their families are developmentally appropriate.

1. Does the hospital (and each pediatric unit) have established policies for entertainment and visits from celebrities?
2. Are they monitored by a team that includes child development or child life specialists, direct care providers, and parents?
3. Does each visiting group receive a copy of the departmental policies concerning such events?
4. Are visiting individuals and groups asked the following questions about their proposed entertainment:
   * Is it appropriate for the developmental age of the children?
   * Could it cause confusion or misconceptions about anything that might happen in the hospital?
   * Might it engender fears or fantasies about being harmed in any way?
   * Does it contain religious themes or content that might trouble some families?
   * Does it avoid any suggestion of violence (including the use of weapons) or death?
   * Does it avoid the use of masks or costumes that might frighten young children?

experience. And because working with children often means working with family members, it is a plus if the artist seems to be comfortable with people of all ages.

Preparing Artists To Work in Pediatric Health-Care Settings

Professionals who work with children generally agree that the special circumstances and needs of children in health-care settings require some sort of preparation beyond a general orientation to the environment for the following reasons (Rollins & Mahan, 1996):

- Children are not simply smaller versions of adults, but are growing and changing constantly.
- Children experience illness and health-care experiences very differently than adults.

- Does it invite children's participation in appropriate and noncompetitive ways?
5. Are visiting groups or celebrities oriented to the needs of children who are hospitalized and their families and how to approach and talk to them?
6. Are these visitors escorted at all times by a staff member who understands the special needs of children who are hospitalized?
   - When accompanied by the media, is there an additional escort?
7. Are parents and patients free to decline visits from celebrities or entertainers, and any related media coverage?
8. Is family privacy and confidentiality protected at all times?
9. Are patients who are confined to their rooms included?
10. Are signed parental consents obtained for all photographs or videotaping?

11. Is the entertainment provided on pediatric units monitored to ensure that it is not disruptive to children and families who may be sleeping, in pain, grieving, or in crisis?
12. If groups are giving away items, will they have enough for all the patients?
    - Are brothers and sisters who are present included?
    - Are items screened for safety?
13. Are visiting groups informed that enough time must be allowed for the visit to occur in a relaxed manner, and that hospital visits with children cannot be planned primarily as publicity opportunities?

Note. Adapted from *Caring for Children and Families: Guidelines for Hospitals* (p. 245–246)), by B. Johnson, E. Jeppson, and L. Redburn, 1992, Washington, DC: Association for the Care of Children's Health. Copyright 1992 by Association for the Care of Children's Health. Adapted with permission.

- Health-care staff members, parents, and even the artists themselves worry that, lacking preparation, artists with even the very best intentions run the risk of hurting children emotionally and perhaps even physically.
- Preparation brings a level of comfort to the artists, and therefore helps them to derive more satisfaction from their work.

What Kind of and How Much Preparation Is Needed?
This depends on several factors:

- *What is the population?* Will artists be working with children in hospitals, in hospice care, in the home, in a community agency? Will artists be working with parents and other family members as well?
- *What role will the artists assume?* Will they be there primarily to entertain and someone will always be with them for supervision? If this is the case, a review of the checklist in the box may be all that is needed. Will artists be conducting groups, working with individual

patients, or both? Will they be working with families, groups of families, staff, or all of the above?

■ *Is it unclear what role the artists will assume?* Often roles evolve or expand once a program is in place. For example, in WVSA arts connection's ART is the heART program, the original intent was to have artists work with children who were ill or dying in home and hospice care and their siblings. Within weeks after the program was implemented, it became clear that another group served by the referral agency (Visiting Nurse Association)—children who had parents or other family members in palliative care—could also benefit from artists' visits. Very quickly the artists' role was expanded and additional training was supplied.

■ *What are some ways to find out what role the artists might assume?* There are informal and formal ways to assess what is needed. The population (including children, families, and staff) can be asked informally or through focus groups and surveys. Having an ongoing advisory group that includes all of these stakeholders also can be helpful.

Conclusion

The current health-care climate insists that all services show just cause for every dollar spent. Because pediatric care costs more to provide than adult care, most pediatric services are faced with justifying their very existence. Particularly at risk are psychosocial services, often referred to as the "soft" services, the "fluff," or the "frills." Arts programs typically are viewed from this perspective. Only when documented research verifies the true benefits of arts programming will such programs become commonplace in children's health-care settings and funding for these services will cease to be such a struggle.

A growing number of health-care professionals share the vision that storytelling, music, painting, poetry, dance, and other forms of the arts will one day be considered essential elements of quality health-care. As we entered the 21st century, costs of managed care plans rose steeply after a period of relative stability, and purchasers are now demanding accountability in both medical outcomes and patient satisfaction. According to Sims (1997), quality is yesterday's buzzword. Today the word is value with a strong emphasis not only on quality and cost, but also on patient satisfaction. Hospitals and other agencies that are adopting and expanding arts programming are finding such collaboration considerably helpful in this regard.

Research on the use of the arts with children in health-care settings must move forward. Sciarillo (1995) spoke of a paradigm shift in children's health care—a change from promoting adaptation to participating in growth. Illness as a "problem" is being transformed to illness as a "challenge" presenting an opportunity for growing in new ways. This subtle distinction is the difference between life as existence and life as being. The arts hold the potential to play a major role in this transformation.

Study Guide

1. Discuss the history and current status of the arts as a healing process.

2. What functions do expressive arts experiences serve for children, and, in particular, children who are ill or hospitalized?

3. Compare and contrast creative arts and play of children, discussing when one or the other might be most beneficial for children in health-care settings.

4. Define expressive therapies and outline their various forms and functions.

5. Explain the processes by which the arts can be tools for (a) coping, (b) reducing stress or pain, (c) adapting, (d) feeling empowered, and (e) learning.

6. Discuss the current status of research on the arts in health care and healing of children.

7. What factors influence selection of type of expressive arts for children?

8. Do specific illnesses or conditions have corresponding appropriate arts activities?

9. What characteristics of artists or arts facilitators prove most effective for working with children in health-care settings?

10. What are the barriers and resources for arts facilitation and arts programs in child health-care settings?

APPENDIX 4.1

Resources for Safety and the Arts

Organizations

Arts, Crafts, and Theater Safety
181 Thompson Street, #23
New York, NY 10012-2586
Phone: 212/777-0062
E-mail: ACTS@CaseWeb.com
www.caseweb.com/ACTS/

The Art & Creative Materials Institute
PO Box 479
Hanson, MA 02341-0479
Phone: 781/293-4100
Fax: 781/294-0808
E-mail: debbief@acminet.org
www.acminet.org/safety.htm

Publications

McCann, M. (1992). *Artist beware: The hazards in working with all art and craft materials and the precautions every artist and photographer should take* (2nd ed.). New York: The Lyons Press.

Rossol, M. (2001). *The artist's complete health and safety guide* (3rd ed.). New York: Allworth Press.

Rossol, M. (1991). *STAGE FRIGHT: Health and safety in the theater.* New York: Allworth Press.

Shaw, S., & Rossol, M. (1991). *Overexposure: Health hazards in photography.* New York: Allworth Press.

APPENDIX 4.2

Resources for Starting Pediatric Arts-in-Health-Care Programs

Consulting Services

Society for the Arts in Healthcare
2437 15th Street NW
Washington, DC 20009
Phone: 202/299-9770
Fax: 202/299-9887
E-mail: mail@the SAH.org
www.theSAH.org

Publications

Breslow, D. (1993). Creative arts for hospitals: The UCLA experiment. *Patient Education and Counseling, 21*, 101–110.

Graham-Pole, J., Rockwoood Lane, M., Kitakis, M., & Stacpoole, L. (1994). Creating an arts program in an academic medical setting. *International Journal of Arts Medicine, 3*(2), 17–25.

Hillman, G., & Gaffney, K. (1996). *Artists in the community: Training artists to work in alternative settings.* Washington, DC: Americans for the Arts, Institute for Community Development and the Arts.

Kable, L. (2004). *Caring for caregivers: A grassroots USA–Japan initiative.* Washington, DC: Society for the Arts in Healthcare.

Kaye, C., & Blee, T. (Eds.). (1997). *The arts in health care: A palette of possibilities.* London: Jessica Kingsley.

Klahr, M., & Oskam, B. (1988). *To open a door: Conducting poetry workshops for populations with special needs.* New York: Poets in Public Service.

Palmer, J., & Nash, F. (1991). *The hospital arts handbook: A resource book for arts and humanities programs in health care settings.* Durham, NC: Duke University Medical Center.

Ridenour, A. (2001). Art for health's sake. A step-by-step approach to developing a facilty arts program. *Health Facilities Management, 14*(9), 21–24.

Rockwood Lane, M., & Graham-Pole, J. (1994). Development of an art program on a bone marrow transplant unit. *Cancer Nursing, 17*(3), 185–192.

Rode, D. (1995). Building bridges within the culture of pediatric medicine: The interface of art therapy and child life programming. *Art Therapy Journal of the American Art Therapy Association, 12*(2), 104–110.

Rollins, J. (2004). *Arts activities for children at bedside.* Washington, DC: WVSA Arts Connection.

Rollins, J., & Mahan, C. (1996). *From artist to artist-in-residence: Preparing artists to work in pediatric healthcare settings.* Washington, DC: Rollins & Associates.

Rollins, J., & Riccio, L. (2001). *ART is the heART: A WVSA arts-in-healthcare program for children and families in home and hospice care.* Washington, DC: WVSA Arts Connection.

References

Atwel, N. (1987). *In the middle—Writing, reading, and learning with adolescents.* Portsmouth, NH: Heinemann.

Bailey, L. (1983). The effects of live music versus tape-recorded music on hospitalized cancer patients. *Music Therapy, 3,* 17–28.

Bailey, L. (1986). Music therapy in pain management. *Journal of Pain Symptom Management, 1,* 25–28.

Banks, S., Davis, P., Howard, V., & McLaughlin, T. (1993). The effects of directed art activities on the behavior of young children with disabilities: A multi-element baseline analysis. *Art Therapy: Journal of the American Art Therapy Association, 10*(4), 235–240.

Bo, L. K., & Callaghan, P. (2000). Soothing pain-elicited distress in Chinese neonates. *Pediatrics, 105*(4), E49.

Bouman, M., Maas, L., & Kok, G. (1998). Health education in television entertainment—Medisch Centrum West: A Dutch drama serial. *Health Education Research, 13*(4), 503–518.

Brounley, N. (1996). Puppet and drama therapy with hospitalized and abused children. In M. Froehlich (Ed.), *Music therapy with hospitalized children* (pp. 177–193). Cherry Hill, NJ: Jeffrey Books.

Brown, C., Chen, A., & Dworkin, S. (1989). Music in the control of human pain. *Music Therapy, 8,* 47–60.

Buttler, K. (Ed.). (1993). *The heart of healing.* Atlanta, GA: Turner.

Calkins, L. (1986). *The art of teaching writing.* Portsmouth, NH: Heinemann Publishers.

Carraro, A., Cognolato, S., Bernardis, A. (1998). Evaluation of a programme of adapted physical activity for ED patients. *Eat Weight Disorders, 3*(3), 110–114

Chetta, H. (1981). The effect of music and desensitization on preoperative anxiety in children. *Journal of Music Therapy, 18,* 88–100.

Chodorow, J. (1992). Sophia's dance. *American Journal of Dance Therapy, 14*(2), 111–123.

Cohen, S., & Walco, G. (1999). Dance/movement therapy for children and adolescents with cancer. *Cancer Practice, 7*(1), 34–42.

Collins, S., & Kuck, K. (1991). Music therapy in the neonatal intensive care unit. *Neonatal Network, 9*(6), 23–26.

Cunningham, M. F., Monson, B., & Bookbinder, M. (1997). Introducing a music program in the perioperative area. *Association of Operating Room Nurses Journal, 66*(4), 674–682.

DiLeo, J. (1983). *Interpreting children's drawings.* New York: Brunner/Mazel.

Dowling, J. (2002). Humor: A coping strategy for pediatric patients. *Pediatric Nursing, 28*(2), 123–131.

Drescher, J. (1993). Murals for healing. *Child Health Design, 7,* 9–10.

Dunn, K. (2004). Music and the reduction of post-operative pain. *Nursing Standard, 18*(36), 33–39.

Edwards, B. (1979). *Drawing on the right side of the brain.* Los Angeles, CA: Tarcher.

Elliott, L., Gruer, L., Farrow, K., Henderson, A., & Cowan, L. (1996). Theatre in AIDS education—A controlled study. *AIDS Care, 8*(3), 321–340.

Express Yourselves. (1997). *Progress Notes, 1*(2), 1.

Ezzone, S., Baker, C., Rosselet, R., & Terepka, E. (1998). Music as an adjunct to antiemetic therapy. *Oncology Nursing Forum, 25*(9), 1551–1556.

Fowler-Kerry, S., & Lander, J. (1987). Management of injection pain in children. *Pain, 30,* 169–175.

Freeman, M. (1991). Therapeutic use of storytelling for older children who are critically ill. *Children's Health Care, 20*(4), 208–215.

Froehlich, M. (1996). Bibliotherapy and creative writing as expressive arts with hospitalized children. *Music therapy with hospitalized children: A creative arts child life approach* (pp. 195–206). Cherry Hill, NJ: Jeffrey Books.

Gappell, M. (1995). Psychoneuroimmunology. In S. Marberry (Ed.), *Innovations in healthcare design* (pp. 115–120). New York: Van Nostrand Reinhold.

Gebreel, A., & Butt, J. (1997). Making health messages interesting. *World Health Forum, 18*(1), 32–34.

Goldstein, A. (1980). Thrills in response to music and other stimuli. *Physiological Psychology, 8*(1), 126–129.

Good, M., & Chin, C. (1998). The effects of Western music on postoperative pain in Taiwan. *Kao Hsiung I Hsueh Ko Hseuh Tsa Chih, 14*(2), 94–103.

Good, M., Picot, B., & Salem, S. (2000). Cultural differences in music chosen for pain relief. *Journal of Holistic Nursing, 18*(3), 245–260.

Goodill, S., & Morningstar, D. (1993). The role of dance/movement therapy with medically involved children. *International Journal of Arts Medicine, 2*(2), 24–27.

Graham, B. (1993). Wounded healers. In N. Vahle (Ed.), *Healing and the mind with Bill Moyers: A resource guide for the field of mind body health.* Sausalito, CA: Institute for Noetic Sciences.

Graham-Pole, J. (2000). *Illness and the art of creative self-expression.* Oakland, CA: New Harbinger.

Grasso, M., Button, B., Allison, D., & Sawyer, S. (2000). Benefits of music therapy as an adjunct to chest physiotherapy in infants and toddlers with cystic fibrosis. *Pediatric Pulmonology, 29*(5), 371–381.

Greaves, B. (1996). Visual expression for the child in hospital. *Children in Hospital, 22*(1), 9–11.

Grimm, D., & Pefley, P. (1990). Opening doors for the child "inside." *Pediatric Nursing, 16*(4), 368–369.

Hanna, J. (1995). The power of dance: Health and healing. *Journal of Alternative and Complementary Medicine, 1*(4), 323–331.

Harding, C., Safer, L., Kaanagh, J., Bania, R., Carty, H., Lisnov, L., & Wysockey, K. (1996). Using live theatre combined with role playing and discussion to examine what at-risk adolescents think about substance abuse, its consequences, and prevention. *Adolescence, 31*(124), 783–796.

Harvey, B., Stuart, J., & Swan, T. (2000). Evaluation of a drama-in-education programme to increase AIDS awareness in South African high schools: A randomized community intervention trial. *International Journal of Sexually Transmitted Disease and AIDS, 11*(2), 105–111.

Heiney, S. (1995). The healing power of story. *Oncology Nursing Forum, 22*(6), 899–904.

Hendricks-Ferguson, V. L. (1997). An analysis of the concept of hope in the adolescent with cancer. *Journal of Pediatric Oncology Nursing, 14*(2), 73–80.

Hilgard, J., & LeBaron, S. (1984). *Hypnotherapy of pain in children with cancer.* Los Altos, CA: William Kaufman.

Howitt, J., & Stricker, G. (1966). Objective evaluation of audio analgesia effects. *Journal of the American Dental Association, 73,* 874–877.

Hudson, C., Leeper, J., Strickland, M., & Jesse, P. (1987). Storytelling: A measure of anxiety in hospitalized children. *Children's Health Care, 16*(2), 118–122.

Johnson, B., Jeppson, E., & Redburn, L. (1992). *Caring for children and families: Guidelines for hospitals.* Bethesda, MD: Association for the Care of Children's Health.

Johnson, L. (1997). *The Life Necklace: Celebrating the creativity of children in hospitals.* Washington, DC: Rollins & Associates.

Kain, Z., Caldwell-Andrews, A., Krivutza, D., Weinberg, M., Gaal, D., Wang, S., & Mayes, L. (2004). Interactive music therapy as a treatment for preoperative anxiety in children: A randomized controlled trial. *Anesthesia & Analgesia, 98,* 1260–1266.

Keller, V. (1995). Management of nausea and vomiting in children. *Journal of Pediatric Nursing, 10*(5), 280–286.

Koshland, L., & Curry, L. (1996). Dance/movement therapy with hospitalized children. In M. Froehlich (Ed.), *Music therapy with hospitalized children* (pp. 161–175). Cherry Hill, NJ: Jeffrey Books.

Kuttner, L. (1988). Favorite stories: A hypnotic pain-reduction technique for children in acute pain. *American Journal of Clinical Hypnosis, 30*(4), 289–295.

Lambert, R., & Lambert, N. (1995). The effects of humor on secretory immunoglobulin A levels in school-aged children. *Pediatric Nursing, 21*(1), 16–19.

Lane, D. (1990). *The effect of a single music therapy session on hospitalized children as measured by salivary immunoglobin A, speech pause time, and a patient opinion Likert scale.* Unpublished doctoral dissertation, Case Western Reserve University, Cleveland, OH.

Laumer, U., Bauer, M., Fichter, M., & Milz, H. (1997). Therapeutic effects of the Feldenkrais method "awareness through movement" in patients with eating disorders. *Psychotherapy and Psychosomatic Medical Psychology, 47*(5), 170–180.

Lewis, R., & Scannell, E. (1995). Relationship of body image and creative dance movement. *Perceptive Motor Skills, 81*(1), 155–160.

Linton, P. (1995). Creating a total healing environment. In S. Marberry (Ed.), *Innovations in healthcare design* (pp. 121–132). New York: Van Nostrand Reinhold.

Macduff, C., & West, B. (2002). Developing the use of poetry within healthcare culture. *British Journal of Nursing, 11*(5), 335–341.

Malchiodi, C. (1993). Introduction to special issue: Art and medicine. *Art Therapy Journal of the American Art Therapy Association, 10*(2), 66–69.

Malchiodi, C. (Ed.). (1999). *Medical art therapy with children.* Philadelphia: Jessica Kingsley.

Marley, L. (1984). The use of music with hospitalized infants and toddlers: A descriptive study. *Journal of Music Therapy, 21,* 126–132.

Massey, M. (1998). Promoting emotional health through haiku, a form of Japanese poetry. *Journal of School Health, 68*(2), 73–75.

McCann, M. (1992). *Artist beware.* Guilford, CT: The Lyons Press.

McCraty, R., Barrios-Choplin, B., Atkinson, M., & Tomasino, D. (1998). The effects of different types of music on mood, tension, and mental clarity. *Alternative Therapies in Health and Medicine, 4*(1), 75–84.

McDonnell, L. (1983). Music therapy: Meeting the psychosocial needs of hospitalized children. *Children's Health Care, 12*(1), 29–33.

McGhee, P. (1979). *Humor: Its origin and development.* San Francisco: Freeman.

McKenna, P., & Haste, E. (1999). Clinical effectiveness of drama therapy in the recovery from neuro-trauma. *Disability Rehabilitation, 21*(4), 162–174.

Micci, N. (1984). The use of music therapy with pediatric patients undergoing cardiac catheterization. *Art Psychotherapy, 11,* 261–266.

Miles, M. (1997). Does art heal? In C. Kaye & T. Blee (Eds.), *The arts in health care: A palette of possibilities* (pp. 241–249). London: Jessica Kingsley.

Molassiotis, A., & Cubbin, D. (2004). Thinking outside the box: Complementary and alternative therapies used in paediatric oncology patients. *European Journal of Oncology Nursing, 8*(1), 50–60.

National Institutes of Health, Office of Alternative Medicine. (1994). *General information.* Bethesda, MD: Author.

Nightingale, F. (1860). *Notes on nursing: What it is and what it is not.* London: Harrison and Sons.

Nolan, P. (1992). Music therapy with bone marrow transplant patients: Reaching beyond the symptoms. In R. Spintge & R. Droh (Eds.), *Music/medicine* (pp. 209–212). St. Louis, MO: MMB Music.

North, A., Hargreaves, D., & O'Neill, S. (2000). The importance of music to adolescents. *British Journal of Educational Psychology, 70* (Pt. 2), 255–272.

O'Callaghan, C. (1996). Pain, music creativity and music therapy in palliative care. *American Journal of Hospice and Palliative Care, 13*(2), 43–49.

Olson, S. (1998). Bedside musical care: Applications in pregnancy, childbirth, and neonatal care. *Journal of Obstetric Gynecology and Neonatal Nursing, 27*(5), 569–575.

Oppenheim, D., Simonds, C., & Hartmann, O. (1997). Clowning on children's wards. *The Lancet, 350,* 1838–1840.

Pert, C., Dreher, H., & Ruff, M. (1998). The psychosomatic network: Foundations of mind–body medicine. *Alternative Therapies, 4*(4), 30–41.

Pfaff, V., Smith, K., & Gowan, D. (1989). The effects of music-assisted relaxation on the distress of pediatric cancer patients undergoing bone marrow aspirations. *Children's Health Care, 18,* 232–236.

Piaget, J. (1962). *Play, dreams, and imitation in childhood.* New York: Norton.

Pinchover, E. (1998). Art therapy for hospitalized children inspired by Elizabeth Kuebler-Ross' approach. *Harefuah, 135*(7–8), 257–262, 336.

Prescott, E., & David, T. (1976). *The effects of the physical environment on day care.* Pasadena, CA: Pacific Oaks College.

Pridmore, P. J., & Lansdown, R. G. (1997). Exploring children's perceptions of health: Does drawing really break down barriers? *Health Education Journal, 56,* 219–230.

Research. (n.d.). Baby-go-to-sleep. Retrieved January 1, 2004, from www.babygotosleep.co.uk/research.html

Rae, W. (1991). Analyzing drawings of children who are physically ill and hospitalized using the ipsative method. *Children's Health Care, 20*(4), 198–207.

Raingruber, B. (2004). Using poetry to discover and share significant meanings in child and adolescent mental health nursing. *Journal of Child and Adolescent Psychiatric Nursing, 17*(1), 13–20.

Robb, S., & Ebberts, A. (2003a). Songwriting and digital video production interventions for pediatric patients undergoing bone marrow transplantation, Part 1: An analysis of depression and anxiety levels according to phase of treatment. *Journal of Pediatric Oncology Nursing, 20*(1), 2–15.

Robb, S., & Ebberts, A. (2003b). Songwriting and digital video production interventions for pediatric patients undergoing bone marrow transplantation, Part 2: An analysis of patient-generated songs and patient perceptions regarding intervention efficacy. *Journal of Pediatric Oncology Nursing, 20*(1), 16–25.

Robinson, A. (2004). A personal exploration of the power of poetry in palliative care, loss and bereavement. *International Journal of Palliative Nursing, 10*(1), 32–39.

Rogers, R. (1995). In need of a guarantee. *Children & Society, 9*(4), 32–51.

Rollins, J. (1990). Childhood cancer: Siblings draw and tell. *Pediatric Nursing, 16*(1), 21–27.

Rollins, J. (1992). *Arts for children in hospitals: A national program of Very Special Arts.* Washington, DC: Very Special Arts.

Rollins, J. (1994). What's making a difference? Studio G. *The ACCH Advocate, 1*(2), 34–35.

Rollins, J. (1995). Art: Helping children meet the challenges of hospitalization. *Interacta, 15*(3), 36–41.

Rollins, J. (2003). *A comparison of the nature of stress and coping for children with cancer in the United States and the United Kingdom.* Unpublished doctoral dissertation, DeMontfort University, Leicester, England.

Rollins, J., & Mahan, C. (1996). *From artist to artist-in-residence: Preparing artists to work in pediatric healthcare settings.* Washington, DC: Rollins & Associates.

Rollins, J., & Riccio, L. (2001). *ART is the heART: An arts-in-healthcare program for children and families in home and hospice care.* Washington, DC: WVSA Arts Connection.

Rollins, J., & Riccio, L. (2002). ART is the heART: A palette of possibilities for hospice care. *Pediatric Nursing, 28*(4), 355–362.

Rory. (1987). The best you can be is you. On *I'm just a kid* [Audiocassette]. Bethesda, MD: Roar Music.

Rubin, J. (1982). Art therapy: What it is and what it is not. *American Journal of Art Therapy, 21,* 57–58.

Rubin, J. (1984). *Child art therapy* (2nd ed.). New York: Van Nostrand Reinhold.

Rubin, J. (1999). Forward. In C. Malchiodi (Ed.), *Medical art therapy with children.* Philadelphia: Jessica Kingsley.

Ryan-Wenger, N. (1992). A taxonomy of children's coping strategies: A step toward theory development. *American Journal of Orthopsychiatry, 62*(2), 256–263.

Ryan-Wenger, N., & Walsh, M. (1994). Children's perspectives on coping with asthma. *Pediatric Nursing, 20*(3), 224–228.

Schiller, T., Bachval, I., Dana, Z., Hadad, S., Gross, J., & Shalev, J. (2003). 2002 APON conference proceedings: Draw me a picture: Children with cancer draw for the nurses. *Journal of the Association of Pediatric Oncology Nurses, 20*(2), 101.

Schirrmacher, R. (1988). *Art and creative development for young children.* Albany, NY: Delmar.

Schroeder-Sheker, T. (1993). Music for the dying: A personal account of the new field of music thanatology—History, theories, and clinical narratives. *Advances, The Journal of Mind–Body Health, 9*(1), 36–48.

Sciarillo, W. (1995). Humanizing health care for children and families: Revitalizing the spirit of our work. *The ACCH Advocate, 2*(1), 4–8.

Seidel, K. (1996). *How the arts contribute to education.* Cincinnati, OH: Association for the Advancement of Arts Education.

Simonds, C. (1999). Clowning in hospitals is no joke. *British Medical Journal, 319,* 792.

Simonton, O. C., Matthews-Simonton, S., & Creighton, J. (1981). *Getting well again.* New York: Bantam Books.

Sims, E. (1997, April). *Managed care creates new opportunities for arts in healthcare.* Paper presented at the Culture, Health and the Arts World Symposium, The Manchester Metropolitan University, Manchester, England.

Spouse, J. (2000). Talking pictures: Investigating personal knowledge through illuminative art-work. *NT Research, 5*(4), 253–261.

Standley, J. (1986). Music research in medical/dental treatment: Meta-analysis and clinical applications. *Journal of Music Therapy, 23,* 56–122.

Standley, J. (1992). Clinical applications of music and chemotherapy: The effects on nausea and emesis. *Music Therapy Perspectives, 10,* 27–35.

Standley, J., & Moore, R. (1995). Therapeutic effects of music and mother's voice on premature infants. *Pediatric Nursing, 21*(6), 509–512, 574.

Stefanatou, A., & Bowler, D. (1997). Depiction of pain in the self-drawings of children with sickle cell disease. *Child: Care, Health and Development, 23*(2), 135–155.

Steinke, W. (1991). The use of music, relaxation and imagery in the management of post-surgical pain for scoliosis. In C. Maranto (Ed.), *Applications of music in medicine* (pp. 141–162). Washington, DC: National Association for Music Therapy.

Sturner, R., Rothbaum, F., Visintainer, M., & Wolfer, J. (1980). The effects of stress on children's human figure drawings. *Journal of Clinical Psychology, 36,* 325–331.

The Pew-Fetzer Task Force. (1995). *Health professions and relationship-centered care.* San Francisco: The Pew Health Professions Commission.

Thompson, R. (1985). *Research on pediatric hospitalization.* Springfield, IL: Thomas.

Thorson, J., Powell, F., Sarmany-Schuller, I., & Hampes, W. (1997). Psychological health and sense of humor. *Journal of Clinical Psychology, 53*(6), 605–619.

Ulrich, R. (1984). View through a window may influence recovery from surgery. *Science, 224,* 420–421.

Ulrich, R., Simons, R., Losito, B., Fiorito, E., Miles, M., & Zelson, M. (1991). Stress recovery during exposure to natural and urban environments. *Journal of Environmental Psychology, 11,* 201–230.

Ulrich, R., Lunden, O., & Eltinge, J. (1993). Effects of exposure to nature and abstract pictures on patients recovering from open heart surgery. *Psycholophysiology: Journal of the Society for Psychophysiological Research, 30,* (Suppl. 1), S7.

Valente, T., & Bharath, U. (1999). An evaluation of the use of drama to communicate HIV/AIDS information. *AIDS Education Preview, 11*(3), 203–211.

Wall, P. (1973). The gate control theory of pain mechanism. A re-examination and restatement. *Brain, 101,* 1–18.

Warren, B., & Coaten, R. (1993). Dance: Developing self-image and self-expression through movement. In B. Warren (Ed.), *Using the creative arts in therapy* (2nd ed., pp. 58–83). London: Routledge.

Watkins, G. (1997). Music therapy: Proposed physiological mechanisms and clinical implication. *Clinical Nurse Specialist, 11*(2), 43–50.

Wisdom Beyond His Years. (2004). Retrieved June 23, 2004, from www.oprah.com/tows/past-shows/tow_past_20011019_b.jhtml

Wolfe, D. (1978). Pain rehabilitation and music therapy. *Journal of Music Therapy, 15,* 162–178.

Wood, T. (2004). *Memories, jokes and respect mark Mattie's services.* Retrieved June 28, 2004, from www.mdausa.org/mattie/remember.cfm

Woodgate, R. (1998). Health professionals caring for chronically ill adolescents: Adolescents' perspectives. *Journal of the Society of Pediatric Nurses, 3*(2), 57–68.

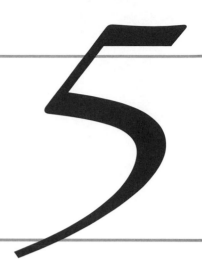

The Child with Special Health-Care Needs

Elizabeth Ahmann and Judy A. Rollins

Objectives

At the conclusion of this chapter, the reader will be able to:

1. Discuss the medical and societal changes that have influenced the mortality rates for children and the supports for sustaining life.
2. Describe the impact of chronic illness or disability in children on the family, society, and the health-care system.
3. List and discuss various theoretical frameworks for understanding and predicting care for children with special health-care needs.
4. Draw implications for prevention and intervention and the various levels of support for assisting families with the care of their children with special health-care needs.

edical and technologic advances have resulted in increased life expectancy for children with chronic and disabling conditions. For example, polio survivors, the first generation of children with technology dependency, have entered the ranks of senior citizens. Advances made during the poliomyelitis era have led to today's progress in neonatology, critical care, and rehabilitation medicine, resulting in the second generation of children with technology dependency. Children with acute or chronic life-threatening illnesses and premature and low birth weight infants never expected to survive in the not-so-distant past now survive to grow into adulthood and, as did many polio survivors, have children of their own.

In many instances, survival has come at a high physical and emotional cost for children and their families. For children with special health-care needs, health-care encounters are not a one-time event but a series of ongoing events. The experiences themselves not only are more numerous but often more invasive, uncomfortable, or painful than those encountered by other children.

The nature of their conditions and ongoing treatments translate into increased and complex psychosocial and family considerations. The effect may be found in several aspects of their lives such as their psychologic well-being and their emotional and behavioral development. This chapter will address psychosocial issues for children with special health-care needs in hospitals, the home, and the community.

The Child with Special Health-Care Needs

Several conceptual approaches have been used to classify children with chronic health problems: condition lists, functional status assessments, an elevated need for health-related services, and limitations in social roles, such as school or play (McPherson et al., 1998; Newacheck et al., 1998). Numerous definitions of the term *chronic illness* have been used, and specific terms such as *disability, impairment*, and *technology dependence* have also been applied to children with special needs. These varied conceptual approaches and definitions have contributed to challenges both in gathering data to describe the population of children with special needs and in planning and advocating for services.

In 1998, in part because eligibility for health and educational services are determined by whether a child is considered to have "special health-care needs," the federal Maternal and Child Health Bureau's Division of Services for Children with Special Health Care Needs developed the following definition:

> Children with special health care needs are those who have or who are at an increased risk for a chronic physical, developmental, behavioral, or emotional condition and who also require health and related services of a type or amount beyond that required by children generally. (McPherson et al., 1998, p. 138)

Because of increased survival rates for prematurely born infants, improved survival rates of trauma victims, improved life-prolonging treatments for previously fatal childhood illnesses (e.g., cystic fibrosis, HIV/AIDS), and improved case-finding, the incidence and prevalence rates of chronic illness have been increasing (Newacheck & Taylor, 1992). Using the Maternal and Child Health Bureau definition above, the National Survey on Children with Special Health Care Needs reported that in 2001, 12.8% of children in the United States under 18 years of age, some 9.4 million children, had a chronic physical, developmental, behavioral, or emotional condition that required health and related services of a type or amount beyond that required by children generally (Maternal and Child Health Bureau/National Center for Health Statistics, 2002). This number does not include children considered "at risk." The researchers found that the prevalence of special health-care needs varied by demographic and socioeconomic categories. For example, the prevalence increased in a step-wise fashion with age; also, one third more boys than girls had a special need. African American children were more likely to have special needs than other racial groups, and children with special needs were more likely to be from low-income and single-parent households. Additionally, an estimated 11% of children with special health-care needs were uninsured and 6% had no usual source of health care.

Today, national data reveal that approximately 20% of all children in the United States have a chronic physical or mental condition requiring services that typically extend beyond those needed by healthy children (McManus, 2000). Common conditions include asthma, attention deficit disorder, sickle cell disease, cerebral palsy, and adolescent depression.

The impact of chronic illness and disability in children is far reaching. Some children may experience effects in developmental, social, and emotional as well as physical realms. Family members—parents, siblings, and even grandparents—often make accommodations and adjustments when a child has special health-care needs. The larger social fabric is also affected. This group of children has an increased use of health-care services and associated higher health-care costs; makes use of special federal programs; and may require specialized local health, developmental, and educational services. In the instance of emergency medical services (EMS), for example, children with special health-care needs who use EMS are more likely to receive advanced life support service, to receive pre-hospital procedures, and to be transferred from one health-care facility to another (Surunda, Vernon, Diller, & Dean, 2000).

Principles of Care and Theoretical Frameworks

The care of children with special needs must be sensitive to the normal and special needs of these children, the central role of the family in care of the child, and cultural considerations. Family-centered care, normalization theories, theories of stress and coping, systems theories, and a comprehensive coordinated multidisciplinary approach all supply useful frameworks for health-care providers working with this population.

Care of the Child

Vessey and Maguire (1999) presented two important principles in the care of children with special needs:

1. Remember that children with special needs are more like their unaffected peers than different from them.
2. Focus on the fact that the concerns and problems faced by children with differing chronic conditions are similar regardless of the chronic condition.

Patterson and colleagues (Patterson & G. Geber, 1991; Patterson & M. Gerber, 1991) articulated the first principle by emphasizing that children with special needs have the same developmental needs as all children. Children's lives can continue to grow and develop beyond a diagnosis or condition (Shelton & Stepanek, 1994). In one mother's words,

> Many professionals seem to forget sometimes that Laura is not only a little girl with Turner Syndrome or congenital heart disease or malformed kidneys or complications of surgery or multiple orthopedic problems ... she is also a Girl Scout, a student of the viola, a reader of great books, a sister who comforts a crying brother, a daughter who sweeps the kitchen, a granddaughter who crafts homemade Valentines, a niece who tickles a cousin—all of the things that are more important about her than the string of diagnoses that we can choose from. (Leff & Walizer, 1992, pp. 209–210)

The second principle—called a noncategorical approach—has a similar thrust and was first suggested by Stein and Jessop (1982). While specific chronic conditions may pose unique challenges and require particular solutions (for example, a child who is deaf may need instruction in sign language, while a child who has asthma may need daily medication), all children with or without chronic conditions face the same general challenges: (a) functioning in developmentally appropriate ways, (b) maintaining self-esteem, and (c) participating in family and community life.

Other principles in planning care and support of the child with special needs emphasize using the child's developmental age, rather than chronologic age, in planning interventions; promoting normal development at each age and stage; encouraging coping and resilience; and focusing on strengths rather than weaknesses.

Family Context for Care

The principles of family-centered care provide an overarching framework for the care of children with or without special needs (see box). The goal of family-centered care is to provide for optimal care of the child. According to Pridham (1995, p. 30),

> Family-centered care refers to nursing care that recognizes the central role of the family, however defined by its members, in the health of children. It is based on a partnership of health professionals, other professionals, the child, and the family. Its goal is to support, respect, encourage, and enhance the strengths and participation of children and families in the child's health care.

Family-centered care is considered the standard in pediatrics and has many demonstrated benefits that are not observed with other models of care (Ahmann & Johnson, 2001; Beach Center on Families and Disability, 1996; Hanson, Jeppson, Johnson, & Thomas, 1997). Although research suggests that health-care providers may fall short in providing family-centered care (Bruce & Ritchie, 1997), it is clearly the approach to care most favored by families of children with critical and chronic illnesses and disabilities (Diehl, Moffitt, & Wade, 1991; McNeil, 1992).

Family-centered care recognizes that family members know their child best. Family members care for their children's health, developmental, social, and emotional needs across settings and over a period of many years (Ahmann, 1999a). Because of this, family members should be active participants in assessing needs, in planning, and in implementing care. Although it is common for health-care providers to focus on an immediate crisis and see the child and family primarily in that limited context, families must balance a child's health-care needs both with the child's other needs and interests and other family members' needs and interests, in the short and long term (Ahmann, 1999a). Health-care providers should assure opportunities for families to

Key Elements of Family-Centered Care

- Incorporating into policy and practice the recognition that the family is the constant in a child's life, while the service systems and support personnel within those systems fluctuate.

- Facilitating family and professional collaboration at all levels of hospital, home, and community care.

- Exchanging complete and unbiased information between families and professionals in a supportive manner at all times.

- Incorporating into policy and practice the recognition and honoring of cultural diversity, strengths, and individuality within and across all families, including ethnic, racial, spiritual, social, economic, educational, and geographic diversity.

- Recognizing and respecting different methods of coping, and implementing comprehensive policies and programs that provide develop-

participate as fully as they wish in decision making and care provision. This requires open, honest, thorough, and supportive sharing of information related to diagnosis, prognosis, options, care strategies, available services, negotiating the system, coping strategies, and the like (Hanson et al., 1997).

Health-care providers also must recognize and accept the fact that family strengths, needs, and coping strategies will vary. Families may be supported in a variety of ways. Dokken and Sydnor-Greenberg (1998) encouraged health-care providers to assist families in mobilizing their own resources. Linking families with community supports is another way to offer valuable support (Shelton & Stepanek, 1994). These supports can include (a) educational, (b) emotional, (c) instructional, (d) financial, (e) environmental, (f) material, (g) emotional, (h) recreational, or (i) respite services. A third approach involves encouraging and facilitating opportunities for family-to-family support and networking (Shelton & Stepanek, 1994). Families traditionally have described this kind of support as helpful; recent research gives evidence that parents of children with special needs are uniquely qualified to help each other (Kerr & McIntosh, 2000). Peer support is not limited to mothers, but includes support for fathers (May, 1996), siblings (Meyer & Vadasy, 1994), and grandparents, especially those in care-providing roles (Ahmann, 1997). See Appendix 5.1 for organizations for family-member peer support.

Cultural Context

Culture and ethnicity have an impact on access to care, use of services, the perceived meaning of illness, health-care practices, and communication (Ahmann, 1994). For example, in a study of 30 urban American Indian family caregivers,

mental, educational, emotional, environmental, and financial supports to meet the diverse needs of families.

* Encouraging and facilitating family-to-family support and networking.

* Ensuring that hospital, home, and community service and support systems for children needing specialized health and developmental care and their families are flexible, accessible, and comprehensive in responding to diverse family-identified needs.

* Appreciating families as families and children as children, recognizing that they possess a wide range of strengths, concerns, emotions, and aspirations beyond their need for specialized health and developmental services and support.

Note. From *Family-Centered Care for Children Needing Specialized Health and Developmental Services* (p. vii), by T. Shelton and J. Stepanek, 1994, Bethesda, MD: Association for the Care of Children's Health. Copyright 1994 by Association for the Care of Children's Health. Reprinted with permission.

one third of the participants thought that their child's providers believed things about their background that were not true and that they were treated less well because of their ethnic or cultural background (Garwick, Jennings, & Theisen, 2002). One fourth of the sample reported that providers were not sensitive to family needs or adequately informed about their child's condition.

Cultural traditions give families guidance, support, comfort, and meaning (McCubbin, Thompson, Thompson, McCubbin, & Kaston, 1993), and can become even more important in stressful or challenging circumstances. Health-care providers should see cultural traditions and culturally derived responses to illness as strengths rather than deficits or challenges (Adams, 1990), and should attempt to understand a family's beliefs and preferences and incorporate them into the plan of care. When a family is not English-speaking, every effort should be made to provide interpretation and translation to enhance communication during health-care visits. For more information regarding cultural issues, see Chapter 10: Cultural Influences in Children's Health Care.

Normalization

Normalization strategies have long been emphasized in the care of children with special needs. Based on a review of the literature, Knafl and Deatrick (1986) outlined four defining characteristics of normalization:

- acknowledging the existence of the illness,
- defining family life as normal,
- defining the social consequences of the illness as minimal, and
- engaging in behaviors consistent with a view of family life as "normal."

Normalization Strategies for Children with Special Needs	Apply the same rules for the child with special need as for other children in the family.
	Foster intrafamily communication.
	Allow the child to participate in decision making according to age and ability.
	Offer the child situational control and choices whenever possible and appropriate.
	Emphasize the child's abilities.
	De-emphasize the child's limitations.
	Prepare the child in advance for medical treatments and side effects or other changes that may occur.
	Encourage self-care appropriate to age and ability.

Normalization has been considered important for the child's optimal development and for encouragement of family stability. Examples of strategies that can be employed to normalize the life of a child with special needs are outlined in the box. Additional strategies to normalize family life include maintaining family routines, planning parental dates, and going on family vacations.

Research by Knafl and colleagues (1996) has examined how families manage a child's chronic condition. Those families in their study considered to be thriving were characterized by a focus on normalcy and a feeling of confidence in their ability to meet illness-related demands. At the same time, normalizing life for a child and family with special needs can pose challenges and require a balance of competing demands on time and energy. Until recently, researchers have focussed little attention on families who do not view normalization as an attainable goal, families who are unable to sustain normalization over time, or families whose social–cultural backgrounds do not support normalization (Knafl & Deatrick, 2002). Families not experiencing normalization tend to reflect one or more of the following qualities in adjusting to their child's chronic illness: (a) parents see the child as very different from his or her peers and their usual parenting style had to change to accommodate this dramatically changed view of their child; (b) the illness is a major focus of family life; (c) the illness is a source of conflict in the family; and (d) the treatment regimen is a significant burden entailing behaviors that make their family different from other families.

Additionally, it may not be reasonable to expect that all families should try to maintain life as "normal" in all phases and circumstances of caring for a child with chronic illness. In particular, during times of upheaval, such as when obtaining a diagnosis, or during a phase of terminal care, deviations from a practice of "normalizing" family life may be quite appropriate (see Case Study 5.1).

Encourage and assist as necessary (e.g., by equipment modification, environmental changes, or therapeutic instruction) to enable the child's participation in age-appropriate activities, whether these be sensory, motor, social, academic, or other.

Expect participation in chores, family activities, and social events as consistent with age and abilities.

Encourage incorporation of care requirements into existing family routines.

Advocate for the child within the school system as necessary.

Provide for age-appropriate extracurricular activities as per the child's interests, including sports, clubs, and camps.

Note. From "Strategies of Normalization Used by Parents of Chronically Ill School Age Children," by E. Bossert, B. Holaday, A. Harkins, and A. Turner-Henson, 1990, *Journal of Comprehensive Pediatric Nursing, 3*(2), pp. 57–61; "Wong's Nursing Care of Infants and Children (7th ed.)," by M. Hockenberry, D. Wilson, M. Winkelstein, and N. Kline, 2003, St. Louis, MO: Mosby; "Chronic Conditions: Effects on the Child," by J. Vessey and M. Maguire, 1999, in M. Broome and J. Rollins (Eds.), *Core Curriculum for the Nursing Care of Children and Their Families* (pp. 243–255), Pitman, NJ: Jannetti Publications.

Case Study 5.1
One Family's Experience

A family presented their 14-month-old son Sam to a hospital emergency department (ED) with an accidental strangulation injury. Sam's first admission to the pediatric intensive care unit (PICU) focused on lifesaving measures and preserving brain and respiratory function. He was discharged after 2 weeks and the family was advised to continue care with the ear, nose, and throat (ENT) surgeon to follow the healing injury to Sam's trachea. The family planned to resume life as usual with their son and his 3-year-old sister, Alice. The child's mother expressed immense feelings of gratitude that her child suffered no brain injury as a result of the accident, and was quite relieved to be able to go on with life as usual.

However, 2 weeks after discharge, the family again presented to the emergency department with their son, who was experiencing increasing breathing difficulties. He was again admitted to the PICU, where the decision was made to urgently perform a tracheostomy. This admission lasted 2 weeks, during which time the family had to learn to care for their child and his new tracheostomy. Sam's mother was very anxious, afraid she would not be able to care for him at home.

During these 2 weeks, Sam's mother learned to care for the tracheostomy, identified other caregivers who needed to be trained, and set up the home to accommodate the new equipment that would be needed to care for Sam. In addition, she identified and sought assistance with a number of developmental issues for both of her children. The child life specialist worked with her to prepare Alice for having a brother with a tracheostomy. Medical, social work, nursing, and case management staff taught the family to provide Sam's care, and helped to arrange the home care he would need. Child life and speech pathology staff worked with Sam and his family to begin using sign language as an alternative means of communicating while this child, at a sensitive age for language acquisition, had a tracheostomy and was prevented from speaking.

As the magnitude of the life changes required for this family became clearer, the mother began to identify areas of her life that could be simplified, and changes she would need to make in her daily routines. Again, the transdisciplinary team helped her work with these issues and become more comfortable with this major life transition. It is anticipated that Sam will have a successful tracheal reconstruction and be decannulated within 18 to 24 months. If that happens, the family will be able to resume life as it was before the accident. If not, they seem to have the skills and the desire to make life as normal as possible for everyone in the family.

This family's experience illustrates the shift from life with healthy children, to life with a child who has special needs. The family appears to be adapting very quickly, but each family will approach this differently, according to their own preferred coping styles. Health-care professionals can help family members identify effective coping strategies and encourage them to use these strategies to manage caring for the family in these new circumstances.

Note: Copyright 2000 by Carmel C. Mahan.

Stress and Coping Theory

Lazarus and Folkman's (1984) stress and coping framework has been widely used in research on children with special needs and their families. In fact, for years, research on this population focused on stressors. As a result, many potential stressors for families of children with special needs have been identified. In broad categories, these include the following (Walker, 1999):

- aspects of the illness trajectory,
- role strain,
- role confusion,
- financial stressors,
- time constraints,
- energy demands,
- psychosocial stressors, and
- sustained uncertainty.

Three distinct theoretical models are often considered when conceptualizing chronic disease and the mechanisms of impact on a child's behavior and emotional functioning: discrete disease, noncategorical, and mixed models (Gartstein, Short, Vannatta, & Noll, 1999). Features of each model and clinical implications can be found in Table 5.1.

At the same time, because individuals and families perceive their own situations differently, what is stressful to one family may not be stressful to another. Additionally, individuals and families bring a variety of coping

Table 5.1

185

Theoretical Models of Psychosocial Adjustment
of Children with Chronic Illness

Model	Features	Clinical Implications
Discrete disease	Focuses on the adaptations of parents, families, and children with one chronic condition Implies that each chronic condition places unique stresses, daily hassles, and demands on the child and the child's family Assumes that each chronic illness is associated with specific social or emotional sequelae	Learning more about a disease-specific sequelae will inform both clinical practice and theory.
Noncategorical	Takes the perspective that children with different chronic conditions experience many common stressors and traumas Views recurring nonspecific disease factors (e.g., chronicity of the illnesses, pain, hospitalizations, lengthy doctor visits, treatment side effects, and limitations imposed by the medical conditions) as stressful and creating hassles for the child and family Recognizes clear differences between chronic conditions, but places more importance on their commonalities Assumes commonalities have the potential for disrupting the child's functioning and development in physical and psychologic domains	Psychosocial services provided for children with chronic illnesses should emphasize the common denominators across diverse medical diagnoses (e.g., develop support groups for adolescents with diverse chronic illnesses because they face a common set of challenges).
Mixed	Blends features of the discrete illness and noncategorical models Recognizes differences between diverse diagnostic categories but also explores similarities across multiple illnesses Attempts to delineate specific disease-related variables that could be responsible for differences or similarities in functioning across different conditions (e.g., any chronic illness that affects the central nervous system may be especially detrimental to academic adjustment)	Groups of children representing certain "clusters" of chronic illnesses are expected to exhibit similarities and differences in functioning on the basis of onset, course, outcome, and incapacitation.

Note. Adapted from "Psychosocial Adjustment of Children with Chronic Illness: An Evaluation of Three Models," by M. Gartstein, A. Short, K. Vannatta, and R. Noll, 1999, *Journal of Developmental Behavior Pediatrics, 20*(3), pp. 157–163. Copyright 1999 by Lippincott, Williams & Wilkins. Adapted with permission.

abilities to a situation, and, despite the stressors they face, most families cope effectively with the demands of raising a child with special needs. Recognizing this, the recent trend in research on children with special health-care needs and their families is to focus on resilience and coping.

Systems Theories

Systems theory suggests that all human systems consist of interdependent, interacting parts characterized by a dynamic steady-state balance between the parts and their environment (Bronfenbrenner, 1979; Feiring & Lewis, 1978; Monane, 1967; VonBertalanffy, 1968). Olson, Sprenkle, and Russell's (1979) circumplex model of family systems suggests that in family life the dynamic balance occurring between cohesion and adaptability determines adjustment. Other applications of systems theory to care of the child with special needs help researchers examine multiple dimensions of child and family life and help clinicians to recognize the interconnections between the child, the family, the health-care system, and the social environment, and to conduct comprehensive assessments. For more on family systems theory, see Chapter 7: Families in Children's Health-Care Settings.

Comprehensive, Multidisciplinary, Coordinated Care

Comprehensive, coordinated, multidisciplinary management facilitates optimal care, especially for the child with multiple, complex problems (Vessey &

Comprehensive Services for Children with Special Health-Care Needs	Outgoing, comprehensive primary, well-child, and preventive care according to American Academy of Pediatrics (AAP) guidelines Periodic primary care for common childhood illnesses and injuries Specialty medical care, including education, training, and consultations as needed Durable and nondurable medical supplies and equipment Durable and nondurable adaptive devices and assistive technology, including equipment for fine and gross motor needs and home adaptation Mental health and social support services for individuals and family Case management Nursing services, including home and school Medications

Maguire, 1999). Care of the child with special needs should be comprehensive and multidisciplinary in that it addresses not only medical concerns and needs but also emotional, developmental, educational, social, financial, and familial concerns and priorities. (A sample listing of comprehensive services is provided in the box.)

Goals should focus not only on short-term management but also on long-term plans. Care coordination serves several purposes: (a) ensuring continuity for the child and family across care settings (i.e., inpatient, outpatient, educational, therapeutic); (b) improving interdisciplinary communication and, thus, reducing fragmentation of care when multiple providers are involved (see box); and (c) both prioritizing and consolidating care requirements, thus reducing the burden of care for the family (Ahmann, 1999b). For the child with multiple and complex needs, care coordination is also important to ensure that health maintenance needs, such as primary care and developmental and emotional support, are not overlooked.

Care coordination is often most effective if a single professional works closely with the family in this role. Because the care coordinator, or case manager, is usually the professional who will have the greatest impact on the child's care, selection of this individual should be based on the child's specific needs, as well as the family's preferences. The professional involved in care coordination *must* support, not usurp, the family's role as primary decision maker (Johnson, Jeppson, & Redburn, 1992; McGonigel, Kaufmann, & Johnson, 1991). This approach will enhance the family's ability to best meet the needs of the child and family unit over time.

Special education from birth through age 21 years

Diagnostic services, including lab work and X-rays

Personal assistance services to aid with activities of daily living

Respite care

Physical, speech, and occupational therapies, including speech, language, vision, and hearing devices

Community recreational programs, including toy-lending libraries and camps

Transportation, including automobile modifications

Vocation, rehabilitation, and habilitation programs

Emergency services

Family planning and genetic counseling for child and other family members

Dental services

Dietary services

24-hour access to medical information

Legal and financial support services

Family-to-family support

Note. From "Chronic Conditions: The Continuum of Care," by W. Nehring, 1999, in M. E. Broom and J. A., Rollins (Eds.), *Core Curriculum for the Nursing Care of Children and Their Families,* p. 334, Pitman, NJ: Jannetti Publications. Copyright 1999 by Jannetti Publications. Reprinted with permission.

*Coordination
of Care*

Interagency collaboration may include links between:

- Primary health-care providers
- Public health programs
- Community and regional hospitals
- Early intervention programs
- Early childhood day care or preschool programs
- Public and private schools
- Special education programs
- Community and special recreational programs
- Medical and university health science centers
- Voluntary agencies and specialized social service agencies across various geographical areas

Chronic Conditions and Child Development

Patterson and G. Geber (1991, p. 150) stated that

> children with chronic illnesses or disabilities are normal children in abnormal situations. They have the same developmental needs as all children. But in many different ways, the accomplishment of their developmental tasks is made more difficult by an extra set of demands and hardships associated with the chronic condition.

Chronic childhood conditions can be classified into three major categories: chronic medical illnesses (e.g., asthma, diabetes), developmental disabilities (e.g., autism, mental retardation), and mental health problems (e.g., depression, conduct disorder; Vessey & Maguire, 1999). Developmental disabilities will have a clear and definable impact on a child's normal development. But, chronic medical illnesses and mental health problems can also have an impact on development by interfering with a child's ability to participate in normal age-appropriate activities or to attain common age-related competencies. These interferences occur as a result of hospitalization, frequent medical appointments, time spent on treatments, side effects of medication, developmental sequelae of treatments, fatigue, physical constraints and activity restrictions, and, occasionally, fears and parental overprotectiveness (Vessey & Maguire, 1999). Table 5.2 offers suggestions for information families can be asked to provide as part of the developmental assessment process.

Composition of the interdisciplinary team may include:

- Child and family members
- Family support members (e.g., extended family, friends, professional friends, clergy)
- Developmental pediatrician
- Nurse
- Physical therapist
- Occupational therapist
- Speech–language pathologist
- Special educator

- Social worker
- Child life specialist
- Other pediatric subspecialists (e.g., orthopedists, ophthalmologists, geneticists, neurologists)

Note. From "Chronic Conditions: The Continuum of Care," by W. Nehring, 1999, in M. E. Broom and J. A. Rollins (Eds.), *Core Curriculum for the Nursing Care of Children and Their Families,* pp. 333–335, Pitman, NJ: Jannetti Publications. Copyright 1999 by Jannetti Publications. Reprinted with permission.

Table 5.2

Assessment Information Families Can Be Asked To Provide

Assessments	Item
Observations regarding child's development	Overall development
	Specific strengths
	Problem areas (explicit observations)
	• motor (gross and fine)
	• cognitive
	• feeding
	• speech and communication
	• social and emotional
Observations regarding developmental impact of child's condition	Environmental limitations
	Tolerance for activity
	Recovery postactivity
Suggestions for intervention plan	Specific activity ideas
	Priorities
	Desired outcomes
	Extent of desire to participate in interventions
	Scheduling suggestions
	Equipment needs
Other family concerns	Information needs
	Preferred methods of sharing information
	Long-term concerns
	Concerns regarding sibling effects

Note. From "Developmental Assessment of the Technology Dependent Infant and Young Child," by E. Ahmann and K. Lipsi, 1992, *Pediatric Nursing, 18*(3), p. 303. Copyright 1992 by Jannetti Publications. Reprinted with permission.

Families may have information needs regarding the growth and development of their child with special needs, such as

- how the condition affects the child's physical growth and development,
- how to provide for the child's emotional needs,
- how to improve communication among all the people caring for the child,
- behavior management/discipline,
- how to plan for the child's future, and
- services available in the community. (Ahmann & Lierman, 1992, p. 147)

Some developmental aspects of chronic conditions are listed, by developmental stage, in Table 5.3, along with potential supportive interventions.

Table 5.3

Developmental Aspects of Chronic Illness or Disability in Children

Developmental Tasks	Potential Effects of Chronic Illness or Disability	Supportive Interventions
Infancy		
Develop a sense of trust	Multiple caregivers and frequent separations, especially if hospitalized Deprived of consistent nurturing	Encourage consistent caregivers in hospital or other care settings. Encourage parents to visit frequently or "room-in" during hospitalization, and to participate in care.
Attach to parent	Delayed because of separation, parental grief for loss of "dream" child, parental inability to accept the condition, especially a visible defect	Emphasize healthy, perfect qualities of infant. Help parents learn special care needs of infant to enable them to feel competent. Expose infant to pleasurable experiences through all senses (touch, hearing, sight, taste, movement).
Learn through sensori-motor experiences	Increased exposure to more painful experiences than pleasurable ones Limited contact with environment from restricted movement or confinement	Encourage age-appropriate developmental skills (e.g., holding bottle, finger feeding, crawling). Encourage all family members to participate in care to prevent over-involvement of one member.

(continues)

Table 5.3 *Continued.* 191

Developmental Aspects of Chronic Illness or Disability in Children

Developmental Tasks	Potential Effects of Chronic Illness or Disability	Supportive Interventions
Begin to develop a sense of separateness from parent	Increased dependency on parent for care Over-involvement of parent in care	Encourage periodic respite from demands of care responsibilities.
Toddlerhood Develop autonomy Master locomotor and language skills Learn through sensori-motor experience, beginning preoperational thought	Increased dependency on parent Limited opportunity to test own abilities and limits Increased exposure to painful experiences	Encourage independence in as many areas as possible (e.g., toileting, dressing, feeding). Provide gross motor skill activity and modification of toys or equipment, such as modified swing or rocking horse. Give choices to allow simple feeling of control (e.g., choice of what book to look at or what kind of sandwich to eat). Institute age-appropriate discipline and limit-setting. Recognize that negative and ritualistic behavior are normal. Provide sensory experiences (e.g., water play, sandbox, finger paint).
Preschool Develop initiative and purpose Master self-care skills Begin to develop peer relationships Develop sense of body image and sexual identification Learn through pre-operational thought (magical thinking)	Limited opportunities for success in accomplishing simple tasks or mastering self-care skills Limited opportunities for socialization with peers; may appear "like a baby" to age-mates Protection within tolerant and secure family may cause child to fear criticism and withdraw Awareness of body may center on pain, anxiety, and failure Sex role identification focused primarily on mothering skills Guilt (thinking he or she caused the illness or disability, or is being punished for wrong-doing)	Encourage mastery of self-help skills. Provide devices that make tasks easier (e.g., self-dressing). Encourage socialization, such as inviting friends to play, day care experiences, trips to park. Provide age-appropriate play, especially associative play opportunities. Emphasize child's abilities; dress appropriately to enhance desirable appearance. Encourage relationships with same-sex and opposite-sex peers and adults. Help child deal with criticisms; realize that too much protection prevents child from learning realities of world. Clarify that cause of child's illness or disability is not his or her fault or a punishment.

(continues)

Developmental Aspects of Chronic Illness or Disability in Children

Developmental Tasks	Potential Effects of Chronic Illness or Disability	Supportive Interventions
School Age		
Develop a sense of accomplishment Form peer relationships Learn through concrete operations	Limited opportunities to achieve and compete (e.g., many school absences or inability to join regular athletic activities) Limited opportunities for socialization Incomplete comprehension of the imposed physical limitations or treatment of the disorder	Encourage school attendance; schedule medical visits at times other than school; encourage child to make up missed work. Educate teachers and classmates about child's condition, abilities, and special needs. Encourage sports activities (e.g., Special Olympics). Encourage socialization (e.g., Girl Scouts, Campfire, Boy Scouts, 4-H Clubs, having a best friend or a club). Provide child with knowledge about his or her condition. Encourage creative activities (e.g., VSA arts).
Adolescence		
Develop personal and sexual identity Achieve independence from family Form heterosexual relationships Learn through abstract thinking	Increased sense of feeling different from peers and less able to compete with peers in appearance, abilities, special skills Increased dependency on family; limited job or career opportunities Limited opportunities for heterosexual friendships; fewer opportunities to discuss sexual concerns with peers Increased concern with issues such as why he or she got the disorder, whether he or she can marry and have a family Decreased opportunity for earlier stages of cognition may impede achieving level of abstract thinking	Realize that many of the difficulties the teenager is experiencing are part of normal adolescence (rebelliousness, risk taking, lack of cooperation, hostility toward authority). Provide instruction on interpersonal and coping skills. Encourage socialization with peers, including peers with special needs and those without special needs. Provide instruction on decision making, assertiveness, and other skills necessary to manage personal plans. Encourage increased responsibility for care and management of the disease or condition, such as assuming responsibility for making and keeping appointments (ideally alone), sharing assessment and planning stages of health-care delivery, and contacting resources. Encourage activities appropriate for age, such as attending mixed-gender parties, sports activities, driving a car.

(continues)

Table 5.3 *Continued.*

193

Developmental Aspects of Chronic Illness or Disability in Children

Developmental Tasks	Potential Effects of Chronic Illness or Disability	Supportive Interventions
Adolescence *(continues)*		Be alert to cues that signal readiness for information regarding implications of condition on sexuality and reproduction.
		Emphasize good appearance and wearing stylish clothes, use of makeup.
		Understand that adolescent has same sexual needs and concerns as any other teenager.
		Discuss planning for future and how condition can affect choices.

Note. From *Whaley and Wong's Nursing Care of Infants and Children–Sixth Edition* (pp. 1006–1007), by D. Wong, M. Hockenberry-Eaton, D. Wilson, M. Winkelstein, and E. Ahmann, 1999, St. Louis, MO: Mosby. Reprinted with permission.

Even a child with serious medical problems who is dependent on medical technology for survival can be assisted to engage in appropriate developmental experiences. Beginning an ongoing discussion with parents about how best to care for their baby and helping them implement a plan for involvement will very likely help them establish the control they need to deal with the early uncertainty of having a baby with special needs (Sydnor-Greenberg & Dokken, 2000). Three principles can be applied to optimize developmental planning for the child with complex medical problems (Ahmann & Klockenbrink, 1996; Ahmann & Lierman, 1992; Glass & Blink-off, 1996). The first principle is to use a full understanding of the child's medical condition to both plan developmental opportunities at a time when the child has the most energy and endurance and, during activities, to observe for signals of stress. The second principle is to flexibly tailor plans to the individual child's abilities, interests, and needs. The third principle is to assure familiarity with the child's medical equipment in order to plan ways to creatively adapt equipment to meet the child's developmental needs. The following examples of developmentally supportive interventions for a child who is ventilator-dependent will demonstrate developmental support at various stages.

Among their various developmental needs, infants need a range of motor experiences and have a strong need to suck. To respond to these needs, health-care providers and parents can vary the ventilated infant's positioning to encourage freedom of movement and, if oral feeding is not tolerated, to encourage non-nutritive sucking as long as the infant shows no signs of distress. As the infant grows and becomes a toddler, needs will change. Freedom and mobility to explore become paramount. A safe environment, including covers on medical supplies and equipment, should be provided for the toddler who is ventilator-dependent, and equipment modifications, such as lengthy oxygen or ventilator tubing, should be made to encourage mobility. Mounting the ventilator on a wheelchair or wheeled wagon or cart will also allow the toddler maximum freedom of movement.

Later, because the preschool-age child begins to master many new skills, providing ways to assist with medical treatments (e.g., opening packages, arranging supplies, holding tubing) can be developmentally supportive. Following on this, the school-age child should increasingly be taught self-care skills, such as suctioning and medication administration under supervision. In addition, the school-age child should carry identification, a medic-alert bracelet, and emergency supplies and equipment, such as saline, portable suction, and a replacement tracheostomy tube, so that attendance at school, visiting friends, and participating in other social activities is safely facilitated. Meeting same-age peers with similar medical conditions, through a camp or support group, may also be beneficial at this age.

Adolescents should begin to master self-care, though some monitoring from afar may still be needed, and should begin to participate in decision making regarding their own medical care. Additionally, during the adolescent years, information about any sexual limitations of the condition (e.g., a spinal cord injury) should be addressed openly, options regarding education, vocation, and employment should be considered, and plans should be made for gradual transition to adult health-care providers (see the following discussion).

Promoting coping and capability can buffer stress and contribute to mental health and self-esteem in a child with special needs (Patterson & G. Geber, 1991). No matter what the age, developmental ability, or medical condition of the child, individualized instruction regarding the condition is essential. Health-care providers and parents can help children understand their medical conditions and can instruct and encourage their participation in self-care. Although the Piagetian framework has been used for several decades to outline children's illness concepts in a stage-based approach (Bibace & Walsh, 1980; Perrin & Gerrity, 1981), Yoos's (1994) more recent research suggests that the illness experience influences one's ability to acquire specific knowledge and reasoning capabilities about the disease and its treatments no matter what developmental stage. Thus, individual assessments of a child's knowledge base and knowledge needs are important. Effective teaching for self-care must be informed by developmental stage, but directed to the child's individual level of understanding, and may be augmented by the use of dolls, models, diagrams, literature, simple explanations, demonstrations, computerized instruction, and repetition (Manworren & Woodring, 1998; Petersen, 1996; Vessey, Braithwaite, & Wiedmann, 1990). In addition to promoting confidence and capability, one-on-one education has been associated with improved outcomes in some illness management approaches (Forshee et al., 1998).

Leadership Model

Kieckhefer and Trahms (2000) developed a Leadership Model, which illustrates the child's and parent's path through a planned and systematic leadership transition. Figure 5.1 shows the directions of systematic, planned shifting of responsibility for the care of the chronic condition from the parent to the child. Bold arrows depict the need for the parent to guide this movement and the important idea that both parent and child have an active

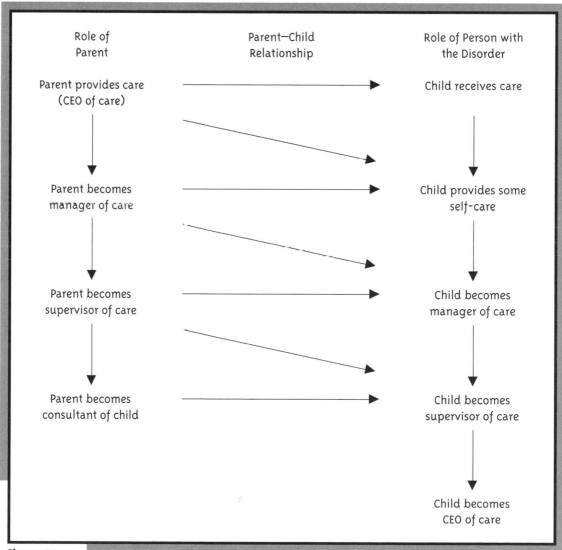

Figure 5.1.

Leadership Model for Systematic Transition of Care. *Note.* From "Supporting Development of Children with Chronic Conditions: From Compliance Toward Shared Management," by G. Kieckhefer and C. Trahms, 2000, *Pediatric Nursing, 26*(4), p. 358. Copyright 2000 by Jannetti Publications. Reprinted with permission.

role to play. The parent–child relationship during effective management of a chronic disorder is dynamic in nature.

> Initially, the parent provides all of the necessary care to the child, regardless of the child's age. As the child grows in cognitive and physical skill development, experience with the condition, and management competence, the parent transfers some of the responsibility for self-care to the child. The parent becomes the "manager" and the child the "provider" for these carefully articulated, skill-appropriate responsibilities. The parent is available to support the child's provider skills and stands ready to re-assume some of these tasks for a short time if it is necessary because the child is ill or other life complications require additional parent support. As the child becomes more confident and competent in self-management, the parent and child negotiate the next step. The parent becomes the "supervisor" and the child becomes the manager of specific tasks. The parent is, again, poised to resume the managerial role or specific tasks for a short time, if necessary. However, the parent and child must both understand and agree that the child does not regress to a previous stage; the parent provides additional support during times of stress and the child continues to progress in self-management skills and self-management responsibility development. Eventually, the parent assumes a "consultant" role in the child's management of the disorder and the child becomes the "supervisor," manager, and provider of care. The parent supplies information, support, decision-making guidance, and resources, but the child assumes ultimate responsibility for his or her health care as the "CEO." (Kieckhefer & Trahms, 2000, pp. 356–357)

Although the child as CEO of his or her own care is often a step that happens in conjunction with emancipation from the family, there is no specific age ascribed to the leadership stages because children progress at an individual cognitive and emotional pace concurrent with their experiences (Kieckhefer & Trahms, 2000). Children may be in a particular stage for a relatively long time as they develop cognitively and emotionally. A premature shift in leadership responsibilities can be just as detrimental to children as delayed progress.

The Leadership Model can be integrated with the developmental model. Table 5.4 lists activities one could expect children of various ages to be able to do and the actions parents could take to support the child's growing capabilities and move the family forward to increasing child leadership.

(text continues on p. 200)

Table 5.4

197

Pragmatic Actions That Support Leadership Skills

Stage/Age	Child Capabilities and Actions That Form the Basis for Leadership Skills	Parent's Leadership Actions To Support the Child's Growing Capabilities
Infant (0–12 months)	Though dependent on parents for care, it is helpful if the child gives clear cues of distress so parents can grow in the recognition of emergent needs and appropriate responses. For example, clear cues of hunger and satiety help the parent understand when to offer formula and when to withdraw it. Similarly, clear cues of increasing respiratory effort (e.g., grunting, use of accessory muscles) provide parents with a sign of respiratory distress in asthma. Clear cues of optimal health (e.g., adequate growth, development, social interaction) also enable parents to identify the positive impact of their actions to promote good management.	Learn ramifications of the condition and how or what resources can help. Learn how to ask questions that can assist managing the condition in the context of an overall healthy living pattern. Participate in support activities to increase knowledge of the disorder and its management. Develop daily treatment routine that fits with family life patterns. Recognize signs of immediate distress and seek emergency care. Recognize signs of early distress and seek evaluation. Learn to acknowledge those challenges that are developmentally typical for most children versus challenges specific to the child's condition. Learn how to share information with extended family and day care providers. See and acknowledge evidence that the child is thriving under attentive management. Assume the role of "repository for condition-specific information" regarding the child's reaction to the treatment.
Toddler (1–3 years) If condition initially diagnosed at this age (e.g., asthma), the earlier child capabilities and parental support actions need to be addressed before attempting to accomplish or master those listed in this section.	Cooperate with routine treatments. Help hold equipment and work with parent to make equipment function as needed (e.g., use of blender to prepare formula for PKU or the nebulizer for asthma medication delivery). Develop a sense that parents are a source of help and comfort. Accept constraints of condition and treatment with limited behavioral acting out (e.g., "yes foods" and "no foods" for PKU or "trigger" avoidance with asthma). Understand firm limits of parents (e.g., "no").	Develop rituals regarding treatment so child knows what to expect and can begin to learn through repetition. Begin to recognize the child needs to have roles in the management of the condition. Identify possible roles the parents are willing to begin to share with the child. Change the established management routine based on the child's growing capabilities and areas of cooperation. Continue to build clinical and community support network.

(continues)

Table 5.4 *Continued.*

Pragmatic Actions That Support Leadership Skills

Stage/Age	Child Capabilities and Actions That Form the Basis for Leadership Skills	Parent's Leadership Actions To Support the Child's Growing Capabilities
Preschool (4–5 years)	Identify body parts important to early identification of a problem or treatment. Test limits of cooperation. Use magical thinking, which may lead to fears. Imitate adult's behaviors. Learn labels for condition-specific "problems" to enable communication about treatment needs. Learn labels for feelings associated with condition and its treatment to enable communication about feelings.	Acknowledge regressions, allow very of brief period of reorganization, and then resume and praise prior skill performance. Set fair and appropriate limits. Model acceptance of the management routines and limits. Encourage some flexibility in rituals of treatment so child begins to experience multiple ways to accomplish same goal. Develop relationships with school personnel regarding specific needs.
Early school age (6–9 years)	Recognize and act on 1 or 2 major internal body cues of a problem. Participate actively in concrete monitoring of condition. Increase understanding of condition, cause and effect, concrete level of what's going on inside the body to necessitate management.	Continue to label cues and give positive reward for child's recognition. Start negotiating with child for what each party will do regarding management and set criteria for forward movement that fits with family life. Be prepared to renegotiate for cause. Establish logical consequences for actions. Negotiate the "rules" for working together to get all necessary treatments completed. Be positive and reinforcing about what needs to get done. Avoid over-emphasis on condition. Support normative activities and integrate treatment needs. Model telling others about the disorder for the child. Discuss the approach to telling teachers, friends, coaches, and others about the disorder and the amount of detail necessary to share.
Late school age (10–12 years)	Increase level of understanding of condition; begin to understand long-term needs. Develop new labels that are medically articulate to enable effective discussion with providers.	Remain present for the child; that is, be involved in care and monitoring decision making. Accept the manager versus CEO role in much of treatment. Ensure that child has told important others (e.g., friends, parents,

(continues)

Table 5.4 *Continued.*

199

Pragmatic Actions That Support Leadership Skills

Stage/Age	Child Capabilities and Actions That Form the Basis for Leadership Skills	Parent's Leadership Actions To Support the Child's Growing Capabilities
Late school age (*continued*)	Learn how and when to respond to peer pressure yet still take care of self. Enact most psychomotor skills associated with treatment with parental support. Learn more sophisticated system for reporting symptoms, management steps, and outcomes. Develop specific set of self-management tasks that are completed independently.	coaches) of the condition and what assistance they could provide if needed. Be there in case of emergencies or new presentation, out-of-the-routine needs, changes and maybe even the doing of some aspects. Provide the tools so the child can self-manage (e.g., get the formula, get the prescriptions). Support the child in actively communicating with his or her provider, encouraging discussion of the child's monitoring system to help the child grow in understanding.
Early adolescent (13–15 years)	Become main manager of daily, routine care. Develop strategies to ensure completion of all necessary routine management tasks. Know how to effectively ask for assistance in complex situations. Know when to be flexible versus not flexible, and be able to enact the flexibility when appropriate.	Shadow, or observe the performance closely to offer immediate corrective feedback. Negotiate and renegotiate who does what. Become the consultant versus remaining the manager Discuss new issues (e.g., sex, drugs, alcohol) for their normative and any special condition effects.
Late adolescent (16–18 years)	Make a commitment to lifetime treatment. Increase understanding of the disorder and its long-term as well as short-term consequences on other aspects of life (e.g., vocations, intellectual achievement, well-being). Achieve sense of self as capable manager of disorder. Integrate the realities of the condition with the invincible nature of their years. Appreciate of benefits that the constraints of the management allow. Continue to develop more independent clinic and community-support network as transition to adult-based care services.	Develop a flexible way of communicating with the child to stay informed while not seen as interfering. Remain "present" for support and problem solving with the youth. Provide support and guidance as the youth transitions from pediatric to adult-care services.

Note. From "Supporting Development of Children with Chronic Conditions: From Compliance Toward Shared Management," by G. Kieckhefer and C. Trahms, 2000, *Pediatric Nursing, 26*(4), pp. 354–363. Copyright 2000 by Jannetti Publications. Reprinted with permission.

Transition Planning

The transfer from pediatric to adult care for adolescents with special health-care needs should be planned individually (Russell, Reinbold, & Maltby, 1996). Age is an arbitrary criterion for transfer. More important considerations include the adolescent's (a) understanding of the condition, related treatments, medications, and precautions; (b) ability to verbalize health-care concerns and needs; (c) compliance with medical regimens; and (d) interest in the transfer. Once parents and the adolescent are ready for a transfer, a meeting between the family and both pediatric and adult providers is sometimes arranged for introductions and an exchange of information. The adolescent and family should also consider visiting the adult-care setting before the transfer so that they do not have to find their way the first time during a crisis or emergency.

Insurance coverage is often decreased or eliminated after age 21, so financial issues should be considered in late adolescence. Some individuals with disabilities will qualify for Supplemental Security Income (SSI) or Medicaid. Educational, vocational, and employment options should all be considered as part of transition planning (Nehring, 1999).

For adolescents with severe disabilities, future planning should also include examining vocational options and training to promote eventual gainful employment, if appropriate. In some cases, families need to investigate independent living arrangements and in-home support services for the transition to adulthood. In other circumstances, residential placement options and advance financial planning should be considered for the time when aging parents may no longer be able to care for the child (Rosenfeld, 1994).

Family Issues

Most families with children with special needs cope reasonably well (O'Brien, 2001). Drawing from theoretical research and clinical literature, Clawson (1996) identified eight adaptive tasks of families having a child with a chronic illness or disability:

- accepting the condition
- providing daily management of the condition
- meeting the normal developmental needs of the child
- meeting the developmental needs of other family members
- coping with ongoing stressors and periodic crises
- helping family members manage feelings
- educating others about the chronic illness or condition
- establishing a support system

Accepting the Condition

Depending on a child's condition, families may face a period of uncertainty prior to obtaining a final or definitive diagnosis. Even if it relieves uncertainty, the time of diagnosis can be challenging to face for parents and professionals alike. Two studies examined parental preferences regarding the "informing interview" (Garwick, Patterson, Bennett, & Blum, 1995; Krahn, Hallum, & Kime, 1993). These studies supported the conventional wisdom that both parents, in a two-parent family, should be together when told of their child's diagnosis; parents should be informed early on; simple, direct language, without medical jargon, should be used; and the informing professional should be both empathetic and supportive of parental emotional expression. Additional considerations raised by these studies included the importance of meeting with parents in person, informing parents in a private setting, emphasizing the child's strengths as well as limitations, and individualizing both the communication style as well as the information shared. It should be recognized that not all parents, often not even both members of one couple, will react similarly to a diagnosis. Additionally, cultural considerations including language, meaning assigned to the diagnosis, and potentially differing treatment preferences should also be addressed during the informing interview (Ahmann, 1998). Parents should be given a way to get in touch with the informing professionals should questions arise once they have digested the initial information presented.

To some individuals, the term *accepting* may carry implications of going beyond adaptation, to being able to say to oneself, for example, "My child has a disability, and this is okay." It may take years before parents are "okay" to that degree with this reality, and there will be times when it isn't "okay." It may be more helpful to think in terms of "acknowledgement," which may be a more accurate term for this task.

Recent research confirms the theory of "parental straddling" (Johnson, 2000). Parents expressed living in the past and the present, striving to view their child as "normal" when, in fact, the child was disabled, and simultaneously dealing with their own and their child's issues and feelings. Health care professionals can prepare parents for anticipated grief work, reassure them that their experiences are expected and normal, reinforce their use of normalization strategies, and help them separate their child's issues and feelings from their own.

Providing Daily Management of the Condition

Parents ultimately are responsible for the day-to-day management of a child's special needs (Sullivan-Bolyai, Knafl, Sadler, & Gilliss, 2003, 2004). Daily management of a child's special needs will vary greatly depending on the diagnosis, condition severity, and therapeutic treatments. Some conditions, such as diabetes, epilepsy, or asthma, require "controlling" as well as managing, and certain nonprogressive conditions, such as cerebral palsy, require vigilance to prevent associated complications (Farley & McEwan, 2000; Palmer, 2001). To varying degrees, parents may need education about the child's condition, education and training in the child's special care requirements, help organizing their time and incorporating the child's care requirements into the family's daily plan, and assistance in developing collaborative working relationships with health-care providers.

Research by Knafl and colleagues (1996) has examined how families manage a child's chronic condition. Aspects of management style include the following:

- how the family understands or defines the illness situation,
- behaviors the family adopts to manage the situation, including changing roles and adapting lifestyle choices, and
- the family's values and beliefs. (Knafl & Deatrick, 1990)

A continuum of five family management styles identified includes (a) thriving, (b) accommodating, (c) enduring, (d) struggling, and (e) floundering (Knafl et al., 1996). Thriving families stressed normalcy and felt confident about being able to handle the demands posed by the illness. Families in between thriving and floundering are characterized by conflict and uncertainty about how to manage the illness. Enduring families have a negative view of the situation and feel burdened even if they are capable. Knafl and Deatrick (1990) stressed that coping patterns and techniques can be learned and supportive; therapeutic interventions are best targeted to a family's individual needs.

Meeting Normal Developmental Needs of the Child

To promote normal developmental in a child with special needs, parents must thoroughly understand the child's condition. Parents of children with special needs typically desire complete and accurate information about their child's condition. Research has documented the confidence and competence that are associated with a thorough understanding (Dixon, 1996).

Parents also need to understand what normal development is for a child of different ages. This will assist them in normalizing opportunities for the child, including (a) emphasizing the child's abilities and de-emphasizing limitations; (b) structuring the environment to provide developmentally appropriate opportunities and activities; and (c) providing appropriate expectations, guidance, and discipline.

An important area of family education addresses how the child's condition may affect activities of daily living, including eating, dressing, toileting, and sleeping. Depending on the complexity of the child's care requirements, families may need assistance in arranging to meet the child's therapeutic needs within the context of family life. For example, whenever possible, medication schedules should be arranged to allow parents to sleep through the night.

Families can be assisted to learn how to accommodate special dietary needs to family menu preferences. Special feeding requirements (i.e., tube feeding), can be scheduled to coincide with family meal time when appropriate. Physical therapy exercises can be incorporated into dressing and other daily routines rather than be scheduled at other times.

Meeting the Developmental Needs of Other Family Members

Over the years, research related to families of children with special needs has identified numerous stressors related to family coping. Many of these fall into the realm of meeting the developmental needs of other family members. Simply making efforts to maintain family rituals and activities that foster cohesiveness and closeness (e.g., celebrating birthdays, sharing meals together) can decrease some of the strains of day-to-day care (Ducharme, 2001).

Parents may face emotional stress due to the diagnosis, changes in the child's condition, unmet developmental milestones, as well as to the impact of managing the condition on a daily basis. Role strain is common as parents learn care procedures, medical terminology, case management tasks, and continue to manage other family and employment responsibilities. Parents may face time constraints in juggling the child's care needs with employment demands and the needs of other family members. Financial stressors can include inadequate insurance coverage, unreimbursed medical expenses, and employment constraints resulting from the need to maintain insurance coverage. Parental health can also be affected by the demands of caring for some children with special needs. Any of these stressors may interfere with parents meeting their own normal developmental needs.

In two-parent families, mothers and fathers may react differently to a child's diagnosis and prognosis, to the demands of daily care, to long-term concerns, and to financial burdens of care. Mothers tend to assume most childcare and family maintenance responsibilities and home-related tasks (Nelson, 2002; Sullivan-Bolyai et al., 2003), while fathers are concerned with balancing work and time with their other children, their spouse, and the care of their child with special needs (Feudtner, 2002). Parents may have different, and sometimes gender-based, coping mechanisms. For example, Heaman (1995) reported that mothers typically have greater needs for social support while fathers more frequently use self-controlling behaviors to cope. Recognizing each others' strengths and contributions to the family and accepting each others' coping mechanisms as valid can assist parents in keeping these various coping differences from becoming a source of conflict. Additionally, the husband–wife relationship needs nurturing. Although finding time to spend alone can be difficult, it often is necessary to prevent marital strain (Nelson, 2002).

Single-parent families may face particular financial, physical, and emotional burdens when providing care for a child with special needs. Research indicates that these burdens may be translated into more stress for the parent and poorer outcomes for the child with special needs when the parent is single. For example, in a study of children with cystic fibrosis (CF), Macpherson, Redmond, Leavy, and McMullan (2000) reported that single mothers experienced more stress-related symptoms than married mothers, and that young CF children of single or teenage mothers have a significantly worse clinical progress. Macpherson and colleagues (2000) and Hogan and Park (2000) stressed the importance of external sources of support.

Research suggests that foster families do not always get the support they need from health-care providers (Barton, 1999). Foster parents need as much information and support as any family to provide optimal care for the child, including information on the child's diagnosis, special needs, available services, warning signs of problems, and sources of support (Rodriguez & Jones, 1996). Foster parent observations, questions, and concerns should be taken seriously by health-care providers.

Research findings about the effects on siblings of a child with special needs are inconsistent and even contradictory (Walker, 1999). While earlier studies suggested greater adjustment problems, many did not use control groups; more recent and better designed studies tend to suggest fewer problems. Gallo and colleagues (1992) reviewed research on sibling adjustment and concluded that effects can be negative, positive, or absent. Some differences in sibling coping are associated with age, birth order, and gender. The box lists potential stressors and coping strategies for siblings. Aware health-care providers and parents can promote coping and positive outcomes.

For more on family issues, see Chapter 7: Families in Children's Health-Care Settings.

Potential Stressors and Coping Strategies for Siblings

Stressors

- Less attention from parents
- Emotional realignments within the family
- Physical and emotional separation from parents and the sibling with special needs
- Lack of information or information that is understandable at their developmental level
- Disrupted family communication
- Perceived sense of guilt over causing the illness or disability
- Negativity between how the ill child and siblings are disciplined
- Assumption of more household responsibilities and chores, often including caregiving functions for the child with special needs
- Fear of the unknown (e.g., fear of what the treatments and hospitalizations are like, fear of death, fear of self or other family members becoming ill)

Coping with Ongoing Stressors and Periodic Crises

Anticipatory guidance for children with special needs and their families can promote coping with ongoing stressors and periodic crises. Some conditions will pose new challenges at different developmental stages, and families can be helped to feel prepared to manage the changes. During these times it is common for parents to experience episodes of recurrent sadness, often termed *chronic sorrow* (Northington, 2000).

Developmental disabilities may have a greater impact on the child's functioning as the child ages and normal developmental expectations change. Anticipatory guidance can help families prepare for potentially difficult or disappointing transitions, such as school entry. Some conditions will have periods requiring crisis management (e.g., acute asthma) and other periods of less intense management. Families can be alerted to signs and symptoms of acute exacerbations and be given protocols to assist decision making in these difficult situations. Still other conditions will have periods of remission and recurrence (e.g., cancer) and families should be prepared in advance for these possibilities as well as for a potential terminal phase. Children with severe disabilities or behavioral problems may eventually require residential placement and these options should be discussed with the family over time as comprehensive advanced planning is necessary (Nehring, 1999).

Periodic ongoing assessment of and with the child and the family is important to ensure optimal outcomes. All planning for the child and family should be undertaken as a collaborative process with the family. Family

---

- Changes in family routines
- Changes in recreation activities

Coping Strategies

- Seeking out information
- Using social support resources
- Having an outlet separate from the ill child and family as a means of distraction and source of self-esteem (e.g., school, recreation activities, clubs, friends)
- Expressing emotions
- Engaging in thought stopping: the forced substitution of positive thoughts for negative ones

- Developing empathy: the ability to assume the perspective of another
- Having other well siblings with whom to share feelings, concerns, and household tasks
- Using available social support network to provide physical and emotional care when needed
- Having open communication within family that promotes expression of feelings

Note. From "Chronic Conditions: Effects on the Child's Family," by C. Walker, 1999, in M. E. Broome and J. A. Rollins (Eds.), *Core Curriculum for the Nursing Care of Children and Their Families.* Pitman, NJ: Jannetti Publications, pp. 262–263. Copyright 1999 by Jannetti Publications. Reprinted with permission.

members should be provided with information and support for decision making as may be necessary on an ongoing or crisis basis. Information should be shared fully and openly and in terms that the family can understand. Additionally, family members can be helped to identify and evaluate their options (Dokken, 1993) and to gain the information and skills they need to sustain their decisions (Mott, 1999). Finally, all support offered in decision making should promote the family's own goals, values, and interests.

Helping Family Members Manage Feelings

Both the professional literature and family reports indicate a wide range of feelings common to families of children with special needs. Some previous research has suggested stages of adaptation, but it is now understood that there is wide variability in how families adjust to a diagnosis in their child.

At the time of diagnosis, shock and denial are common. Denial may last for some time and is not always maladaptive. In fact, it can be a useful protective mechanism for some families who continue to provide appropriate care for their children, allowing the family to adjust over time to a diagnosis while they mobilize their energies and coping resources.

Adjustment to the diagnosis may involve feelings of guilt, bitterness, and anger as the family acknowledges the presence of the diagnosed condition (Ahmann [revision], 1999). Understanding family, friends, and professionals can provide the support needed for family members to process these strong feelings as they acclimate to the new family circumstances.

As families adjust and gather information, realistic expectations for the child can be formed and family life can be reintegrated with the new perspective imposed by the illness or disability (Ahmann [revision], 1999). A focus on family strengths, the promotion of normalization, encouragement and promotion of family cohesion, and involvement of the family as collaborators in assessment and planning related to health care of the child can support family empowerment.

Patterson and M. Geber (1991) stressed that cognitive, behavioral and emotional tasks all comprise the adaptive coping process. Cognitive tasks include learning about the condition, the prognosis, and the care requirements. Behavioral tasks include providing for the child's therapeutic needs, monitoring the child's condition, and day-to-day management. Emotional tasks include grieving the loss of the "perfect child," managing anger, and addressing the limitations the condition places on the parents and the family as a whole.

Educating Others About the Chronic Illness or Condition

Parents face the task of gaining an accurate and complete understanding of the child's condition both for themselves and so they can educate the child, the siblings, extended family members, friends, neighbors, teachers, and sometimes health-care providers with whom the child may come in contact (Canam, 1993).

Parents may want help knowing how to explain a disability or illness to the child or siblings of various ages. They may want guidance on how much to tell and how to tell friends and neighbors about a condition so that the child can be understood but not teased or stigmatized. The child may also need similar guidance. Parents may also need to be prepared so they are able to train home care nurses and respite workers in how to meet their child's special needs. They may need to be prepared to explain an uncommon condition to either physicians providing emergency care or other physicians who may not be knowledgeable about their child's diagnosis and care requirements. All of this should be considered when educating families and providing anticipatory guidance.

Establishing a Support System

Social support has repeatedly been shown to positively influence coping and health-care outcomes. Families can benefit from professional support, support from family and friends, and from the unique support of peers.

Support provided by peers, also known as family-to-family support, can provide families with information, emotional support, a sense of being understood, friendship, mentoring, role modeling, assistance with problem solving, and a base for advocacy efforts (Ahmann, 1999a). Professionals can facilitate family-to-family support by (a) making referrals to local and national support groups (see Appendix 5.1); (b) facilitating meetings by providing space, transportation, and child care; (c) developing peer support networks; and (d) linking interested parents one-on-one when no formal support group is available.

While peer support for fathers is less common than that for mothers, it can be very beneficial either in a group or one-on-one setting (May, 1996). Children with special needs and their siblings can also benefit from peer support provided in a fun, engaging manner (Meyer & Vadasy, 1994). Referrals to condition-specific camps may also be offered to children. Finally, grandparents and extended family members caring for the child (kinship care) have unique issues to face and may also benefit from peer support (Ahmann, 1997).

Community Supports

Children with special needs are not only part of their families, they are part of their communities. Comprehensive, coordinated care, based in their communities, is essential for promoting their optimal development. Considerations include educational issues, developmental support, home care services and other community resources, and financial support.

Educational and Developmental Issues

One important aspect of normal childhood activity is formal education. The Education for All Handicapped Children's Act (PL 94-142), passed in 1975, emphasizes the right of all children, ages 5 to 21 years, to a free public education in the "least restrictive environment," and provides for related services such as physical and occupational therapy, as necessary, for the child to obtain maximum benefit from the educational program. In 1986, PL 99-457, the Education of the Handicapped Amendment, extended PL 94-142 to children with disabilities between the ages of 3 and 5 years. The title of the Act was later changed to the Individuals with Disabilities Education Act (known as IDEA). In 1993, Part H of PL 103-382, amendments to IDEA, strengthened the federal commitment to provision of early intervention services by extending services to infants and toddlers ages birth to 3 years. The most recent renewal of IDEA, in 1997, required new regulations (available online at www.fape.org) but keeps most major aspects of IDEA intact.

As part of IDEA, children ages 0 to 3 years old with or at risk of disabilities are entitled to a comprehensive evaluation and, if the child is eligible for early intervention services, the development of an individualized family service plan (IFSP). When a child approaches 3 years of age, he or she can be referred to community programs, or, if intervention services are still needed, can be transitioned to Part B of IDEA, serving children ages 3 to 21 years with special needs, and an individualized education plan (IEP) will be developed.

Over the years, states have interpreted the provisions of IDEA variously, in particular the meaning of "related" services. In a recent Supreme Court case (The Garret F case), the family of a ventilator-dependent child wanted the school district to pay for a registered nurse to care for the child at school, but the school district did not think that was required by IDEA. The Supreme Court ruled that IDEA requires schools to provide health supports for students who need them as long as the care is not medical and not performed by doctors (Questions and Answers, 1999).

In many cases, children with special educational or developmental needs can easily be incorporated into the general education classroom. Some may be "pulled out" of the classroom to be provided special services such as occupational, physical, or speech therapy. In certain situations, preparation of the child for the school experience or for school re-entry after a hospitalization may be helpful. Preparation of classmates and teachers can also be helpful when a child has noticeable physical changes or differences (e.g., loss of hair due to chemotherapy, use of a wheelchair). Other planning and preparations to ensure the child's safety and appropriate care may be necessary when a child requires complex health-care services (e.g., a child dependent on oxygen or a ventilator; Porter, 1997). Children with severe cognitive or behavioral problems often require placement in specialized educational settings (Nehring, 1999). Additionally, parents may need assistance to develop the skills required to effectively advocate for their child in the educational setting (DiGregorio-Hixson, Stoff, & White, 1992).

Home Care Services and Other Community Resources

Some children with special health-care needs will require home-care nursing and therapeutic services. In fact, pediatric home care has been among the fastest growing components of the home care industry in recent years. Plans to transition a child from hospital to home should begin early during a hospitalization to allow family members to learn and demonstrate all aspects of the child's care.

Principles of family-centered care must apply in the home setting. The home is the family's domain and home care providers must respect family choices and values, and work in collaboration with the family in efforts to care for the child. The family should be seen as a partner in care. Bishop, Woll, and Arango (1993) characterized collaborative relationships by five key features: (a) communication, (b) dialogue, (c) active listening, (d) awareness and acceptance of difference, and (e) negotiation.

Part of the collaborative process should involve establishing "house rules" that allow the family to maintain a feeling of control over their environment when health-care providers are present (Klug, 1993). House rules, or guidelines with which families and professionals are comfortable, also serve to frame, from the beginning, the working relationship between the family, home health agency, nurses, and other professionals who come into the home (Wegener, 1996). For example, one mother of a child who is ventilator dependent, designated a place in the home that belonged only to her (Creasser, 1996, p. 42):

> As a parent, sometimes it seems as though nurses are everywhere calling your name and asking questions ... When I am in my bedroom, everyone knows that I want to be left alone. The nurses know it, and so does my child. Unless there is an emergency, no one bothers me when I am in my bedroom.

Establishing these guidelines helps ease the potential tension between parents and professionals around boundary and authority issues.

A variety of therapeutic and other community resources may benefit individual children and families. A good case manager should be able to assist a family in accessing needed services, including the following (Davis & Steele, 1991; Scher & Ahmann, 1996):

■ primary, secondary, and tertiary health-care services
■ nutrition services, speech, hearing, language, and vision resources

- respite services
- developmental and educational services
- special pharmacy services
- financial support programs
- durable medical equipment suppliers
- transportation services
- parent groups
- advocacy groups
- local, state, and federal officials' services

Increasingly, many families are finding it necessary or desirable for both parents to work, or want their preschool child with special needs to benefit from the socialization with other children offered by day care services. Findings from research in one large metropolitan area on the availability of day care services for preschool children with special health-care needs indicate that although 65% of the area's day care centers had a provision to enroll preschoolers with special health-care needs, less than 5% of children enrolled had special care needs, and few had disabilities or conditions that required special interventions (Markos-Capps & Godfrey, 1999). Restrictive admittance requirements, lack of staff, fear of not meeting the child's need, and lack of trained personnel were cited as barriers to admission. Despite the fact that more than half of the directors expected benefits from enrollment of these children, few knew the requirements of the Americans with Disabilities Act for inclusion of children with special health-care needs. Although limited to a single metropolitan area, data from this study suggest that quality day care services are not as available as needed for infants and young children with special health-care needs.

Financial Considerations

Financial concerns can pose a challenge for many families having children with special needs. Expenses exceeding basic costs of living can include the

Potential Sources of Funding	• Private insurance • HMOs • Medicaid • Supplemental Security Income (SSI) • Women, Infants, and Children (WIC) programs • Food stamps • State crippled children's services (may also be known by other names, e.g., Children's Special Health Services)

costs of evaluations, nonstandard therapies, special supplies and equipment, medications, special formulas or foods, transportation, insurance co-pays, and unreimbursed bills. (Scher & Ahmann, 1996)

The National Health Interview Survey (NHIS) and current census data show that 8% of children in this country have significant disabilities, many of whom do not have access to critical health-care services they need (Manley, 2000). For these families to get needed health services for their children, many are forced to stay impoverished, become impoverished, put their children in out-of-home placements, or simply give up custody of their children—so that their child can maintain eligibility for health coverage through Medicaid. Many employer health plans and a number of federal and state programs do not cover essential services that these children need to maintain and prevent deterioration of their health status. Medicaid can provide these comprehensive services.

In a recent family survey of 20 states, 64% of families with special-needs children reported that they are turning down jobs, turning down raises, turning down overtime, and are unable to save money for the future of their children and family—so that they can stay in the income bracket that qualifies their child for SSI or Medicaid. Currently, less than 4% of the 850,000 children receiving Social Security benefits leave the Social Security rolls due to increased family income; however, many would leave if access to needed health services was available. More than half the states in the United States are reporting increasing rates of families giving up custody of their children in order to secure needed health-care services and supports. The Family Opportunity Act of 2000 is intended to address the two greatest barriers preventing families from staying together and staying employed: (a) lack of access to appropriate services and (b) lack of access to the advocacy and assistance services they need to help cut the "red tape" to meet their children's health care needs.

Families may need help to understand and advocate for the maximum benefits from their insurance company or managed care organization. "Evaluating Managed Care Plans for Children with Special Health Needs: A Purchaser's Tool" is an excellent resource for families (available online at www .ichp.edu/managed/materials/purchaser/). Potential sources of funding are listed in the box.

- Part H of the Individuals with Disabilities Education Act (IDEA)
- State and local social service agencies
- Community organizations
- Disease-specific organizations
- Religious organizations
- State and local public health departments
- State and local departments of education

- Private contributions

Note. From "Community Resources for the Family," by A. Scher and E. Ahmann, 1996, in E. Ahmann (Ed.), *Home Care for the High Risk Infant: A Family-Centered Approach* (pp. 77–78). Subbury, MA: Jones and Bartlett. Copyright 1996 by Jones and Bartlett. Reprinted with permission.

Conclusion

Over the past 2 decades, survival of youth with special health-care needs has markedly improved. Today, over 90% of these children will survive past their 20th birthday (White, 1999). With a community-based commitment to family-centered care—a seamless system that offers continuity of care from birth through the childhood years and bridges medical, educational, and social services—quality of life, rather than merely survival, can be our goal.

Study Guide

1. Discuss factors that have contributed to decreased mortality for children with major chronic illnesses or special health-care needs.

2. What are the demographic characteristics of children with special health-care needs?

3. Describe the impact of chronic illness or disability in children on family, society, and the health-care system.

4. List and discuss various theoretical frameworks for understanding and predicting care for children with special health-care needs.

5. What are the major principles for parenting a child with special health-care needs?

6. Does the research support any one approach to assisting families of children with special health care needs?

7. Explain Home Care Services and other community resources essential to support for children with special health care needs and their families.

8. There are several legal or policy requirements in the care and schooling of children with special health-care needs. Cite these acts and explain the implications for health-care providers.

9. What quality of life issues for children with special needs are under-addressed either in the research or in support systems?

10. Hypothesize future health-care advances that might create an increase in the number of children with special needs or change the course of the lives of children with those conditions existent today.

APPENDIX 5.1

Resources for Family-Member Peer Support

American Association for Premature Infants
PO Box 46371
Cincinnati, OH 45246-0371
Phone: 513/956-3046
www.aapi-online.org

Family Voices
Box 769
Algodones, NM 87001
Phone: 505/867-2368
Fax: 505/867-6517
E-mail: kidshealth@familyvoices.org
www.familyvoices.org

National Father's Network
Kindering Center
16120 NE Eighth Street
Bellevue, WA 98008
Phone: 425-747-4004 ext. 218
E-mail: jmay@fathersnetwork.org
www.fathersnetwork.org

National Perinatal Association
3500 East Fletcher Avenue, Suite 205
Tampa, FL 33613-4712
Phone: 813/971-1008
Toll Free: 888/971-3295
Fax: 813/971-9306
E-mail: npa@nationalperinatal.org
www.nationalperinatal.org/

National Resource Center for Family Centered Practice
The University of Iowa
School of Social Work
100 Oakdale Campus #W206 OH
Iowa City, IA 52242-5000
Phone: 319/335-4965
Fax: 319/335-4964
www.uiowa.edu/~nrcfcp

Partners in Intensive Care
504 North Drive
Tracy's Landing, MD 20779
Phone: 301/681-2708

ROCKING, Inc. (Raising Our Children's Kids: An Intergenerational Network of Grandparenting, Inc.)
PO Box 96
Niles, MI 49120
Phone: 616/683-9038

Sibling Information Network
The University of Connecticut
A. J. Pappanikou Center on Special Education and Rehabilitation
249 Glenbrook Road, Box U64
Storrs, CT 06269
Phone: 860/486-5035
Fax: 860/486-5037

The Institute for Family-Centered Care
7900 Wisconsin Avenue, Suite 405
Bethesda, MD 20814
Phone: 301/652-0281
Fax: 301/652-0186
E-mail: Institute@iffcc.org
www.familycenteredcare.org

References

Adams, E. V. (1990). *Policy planning for culturally comprehensive special health care services.* Washington, DC: Bureau of Maternal and Child Health, Department of Health and Human Services.

Ahmann, E. (1994). "Chunky Stew:" Appreciating cultural diversity while providing health care for children. *Pediatric Nursing, 20*(3), 320–324.

Ahmann, E. (1997). Kinship care: An emerging issue. *Pediatric Nursing, 23*(6), 598–600.

Ahmann, E. (1998). Review and commentary: Two studies regarding giving "bad news." *Pediatric Nursing, 24,* 554–556.

Ahmann, E. (1999a). Family-centered care. In M. E. Broome & J. A. Rollins (Eds.), *Core curriculum for the nursing care of children and their families* (pp. 373–392). Pitman, NJ: Jannetti.

Ahmann, E. (1999b). Pediatric patient issues. In L. A. Gorski (Ed.), *Best practices in home infusion therapy* (pp. 5:1–5:16). Gaithersburg, MD: Aspen.

Ahmann, E. (revision, 1999). Family-centered care of the child with a chronic illness or disability. In D. Wong, M. Hockenberry-Eaton, D. Wilson, M. Winkelstein, & E. Ahmann (Eds.), *Whaley & Wong's nursing care of infants and children* (pp. 1000–1041). St. Louis, MO: Mosby.

Ahmann, E., & Johnson, B. (2001). New guidance materials promote family-centered change in health care institutions. *Pediatric Nursing, 27*(2), 173–175.

Ahmann, E., & Klockenbrink, K. L. (1996). Developmental assessment and intervention in the home. In E. Ahmann (Ed.), *Home care for the high risk infant: A family-centered approach* (pp. 293–304). Gaithersburg, MD: Aspen.

Ahmann, E., & Lichman, C. (1992). Promoting normal development in technology dependent children: An introduction to the issues. *Pediatric Nursing, 18*(?), 143–148.

Ahmann, E., & Lipski, K. (1992). Developmental assessment of the technology dependent infant and young child. *Pediatric Nursing, 18,* 294, 299–305.

Barton, S. J. (1999). Promoting family-centered care with foster families. *Pediatric Nursing, 25*(1), 57–59.

Beach Center on Families and Disability. (1996). *What research says: Family-centered service delivery.* Lawrence: The University of Kansas.

Bibace, R., & Walsh, M. (1980). Development of children's concept of illness, *Pediatrics, 66,* 912–917.

Bishop, K. K., Woll, J., & Arango, P. (1993). *Family-professional collaboration.* Burlington: Department of Social Work, University of Vermont.

Bossert, E., Holaday, B., Harkins, A., & Turner-Henson, A. (1990). Strategies of normalization used by parents of chronically ill school age children. *Journal of Comprehensive Pediatric Nursing, 3*(2), 57–61.

Bronfenbrenner, U. (1979). *The ecology of human development.* Cambridge, MA: Harvard University Press.

Bruce, B., & Ritchie, J. (1997). Nurses' practices and perceptions of family-centered care. *Journal of Pediatric Nursing, 12*(4), 214–222.

Canam, C. (1993). Common adaptive tasks facing parents of children with chronic conditions. *Journal of Advanced Nursing, 18*(1), 46–53.

Clawson, J. (1996). A child with chronic illness and the process of family adaptation. *Journal of Pediatric Nursing, 11*(1), 52–61.

Creasser, C. (1996). A family perspective. In K. Gunter & R. Manago (Eds.), *Beyond discharge: Interdisciplinary perspectives for transitioning children with complex medical needs from hospital to home* (pp. 39–44). Bethesda, MD: Association for the Care of Children's Health.

Davis, B. D., & Steele, S. (1991). Case management for young children with special health care needs. *Pediatric Nursing, 17*, 15–19.

Diehl, S. F., Moffitt, K. A., & Wade, S. M. (1991). Focus group interview with parents of children with medically complex needs: An intimate look at their perceptions and feelings. *Children's Health Care, 20*(3), 170–178.

DiGregorio-Hixson, D., Stoff, E., & White, P. H. (1992). Parents of children with chronic health impairments: A new approach to advocacy training. *Children's Health Care, 21*(2), 111–115.

Dixon, D. M. (1996). Unifying concepts in parents' experiences with health care providers. *Journal of Family Nursing, 2*(2), 111–132.

Dokken, D., & Sydnor-Greenberg, N. (1998). Helping families mobilize their personal resources. *Pediatric Nursing, 24*(1), 66–69.

Dokken, D. (1993, summer). The physician as enabler. *Ethiscope* (pp. 3–4). Washington, DC: Children's National Medical Center.

Ducharme, F. (2001). Development process and qualitative evaluation of a program to promote the mental health of family caregivers. *Clinical Nursing Research, 10*, 182–201.

Farley, J., & McEwan, M. (2000). Epilepsy. In P. Jackson & J. Vessey (Eds.), *Child with a chronic condition* (pp. 475–494). St. Louis, MO: Springer.

Feiring, C., & Lewis, M. (1978). The child as a member of the family system. *Behavioral Science, 23*, 225–233.

Feudtner, C. (2002). Grief-love: Contradictions in the lives of fathers of children with disabilities. *Archives of Pediatric and Adolescent Medicine, 156*, 643.

Forshee, J. D., Whalen, E. B., Hackel, R., Butt, L. T., Smeltzer, P. A., Martin, J., Lavin, P. T., & Buchner, D. A. (1998). The effectiveness of one-on-one nurse education on the outcomes of high-risk adult and pediatric patients with asthma. *Managed Care Interface, 11*(12), 82–92.

Gallo, A., Breitmayer, B., Knafl, K., & Zoeller, L. (1992). Well siblings of children with chronic illness: Parents' reports of their psychological adjustment. *Pediatric Nursing, 18*(1), 23–27.

Gartstein, M., Short, A., Vannatta, K., & Noll, R. (1999). Psychosocial adjustment of children with chronic illness: An evaluation of three models. *Journal of Developmental Behavior Pediatrics, 20*(3), 157–163.

Garwick, A., Jennings, J., & Theisen, D. (2002). Urban American Indian family caregivers perceptions of the quality of care provided by health-care providers. *Children's Health Care, 31*, 185–198.

Garwick, A. W., Patterson, J., Bennett, F. C., & Blum, R. W. (1995). Breaking the news: How families first learn about their child's chronic condition. *Archives of Pediatric and Adolescent Medicine, 149*(90), 991–997.

Glass, P., & Blinkoff, R. (1996). Overview of developmental issues. In E. Ahmann (Ed.), *Home care for the high risk infant: A family-centered approach* (pp. 285–292). Gaithersburg, MD: Aspen.

Hanson, J. L., Jeppson, E. S., Johnson, B. H., & Thomas, J. (1997). *Newborn intensive care: Resources for family-centered practice.* Bethesda, MD: Institute for Family-Centered Care.

Heaman, D. J. (1995). Perceived stressors and coping strategies of parents who have children with disabilities: A comparison of mothers with fathers. *Journal of Pediatric Nursing, 10*(5), 311–320.

Hockenberry, M., Wilson, D., Winkelstein, M. L., & Kline, N. (2003). *Wong's nursing care of infants and children* (7th ed.). St. Louis, MO: Mosby.

Hogan, D., & Park, J. (2000). Family factors and social support in the developmental outcomes of very low-birth weight children. *Clinical Perinatology, 27*(2), 433–459.

Johnson, B. (2000). Mothers' perceptions of parenting children with disabilities. *American Journal of Maternal and Child Nursing, 25*(3), 127–132.

Johnson, B. H., Jeppson, E., & Redburn, L. (1992). *Caring for children and families: Guidelines for Hospitals.* Bethesda, MD: The Association for the Care of Children's Health.

Kerr, S., & McIntosh, J. (2000). Coping when a child has a disability. Exploring the impact of parent-to-parent support. *Child Care Health and Development, 26,* 309–322.

Kieckhefer, G., & Trahms, C. (2000). Supporting development of children with chronic conditions: From compliance toward shared management. *Pediatric Nursing, 26*(4), 354–363.

Klug, R. M. (1993). Clarifying roles and expectations in home care. *Pediatric Nursing, 19,* 374–376.

Knafl, K., & Deatrick, J. (1986). How families manage chronic conditions: An analysis of the concepts of normalization. *Research in Nursing and Health, 9,* 215–222.

Knafl, K., & Deatrick, J. (1990). Family management style: Concept analysis and development. *Journal of Pediatric Nursing, 5*(1), 4–14.

Knafl, K., & Deatrick, V. J. (2002). The challenge of normalization for families of children with chronic conditions. *Pediatric Nursing, 28*(1), 49–52, 56.

Knafl, K., Breitmayer, B., Gallo, A., & Zoeller, A. (1996). Family response to childhood chronic illness: Description of management styles. *Journal of Pediatric Nursing, 11*(5), 315–326.

Krahn, G. L., Hallum, A., & Kime, C. (1993). Are there good ways to give "bad news"? *Pediatrics, 91*(3) 578–582.

Lazarus, R. S., & Folkman, S. (1984). *Stress, appraisal and coping.* New York: Springer.

Leff, P., & Walizer, E. (1992). *Building the healing partnership: Parents, professionals, and children with chronic illnesses and disabilities.* Cambridge, MA: Brookline Books.

Macpherson, C., Redmond, A., Leavy, A., & McMullan, M. (1998). A review of cystic fibrosis children born to single mothers. *Acta Paediatrics, 87*(4), 397–400.

Manley, J. (2000). *Summary of the major provisions of the Family Opportunity Act of 2000.* Retrieved August 2000, from www.senate.gov/~kennedy/statements/00/03/2000327511.html

Manworren, R. C., & Woodring, B. (1998). Evaluating children's literature as a source for patient education. *Pediatric Nursing, 24*(6), 548–553.

Markos-Capps, G., & Godfrey, A. (1999). Availability of day care services for preschool children with special health care needs. *Infants and Young Children, 11*(3), 62–78.

Maternal and Child Health Bureau, U.S. Dept. of Health and Human Services/National Center for Health Statistics. (2002). *National survey of children with special health care needs.* Retrieved August 10, 2004, from cshcndata.org

May, J. (1996). Fathers: The forgotten parent. *Pediatric Nursing, 22*(3), 243–246, 271.

McCubbin, H. I., Thompson, E. A., Thompson, A. I., McCubbin, M., & Kaston, A. J. (1993). Culture, ethnicity, and the family: Critical factors in childhood chronic illness and disabilities. *Pediatrics, 91*(50), 1063–1070.

McGonigel, M., Kaufmann, R., & Johnson, B. (Eds.). (1991). *Guidelines and recommended practices for the individualized family service plan* (2nd ed.). Bethesda, MD: Association for the Care of Children's Health.

McManus, M. (2000). *A purchaser's tool.* Gainesville, FL: Institute for Child Health Policy.

McNeil, D. (1992, March). *Uncertainty, waiting and possibilities: Becoming a mother in the NICU.* Paper presented at the National Association of Neonatal Nurses' Preconference Research Symposium, Washington, DC.

McPherson, M., Arango, P., Fox, H., Lauver, C., McManus, M., Newacheck, P. W., Perrin, J. M., Shonkoff, J. P., & Strickland, B. (1998). A new definition of children with special health care needs. *Pediatrics, 102*(1), 137–140.

Meyer, D. J., & Vadasy, P. F. (1994). *Sibshops: Workshops for siblings of children with special needs.* Baltimore: Brookes.

Monane, J. H. (1967). *A sociology of human systems.* New York: Appleton-Century-Crofts.

Mott, S. R. (1999). Chronic conditions: Intervention strategies. In M. E. Broome & J. A. Rollins (Eds.), *Core curriculum for the nursing care of children and their families* (pp. 305–317). Pitman, NJ: Jannetti.

Nehring, W. M. (1999). Chronic conditions: The continuum of care. In M. E. Broome & J. A. Rollins (Eds.), *Core curriculum for the nursing care of children and their families* (pp. 331–341). Pitman, NJ: Jannetti.

Nelson, A. (2002). A metasynthesis: Mothering other-than-normal children. *Qualitative Health Research, 12*, 515–530.

Newacheck, P. W., & Taylor, W. (1992). Childhood chronic illness: Prevalence, severity and impact. *American Journal of Public Health, 82*(3), 364–371.

Newacheck, P. W., Strickland, B., Shonkoff, J. P., Perrin, J. M., McPherson, M., McManus, M., Lauver, C., Fox, H., & Arango, P. (1998). An epidemiologic profile of children with special health care needs. *Pediatrics, 102*(1), 117.

Northington, L. (2000). Chronic sorrow in caregivers of school age children with sickle cell disease: A grounded theory approach. *Issues in Comprehensive Pediatric Nursing, 23*, 141–154.

O'Brien, M. (2001). Living in a house of cards: Family experiences with long-term childhood technology dependence. *Journal of Pediatric Nursing, 16*, 13–22.

Olson, D. H., Sprenkle, D., & Russell, C. S. (1979). Circumplex model of marital and family systems: I. Cohesion and adaptability dimensions, family types, and clinical applications. *Family Process, 18*, 3–28.

Palmer, E. (2001). Family caregiver experiences with asthma in school-age children. *Pediatric Nursing, 27*, 75–81.

Patterson, J. M., & Geber, G. (1991). Preventing mental health problems in children with chronic illness or disability. *Children's Health Care, 20*(3), 150–161.

Patterson, J. M., & Gerber, M. (1991). Family resilience to the challenge of a child's disability. *Pediatric Annals, 20*(9), 491–499.

Perrin, E. C., & Gerrity, P. S. (1981). There's a devil in your belly: Children's understanding of illness. *Pediatrics, 67*, 841–849.

Petersen, M. (1996). What are blood counts? A computer-assisted program for pediatric patients. *Pediatric Nursing, 22*(1), 21–25.

Porter, S. (Ed.). (1997). *Children and youth assisted by medical technology in educational settings: Guidelines for care* (2nd ed.). Baltimore: Brookes.

Pridham, K. F. (1995). *Standards and guidelines for prelicensure and early professional education for nursing care of children and their families.* (Project #MCJ-559327) Washington, DC: Maternal and Child Health Bureau.

Questions and Answers about the Garret F. Supreme Court Case. (1999, March-April). *Family Voices* (newsletter). Algodones, NM: Family Voices.

Rodriguez, J. A., & Jones, E. G. (1996). Foster parents' early adaptation to the placement of a child with developmental disabilities in their home. *Journal of Pediatric Nursing, 11*(2) 111–118.

Rosenfeld, L. (1994). *Your child and health care: A "dollars and sense" guide for families with special needs.* Baltimore: Brookes.

Russell, M. T., Reinbold, J., & Maltby, H. J. (1996). Transferring to adult health care: experiences of adolescents with cystic fibrosis. *Journal of Pediatric Nursing, 11*(4), 262–268.

Scher, A., & Ahmann, E. (1996). Community resources for the family. In E. Ahmann (Ed.), *Home care for the high risk infant: A family-centered approach* (pp. 77–80). Gaithersburg, MD: Aspen.

Shelton, T. L., & Stepanek, J. S. (1994). *Family-centered care for children needing specialized health and developmental services.* Bethesda, MD: Association for the Care of Children's Health.

Stein, R. E. K., & Jessop, D. J. (1982). A noncategorical approach to chronic childhood illness. *Public Health Reports, 97,* 354–362.

Sullivan-Bolyai, S., Knafl, K., Sadler, L., & Gilliss, C. (2003). Great expectations: A position description for parents as caregivers: Part I. *Pediatric Nursing, 29,* 457–461.

Sullivan-Bolyai, S., Knafl, K. Sadler, L., & Gilliss, C. (2004). Great expectations: A position description for parents as caregivers. Part II. *Pediatric Nursing, 30*(1), 52–56.

Surunda, A., Vernon, D., Diller, E., & Dean, J. (2000). Usage of emergency medical services by children with special health care needs. *Prehospital Emergency Care, 4*(2), 131–135.

Sydnor-Greenberg, N., & Dokken, D. (2000). Coping and caring in different ways: Understanding and meaningful involvement. *Pediatric Nursing, 26*(2), 185–190.

Vessey, J. A., & Maguire, M. C. (1999). In M. E. Broome & J. A. Rollins (Eds.), *Core curriculum for the nursing care of children and their families* (pp. 243–256). Pitman, NJ: Jannetti.

Vessey, J. A., Braithwaite, K. B., & Weidmann, M. (1990). Teaching children about their internal bodies. *Pediatric Nursing, 16,* 29–33.

VonBertalanffy, L. (1968). *General systems theory.* New York: Braziller.

Walker, C. L. (1999). Chronic conditions: Effects on the child's family. In M. E. Broome & J. A. Rollins (Eds.), *Core curriculum for the nursing care of children and their families* (pp. 257–266). Pitman, NJ: Jannetti.

Wegener, D. (1996). A social work perspective. In K. Gunter & R. Manago (Eds.), *Beyond discharge: Interdisciplinary perspectives for transitioning children with complex medical needs from hospital to home* (pp. 19–24). Bethesda, MD: Association for the Care of Children's Health.

White, P. (1999). Transition to adulthood. *Current Opinion in Rheumatology, 11*(5), 408–411.

Wong, D., Hockenberry-Eaton, M., Wilson, D., Winkelstein, M., & Ahmann, E. (1999). *Whaley and Wong's nursing care of infants and children* (6th ed.). St. Louis, MO: Mosby.

Yoos, H. L. (1994). Children's illness concepts: Old and new paradigms. *Pediatric Nursing, 20*(2), 131–140.

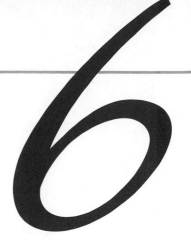

The Child Who Is Dying

Lois J. Pearson

Objectives

At the conclusion of this chapter, the reader will be able to:

1. Discuss the theories and research on grief and the implications for understanding and supporting children and families.
2. Delineate children's understanding of death at various stages of development and the typical responses at each stage.
3. Relate the historical and current views of health-care professionals on supports for children who are dying and their families, citing social, economic, medical, cultural, and religious factors that have contributed to changing ideas.
4. Summarize preparation and support strategies for children and their families.

*T*he birth of a child represents fulfillment in the creation of a family, not only for the present but also for the future. The attachment between a parent and child is stronger than any other relationship (Doka, 1995). The connecting bond formed at conception is intensely developed before the child is born, not only in the life of each parent, but also in the life of the child who will soon become a big brother or big sister. Grandparents also anticipate new life as the fulfillment of hope into a new generation. The family is forever changed with each addition of a new member and relationship. It is for all of these reasons that the event of critical illness or injury and death of an infant, child, or adolescent can be a devastating experience.

Health-care professionals are in a critical position to support families in a time of such great stress. This may be either at the time of diagnosis with a serious and potentially terminal illness or at the time of catastrophic injury or sudden illness with little hope for survival. Knowledge of the characteristics of grief for each member of the family and interventions that may promote positive coping are essential for the provision of family-centered care. This sensitive caring should be a component of health care intended to cure, but also care that is provided when no cure is possible. Irving (1992) wrote of working with grieving parents on the obstetric unit, stating "Bereaved parents remember such caretakers as people who helped them live with death, not as people who failed to bring life" (p. 10). A growing number of health-care facilities are providing death and bereavement seminars to prepare clinicians and increase their confidence in caring for seriously ill and dying children and their families (Bagatell, Meyer, Herron, Berger, & Villar, 2002; Serwint et al., 2002).

This chapter will look at the unique characteristics of grief for parents, siblings, grandparents, and others. The impact of death at home or in the hospital will be explored within the context of palliative care. The particular needs and issues of the dying child will also be considered. In each circumstance, special attention will focus on interventions by health-care professionals that may have lasting effects for families facing the loss of a child.

The Grief of Parents

For parents, the agony of losing a child is unparalleled. When their child dies, a vital part of time has been severed. Parents grieve the lost child for the rest of their lives, never to be whole again. A parent's grief is forever. Only memories remain.
—Rando, 1986, p. 11

Much research has been done on the impact of the loss of a child. Rando's classic work identified the loss of a child as "severe, complicated and long-lasting" (Rando, 1986). It does not matter at what age a child dies, for the loss of a child is always unnatural. For a parent, the loss of a child reflects the loss of part of the parent and the parent's hopes and dreams for the future. It is an assault on the parent's role as protector and provider and results in a diminished sense of self. The loss of a child even has an impact on the promise that children will be the caregivers for the parent in his or her old age. In the instance of genetic factors responsible for a child's death, a parent may experience guilt about not being able to produce a child that could survive to old age (Rando, 1986).

Grief is defined as "the thoughts and feelings that are experienced when someone they love dies. Grief is the internal meaning given to the experience of bereavement" (Wolfelt, 1996, p. 322). Mourning is "grief gone public," and involves taking the internal experience of grief and expressing it outside oneself (Wolfelt, 1996, p. 322).

The grief of a parent is described as "the most difficult, painful, and time-consuming loss anyone can survive" (Doka, 1995, p. 73). It is a grief that comes in overlapping phases, the first of which is shock. It includes devastating disbelief, helplessness, and bewilderment, which cause a state of physiologic and emotional alarm (Doka, 1995). The second phase begins when the state of shock wears off and the actuality of the absence of the child is realized. Rando (1986) described the emotion of this phase as "angry sadness." This may include feelings of panic and extreme fear, guilt, and anger directed at God, medical personnel, or even the dead child for leaving. During this phase of increased awareness of the loss, there are often acute physical feelings of emptiness and longing with vivid visual and auditory recall or dreams (Rando, 1986). The third phase is often the longest phase of the grieving process, that of conservation and withdrawal (Doka, 1995). It is a time characterized by despair when grieving parents finally realize the loss and that life will be forever changed. Parents may withdraw from external activities to regain strength and energy. Strengthened by this renewed energy, bereaved parents enter the phase of "searching for meaning" characterized by attempts to put the loss of a child into some natural order, which begins the process of healing. Rando (1986) described a similar "reestablishment phase," when parents are finally able to reengage in everyday activities and begin "growing up" with the loss.

Despite what we know about parental grief, research indicates that many feelings and experiences of parental grief remain unidentified by health-care professionals (Laakso & Paunonen-Ilmonen, 2001). Parental loss affects the marital relationship as severe grieving takes emotional energy away from the relationship. Grief responses may be very dissimilar between spouses, and reactions to the loss will have different effects based on specific marital roles.

Parental loss of a child also has tremendous societal impact as the devastating grief of parents is out of all proportion to the expectations of society based on responses to other losses. Rando (1986) highlighted the fact that while a grieving spouse is referred to as "widow" or "widower" and a child who has lost parents as an "orphan," there is no accepted specific term in reference to a grieving parent. Perhaps this omission reflects the challenge experienced in trying to be supportive of grieving parents. And finally, the ability to be supportive of grieving parents often is difficult when society members fear even contemplating the loss of their own child.

Children's Understanding of Death

For the past half-century, researchers have attempted to study the child's understanding of death. Classic studies of Spitz (1945) and Bowlby (1980) described the effects of separation on children and their associated responses. Certainly the concept of death is complex and acquired over a lifetime (see Figure 6.1). To be able to support a child facing his or her own death or the death of a sibling requires knowledge of the degree to which a child's understanding of death differs from that of adults. The provision of family-centered care requires not only the ability to answer children's questions, but more important, an understanding of what questions a child may ask and why (see Table 6.1. Children's Understanding of Death, by Age).

Age-appropriate attention to a child's understanding of death is found in Piaget's work detailing cognitive development (Piaget, 1960). His classic study of the way children acquire and process information helps adults realize what children are capable of understanding about death at each developmental level.

The first stage, sensorimotor, describes an infant's ability to respond to feelings associated with separation from those who love them, rather than understanding death itself. Attention to comfort and care routines are important in this stage. Piaget described the next period in two stages, preoperational and concrete operational. In the preoperational stage, children 2 to 6 years of age do not process thought logically, but instead function within an egocentric world. Children in this stage perceive death as temporary and reversible, somewhat like the concept of sleep. Questions in this stage often

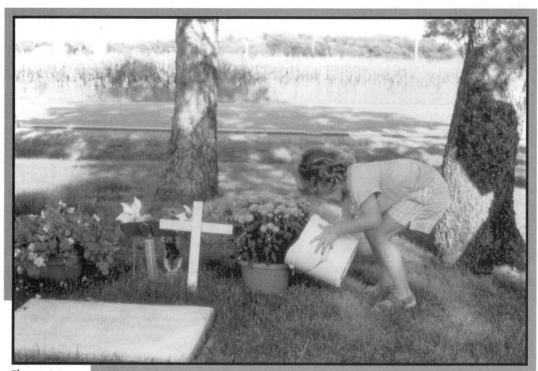

Figure 6.1.
The concept of death is complex and is acquired over a lifetime.

center on issues of the dead person's ability to eat, sleep, stay warm under the ground, and so on. In the second stage, concrete operational, children 7 to 12 years of age begin to think more logically. They are increasingly able to process events less egocentrically and learn by observation. Their understanding of death also is affected by their experience. Questions may relate to physiologic processes of dying as their knowledge of the body and its function increases. In this developmental stage, children begin to role-model adult behaviors related to grief while also gaining support from religious beliefs and practices shared within the family (Piaget, 1960).

Finally, in Piaget's formal operational stage, children over the age of 12 years begin to integrate adult concepts of death. They can differentiate causes with increased intellectual capacity, and also are able to acknowledge feelings and beliefs about death and life after death based on their ability to handle abstract concepts (Davies, 1999).

A comprehensive review of more than 100 research studies done between 1934 and 1990 examined and contrasted age and developmental stages of a child's concept of death (Speece & Brent, 1996). This review concluded that a child's concept of death does not consist of a single complex concept, but rather may be broken down into three components or subconcepts (Davies, 1999). The first component, which describes the understanding that once

(*text continues on p. 228*)

Table 6.1

Children's Understanding of Death, by Age

Age	Understanding of Death	Characteristic Behaviors
Newborn to 3 Years A 2-year-old has begun having temper tantrums each morning 2 weeks after the death of her 1-week-old sister. Her mother admits that she cries each morning upon awakening to another day of grieving. When questioning the 2-year-old about why she is acting that way, the daughter replies that she "wants Mommy not to be sad anymore!"	• Does not comprehend death • Aware of a constant buzz of activity in the house • Aware of Mom and Dad looking sad and teary-eyed • Aware that someone in the home is missing	• Has altered eating and sleeping patterns • Is irritable • Clings
3 to 5 Years A 4-year-old was thought to not know anything about the anticipated death of her soon-to-be-born baby brother until she was observed playing "dead baby" with her dolls. It was only then that the family realized how perceptive this 4-year-old was to the surrounding grief.	• Sees death as temporary and reversible; child continually asks if person will return • May feel ambivalent • Through magical thinking, may assume responsibility for the death	• Is concerned about own well-being • Feels confused and guilty • May use imaginative play, reenacting scene of CPR, etc. • Withdraws • Is irritable • Regresses
6 to 9 Years A 6-year-old boy who has just returned from the bedside of his dying newborn sister explains in a matter-of-fact style to his 5-year-old sister, "We cannot go to heaven after Mindy goes there, because you would have to have a spaceship. Heaven is way farther away. You have to go past Mars."	• Begins to understand concept of death • Feels it happens to others • May be superstitious about death • May be uncomfortable in expressing feelings • Worries that other important people will die	• May seem outwardly uncaring, inwardly upset • May use denial to cope • May attempt to "parent" parent • May act out in school or home • May play death games
9 to 12 Years A 10-year-old girl describing her feelings following the unexpected death of her father: "Sure I thought he would die before me. He was older than I am. But I certainly didn't expect him to die when I was only 10 years old!" A 9-year-old boy, in explaining why his baby sister did not look like herself at the open casket visitation, stated, "Her soul is gone, and that's what gives people their light."	• Accepts death as final • Has personal fear of death • May be morbidly interested in skeletons, gruesome details of violent deaths • Concerned with practical matters about child's lifestyle	• May appear tough or funny • May express and demonstrate anger or sadness • May act like adult, but regress to earlier stage of emotional response

Table 6.1 *Continued.*

227

Children's Understanding of Death, by Age

Language/ Approach	Interventions
Newborn to 3 Years • Use the *D* words: *dying, death, dead.* • Avoid euphemisms like "lost, passed away, gone to sleep," which confuse young children. • Explain in physiologic terms (i.e., person who is dead does not eat or drink, or feel feelings, like being cold after burial in the ground). • Expect questions to change. • Expect repeated questioning and testing to confirm information.	• Maintain routines but allow for flexibility. • Choose familiar and supportive caregivers. • Assign a support person for each child during funeral, burial, and other rituals. • Acknowledge all feelings of child and adult by naming feelings and giving permission to express anger and sadness in developmentally appropriate ways. • Give extra hugs when needed to help child feel secure.
3 to 5 Years • Explain cause of death factually; that which is mentionable is manageable. • Answer questions honestly (e.g., clarify wellness of sibling, unlike that of dying child). • Avoid abstracts. • Diffuse magical thinking. • Be consistent and persistent.	• Reinforce that when people are sad, they cry; crying is natural. • Read stories (see bibliography of children's books). • Provide materials for child to draw pictures. • Encourage dialogue and family meetings. • Expect misbehavior as child struggles with confusing feelings and issues. • Offer play with themes of death while providing supportive guidance.
6 to 9 Years • Look for questions within questions. • Expect a more global view. • Encourage child to answer own questions. • Explore feelings by asking questions such as "What do you think?"	• Listen to determine what kind of information the child is seeking. • Increase physical activity while role-modeling stress-reducing behaviors. • Work on identifying feelings, which are becoming more sophisticated (i.e., frustration, confusion). • Encourage creative outlets for feelings (i.e., drawing, painting, clay, blank books).
9 to 12 Years • Provide more detail as needed, especially to explain cause of death in physiologic context. • Probe for thoughts and feelings. • Allow for spiritual development. • May answer questions about an afterlife by stating, "We don't really know but we believe that…"	• Encourage creative expressions of feelings. • Explore support group and peer-to-peer connection. • Establish family traditions and memorials. • Incorporate children into rituals not just at time of death, but at important anniversaries (e.g., taking balloons to the cemetery; creating a special ornament for the Christmas tree, which is always hung first; having birthday dinners and memory nights).

(continues)

Table 6.1 *Continued.*

Children's Understanding of Death, by Age

Age	Understanding of Death	Characteristic Behaviors
Adolescents An adolescent girl wrote these words after her father died and her mother was diagnosed with cancer: "While I was tending to my mom, all I felt was anguish and despair. I tried to kill myself in an adverse way by driving my Firebird at 100 mph on a winding road. It was stupid, but it was the only way to rid myself of my anger. I had bad feelings that my mom was going to leave me alone and I would be without the two people I loved the most, my mom and dad." (Snoddy, 1992, p. 13)	• Has adult concept of death, but ability to to deal with loss is based on experience and developmental factors • Experiences thrill of recklessness • Focuses on present • Is developing strong philosophical views • Questions existence of an afterlife	• Increased reliance on peers instead of family • Moodiness and irritability • May engage in risk-taking behaviors • Appears rebellious and tests limits • May act impulsively or without common sense

something is dead it will not come alive again, is termed *irreversibility*. Before grasping the concept of irreversibility, a child thinks that a sibling who dies today will be back tomorrow, similar to the idea of waking from sleep. The 4-year-old at the bedside of her dead newborn brother, shaking a stuffed animal energetically as if attempting to wake him from his sleep, has not yet developed the concept of irreversibility.

Nonfunctionality, as described by Speece and Brent (1996), refers to a child's understanding that all external and internal functions have stopped (i.e., breathing, thinking, moving). The child who is capable of understanding nonfunctionality will be supported by attention to the physiological explanations of dying (i.e., the heart stops beating, the lungs stop breathing and the brain stops thinking). The child no longer questions what the body will feel or do when buried under the ground.

The third component is *universality*, the understanding that all living things eventually die. At this level a child will understand that they, too, will one day die. Magical thinking or the belief that one may avoid dying by being smart or lucky no longer protects children in this stage. Death is universal.

Two other components emerged from the review by Speece and Brent (1996), but are not as clear. One component is *causality*, the ability to understand both internal and external events that may bring about a death. The last component of death identifies the belief in some form of life after death, which characterizes a child's and adult's concept of death. However, this belief in an afterlife is still the subject of discussion among researchers (Davies, 1999).

Table 6.1 *Continued.*

229

Children's Understanding of Death, by Age

Language/ Approach	Interventions
Adolescents	
• Treat as adult with information, respect, and responsibility.	• Allow for informed participation.
• Role-model adult behaviors.	• Encourage peer support.
• Allow to make informed choices.	• Suggest individualized and group expressions of grief (i.e., school memorials).
	• Support group advocacy for causes (e.g., Students Against Drunk Driving [SADD]).
	• Recommend creative outlets (e.g., writing, art, music).

Note. From "Separation, Loss, and Bereavement," by L. Pearson, 1999, in *Core Curriculum for the Nursing Care of Children and Their Families* (pp. 77–92) by M. Broome and J. Rollins (Eds.), 1999, Pittman, NJ: Jannetti. Copyright 1999 by Jannetti. Reprinted with permission.

Speece and Brent (1996) concluded that the "model age" for acquiring all three concepts is at about the age of 7 years. They report that 60% of children achieve a mature understanding of all three concepts between 5 and 7 years of age (Davies, 1999). Perhaps the most helpful aspect of this research for health-care professionals is the knowledge that what is happening when a child is dying must be explained in terms of death as universal, and more important, must focus on the differences between being alive and being dead.

Talking to Children About Death

The responsibility of explaining death to children is critical. Like all grief work with families, it carries great significance for a child and family's future grief work. Role-modeling appropriate language and behavior may make the critical difference when a child is dying. When the medical environment describes a critical illness or injury as "incompatible with life," it is up to child life professionals, nurses, social workers, and pastoral care staff to provide age-appropriate explanations for children. At times it may be necessary to begin a conversation with parents by acknowledging their grief, while identifying the need to be honest and accurate in talking to children. The reality of the *D* words, *dying, dead, death,* may seem insensitive to grieving parents without preparatory explanations.

The most important consideration is that children hear the words from people they trust, or in the presence of people they trust. Often times a parent may be too emotionally distraught or exhausted to actually say the words telling of a child's death, but may be able to provide their physical presence and supportive touch while a health-care professional, extended family member, or friend actually says the words. It is doubtful that children will remember who said the words, but will remember in whose lap they were sitting at the time. Words will need to be repeated and a child's questions may be repeated to many people as the child continually seeks to integrate what is happening and being communicated.

Keeping in mind the research of Speece and Brent (1996), the most important aspects of communication should be focused on physiologic happenings. Explaining present medical conditions age-appropriately will help children to understand impending death in terms of what is happening to a person's body. Explaining the inability of a person's heart to work or an injury to someone's brain that cannot be fixed with medicines helps a child understand the impossibility of continuing to live.

Communication often may be enhanced by first asking a child what is happening. A child's explanation of the present situation will help health-care professionals to begin preparation at the level of the child's understanding. This approach also helps to identify information that has already been conveyed to the child directly by other family members, or indirectly, by overhearing telephone conversations or observing family members' behaviors. Many families truly believe that they have protected a child from the tragic events that are happening to the family, only to witness the child's explanation of all that they know in response to a staff member's assessment and initial intervention.

The next step in communicating an impending death includes the ability to reframe explanations more developmentally appropriately while clarifying misconceptions. A young school-age child who has been told that his or her sibling is going to heaven so great-grandma can take care of him may have difficulty. It is not necessary to deny those concepts that bring comfort to a family in the acceptance of the loss, but rather to contrast this information with more age-appropriate explanations. "Because baby brother's heart did not grow right inside Mom's tummy, and the doctors and nurses are not able to fix it, his body may stop working and he will die. Mommy and Daddy believe he will be in heaven with great-grandma." The ability to process the abstract concept of heaven is one that the child may need to "grow into" as he or she matures in developmental understanding of death, but does not take away the comfort of family beliefs.

It is important to avoid euphemisms in communicating with children of all ages. Using words that relate to sleep, journeys, or being lost often confuse young children and may cause difficulties after the death. Children's drawings illustrate how easily children confuse death with sleep, drawing coffins that look like beds under the ground. Even the concept of an open casket at a funeral visitation may confuse a child unless statements are clear (e.g., "She may look like she is sleeping, but she is dead. Her head and body are cold because no parts of her body are working."). Using appropriate words helps children clarify these misconceptions. For example, a child life specialist relates the confusion over terminology at the death of her uncle when she was 4 or 5 years old. Her parents told her that her Uncle Bob had been killed in a car crash, but she recalls asking over and over again during the long trip to her grandparents' home, "Was Uncle Bob killed?" While her parents' frustration level continued to escalate, what she really needed to know was if the term "killed" meant the same as "died."

The ability to identify a cause for the death, again using age-appropriate language, is another important aid to children's understanding of death. If the death is a result of an illness, it is important to address the child's basic and often unspoken questions:

- Did I cause it to happen?
- Can it happen to me?
- Who will take care of me now?

The young child's belief in magical thinking means that they believe that their thoughts, wishes, or actions may have caused the illness, injury, or accident. Clarification of the cause of illness or injury often helps, if an explanation is possible. If not entirely possible, for example, if the cause of the death is not known, reassurance of the known factors should help (e.g., "Usually children get special medicine to make them better and go home from the hospital, but the medicine that doctors have didn't work for the kind of illness your brother had."). Since death from an unexplainable illness complicates grieving for adults, it is even more complex for children with less developmental understanding. Reassurance that the dying child's illness is much different than the kind of illness that a child brings home from day care or school includes attention to the magnitude of how sick the child is, and how medicine that doctors have does not work for this kind of illness. Even with this reassurance, children may be expected to react differently the first time that they are ill or a parent is ill after the death of a family member. Finally, it is most important while communicating with children about any death, to provide a caring presence for reassurance, extra love and support, availability of trusted adults to answer questions, and time to integrate information.

The Grief of Siblings

"The experience of sibling bereavement is a life long process requiring ongoing integration into the lives of those touched by such a loss" (Davies, 1997, p. 595). The death of a brother or sister represents a double loss because grieving parents are often unavailable to surviving children. No life experience prepares a sibling for a death. A young girl sitting with a child life specialist in the ICU where her teenage brother had just died remarked, "Ah, Buddy (her pet name for him), we had such great times together, but he never died before!" The bond between siblings begins before birth as the family eagerly anticipates the new baby and a child prepares to become a big brother or sister; it strengthens as the siblings spend time together, more time than they will spend with any other family members (Grollman, 1995).

The child in a family with a sibling who has a life-threatening illness often experiences more distress than the parent due to social isolation, while the parent spends long hours with the ill child during treatment. Healthy children may view parents as overprotective of the ill child and then feel guilty about such negative feelings. They also may become preoccupied with their own health, either because of a fear that they also are vulnerable to illness, or because of excessive family concerns over the sick child's lack of immunity to common childhood illnesses (Davies, 1999).

A study by Sourkes (1980) described siblings' own private versions of the causation of illness. Misconceptions about the nature of treatment resulted from observable disease symptoms. Further misconceptions centered on the hospital, clinic, and routines of the treatment protocol. Siblings also feared developing the same illness or felt guilt and shame in their relief at not having the illness. Shame may also be a factor if the sick child's illness has caused any disfigurement, which the child may perceive as identifying the family as different. Finally, Sourkes identified decreased academic and social functioning due to preoccupation and stress about the illness.

Davies (1997, 1999) has extensively researched the grief of siblings. She identified important situational, individual, and environmental factors that have an impact on sibling bereavement. Situational factors include the cause of death, sudden death versus long-term illness, and accident or homicide. Individual factors include age, gender, past experiences, and coping styles. The involvement of an extended support network of family and friends, and communication among family members of both factual and emotional responses constitute environmental factors (Davies, 1999).

Even after a long-term illness, the actual death still may be perceived as a surprise (Davies, 1999). While parents continue to hope that their child will be the one to survive, the timing of the death may be unexpected (e.g., "We expected him at least to live through Christmas."). Siblings tend to revise their appraisal of the sick child's state of health in a positive direction unless they continue to be exposed to negative reminders. For example, a 9-year-old girl visited the bedside of her dying newborn baby brother in the ICU. The child life specialist often asks siblings if they would like to create memory books (see Figure 6.2). After several sad visits to the bedside in the presence of her grieving family, the girl remarked to the child life specialist that she was going to leave a few blank pages in the memory book she was creating for her brother, stating that her brother could then "tell his own story when he grows up." Whether this reflected wishful thinking or her inability to process the events that indicated the infant's death was imminent

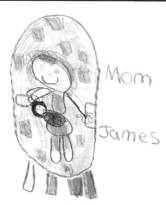

My mom had a baby in her tummy. We didn't know the baby was very sick.

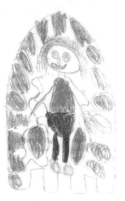

My mom had to go to get her pictures checked for her tummy once in a while. The baby got bigger and bigger.

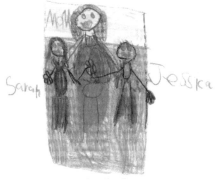

We felt him kicking and then we made up his name. His name was James. He was very sick.

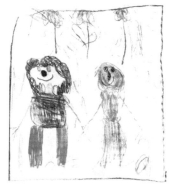

When mama had the baby, he felt even sicker. Somebody said if he goes up to heaven he would feel much better. We only got to stay with him for two days. The next day he died at 1:00.

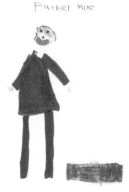

Then Father Mike, who is always our priest in the church. He had a box where James was in and somebody buried him up.

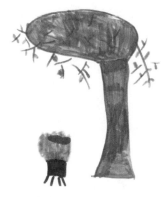

We put a wreath by his grave and it was very pretty. We still have the wreath on. We put snow on it to make it look very pretty. We always go and see James Louis.

Figure 6.2.

"My Brother," by Sarah, age 6 years.

is unknown, but her comment identified the need to gently clarify this expectation: "Everybody wishes that your baby brother would grow up to write his own book, but we do not think that he will be alive much longer. When his heart stops working, he will die. That is why everyone is very sad."

Helpful Interventions for Siblings When a Child Has a Life-Threatening Illness

The responsibility of parenting both healthy and ill children can be an overwhelming task. Health-care professionals can help parents by encouraging the inclusion of siblings during the stages of illness. Interventions that health-care professionals can use to help parents and siblings include the following (Davies, 1999):

- Encourage siblings to participate in family meetings with health-care professionals.
- If siblings are not able to be included, inquire about their coping.
- Allocate time to be spent alone with siblings. (In one hospital, physicians in the ICU have been known to sit alone with a sibling in the playroom to answer questions and provide information and support for the sibling without the presence of other adult family members.)
- Encourage siblings to participate in bedside cares.
- If siblings cannot be at the hospital, include them in indirect participation (e.g., phone calls, letters, e-mails).
- Offer age-appropriate teaching sessions that help siblings understand the process of illness.
- Develop sibling groups and special sibling events, when possible, so that support may be gained from peers. (Sibling Day for oncology families is held twice a year at one Midwestern hospital. Coordinated by child life and social work, the day features activities that focus on siblings' coping, expression of feelings, and inclusion in medical treatment. It is the one activity that the ill child does not attend.)
- Provide positive reinforcement for siblings' coping behaviors.
- Encourage open discussion between parents and their well children.
- Facilitate healthy children's relationships with their peers, encouraging hospital visiting and school involvement.

Sibling Responses at the Time of Death

Nearly all children, regardless of the circumstances of a sibling's death, experience certain characteristic responses. Davies' studies (1999) indicated that the greatest incidence of behavioral problems after the death of a sibling was noted in preschool and young school-age children. Attention-seeking behavior and irritability were common. One fourth of siblings in the study reported "crying a lot." Generally, crying or not crying was attributed to individual coping styles and the attitude of a family toward tears as emotionally and physiologically healing (Davies, 1999). Forty-four percent of siblings reported an inability to concentrate in school, and went on to report that the longer they stayed away from school, the harder it was to re-enter the school routine. Siblings reported that a week was the right amount of time before returning to school.

Sleeping difficulties were frequent in the study group, especially in the ability to fall asleep, although insomnia is uncommon in children (Davies, 1999). Guilt also was universal, in terms of siblings' perceptions of the cause of death. Some siblings feel survivor guilt that perhaps they should have died instead of the one who did. These feelings may be difficult to resolve if the surviving child feels as though he or she is competing with the dead child's memory within the family (Grollman, 1995). Health complaints are often reported and, like other responses, may be observed up to 3 years after the death. Aches and pains are common in siblings, and may be similar to the symptoms or medical condition of the ill sibling (Grollman, 1995). Finally, there is frequently confusion on the part of surviving siblings as to their role in the changed family. Becoming the oldest child or only child often challenges the sibling's perception of his or her own identity (Grollman, 1995).

Helpful Interventions at the Time of Death

Despite the research examining the difficulty of reconciling children's grief, there have been factors identified in the literature that may prove beneficial. As health-care professionals, it is important to support these behaviors at the time of death and help families access known resources and supports. Siblings who are included at the time of death and in the rituals following the death are better able to reconcile the loss (Davies, 1999). Providing stable caregivers and supportive extended family during the first days of a parent's acute grief also helps. Often at the bedside of a dying child in the ICU, the child life specialist or other staff members may gently enlist the strong arms of an uncle, aunt, or other family member to hold a younger sibling who may be lost in the group of mourners at the bedside. Being the recipient of a child's trust at that time will certainly help the adult in whose care a sibling might be placed, as well as helping the child.

Role-modeling feelings is another area where caregivers begin the process of helping children and adults. "Daddy is having a hard time talking right now because he is feeling very sad. People express sadness in many ways, and they are all okay ways to help get feelings out." Suggesting appropriate ways to express anger is also important at the start of grief work. Being able to identify particular behaviors that help reduce stress is important for staff and families. For example, an ICU staff member obtained a pass to a nearby athletic club, so that an adolescent boy and his cousin could go over to shoot baskets while the rest of the family sat at the bedside of his dying younger brother.

For younger children, the ability to retreat to a playroom and draw, write, play with toy emergency vehicles, or simply feel comfortable is a significant factor in helping family members meet the needs of children. The theoretical base of all psychosocial care is that child's play is the mode of expression and communication. Acknowledging the importance of play within the critical care setting begins the long process of helping children heal though play opportunities. Wolfelt (1996) wrote: "For bereaved children to 'play out' their grief thoughts and feelings is a natural and self-healing process" (p. 150).

Siblings who are included in caretaking during illness, are prepared and present at the time of death, participate in family rituals, and are supported by family in their grief work demonstrate higher self-concepts. They also demonstrate psychologic growth and move on in life with the ability to reach out to others with greater sensitivity while valuing life and people (Davies, 1999). Sensitive and age-appropriate preparation is required before a child visits his or her sibling who is dying. For guidance, see the following box and Case Study 6.1, Fulfilling a Family's Wishes.

Case Study 6.1
Fulfilling a Family's Wishes

The anticipated birth of a new baby into the family was filled with happy preparation because an early ultrasound documented that this new infant would not be born with the same congenital kidney disease that had caused the death of a baby girl 7 years earlier. That baby had lived only 4 hours, and her mother's grief had been complicated by the fact that she did not reach the tertiary care hospital where the baby died until after her death. Their 9-year-old son, though only 2 years old at the time of his sister's birth and death, grew up in the midst of the family's grief. Their daughter, born 5 years ago, understood less of the circumstances of the earlier loss experience, but was able to state that she "had a sister in heaven."

When this fourth infant was born in severe respiratory distress, he was immediately transported by helicopter to a metropolitan hospital and placed on a ventilator. The two older children were able to see and touch him before he was flown again to a children's hospital in a city about 2 hours from home. Efforts at this third hospital focused on diagnosing his medical condition and placing him on ECMO, a high-tech system that allows the heart and lungs to be supported mechanically, not unlike cardiac bypass used during surgery.

The family was devastated to hear that their newborn did indeed have the same disease as his sibling and his survival was unlikely. Yet this time the family knew what they wanted—to be with the baby and hold him as much as possible while photographing every moment of his short but significant life. The siblings were prepared by the child life specialist, and were able to spend much valuable sibling time at the bedside, reading books, singing lullabies, and making dolls.

The fourth-grader was able to understand what was wrong with the baby when given age-appropriate information about the infant's kidneys and lungs. He amazed the physicians by appearing to understand the reason why the mechanical support needed to be discontinued after the baby suffered bleeding in his head. The 5-year-old daughter was less able to process so much information, but took her cues from the tears and coping of her mother.

For many hours, each family member held the precious baby. Although only his parents were at the bedside when the baby died, the siblings and extended family returned to the bedside for more holding and picture taking. While staff people were somewhat uncomfortable with this extended time at the bedside, especially for the children, every family member expressed gratitude that "this time" at least they had been allowed the experience of holding their baby. And they were certain that their grief work would be helped by the collection of photographs. The older son took one of the baby's pictures to school so his classmates might see "how his baby brother should have looked without all those tubes."

Ultimately, this family, whose members supported one another and did what felt right for them, told the hospital staff that the infant's father, grandfather, uncle, and big brother actually dug the grave together in a final expression of their love.

Note. Courtesy of James and Catherine Hackbarth.

The Grief of Adolescents

On a cognitive level, adolescents may be able to integrate the death of a loved one like an adult, yet their response will be influenced by additional developmental tasks of adolescence. Adolescents feel invincible and may react to a death by increasing risk-taking behaviors. Anger at life's unfairness may encourage acting-out behaviors. Other teens may withdraw, using art, writing, or music to express complex feelings.

Of interest is the effect of recent terrorism on teenagers' perceptions of dying. Halpern-Felsher and Millstein (2002) found that adolescents assessed after the September 11, 2001, terrorist attacks in the United States perceive the risk of dying from general causes, a tornado, and an earthquake as dramatically higher than did adolescents assessed years before the attacks. Further, their heightened perceptions of vulnerability to death extended beyond the terrorist acts and were generalized to unrelated risks.

Teens frequently struggle in finding support systems. At a time when adolescents are pulling away from the family structure and relying on the support of peers, the experience of loss and its associated emotions may frighten friends away. In addition, family members also may be unavailable due to their personal grief (Wolfelt, 1996). Wolfelt has described both "normal" behaviors of grieving adolescents and "red flag" behaviors that indicate when a teen needs help (see Table 6.2, Behaviors of Grieving Adolescents).

(*text continues on p. 240*)

Preparing Children for the Death of a Sibling in the ICU

Choices related to the ICU experience:

- To visit or not to visit
- With whom and for how long
- Required preparation
- Availability of support persons other than parents

Information to be gathered from parents, if possible:

- Desire to have siblings visit
- Ages and stages of siblings
- Present understanding of situation
- Previous experience with hospitalization or loss
- Person(s) to bring children to hospital and relationship to child
- Availability of person(s) for follow-up
- Members of hospital staff parents want present
- Role of hospital staff at visit

Before the visit:

- Identify cause of accident, nature of illness, and other important factors for siblings.
- Determine present medical condition.
- Know immediate medical and family plans, expected outcomes.
- Find quiet place with privacy but easy access to unit.
- Identify and assemble all who will be present.
- If possible, have one staff person for children, another for adults.
- Have children's resources available:
  - Preparation photographs
  - Paper and markers
  - Cloth dolls
  - Blank books
- Look at patient from visiting child's perspective.
- Arrange to reduce scary details, if possible.

During the visit before going to ICU:

- Arrange seating of children to be close to supportive person.
- Introduce self and meet children.
- Begin by acknowledging frightening nature of situation.
- Acknowledge tears and grief behaviors of surrounding adults.
- Explain present situation by first asking if children understand what has happened so far.
- Respond to child's comments, remembering the three biggest fears of children:
  - Did I do anything to cause this to happen?
  - Could it happen to me?
  - What will happen to me now?
- Clarify cause of injury or illness.
- Explain where sibling is and what is being done.
- Be honest but do not take away family's hope.
- Explain medical details in simple physiologic terms.
- Describe physical environment of ICU: size, windows, number of doctors and nurses, presence of other children and families, some very sick.

- Briefly and simply describe medical equipment—function, look, and sound.
  - Ventilator, IVACs, catheter bag, chest tubes. Reassure that although scary-looking, are helping sibling.
  - Monitors and alarms. Describe place where attached to body, as well as sounds and meanings.
- Describe neurologic condition of patient. Describe coma unlike sleeping, cannot walk or talk, can hear.
- Identify what child can do at bedside (i.e., talk, touch).
- Incorporate decorating cloth doll, drawing, or journaling in blank book.

At the bedside:

- Encourage child's entrance into room.
- Facilitate child's easy viewing (e.g., step stool, chair, parent lifting).
- Review equipment that is present. Point out important pieces, especially ventilator.
- Identify familiar or comforting objects (e.g., photographs, stuffed animal).
- Be sure that child is physically supported by adult family member or yourself.
- Allow family time alone in rooms if members are handling situation well.
- Observe family members, especially children, for cues that the visit has been long enough. Intervene if necessary.

After visit to the room:

- Sit with the children while they process the visit.
- Listen for questions within questions.
- Turn questions back if needed to clarify concerns.
- Acknowledge feelings of all.
- Continue to build trust by being honest and caring.
- Attend to physical needs of children. Offer juice, crackers.
- Be prepared, and help adults understand that children grieve in different ways.

If patient dies:

- Continue interventions in same style that has allowed children to place their trust in you.
- Be honest and explain using physiologic terms.
- Clarify cause of death according to original explanation.
- Ask if children want to see sibling again.
- Acknowledge spiritual beliefs if proffered by family and clergy. Avoid abstract images if not age-appropriate.
- Encourage drawing and writing in blank books to help children express feelings.
- Offer children a chance to leave the bedside if adults are not ready. Maintain a presence with the children.
- If you knew the child, recall characteristics you liked.
- Reinforce what a great brother or sister the survivor has always been.
- Encourage child to leave something with the patient if desired (e.g., cloth doll, book, drawing).
- Provide for sibling a comfort object that was with the patient (e.g., stuffed animal, quilt—one for each surviving sibling).
- Always accompany family when leaving the hospital after a death.
- If possible, follow up with the surviving siblings by attending the visitation or funeral, writing a note, or calling the children.

Note. From "Separation, Loss, and Bereavement," by L. Pearson, in Core Curriculum for the Nursing Care of Children and Their Families (pp. 77–92), by M. Broome and J. Rollins (Eds.), 1999, Pittman, NJ: Jannetti Publications. Copyright 1999 by Jannetti. Reprinted with permission.

Table 6.2

Behaviors of Grieving Adolescents

Type	Behaviors
Normal	Some limit-testing and rebellion
	Increased reliance on peers for problem solving
	Egocentrism
	Increased sexual awareness
	Increased moodiness
	Impulsiveness, lack of common sense
Red Flag	Suicidal thoughts or actions
	Chronic depression, sleep problems, low self-esteem
	Isolation from family and friends
	Academic failure or overachievement
	Dramatic changes in attitude
	Eating disorders
	Drug or alcohol abuse
	Fighting or legal problems
	Inappropriate sexual behaviors

Note. Adapted from *Healing the Bereaved Child* (pp. 281–282), by A. D. Wolfelt, 1996, Fort Collins, CO: Companion Press. Copyright 1996 by Companion Press. Adapted with permission.

In a study conducted through the Compassionate Friends Organization, Hogan and DeSantis (1994) asked 157 adolescents in 223 families what helped and what made their grief work harder. Each had experienced the death of a sibling within the last 5 years. Things that helped adolescents cope with the death of a sibling were related to themes of self, specific individuals, and a social network. Having a personal belief system and being able to engage in activities that were known to reduce stress were helpful. Parental support, sharing memories, and the support of friends were identified as important. Things that hindered their efforts to cope included intrusive thoughts, feelings of guilt, loneliness, insensitivity in the actions or words of others, and parental discord. Researchers noted that these resilient teens were able to identify both family and friends who helped them cope, but also noted the lack of school personnel or community resources in providing support for these grieving adolescents.

The Grief of Grandparents

The loss of a grandchild presents particular concerns. It is a grief that is unique and complex, as a grandparent mourns the loss of the grandchild but also feels helplessness in witnessing the grief of their adult child (Ponzetti & Johnson, 1991). Grandparents grieve as do parents over the loss of future experiences of the child and the natural order of life, which assumes that young children do not die. Survivor guilt is common, wherein grandparents question why they should go on living in old age, and why a young child should die.

Secondly, grandparents feel intense sadness for the loss felt by their adult children. Often they do not know how to support the child's parents in the face of such overwhelming sadness (Ponzetti & Johnson, 1991). They may feel as though they have failed by not protecting the family or recognizing symptoms or hazards leading to the death. Communication between parents and grandparents may be strained as the strong feelings of acute grief are expressed. Feelings of helplessness may be exaggerated if grandparents are excluded from the grieving family. If grandparents are physically or emotionally unhealthy, bereavement may be more complex.

The ability of health-care professionals to include grandparents in the support of families is important to consider. Assessing the role and availability of grandparents within the family structure helps identify particular strengths that may be used to support parents. Sharing information with grandparents as well as parents helps the family to process events together, relying on mutual support. Encouraging families to use the wisdom and solid presence of extended family, including grandparents, aids in coping while reducing feelings of helplessness. The comforting care of grandparents is often critical to the coping of siblings who are not able to maintain a continuous presence at the bedside. Finally, bereavement programs need to address the particular grief of grandparents. Resources and support services, such as support groups for grandparents, make an important contribution to a family's reconciliation of loss.

Anticipated Versus Sudden Grief

Anticipatory grief is defined as "grief expressed in advance when the loss is perceived as inevitable" (Sourkes, 1996, p. 56). The concept may be applied to the behaviors of parents or the child facing death. Much of Rando's (1986) research suggests that support to parents during a child's illness facilitates anticipatory grief and may be associated with fewer abnormal responses to grief after the death. This is important information for health-care professionals, who often feel helpless in terms of assisting parents in facing the death of a child. However, Rando cautioned that there are two variables that place parents at higher risk in terms of adaptation to the loss. Parents whose child has been ill for longer than 18 months may have a more difficult adaptation to their loss. Rando attributed this to the possibility that the stress of long-term illness lessens parents' ability to cope in all aspects. The sequence of remissions and relapses occurring in the course of chronic illness, and the resulting parental denial, may counteract the positive aspects of anticipatory coping. Other parents who are at higher risk for complicated grief are those who have experienced previous losses (Rando, 1986).

Cancer is the number one cause of childhood death caused by disease, while accidents are the leading cause of all childhood deaths (National Center for Health Statistics, 2004). Medical advances including new drugs and treatment options have turned cancer from a terminal illness to a chronic illness. The impact of cancer on families includes long or repeated hospital stays with resultant close relationships developing between families and staff. Consequently, the majority of research has looked at cancer-related deaths in terms of both parental and sibling grief. It is only recently that research has begun to look at responses to sudden death.

The sudden and unexpected death of a child due to tragic accident or injury throws the entire family into chaos. For parents, sudden accidental death usually carries with it some implication of fault or preventability that may or may not be resolved within the family. Violent and traumatic deaths raise anxiety levels and may negatively affect the grief process (Davies, 1999). Siblings involved in a traumatic death often feel much more vulnerable and require additional support before achieving a sense of being safe in similar circumstances. The inability to provide factual information regarding accidental deaths (e.g., the drowning death of a strong swimmer) may cause greater confusion for children.

The response of grieving siblings may be different if the death has been sudden and unexpected. According to Wolfelt (1996), the more sudden the death, the more likely the child is to mourn in doses and to push away the pain at first. Caring adults may be concerned by the siblings' apparent lack of feeling. In fact, there may be fewer outward expressions of grief. A pilot study by Davies and Kalischuk in 1997 looked at the bereavement responses of siblings experiencing a sudden versus a long-term death. Preliminary results support the view that sudden death is far more disruptive to survivors. In addition, children who have experienced the traumatic and sudden death of a sibling scored consistently lower on self-esteem tests (Davies, 1999).

Johnson and Mattson (1992) identified three major variables in a family's response to crises. These include severity of the event causing the crisis, personal resources of the individual or family, and social resources (i.e., who is available and what assistance they are able to provide). For health-care professionals, therapeutic interventions should be aimed at assessing the patient and family situation, mobilizing coping resources, and discovering coping strategies. The presence of a trauma response team to provide a total psychosocial assessment should include social work, pastoral care, and child life to help meet the needs of all family members. Team members should use an empathetic approach, which Johnson and Mattson (1992) defined as the ability to identify feelings, restate and clarify responses of family members, listen quietly, and validate a family's loss.

Because even a few hours of time spent in a critical care unit following a sudden and traumatic injury gives families time to begin integrating what is happening, health-care professionals have been able to identify supportive measures that assist families in coping. But what about the family whose child dies in the emergency department?

A study by Jones (1978) helped to identify four major areas of intervention at the time of sudden death. The first intervention occurs at the time of the family's arrival at the hospital. Family members should be met immediately, and escorted to a private area where a staff member stays with the family. All known information is shared, especially the extent of the child's injuries. Additional updates on medical conditions should be provided at pre-arranged intervals of time.

Notification of the death is the next crisis intervention point. A physician who is honest and compassionate should do it. Nonverbal communication is also significant, with physical touch important, if a family will accept it. Clarification of misconceptions and feelings of guilt should be included in the interaction, with adequate time for questions by parents and other family members. It is crucial to give reassurance that everything was done that could be done (Jones, 1978). A study by Owens, Fulton, and Markhusen (1982) reported that the single greatest effect on grief responses identified by families was the manner in which parents were informed of the death.

Following notification of the death, the next area of critical intervention is viewing of the body (Jones, 1978). Generally, it is accepted that the long-term outcomes are better for those who are able to see the body of a loved one as it helps people who are grieving come to terms with the death (Haas, 2003). Family members need to be prepared for changes in the body. A single staff member should provide a supportive presence during viewing of the body while allowing some private time. No time limits need apply. Each family determines their own schedule. Studies indicate that for most families the opportunity to see and touch the body helps actualize the death and is reported by grieving families as a choice they were glad to have made (Back, 1991).

Finally, Jones (1978) identified the concluding process as the last important intervention following death in the emergency department. A formalized sequence of signing papers, including the body release form, helps to bring closure to this initial portion of grief. Families should be directed in the process of funeral home notification, if appropriate, and told what needs to happen in the following hours or days. It is also beneficial to provide informational resources about initial grief responses and available support services. (The inclusion of siblings in the initial response to traumatic death is covered in the segment on sibling grief.)

Supportive Interventions at the Time of Death in the Hospital

In a recent study of age-specific death rates for all deaths in the United States that occur in intensive care units in hospitals, the highest rate (43%) was for infants; rates ranged from 18% to 26% among older children and adults (Angus et al., 2004). Supportive interventions at the time of a child's death on any unit within the hospital should be detailed in policies that reflect the philosophy of family-centered care. The ability of parents to make as many choices as possible is of ultimate importance, as it restores parenting roles in a situation where everything may appear to be out of control. The word *choices*, rather than *decisions*, may be helpful to indicate that the parent did not have to "decide" about ending treatment, only the manner and timing. This may help to reduce grieving parents' guilt about giving up too soon, which is a common concern in later grief work.

Health-care professionals may help parents identify significant support persons and encourage their presence at the bedside when a child is dying. Providing a private place close to the unit but away from the bedside allows family members opportunities to talk, support one another, and make necessary phone calls. A staff person should check frequently to answer questions and respond to needs, while giving the family time to grieve together. The ability to voice empathy by acknowledging feelings of family members is important while listening a lot and talking less (Pearson, 1999).

Providing access to available resources is also important: (a) social work for crisis intervention and support; (b) pastoral care to offer spiritual support; (c) child life to address issues of surviving siblings and other children involved in the death; (d) bereavement counselors for complex needs of particular family members; and (e) hospice or palliative care staff, if appropriate. The process at the time of death should be described, as well as choices the family may have about saying good-bye, either at the bedside or in another suitable place. Parents should be encouraged to participate in cares at the time of the death (e.g., holding, bathing, dressing). Including siblings and extended family, especially grandparents, should be discussed by staff and parents. Some families may need reassurance that all requests, rituals, or plans at the time of the death are acceptable and based only on the parents' needs and wishes.

The concept of memory making is a critical part of supportive caring at the time of the death. This may include

- a lock of hair,
- an ink or plaster hand or foot prints (see Figure 6.3),
- photographs of family and child before and/or after the death,
- comfort objects used at the time of the death (e.g., stuffed animals, quilt), and
- the gown worn at time of the death.

One child life specialist is careful to place an extra stuffed animal at the bedside for each surviving sibling so that they have their own comfort objects to cherish after the death. Clergy members sometimes use a seashell for baptisms and blessings, thus providing another memento for the family to keep.

Private time at the bedside following the death of a child may vary greatly, depending on the family's needs. Providing this may seem troublesome for staff of busy critical care units, but accommodations need to be made for this critical time. Sometimes a family also may need staff help to actually conclude this final visit. One mother described her feelings of knowing that

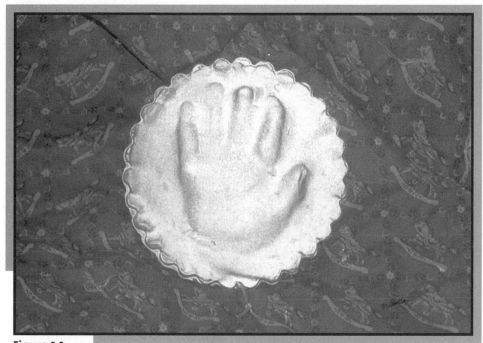

Figure 6.3.
A plaster cast of the child's hand provides a treasured keepsake for the family.

it was time to leave her child, but of not being able to actually lay the child back in bed. She recalls, years after the death, the precious memory of the ICU physician holding her child and rocking quietly as the family left the unit. Similarly, it may help the family a great deal if they are reassured that a favorite staff member will accompany the child to the morgue after the family has left.

Finally, parents need to be accompanied out of the hospital when leaving after their child's death. After all personal belongings, photos, and so on have been gathered and packed, and good-byes said to unit staff, the actual process of leaving may be extremely difficult for family members. Walking the family to the car offers physical and emotional support. Pastoral care staff members in one hospital provide a new teddy bear for mothers to clutch when leaving the hospital after her infant has died. This object of physical touching may help fill the void of empty arms and is reported to be especially comforting for some parents.

The Dying Child

For many years, child development experts believed that children younger than 10 years of age did not have the cognitive ability to express feelings or experiences related to their own death. Research into the fatally ill child's awareness of death began with Waechter's classic study in 1971. Results of her study indicated that children who are terminally ill are most often protected by adult silence, but, if given both the encouragement and the opportunity, they will talk about their understanding of their illness and fears (Waechter, 1971).

In 1978, Bluebond-Langner studied the interactions of children who were patients on an oncology unit. Her observations and interviews published in her book, *The Private Worlds of Dying Children*, provide great insight into how children learn about their illness, treatment, and prognosis in stages, each marked by the acquisition of important information. The stages are as follows:

1. Realization that "it" is a serious illness
2. Understanding of the names of the drugs, uses, and side effects
3. Knowledge of the procedures and treatments, relationships between symptoms and procedures, each viewed as unique and isolated events
4. Realization that the disease is a series of remissions and relapses
5. Understanding that the disease will cause death when drugs are no longer effective

As a child passed through each of the above stages, Bluebond-Langner observed that the child went through similar stages related to differing self-concepts.

1. Well at diagnosis
2. Seriously ill and will get better (evidenced by responses of family and friends, and physical changes in themselves)
3. Always ill and will get better
4. Always ill and will never get better (relapses and drug complications threatened child's sense of well-being)
5. Dying (only realized when child heard of the death of a peer)

Stages of acquisition of information and stages of changes in self-concept correspond and may be charted on a continuum (see Figure 6.4). Points on the continuum depict catalytic experiences and events in the child's illness journey.

Despite the parent's refusal to acknowledge the impending death and engage the child in preparation, the behaviors of the children provided clues that they did actually realize their imminent death. The children Bluebond-Langner observed exhibited nine types of behavior (Bluebond-Langner, 1978, p. 234):

1. Avoidance of deceased children's names and belongings
2. Lack of interest in non–disease-related conversations or play
3. Preoccupation with death and disease imagery in play, art, and literature

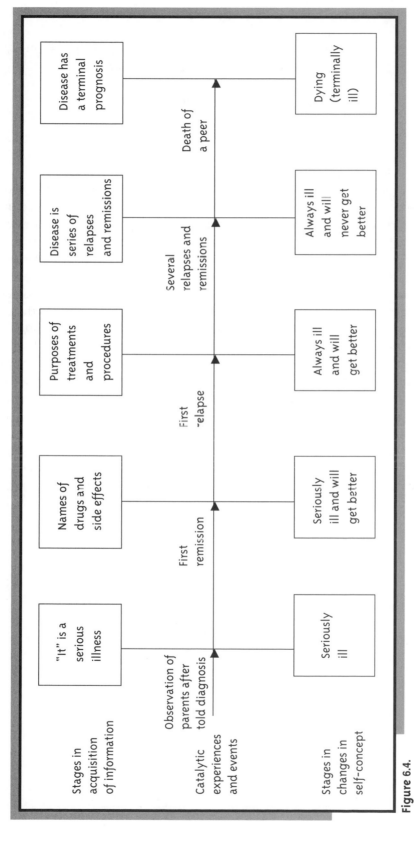

Figure 6.4.

Children acquire knowledge of their disease's process, treatment, and prognosis in stages. *Note.* From *Children Mourning; Mourning Children* (p. 117), by K. J. Doka, 1995, Bristol, PA: Hospice Foundation of America. Copyright 1995 by Hospice Foundation of America. Reprinted with permission.

4. Engagement of selected individuals in either disclosures, conversations, or disclosure speeches
5. Anxiety about increased debilitation and about going home, but for different reasons than earlier on in the disease process
6. Avoidance of talk about the future
7. Concern that things be done immediately
8. Refusal to cooperate with relatively simple, painless procedures
9. Establishment of distance from others through displays of anger or silence

The children in her study exhibited a complex form of mutual pretense between themselves and their parents, and between themselves and medical personnel. The author challenges health-care professionals to develop a policy that allows children to talk openly about their illness or prognosis with those whom they choose while still protecting those people, such as their parents, whom they may wish to protect in order to keep them close. Additionally, the child who is terminally ill may not directly disobey societal restrictions to talk openly about the death, but rather will approach the process of gaining information through highly symbolic questions and interactions (Bluebond-Langner, 1978; Sourkes, 1995).

The spiral of grief and anticipatory grief often begins when another child patient dies. Previously unexpressed fears and thoughts of separation begin to be more openly evident or observed. Children may become increasingly sensitive to the effects of separation as though in preparation for the separation caused by death. Play themes may focus on disappearance and return, or elaborate games of hide and seek, which test whether the child's absence would be noticed or missed (Sourkes, 1995). More recent study has been made of the effects of anticipatory grief in the dying child. Sourkes (1995) stated, "The child's view of his or her own illness is irrevo-

Guidelines for Intervention with a Child Who Is Dying	1. Do not underestimate the child's capacity to understand.
	2. Create open communication but do not force it.
	• Listen first, then offer support.
	• Provide honest information.
	• Remember that it is okay to say, "I don't know."
	• Answer only what the child wants to know.
	3. Provide creative outlets for anger, such as art.
	4. Follow the child's lead.
	5. Be honest with the child about impending death.
	6. Allow the child time to say good-byes.
	7. Permit the child to decide when he or she wants to share the pain of grief.

cably changed by the evidence that the possibility of death can be transformed into actuality. This is especially true of the first death that the child encounters" (p. 147).

The terminal phase is described as the point when the child's illness no longer responds to conventional treatment. The child becomes aware that there are few remaining options, and attention turns from cure to palliative care. This phase may last for days or weeks or months with experimental treatment or no treatment. During this phase, the most important choices may be related to pain management and the exploration of palliative care options (Sourkes, 1995). (See section on palliative care.)

The end of the terminal phase is marked by the child gradually turning inward. His or her physical energy is directed toward physical survival and there may be few opportunities for talking. The child may retreat from physical contact and pull into himself or herself and away from others. Preparing parents for these new behaviors as normal and expected as the child nears death will help avoid feelings of rejection often felt by the parents. Rephrasing this concept as the child pulling "into" himself or herself rather than "away" from others may also lessen a parent's reaction to this experience (Sourkes, 1995). For other guidelines on intervening with a child who is dying, see box.

It is not unusual for children who are dying to continue to fight death long beyond their expected endurance. This process can be exhausting for the child and for the family and staff at their side. One explanation for this struggle is that the child is trying to stay alive for some particular reason: There may be a misunderstanding of terms or the child knows how sad Mom and Dad will be when death finally arrives, and wants to postpone the event. Usually all that the child needs is permission from Mom or Dad or someone else on the parents' behalf—the struggle ends, and the child goes peacefully (see Case Study 6.2, Permission to Say Good-Bye).

---

8. Remember the child may choose to protect the parent (mutual pretense).
9. Help the dying child to live.
   - Make the child comfortable
     — Arrange physical setting for the child to be with family.
     — Create space for the child in family living area.
     — Plan family activities for the child to participate in or observe.
     — Arrange for medical equipment only as needed.

- Create special memorable moments.
- Continue some routine.
- Surround the child with people who mean the most to the child.
- Help the child maintain peer friendships.

Note. From "Separation, Loss, and Bereavement," by L. Pearson, in *Core Curriculum for the Nursing Care of Children and Their Families* (p. 87), by M. Broome and J. Rollins (Eds.), 1999, Pittman, NJ: Jannetti. Copyright 1999 by Jannetti. Reprinted with permission.

Case Study 6.2
Permission To Say Good-Bye

A 12-year-old boy had been in the Intensive Care Unit for the past 4 weeks. Admitted to the hospital for seizures following a brief viral illness, his medical course had been incredibly complex. Each test, treatment, and surgery resulted in a further decline in his condition, leaving him with multisystem failure. His parents and adolescent brother sat by his bedside almost continuously and had come to realize that he would not survive. The choice to provide supportive care until his death is one that this family approached with the same control and information-based approach that they used since his very first hospital day.

After discussing the details of supportive care, especially the concerns of pain control, his mother turned her attention to meeting the needs of extended family and friends. She invited four of John's best friends to gather at the bedside to say good-bye to John. Staff and John's parents prepared these sixth-graders in the supportive presence of their parents for this difficult bedside visit. The boys undertook their task with age-appropriate style, talking and laughing about shared experiences while looking at the many photographs surrounding John's bedside. Following the modeling of John's parents, the friends gained strength and comfort from the belief that John was able to hear their expressions of friendship and love, despite his unresponsiveness. As is often the case, this touching scene was extremely emotional for gathered adults and staff while the boys managed the visit in an easy style.

Supportive care without aggressive treatments began on Thursday, and John died 2 days later. In the words of John's mother, "We had been telling John that he would be going home soon. Our interpretation of 'home' was heaven. It wasn't until we talked to Dr. P., one of John's physicians, in the ICU on Saturday morning that we realized what we were telling John was probably being interpreted differently by John. Our son was an incredible fighter, as he had demonstrated over the weeks of his hospitalization. We realized that John was fighting to stay alive so that he could go home from the hospital. Dr. P. asked us if we would feel comfortable talking to John and giving him permission to stop fighting. We went back to John's room and told him that it was okay to stop fighting. We told him that he would be going to heaven to be with God, and we would be with him again one day. Within minutes after having this conversation with John, his breathing pattern changed, and he became diaphoretic. Family was called back to his bedside, and within a few hours John died. That moment when his respirations changed and he broke out in a sweat will be forever engrained in my memory. It was a powerful moment for his father and me. We were sure he heard us, and he was relieved to have Mom and Dad's permission to say good-bye."

Note. Courtesy of Kris and Bob Koebele.

The Dying Adolescent

A characteristic of a typical teenager's developmental level is the sense of invincibility and subsequent risk-taking behaviors. Additionally, teens often are acutely aware of their newly changing body and self-image as they develop a psychosexual identity. They develop a set of values, resolve conflicts related to dependence and independence, and start making vocational choices and setting goals (Buckingham, 1989). Buckingham pointed out the contrast between these developmental milestones with the implications of terminal illness: (a) alteration in self-concept, (b) threats to body image caused by disease, (c) differences in interpersonal relationships, and (d) interference with future plans.

For an adolescent, the experience of living with a life-threatening illness requires the development of ongoing coping skills. While many adolescents demonstrate resilience and the ability to face new challenges despite setbacks, other adolescents may have difficulty in coping, as evidenced by increased noncompliance, behavioral problems, and disruptions in peer relationships (Morgan, 1990). One intervention that is often effective is involvement in peer support groups. Because the dependence on peers is a natural developmental task, using the peer group as a way to encourage the exchange of ideas and information may be valuable (Morgan, 1990). Opportunities to share common experiences and explore coping strategies may help boost an adolescent's self-esteem and facilitate adjustment to treatment. Giving permission to express fears and concerns as well as difficulties in daily living related to diagnosis and prognosis is found in peer support within the group setting. Providing a social structure within which adolescents are able to develop coping skills and respond proactively to illness-related causes also helps teens to feel empowered and in control of their lives and their future.

When an adolescent realizes that a cure is no longer possible and begins the process of saying good-bye, health-care professionals may make a difference by using techniques of empathetic listening. To be the person that the adolescent chooses to help prepare others for his or her upcoming death is indeed a privileged role. Pazola and Gerberg (1990) developed guidelines for talking with a dying adolescent while supporting the developmental tasks of fostering independence and control (see next box).

Hospice and Palliative Care

The task of understanding the complexity of the child and family as they live through the experience of a child's dying is enormous. The need to give care and attempt the relief of suffering is just as great as the need to cure and should be no less an ultimate goal of medicine.

—Liben, 1996, p. 28.

Guidelines for Communicating with the Adolescent Who Is Dying	1. Tell the adolescent he or she is dying.
	  • When disease is progressing and treatment is not working, the adolescent needs to be given the permission to talk about death.
	  • Plan for the supportive presence of parents, physician, nurse, and significant others.
	  • Answer questions such as "Why?" and "What will happen next?" with honesty, sensitivity, and directness.
	  • Adolescents will confide in caregivers who are able to tolerate the overwhelming sadness of impending death.
	2. Acknowledge sadness of this news on patient, parents, and caregivers.
	3. Allow adolescent time to make plans, bring closure.
	4. Intervene if denial occurs.
	  • The adolescent who states she's going to be an Olympic swimmer may be expressing wishes of what she had hoped would be her future.

The Hospice Movement

The concept of hospice dates back to ancient times. The U.S. hospice movement began in the 1960s. Although there are free-standing hospices, hospice care is primarily provided in the patient's home to maintain peace, comfort, and dignity. Hospice care relies on the combined knowledge and skill of an interdisciplinary team of professionals—physicians, nurses, medical social workers, therapists, counselors, and volunteers—who coordinate an individualized plan of care for each patient and family. Hospice reaffirms the right of every person and family to participate fully in the final stage of life. Components of hospice care include physical, psychological, social, and spiritual support for the child and family with a life-threatening illness (Grollman, 1995). One study indicates that approximately 64% of disease-related children's deaths occur in the home with support from home care or hospice (Klopfenstein, Hutchison, Clark, Young, & Ruymann, 2001).

Martinson established one of the earliest hospice-like programs in the United States in 1972 for children with cancer (Buckingham, 1983). It was developed as an alternative to hospital care and its associated costs at a time when the overwhelming effects of hospitalization on children were being extensively examined. The program helped to focus on the importance of patients' rights and the ability of parents to maintain control with the continuous availability of medical and nursing resources. Procedures were fully explained to parents, who then provided cares as much as possible. Parents were given information as to potential complications and possible scenarios. Parents also were able to employ those comfort measures that seemed most helpful to their child and appeared to reduce the child's perception of pain.

Martinson's program proved to be cost-effective while demonstrating psychosocial benefits for families as well. Children with cancer reported

- Redirect communication: "You wish that you could be well enough to do that."
- Reframe the situation with reassurance that the adolescent will not be alone.

5. Respond to indirect pleas for support.
   - Adolescent may need confirmation from caregivers that death is imminent or treatment is no longer working.
   - Last wishes may be made of caregivers to protect family members; teens are often especially protective of their parents' feelings.

6. Enable expression of needs and wishes to pursue unfinished business (i.e., make ac- commodations for teen to travel to say good-bye to close friends).

7. Advocate for the adolescent in ethical dilemmas of treatment and end of treatment choices.

8. Support decisions on how and where the adolescent wants to die.

Note. From "Separation, Loss, and Bereavement," by L. Pearson, in *Core Curriculum for the Nursing Care of Children and Their Families* (pp. 77–92), by M. Broome and J. Rollins (Eds.), 1999; adapted from "Privileged Communication: Talking with the Dying Adolescent," by K. S. Pazola and A. K. Gerberg, 1990, *Maternal Child Nursing, 19,* pp. 16–21. Copyright 1999 by Jannetti. Reprinted with permission.

feeling more secure in the comfortable setting of home and more involved in the activities of all members of the family. Of the children with cancer in her study who were old enough to express an opinion, all preferred being at home to being in the hospital. Parents reported that they felt more in control and less stressed in meeting the needs of all family members when not forced to spend time at the hospital and at home (Grollman, 1995).

Following the death of a child at home rather than in the hospital, Martinson's study demonstrated that parents whose child died at home went through the same grieving process as other parents but were able to return to work and other responsibilities sooner (Grollman, 1995). Research indicated that these parents also were able to focus more often on positive aspects of the child's life and minimize feelings of guilt or bitterness about the loss of their child.

Another study of children who died at home looked specifically at the effects of home deaths on siblings. Mulhern, Lauer, and Hoffman (1983) concluded that siblings of patients who received hospice care at home felt less isolated and fearful and more socially valued than siblings of patients who died in the hospital. In addition, siblings included in home care exhibited fewer neurotic and somatic behaviors and returned to school with less disruption than the siblings of hospitalized patients.

Trend to Palliative Care

In recent years, the term *palliative care* has been gradually replacing the term *hospice care*. Palliative care is a broad philosophy of total, compassionate care that meets the physical, social, psychological, and spiritual needs of the patient and family when cure is no longer possible. This includes care of children with life-limiting illnesses through to those in the terminal phase of their illness (World Health Organization & International Association for the Study of Pain, 1998). The term *palliative care* extends the concept of care beyond the sometimes negative connotation of hospice, meaning "imminent" death, to include a longer timeframe when new treatment options are no longer available, but there is still quality of life for a family. In addition, palliative care broadens the scope to apply to other illnesses that are life limiting (i.e., neuro-degenerative and metabolic disorders, severe congenital abnormalities, muscular dystrophy, organ failures, HIV/AIDS; Goldman, 1996). Palliative care is defined as care for a child who has a high potential for death within a less precise timeframe. The term *palliative care* helps reduce the assumption that death will occur soon, and for children this is especially important, as it is more difficult to predict length of life. Palliative care focuses on pain and symptom management with the possibility of death. It also looks at the grieving process across the span of life, regardless of when death occurs. Palliative care may be provided in the hospital or at home, and serves as a complement to primary care medicine.

In the hospital setting, palliative care may not mean stopping all technologic support, but rather, it may mean changing the focus to less active and technologically intense forms of medical care. Even in the neonatal intensive care unit, families may be provided privacy, a comfortable environment that is physically removed from the sounds of high-tech equipment alarms and the demands of intensive care. It is important to shift the focus from the needs of the patient to the needs of the grieving family. A less restrictive visiting policy, especially for siblings, should be encouraged. Attention to requested wishes of parents is part of family-centered care and may require some accommodations on the part of staff to support family choices. For example, after making the difficult decision to withdraw ventilator support from their infant born with a devastating genetic abnormality, a family was moved from the private room in the neonatal intensive care unit to a larger room on another unit. This move accommodated the family's wish to videotape the final hours of the infant's life with the surrounding presence of extended family.

Although at times staff may struggle with family wishes for supportive end-of-life care, at other times sensitive and caring staff may make critical decisions that provide great support for families. A mother and father whose newborn infant son was dying in the intermediate intensive care unit of a hospital recall "the one good night" they shared as a couple with their newborn son. An insightful nurse rearranged the room to accommodate two day beds pushed together to form a double bed and allowed both parents to sleep there with the baby between them (Pearson, 1997).

Death at Home Versus Death in the Hospital

How do families decide on care in the hospital or at home for their terminally ill child? The realization that curative treatments are no longer possible is often devastating to family and health-care professionals. In the case of cancer, the child who relapses, as well as the child's family, suffers the same feelings of grief, shock, and depression that were present at diagnosis (Stevens, Smith, & O'Riordan, 1996). The difference is that this time these same feelings are heightened when combined with a sense of lost hope. For families, Stevens and colleagues noted,

> transition to palliative care becomes a confirmation of an earlier fear and there may even be a sense of relief expressed that the worst has happened, or knowing that the child's death will definitely occur, that now the uncertainty is gone and preparations can be made. (p. 54)

Families must turn from hope for a cure to hope for a death without pain, and in a setting that is right for their unique wishes and needs. Health-care providers are responsible for helping the child and family by communicating necessary information with empathy and sensitivity. A positive approach includes the responsibility to listen to the child's questions and concerns as well as their choices. It may be important to look not only at how the family will handle the palliative care phase, but also life after the child's death.

Although the hospital setting offers greater security for managing potentially frightening complications at time of death, and older children, teen patients, and parents may feel safer with trusted staff available, Stevens et al. (1996, p. 52) listed the following advantages to dying at home:

- less disruption of family life
- nursing care by parents
- sibling participation
- ability to provide child's food preferences
- greater privacy
- freedom from hospital routines
- ready access to all family members, friends, possessions, and pets

Some disadvantages would include the following (Stevens et al., 1996, p. 52):

- watching child's physical decline
- coping with nights
- handling fears of what may happen at time of death
- dealing with medical complications (e.g., seizures, hemorrhaging)
- domestic difficulties, including care of siblings

A decision to provide care for a child who is dying at home will require a simple management plan that addresses all parental concerns. Information should include attention to all practical details that help to give parents confidence and control. Knowing the possible progression of the disease, available pain medications, how death is likely to occur, and what will be required at the time of death will add to parents' ability to cope (Goldman, 1996; Stevens et al., 1996). Pain management can be accomplished by making the prevention and alleviation of pain a primary goal, partnering with the patient and parents, and aggressively using appropriate pharmacologic and non-pharmacologic interventions (Hooke, Hellsten, Stutzer, & Forte, 2002). Perhaps the most important component of palliative care in the home setting is focused on the supportive presence or readily accessible support of members of the health-care team. When families face the most difficult aspects of a child's death in any setting, dedicated professionals often provide the information, reassurance, and resources for families to face what is to come with confidence and courage. As physicians frequently affirm, families may not remember or even acknowledge explicit details of medical care, but they remember vividly the names and faces of those staff members who were present, supportive, and caring at the time of their child's death.

Although no one individual or group can provide all of the necessary services, institutions and agencies that provide palliative care services should develop a comprehensive palliative care package to ensure that the certain ingredients are available, and that the child, family, and health professionals have access to them. The following services can be achieved by combining available resources and sharing established expertise through partnerships among various individuals and agencies (Frager, 1996):

- ongoing supportive care linked to the child and family at the time of diagnosis
- early and continuing intervention for psychosocial and spiritual support
- management of pain and other symptoms
- liaison between tertiary care center and local health community
- a sibling support program
- support for staff in dealing with critically ill children
- a school reintegration program
- a humanistic approach within high-tech arenas of care
- a school visitation program for schoolmates and teachers of terminally ill children
- an ethics committee approachable by any concerned member of the caregiving team
- anticipatory grief counseling and bereavement follow-up
- a speakers bureau to share information about palliative care with the medical and lay communities

Spiritual Care of the Dying Child

"Children try to understand not only what is happening to them but why, and in doing that, they call upon the religious life they have experienced, the spiritual values they have received, as well as other sources of explanation" (Coles, 1990, p. 100). The development of children's awareness of their own illness and dying has been examined in the literature (Bluebond-Langner, 1978). Knowledge of this capacity of children prompts close attention to their spiritual needs. Because a child's body is connected to all that a child is and will become psychologically, behaviorally, socially, and intellectually, the experience of illness threatens a child's total being (Attig, 1996). It not only interrupts his or her ongoing life, with the impact of hospitalization and treatment, but it often disturbs the child's sense of invulnerability. The child who is ill may feel different, which may disturb relationships between the child and the rest of his or her world. The experience of being ill or facing death challenges a child's system of beliefs.

Seeking answers to questions about the meaning of their experience, children rely on their particular spiritual development to provide explanations and offer support (Attig, 1996). Fears of children who are dying may focus on the threat of pain and the possibility of being alone, as well as needing to know how they will be remembered after their death. Health-care professionals may reassure children who are dying that they will never be alone unless they choose to be. Including the children in planning cares and making treatment decisions may help them feel less powerless and helpless. Providing a listening presence often encourages them to talk about spiritual concerns, which may be expressed directly or symbolically. Drawing, writing, or play may help in expressing spiritual concerns. Asking children to explain their creative work in their own words helps to prevent misinterpretation.

An assessment of spiritual needs of the child and family helps to identify issues as well as strengths of a family's religious beliefs. Addressing the spiritual needs of parents must be a priority, and is necessary in order for parents to support their dying child. In a national survey of pastoral care services in children's hospitals, pastoral care providers identified three barriers to providing spiritual care: (a) inadequate staffing of the pastoral care office; (b) inadequate training of health-care professionals to detect patients' spiritual needs; and (c) being called too late to provide all of the care that could have been offered (Feudter, Haney, & Dimmers, 2003). The resources provided by pastoral care or a family's own spiritual leader as part of the health-care team may be a positive contribution to family-centered care of the whole family. Core activities of the hospital pastoral care staff include (a) resolving hopelessness, despair, anger, fear, and anxiety; (b) promoting hope and celebration; (c) resolving actual loss; (d) providing ministry of company; (e) maintaining an intact identity; and (f) providing specialized pastoral interventions (Gibbons, Retsaas, & Pinikahana, 1999). Within many hospitals, the presence of pastoral care provides another caring person to listen to the child and family, and respond supportively using particular gifts of ministry.

For more on spirituality, see Chapter 9: Spiritual Issues in Children's Health-Care Settings.

Culturally Sensitive Grief Work

"What people who have experienced a loss believe, feel and do, varies enormously from culture to culture" (Irish, Lundquist, & Nelsen, 1993, p. 114). Culturally sensitive grief work requires particular attention to the needs of every family and the unique cultural heritage of which members are a part. Initially, a simple awareness of cultural differences was broadly generalized into categories as if all members of a certain heritage believed and practiced the same rituals. This approach is limited and inconsistent with a policy of family-centered care. There is a great deal of diversity within common ethnic groups and children may represent a new generation that is partially assimilated into the dominant culture (Grollman, 1995).

For many families, the practices associated with medical care and decision making in the critical care settings may be difficult. Family culture may not encourage assertiveness in relation to medical authority (Shapiro, 1994). Family and extended family support for a child may require leniency in terms of restricted visitation and hospital policies. Treatment decisions may have both medical and moral consequences and tremendous impact on a family's subsequent grief or their ability to come to terms with the death. Translators must be provided to help families understand not just the present medical treatment, but also the family's options to say "no" to medical treatments that are not consistent with religious or cultural beliefs (Shapiro, 1994).

To provide culturally supportive care requires the realization that normal indicators of previous experience with death may not apply. People from different cultural backgrounds may be grieving significant losses on a chronic basis (i.e., loss of homeland, loss of possessions, loss of native language, tradition; Grollman, 1995).

A series of questions has been developed for health-care professionals to address in making plans for supporting parents and families facing the death of a child (McGoldrick et al., 1991):

- What are the prescribed rituals for handling dying, the dead body, the disposal of the body, and rituals to commemorate the loss?
- What are the group's beliefs about what happens after death?
- What do people believe about appropriate emotional expression and integration of a loss experience?
- What are the gender rules for handling a death?
- Are certain deaths particularly stigmatized (e.g., suicide) or traumatic for the group?

A recent experience in one setting illustrates the changing awareness and respect for culturally diverse grief practices. A Native American adolescent died in the Intensive Care Unit of a pediatric hospital. A large group of family and friends were gathered at the bedside. The family's religious beliefs required that a shaman perform a ceremony using eagle feathers to fan smoke from a fire to ensure the passage of the teen's soul beyond death. Nurses at the hospital recalled an incident more than 10 years earlier when a staff person discovered a similar ceremony being conducted in the Parent Waiting Room just outside the Intensive Care Unit. That ceremony had been stopped abruptly due to the overwhelming risk to the safety of all patients and staff. But this time, with staff and hospital administrators much more sensitive to the great variety of cultural practices of grieving families, arrangements were made to allow this ceremony to occur in an undeveloped building space close to the ICU but with safety factors also considered.

In a far more unsettling acquiescence to cultural demands and differences, a child life specialist in the same unit spent several hours working with two school-age siblings whose younger brother had become suddenly and seriously ill and was not expected to survive. The children in the playroom were interactive and quite knowledgeable about the beliefs of their Middle Eastern heritage in terms of a life after death for their brother who had chronic health concerns and special needs. They engaged in creating a memory book about their brother and were allowed to visit at the bedside in the presence of both parents and many young uncles and male family friends. After a period of time, the children returned to tell the child life specialist that they would be leaving the hospital soon. Conversations between the child life specialist and the uncle who had emerged as the spokesperson for the family failed to convince him that the children might better handle the sad nature of the sibling's death if allowed to stay with the family at the hospital. The children left a short time later. When the mother and all of the female relatives were also sent home before the anticipated death of the young son, it became clear to the child life professional that the decisions to send both the children and the mother home were not made out of failure to understand the grief needs of children, but rather in accordance with strict cultural beliefs about the death of a child.

Ethical Issues and End-of-Life Decisions

No issue is more difficult in the scope of meeting the psychosocial needs of children and families than the decisions related to end-of-life care. To recognize that a child is dying requires consummate energy and emotional investment on the part of families and caregivers. The realization that the intensity of high-tech medical care might be more appropriately replaced by supportive care signifies the abandonment of hope for a cure. It is at this most stressful time that decisions must be made and it is a time that is filled with ethical and moral conflicts. The goals of decision making require that any decision be made with the child's best interests in mind, and that decisions must be shared—a philosophy that has evolved with the focus of family-centered care.

According to Rushton and Glover (1990),

> To respect a child is to acknowledge the importance of his or her world and the relationships that are central to it. Unilateral decision-making by health care professionals based solely on "medical indications" would deny the fullness of a child's life and the value of the relationships that also benefit to sustain the child. (p. 207)

Thus, it is most important to create a partnership between the family, nursing staff, and physicians. Parents need professional guidance to face the issues of quality of life, knowing that the results of these decisions will have lifelong effects on the family. The ability to participate actively in decision making is often complicated by feelings of shock and disbelief when a child suddenly becomes critically ill or severely injured. Parents struggle with the transition from parenting a well child to parenting a critically ill child. Other factors having impact include inadequate information, emotional upheaval, uncertainty of diagnosis or prognosis, and distrust of medical professionals (Rushton & Glover, 1990).

One of the most difficult decisions health-care providers and parents may face involves life-support withdrawal (LSW). Votta and colleagues (2001) examined whether parental involvement in an LSW decision had an impact on the perceptions and adjustment of parents whose child died in a pediatric critical care unit. Responses of parents whose child died with an LSW decision were compared with those of parents whose child died without an LSW decision. Findings revealed that in comparison to parents whose child died without an LSW decision, a significantly greater number of parents whose child died following an LSW decision were certain about their child's future health; believed that their child's quality of life would have been unacceptable; and reported less dissatisfaction with time spent with their child, fewer negative changes in family functioning, and more positive changes in feelings toward staff.

Certain strategies have been identified as helpful for parents. The first is to provide an environment that may facilitate the family's ability to integrate information at this stressful time. This may be accomplished by taking the family away from the noises of medical monitors and alarms. Physicians should be unhurried and uninterrupted at this critical time, not only providing clear and honest information, but also listening and encouraging questions on the part of the family (Vose & Nelson, 1999). Asking the family to describe their perception of the present situation is helpful, and identifying the roles of various physicians involved in their child's care may reduce confusion. The longer a child stays in the Intensive Care Unit, the more opportunity there is for confusion as parents seek out information about their child's medical condition (Vose & Nelson, 1999). Providing continuity in caregivers, both nurses and primary physicians, will help families gather information while demonstrating clinical competencies, which helps in trust building.

Enhancing communication is the second strategy, which helps families process information vital to decision making. Asking parents to share their goals and desires for their child, as well as their values related to life, death, disability, and suffering, will encourage shared decision making (Rushton & Glover, 1990). Information should be provided about the details of the child's present condition, diagnosis, prognosis, risks, and benefits of further treatment. Nursing staff may play a critical role in helping present information clearly and objectively, yet with sensitivity. Often it is helpful to have several staff people hear the information with the family to enable clarification in areas of confusion. Providing written materials may help some families feel a greater sense of control (Vose & Nelson, 1999).

Discussion of pain and suffering helps parents explore their beliefs and what they feel would be the wishes of their child. Clarifying misconceptions is always crucial. Explaining observable or expected responses of the child to medical interventions such as suctioning helps reduce anxiety. Perhaps the most important concern of parents is the ability to keep their child comfortable and experiencing as little pain as possible.

In addition, assessment of the family's support systems and previous experiences with loss helps identify needs. Inadequate support systems may have a negative effect on family decision making (Rushton & Glover, 1990). Connecting at-risk families with hospital-based resources and supports should be a priority. Social services, child life, pastoral care, palliative care, and nursing bring different perspectives to total family-centered care and decision making and should be incorporated as available. Professionals who have greater knowledge of ethics, policies, and legal issues often feel more empowered as advocates for patients and families. It is important to realize that the process of decision making may have multiple steps, and assisting families from one level to the next often takes time. Information about particular responses to treatments or observations of the child's responses may help parents to think further about the implications of ongoing aggressive treatment.

Although the federal Patient Self-Determination Act (PSDA) supports the right of adults age 18 years and older to information regarding the execution of advanced directives, the spirit of PSDA creates opportunities for minors to participate in treatment decisions and rights to determine the circumstances of their death (Rushton & Lynch, 1992). Many children and teens do have the capacity to assist in making decisions about what is in their best interests. Rushton and Lynch (1992) suggested that children, by 11 or 12 years of age, should be assessed by the same criteria as is used for adults: (a) ability to comprehend essential information about their diagnosis and prognosis; (b) ability to reason about their choices in accordance with their values and life goals; and (c) ability to make an informed decision based on recognizing the important consequences of various courses of action. Further, it is felt that in the case of chronic illness, parents need to be supported throughout the process of illness and treatment to explore the wishes and beliefs of their child related to life-supporting medical technology (Vose & Nelson, 1999).

The standard of care in the "best interests of the child" focuses on the presumption of life, and when life can be saved, it should be. But when life cannot be saved, or the chance of survival is minimal and treatment would include repeated pain and suffering; invasive procedures; immobilization; and prolonged hospitalization and isolation from parents, family, and friends, then the decision of treatment should focus on comfort care while dying (Rushton & Glover, 1990).

Participation of Children at Funerals

One of the most frequently asked questions at the time of a child's death concerns the participation of siblings, cousins, and other children at funerals or memorial services. Because the experience of loss is so overwhelming, concerned family members often want to protect children from these feelings of sadness and loss. Yet children and teens that are included in rituals following the death of a loved one often demonstrate better coping skills and more favorable adjustment. The health-care professional may be the first person that families turn to for advice as they begin the experience of mourning the loss of a member of the family.

Wolfelt (1994, p. 13) described rituals as "symbolic activities that help us, together with our families and friends, express our deepest thoughts and feelings about life's most important events." He went on to describe the funeral ritual in the following manner:

> Rich in history and rife with symbolism, the funeral ceremony helps us acknowledge the reality of death, gives testimony to the life of the deceased, encourages expression of grief in a way consistent with the culture's values, provides support to mourners, allows for the embracing of faith and beliefs about life and death, and offers continuity and hope for the living. (p. 14)

For children to be invited to participate in funeral or memorial rituals requires preparation. If parents are unable either physically or emotionally to provide such preparation, then another trusted adult may do so. Children need to know what they will see, hear, feel, and be expected to do, as well as understand how adults may be expressing their feelings of loss. Attention to the physical presence of the body of the person who has died should address the state of being dead, the end of all physiological processes of life, opportunities to touch the body, and accepted behaviors. A child should never be forced to attend a funeral or do anything that may be uncomfortable.

Many funeral directors are becoming more knowledgeable about the needs of surviving children and may offer opportunities for grieving family members to be together at the funeral home or church before the arrival of extended family and friends. As intense as are the feelings of sadness for families is the need for children to grieve in manageable doses. It is also important to have appropriate play and art activities available for children during the long hours of visitation. Many families find that encouraging children to create memory photo displays, select favorite toys for the casket, or assume helpful roles during the public rituals also is supportive.

Assigning responsibility of young children to a trusted adult or family member other than the grieving parent also helps families. For older children and teens, actual participation in the rituals may be healing (i.e., reading scripture or original poetry, sharing an anecdote, or taking part in rituals of particular religious symbolism). Whatever roles families choose for incorporating children are good, as long as the child is prepared and supported throughout the experience. It is not essential or even developmentally possible for a child to understand exactly what is happening at every point. What is important is that the child is included in the family's expression of grief. Part of the healing process will be helping the child "grow into" understanding as they grow up with the loss within the context of their own family.

Memorial Programs and Bereavement Programming

The work of bereavement by definition begins at the moment of death. For health-care professionals, follow-up care constitutes bereavement programming. Goals of such programs are threefold: (a) to help families through the immediate crisis of their child's death, (b) to offer ongoing support and resources to bereaved families for a period of time after the death of a child, and (c) to provide support, education, and resources for staff (Brown & Sefansky, 1995).

Although availability of services varies greatly in different settings in terms of how support is given and by whom, certain elements of programming are assumed. Initially a family may need resources to help arrange for their child's funeral, with questions arising related to expenses, legal requirements, transport of the body, autopsy, and burial. Referral to appropriate resources within the family's home community may help the family find local supportive services. Pastoral care and social workers may be most helpful in addressing these first concerns. Physicians and other medical staff may be able to expedite concerns related to autopsy or organ donation. Child life should be available to answer questions related to the involvement of children and adolescents in rituals following a death. In the absence of child life services, a nurse, social worker, or other member of the health-care team who is highly skilled in the developmental and psychosocial needs of children should be available. Other members of the multidisciplinary bereavement committee may respond immediately or after initial plans are made. For some families with complicated grief or issues of violent and tragic death, mental health counselors may be especially helpful in the hours soon after death to help diffuse anger and address mental health needs.

In the days following the death, many health-care professionals support grieving families by their participation or presence in the planned funeral and memorial rituals. The presence of someone who cared for the child in the final hours of his or her sudden death or staff who knew the child for months or years during the struggle of a chronic life-threatening illness can be invaluable. It often helps families to find comfort in the realization that their child's life, if short or long, had importance to others. Many times a family's hospital stay may have occurred a long distance from home, especially in these days of high-tech treatment at tertiary care centers of excellence. For families who have traveled great distances for a child to have a bone marrow or organ transplant, the details and intensity of the medical experience may be simply incomprehensible to those family and friends who were not able to share in the experience of hospital treatment or be present at the time of death.

Sympathy notes by caregivers, follow-up phone calls, and the opportunity for families to return to the medical setting after the death all help families begin their grief work. Many bereaved parents return on special days, such as birthdays or anniversaries, to visit with staff or to bring memorial gifts to other patients in honor of their child who died. These expressions of helping others are often healing to families and health-care professionals. Recently a gentleman was found standing at the door to one of the empty rooms in an ICU. When asked if he needed help to find the patient he had come to visit, he replied, "No, my son died in this room 6 years ago, and I just needed to come by."

Hospitals have different ways to accomplish the overwhelming task of keeping records on the dates of death, birthdays, and significant dates in the lives of all the children who have died within the year. In some instances, bereavement counselors are the sole handlers of these follow-up contacts. In other places, staff nurses and others may be enlisted to accomplish the task of remembering for those families with whom they worked. The number of years that a family is followed also may vary. For many health-care professionals, there are certain families with whom lasting friendships have been made during the dying of a child, and the relationship with the family continues for long periods of time. The more challenging aspect of bereavement care is providing the same standard of caring for all families. The ability to provide this sensitive care for all families who have experienced a death is affected by cultural practices of grief, geographical distances, nontraditional family relationships, and the turnover of staff.

In some medical settings, memorial programs may be sponsored by the hospital for children whose death affected many caregivers and other personnel. The death of one young toddler who spent more than 2 years in a hospital affected many personnel, housekeeping, maintenance staff, dietary aides, nurses, physicians, and parents of other patients. The ability to hold a nonreligious memorial in the hospital auditorium was significant to honor this patient and helped many hospital personnel recognize their loss.

Many hospitals also provide memorial programs for families during the year. These programs are designed to help families who have lost a child to recognize their loss and share positive memories with other families who have had similar experiences. These programs usually include rituals to increase coping, such as reading the names of the children who have died, lighting candles, and encouraging conversation with health-care staff and other families. Particular issues such as coping with holidays and anniversaries may be included in programming. The provision of age-appropriate activities for siblings should be part of memorial programming as families mourn the loss together. Allowing families to create a memory symbol, light a candle, plant a flower, or create a quilt square may help to acknowledge their participation and continue the healing process in the days, weeks, and months to come.

Resources for grieving families include printed materials, which should be available in several languages, as well as lists of resources with the names of counselors and support groups within the family's community. Resources for parents to help siblings should also be included, with suggested activities and a bibliography of books for grieving children (see Appendix 6.1).

Hospitals with a pediatric trauma center may also provide resources particular to traumatic death for families and for schools. Including health-care personnel who were involved in the initial on-site treatment of a child or the transport to the hospital is often helpful for families, especially siblings who may have been present at the scene of the injury or accident but not able to accompany parents to the tertiary medical center. At one children's hospital in the Midwest, the Flight for Life crew welcomes the opportunity to take siblings and other family members up to the helicopter landing area. Talking with a flight crew nurse or helicopter pilot frequently helps siblings sequence the events of the trauma while reassuring family that the child was well cared for and supported during those first critical hours after the traumatic event. A photograph of a sibling sitting in the pilot's seat of the helicopter helps a child master feelings of insecurity and vulnerability in addition to being the source of much discussion when the child returns to school.

Support to communities may include visits by bereavement or trauma team members to help children who have experienced the death of a classmate, or children who have witnessed a traumatic injury or death. Helping children understand the death of another child caused by accidental injury may require the combined skills of social work, nursing, pastoral care, and child life as children struggle with the sudden nature of loss and with their own vulnerability and loss of feelings of safety. Injury prevention for school-age children may be an important part of integrating a death and moving forward with an increased sense of control and security. In one intervention in a local community, a nurse, chaplain, social worker, and child life specialist visited several classrooms after the preschool sister of one of the students was struck by a motor vehicle in the crosswalk in front of the school's entrance. Helping the children to understand what they had seen, facilitating discussion of feelings related to the incident, reassuring children while reviewing issues of safety, and encouraging age-appropriate processing through art and journaling helped students and teachers cope. The school crossing guard, whose feelings of guilt were overwhelming, was a welcome participant in the debriefing process.

Support groups for parents, grandparents, and siblings are another important element of bereavement programming. For parents to work together with other parents who have experienced the untimely death of a child often is crucial to beginning grief work. Facilitated by bereavement counselors, these parent groups allow parents to express feelings, vent anger and frustration, share ideas for coping, and help reduce feelings of isolation and utter hopelessness.

Support groups for grieving children accomplish similar goals within the context of age-appropriate activities. For children, the opportunity to know other children who have experienced similar losses is significant to gain peer understanding and normalize experiences. Groups provide a safe and appropriate place to express many scary issues and feelings. Because the grieving parent may be emotionally unavailable for the grieving child, a peer group may provide alternative ways to enhance a child's sense of competence and self-esteem. Children's support groups may include discussion of problem areas of coping, art activities to facilitate expression of feelings and concerns, and social time to reassure grieving children and teens that it is still okay to laugh and have fun. Many of the tasks of childhood described by Wolfelt (1996), in terms of reconciling the loss and moving forward with memories and a changed self-identity, are easily addressed within the context of a support group. Grieving children often demonstrate less resistance to group work than to individual counseling. Participants are extensively screened to be certain that the work of a peer group program is appropriate for each child or teen. And the ongoing presence of a group helps children and teens continue to learn new coping styles as their developmental or family needs change. Many child life specialists are specially trained in the skills of supporting grieving children and are excellent facilitators of groups, incorporating knowledge of normal developmental needs of children and teens, the impact of grief, and the therapeutic expression of feelings through play and art.

Disengagement Versus Continuing Bonds

The view of grief most accepted during the past century holds that for successful mourning to take place the mourner must disengage from the deceased, and let go of the past. It has only been in these past 100 years that continuing bonds have been denied as a normal part of bereavement behavior. Klass, Silverman, and Nickman (1996) suggested that we need to consider bereavement as a cognitive as well as an emotional process that takes place in a social context of which the deceased is a part. The process does not end, but bereavement affects the mourner in different ways for the rest of his or her life. People do not "get over" the experience; rather, they are changed by it. Part of the change is a transformed but continuing relationship with the deceased. According to Klass and colleagues (1996),

> Accommodation, in its full Piagetian sense, may be a more suitable term than recovery, closure, or resolution. Accommodation in this context is not a static phenomenon. People do not change in some time-limited bereaved condition and then remain unchanging until their next bereavement. Accommodation is a continual activity, related both to others and to shifting self-perceptions as the physical and social environment changes and as individual, family, and community developmental processes unfold. It is a continual process because individuals and communities continually construct meaning in the interchanges between themselves and their world. Accommodation does not disregard past relationships, but incorporates them into a larger whole. In this process, people seek to gain not only an understanding of the meaning of death, but a sense of the meaning of this now dead or absent person in their present lives. (p. 19)

The deceased becomes part of a child's inner world. He or she continues the relationship by dreaming, by talking to the deceased, by believing that the deceased is watching, by keeping things that belonged to the deceased, by visiting the grave, and by frequently thinking about the deceased. These connections are not static, but are developmentally appropriate to the child and to the child's present circumstances.

Bereaved parents undergo a similar process to develop a set of memories, feelings, and actions to keep them connected to the deceased child (Klass et al., 1996). A study of a self-help group of bereaved parents revealed that the processes by which parents resolved their grief involved intense interaction with their dead children. They sustained these interactions using similar means to those of the bereaved children.

These findings cause us to rethink the way we talk about the resolution of grief. The concept of a continuing relationship presents a challenge to the idea that the purpose of grief is to sever the bonds with the deceased in order for the survivor to be free to make new attachments and to construct a new identity. According to Klass et al. (1996), these bonds do not end, they simply change.

Conclusion

Working with families during the death of a child can be an overwhelming and emotionally exhausting task for any health-care professional. Research in recent years has identified the impact of a child's death upon a family system, including parents, siblings, grandparents, and other extended family members. Long-term studies have demonstrated both the struggles and the resiliency of individuals affected by the loss of a child, sibling, or grandchild. Knowing the enormity of the issues facing the grieving family, research has also helped to identify those areas where the skills and expertise of health-care professionals may be supportive to families anticipating the death, experiencing the death, and facing the changed future. The ability to provide family-centered care in the midst of great sadness is a challenging but necessary role. Encouraging family participation in end-of-life cares and choices, preparing family members of all ages for imminent death at home or in the hospital setting, and fostering open communication within families and between families and medical staff have documented value for a family's ability to live beyond the loss (Walsh & McGoldrick, 1991).

Developing the professional skills and confidence to provide specific interventions to address the unique needs of each family when a child is dying is a challenging task. When asked what he would teach all new medical students and residents about caring for families at the time of death, one pediatric physician responded that it is a true privilege to be present at the time of a child's death. Another described that moment as a gift. Both went on to say that parents want to know that you knew what to do medically, but more important, that you cared about their child. Years after the death, families may not remember what medical interventions were used in an attempt to save their child, but they remember those health-care staff who were supportive by their presence at the time of death and afterward. "The way a child dies will remain in the memory of his parents forever" (Postovsky & Arush, 2004, p. 67). Another physician has written, "Many of us are not as comfortable in assuming a passive role—listening, sitting in silence, being supportive by our presence—as we are in taking on a specific action" (Schulman & Rehm, 1983, p. 993). It is also important to remember that there are critical roles for each member of the health-care team. As important as the respirator or the administration of pain-relieving medications is the placement of a beloved teddy bear in the dying child's hand.

Study Guide

1. Describe the impact of a child's death on parents, siblings, and other family members.

2. What are the phases of grief that parents experience?

3. How does grief affect marital and other relationships?

4. What factors influence children's understanding of death?

5. Describe responses of children to death and dying at various stages of development.

6. Why should death and dying be discussed with children?

7. In talking about death, what are the things to avoid saying or implying?

8. What are some interventions health-care providers can use to help parents and siblings?

9. Describe four areas for intervention in sudden death situations.

10. Describe various forms of end-of-life care and their functions and usefulness for children.

APPENDIX 6.1

Resources for Grieving Family Members

Organizations

A Place to Remember
De Ruyter-Nelson Publications, Inc.
1885 University Avenue, Suite 110
St. Paul, MN 55104
Toll-Free: 800/631-0973
Phone: 651/645-7045
Fax: 651/645-4780
www.aplacetoremember.com

Center for Loss and Life Transition
3735 Broken Bow Road
Fort Collins, CO 80526
Phone: 970/226-6050
Fax: 800/922-6051
www.centerforloss.com

Centering Corporation
1531 Saddle Creek Road
Omaha, NE 68104
Phone: 402/553-1200
Fax: 402/553-0507
www.centering.org

Children's Hospice International
2202 Mount Vernon Avenue, Suite 3C
Alexandria, VA 22301
Phone: 703/684-0330
Fax: 703/684-0226
www.chionline.org

The Compassionate Friends
National Headquarters
PO Box 3696
Oak Brook, IL 60522
Phone: 630/990-0010
Fax: 630/990-0246
www.compassionatefriends.org

National SHARE Office
Infant and Pregnancy Loss
St. Joseph's Health Center
300 First Capitol Drive
St. Charles, MI 63301
Toll-Free: 800/821-6819

Rainbow Connection
477 Hannah Branch Road
Burnsville, NC 28714
Phone: 704/675-5909
Fax: 704/675-9687

RTS Bereavement Services
1910 South Avenue
La Crosse, WI 54601
Toll-Free: 800/362-9567 ext. 4747

Books for Young Children

Aliki. (1991). *Christmas tree memories.* New York: HarperCollins.
    Family members admire the ornaments on their Christmas tree and share memories of previous holidays as evoked by the ornaments.

Carson, J. (1992). *You hold me and I'll hold you.* New York: Orchard Books.
    When a great-aunt dies, a young child finds comfort in being held and in holding, too.

Clifton, L. (1982). *Everett Anderson's goodbye.* New York: Henry Holt.
    Everett has a difficult time coming to terms with his grief after his father dies.

DePaola, T. (1973). *Nana upstairs and Nana downstairs.* New York: Putnam.
    A small boy enjoys his relationship with his grandmother and great-grandmother, but he learns to face their inevitable death.

Douglas, E. (1990). *Rachel and the upside down heart.* Los Angeles: Price, Stern, Slogan.
    The death of a little girl's father causes her to draw all her hearts upside down, but as she grows, she finds joy in her father's memory and begins to draw her hearts right side up.

Johnson, J., & Johnson, M. (1982). *Where's Jesse?* Omaha, NE: Centering Corp.
    A very young child tries to understand the death of his baby brother.

Lawton, S. (1990). *Daddy's chair.* Rockville, MD: Ken-Ben Copies.
    When Michael's father dies, his family sits Shiva, observing the Jewish week of mourning, and remembers the good things about him.

Melanie, B., & Kingpin, R. (1983). *Lifetimes: A beautiful way to explain death to children.* New York: Bantam Books.
    Explains life and death through plants, animals, and people living and dying in their time.

Miller, M. (1987). *My grandmother's cookie jar.* Los Angeles: Price, Stern, Sloan.
    Grandma passes on stories of her native people to her grandchild as they eat cookies together from the cookie jar.

Viorst, J. (1971). *The tenth good thing about Barney.* New York: Athenaeum.
    Young children learn about funeral rituals after the death of their cat named Barney.

Wilhelm, H. (1985). *I'll always love you.* New York: Athenaeum, Crown.
    A child's sadness at the death of a beloved dog is tempered by the remembrance of saying every night, "I'll always love you."

Books for Older Children and Teens

Blackburn, L. B. (1991). *The class in room 44: When a classmate dies.* Omaha, NE: Centering Corp.
    A story to help children understand their feelings related to the death of a classmate.

Bunting, E. (1990). *The wall.* New York: Clarion Books.

A boy and his father come from far away to visit the Vietnam Veteran's Memorial in Washington, DC, and find the name of the boy's grandfather, who was killed in the conflict.

Grollman, E. (1993). *Straight talk about death for teenagers.* Boston: Beacon Press.

Offers advice and answers the kinds of questions that teens are likely to ask themselves when grieving the death of someone close.

Hanson, W. (1997). *The next place.* Minneapolis, MN: Waldman House Press.

Suitable for all ages.

Krementz, J. (1976). *How it feels when a parent dies.* New York: Macmillan.

Eighteen children ages 7 to 16 years speak openly, honestly, and unreservedly of their experiences and feelings after a parent has died.

LeShan, E. (1976). *Learning to say good-bye: When a parent dies.* New York: Macmillan.

Text discusses the questions, fears, and fantasies many children feel when a parent or someone close to them dies.

LeShan, E. (1972). *What makes me feel this way?* New York: Macmillan.

Advice to school-age children about feelings of grief.

Romond, J. (1989). *Children facing grief: Letters from bereaved brothers and sisters.* St. Meinrad, IN: Abbey Press.

A collection of letters written by children and teens who have experienced the death of a sibling.

Rylant, C. (1992). *Missing May.* New York: Doubleday/Dell.

For older readers; winner of the 1993 Newbery Award. A 12-year-old girl and her uncle struggle to accept the death of Aunt May, who has raised her.

Traisman, E. (1992). *Fire in my heart, ice in my veins: A journal for teenagers experiencing a loss.* Omaha, NE: Centering Corp.

A write-in journal for teenagers experiencing a loss.

References

Angus, D., Barmata, A., Linde-Zwirble, W., Weissfeld, L., Watson, R., Rickert, T., & Rubenfeld, G. (2004). Use of intensive care at the end of life in the United States: An epidemiologic study. *Critical Care Medicine, 32*, 638–643.

Attig, T. (1996). Beyond pain: The existential suffering of children. *Journal of Palliative Care, 12*(3), 20–30.

Back, K. J. (1991). Sudden, unexpected pediatric death: Caring for parents. *Pediatric Nursing, 17*(6), 571–575.

Bagatell, R., Meyer, R., Herron, S., Berger, A., & Villar, R. (2002). When children die: A seminar series for pediatric residents. *Pediatrics, 110*(2, Pt. 1), 348–353.

Bluebond-Langner, M. (1978). *The private worlds of dying children.* Princeton, NJ: Princeton University Press.

Bowlby, J. (1980). *Attachment and loss, Vol. III: Loss.* New York: Basic Books.

Brown, P. S., & Sefansky, S. (1995). Enhancing bereavement care in the pediatric ICU. *Critical Care Nurse, 15*, 59–64.

Buckingham, R. W. (1983). *A special kind of love: Care of the dying child.* New York: Continuum.

Buckingham, R. W. (1989). *Care of the dying child: A practical guide for those who help others.* New York: Continuum.

Coles, R. (1990). *The spiritual life of children.* Boston: Houghton Mifflin.

Davies, B. (1997). Commentary on Van Riper's article on sibling bereavement. *Pediatric Nursing, 23*(6), 594–595.

Davies, B. (1999). *Shadows in the sun: The experience of sibling bereavement in childhood.* Philadelphia: Taylor & Francis.

Davies, B., & Kalischuk, R. (1997). *Sibling bereavement responses to death from long-term illness and trauma.* Unpublished manuscript.

Doka, K. (1995). *Children mourning, mourning children.* Washington, DC: Hospice Foundation of America.

Feudtner, C., Haney, J., & Dimmers, M. (2003). Spiritual care needs of hospitalized children and their families: A national survey of pastoral care providers' perceptions. *Pediatrics, 111*(1), 67–72.

Frager, G. (1996). Pediatric palliative care: Building the model, bridging the gaps. *Journal of Palliative Care, 12*(3), 9–12.

Gibbons, G., Retsaas, A., & Pinikahana, J. (1999). Describing what chaplains do in hospitals. *Journal of Pastoral Care, 53*(2), 201–209.

Goldman, A. (1996). Home care of the dying child. *Journal of Palliative Care, 12*(3), 16–19.

Grollman, E. (1995). *Bereaved children and teens: A support guide for parents and professionals.* Boston: Beacon Press.

Haas, F. (2003). Bereavement care: Seeing the body. *Nursing Standard, 17*(28), 33–37.

Halpern-Felsher, B., & Millstein, S. (2002). The effects of terrorism on teens' perceptions of dying: The new world is riskier than ever. *Journal of Adolescent Health, 30*(5), 308–311.

Hogan, N. S., & DeSantis, L. (1994). Things that help and hinder adolescent sibling bereavement. *Western Journal of Nursing Research, 16*(2), 132–153.

Hooke, C., Hellsten, M., Stutzer, C., & Forte, K. (2002). Pain management for the child with cancer in end-of-life care: APON position paper. *Journal of Pediatric Oncology Nursing, 19*(2), 43–47.

Irish, D. P., Lundquist, K. F., & Nelsen, V. J. (1993). *Ethnic variations in dying, death and grief: Diversity in universality.* Washington, DC: Taylor & Francis.

Irving, L. G. (1992). Perinatal loss: Choreographing grief on the obstetric unit. *American Journal of Orthopsychiatry, 62*(1), 7–8.

Johnson, L., & Mattson, S. (1992). Communication: The key to crisis prevention in pediatric death. *Critical Care Nurse, 12*(8), 23–27.

Jones, W. H. (1978). Emergency room sudden death: What can be done for survivors? *Death Education, 2*, 231–245.

Klass, D., Silverman, P., & Nickman, S. (1996). *Continuing bonds: New understanding of grief.* Philadelphia: Taylor & Francis.

Klopfenstein, K., Hutchison, C., Clark, C., Young, D., & Ruymann, F. (2001). Variables influencing end-of-life care in children and adolescents with cancer. *Journal of Pediatric Hematology Oncology, 23*(8), 481–486.

Laakso, H., & Paunonen-Ilmonen, M. (2001). Mothers' grief following the death of a child. *Journal of Advanced Nursing, 36*(1), 69–77.

Liben, S. (1996). Pediatric palliative medicine: Obstacles to overcome. *Journal of Palliative Care, 12*(3), 24–28.

McGoldrick, M., Almeida, R., Hines, P. M., Rosen, E., Garcia-Preto, N., & Lee, E. (1991). Mourning in different cultures. In F. Walsh & M. McGoldrick (Eds.), *Living beyond loss: Death in the family* (pp. 176–206). New York: Norton.

Morgan, J. D. (1990). *The dying and the bereaved teenager.* Philadelphia: The Charles Press, Publishers.

Mulhern, R. K., Lauer, M. E., & Hoffman, R. G. (1983). Death of a child at home or in the hospital: Subsequent psychological adjustment of the family. *Pediatrics, 71*(5), 743–747.

National Center for Health Statistics, Division of Vital Statistics, Centers for Disease Control. (2004). *Ten leading causes of death, by age and sex, 2002* (U.S. Mortality Public Use Data Tapes). Retrieved February 5, 2005, from http://www.cdc.gov/nchs/htm

Owens, G., Fulton, R., & Markhusen, E. (1982). Death at a distance: A study of family survivors. *Omega, 13*(3), 191–225.

Pazola, K. S., & Gerberg, A. K. (1990). Privileged communication—Talking with a dying adolescent. *Maternal Child Nursing, 15*, 16–21.

Pearson, L. (1999). Separation, loss and bereavement. In M. Broome & J. Rollins (Eds.), *Core curriculum for the nursing care of children and their families* (pp. 77–92). Pitman, NJ: Jannetti.

Pearson, L. (1997). Family-centered care and the anticipated death of a newborn. *Pediatric Nursing, 23*(2), 178–182.

Piaget, J. (1960). *The child's concept of the world.* Patterson, NJ: Littlefield, Adams.

Ponzetti, J. J., & Johnson, M. A. (1991). The forgotten grievers: Grandparents' reactions to the death of grandchildren. *Death Studies, 15*, 157–167.

Postovsky, S., & Arush, M. (2004). Care of a child dying of cancer: The role of the palliative care team in pediatric oncology. *Pediatric Hematology Oncology, 21*(1), 67–76.

Rando, T. (1986). *Parental loss of a child.* Champaign, IL: Research Press.

Rushton, C., & Glover, J. (1990). Involving parents in decisions to forgo life-sustaining treatment for critically ill infants and children. *AACN Clinical Issues in Critical Care Nursing, 1*(1), 206–214.

Rushton, C. H., & Lynch, M. A. (1992). Dealing with advance directives for critically ill adolescents. *Critical Care Nurse, 12*(5), 31–37.

Schulman, J. L., & Rehm, J. L. (1983). Assisting the bereaved. *Journal of Pediatrics, 102*(6), 992–998.

Serwint, J., Rutherford, L., Hutton, N., Rowe, P., Barker, S., & Adamo, G. (2002). "I learned that no death is routine": Description of a death and bereavement seminar for pediatrics residents. *Academic Medicine, 77*(4), 278–284.

Shapiro, E. R. (1994). *Grief as a family process: A developmental approach to clinical practice.* New York: Guilford Press.

Snoddy, A. (1992). A teenager's personal account of tragedy. *Thanatos, 17*(2), 13–15.

Sourkes, B. M. (1980). Siblings of the pediatric cancer patient. In J. Kellerman (Ed.), *Psychological aspects of childhood cancer* (pp. 47–69). Springfield, IL: Thomas.

Sourkes, B. M. (1995). *Armfuls of time: The psychological experience of the child with a life-threatening illness.* Pittsburgh, PA: University of Pittsburgh Press.

Sourkes, B. M. (1996). The broken heart: Anticipatory grief in the child facing death. *Journal of Palliative Care, 12*(3), 56–59.

Speece, M. W., & Brent, S. B. (1996). The development of children's understanding of death. In C. A. Corr & D. M. Corr (Eds.), *Helping children cope with death and bereavement* (pp. 29–51). New York: Springer.

Spitz, R. (1945). Hospitalism: An enquiry into the genesis of psychiatric conditions in early childhood. *Psychoanalytic Study of the Child, 1,* 53–74.

Stevens, M. M., Jones, P., & O'Riordan, E. (1996). Family responses when a child with cancer is in palliative care. *Journal of Palliative Care, 12*(3), 51–55.

Vose, L. A., & Nelson, R. M. (1999). Ethical issues surrounding limitation and withdrawal of support in the pediatric intensive care unit. *Journal of Intensive Care Medicine, 14*(5), 220–230.

Votta, E., Franche, R., Sim, D., Mitchell, B., Frewen, T., & Maan, C. (2001). Impact of parental involvement in life-support decisions: A qualitative analysis of parents' adjustment following their critically ill child's death. *Children's Health Care, 30*(1), 17–25.

Waechter, E. H. (1971). Children's awareness of fatal illness. *American Journal of Nursing, 71*(6), 1168–1172.

Walsh, F., & McGoldrick, M. (Eds.). (1991). *Living beyond loss: Death in the family.* New York: Norton.

Wolfelt, A. D. (1994). *Creating meaningful funeral ceremonies: A guide for caregivers.* Fort Collins, CO: Companion Press.

Wolfelt, A. D. (1996). *Healing the bereaved child.* Fort Collins, CO: Companion Press.

World Health Organization & International Association for the Study of Pain. (1998). *Cancer pain relief and palliative care in children.* Geneva, Switzerland: WHO.

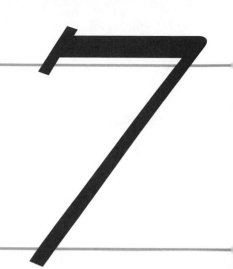

Families in Children's Health-Care Settings

Teresa W. Julian and David A. Julian

Objectives

At the conclusion of this chapter, the reader will be able to:

1. Discuss the functions of "family," specifically in health-care encounters.
2. Describe factors and influences on effective family health care.
3. Relate the historical, cultural, and research factors that have affected society's perspective on family involvement in health care.
4. Compare and contrast various approaches to involving families in health care and the relative influence of each approach.

*W*hen one traditionally thinks of working with families in health-care settings, one pictures a health-care professional who works in a hospital. In this picture, the health-care professional is tending to a mother, father, and sick child. This traditional view is inadequate for at least three reasons: (1) the definition of family is more inclusive than mother, father, and child; (2) health-care settings are more diverse than hospitals; and (3) many health-care professionals intervene before families find themselves in crisis with sick family members. In this chapter, we will attempt to discuss some of the issues that health-care professionals need to consider when working with families in a variety of health-care settings. We will also stress the health-care professional's need to recognize that the family is the constant in a child's life, while service systems and personnel within those systems fluctuate.

First, we will describe several perspectives that might be useful to health-care professionals who work with families. These perspectives include (a) adopting prevention as a guiding principle, (b) viewing families as unique systems, and (c) using principles of caring practice. Second, we will describe several skills essential to effective health-care delivery, including teaching, communication, and relationship building. Third, we will describe several systemic conditions that have the potential to make health-care provision for families more or less effective. These conditions include (a) adherence to scientific and biomedical beliefs about health care; (b) poverty and inadequate access to health-care resources; (c) the proliferation of technology and broad access to health-care information; and (d) home care and other alternative practice settings. The health-care professional as change agent is infused throughout the discussion of perspectives, skills, and systemic issues.

This chapter is not intended to be the definitive treatment of any of these subjects. The reader is encouraged to seek out more specific materials according to their needs and interests. Rather, this chapter is intended to provide an overview of many issues that can affect family health care and contribute to a holistic approach. As the reader will see, the subjects discussed in this chapter have the potential to have a dramatic impact on the success of clinical interventions and, ultimately, to enhance the physical and psychosocial health of children and their families. Further, it is clear that, early in this century, health policy makers will be forced to struggle with most of the systemic questions described below.

Overview of Practice with Families

Figure 7.1 provides an overview of the theory of family practice espoused in this chapter. Four major factors are represented. First, adopting prevention as a guiding principle, viewing families as unique systems, and using principles of caring practice provide a strong basis for effective service delivery. Second, the effects of skills such as teaching, communication, and relationship building are likely to be enhanced to the extent that these perspectives influence the health-care professional. Third, the provision of health-care services to families is affected by a number of systemic conditions that describe the environment within which the health-care professional must operate. Fourth, successful work with families is strongly related to the extent to which health-care professionals adopt the role of change agent. For example,

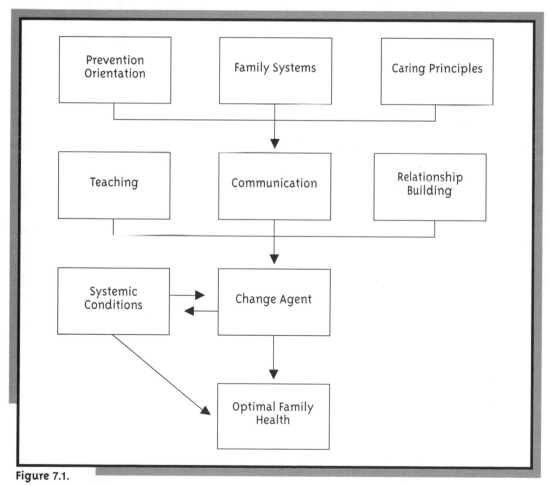

Figure 7.1.

Interaction between perspectives, skills, roles, and systemic issues that influence partnerships toward optimal family health.

simply providing a prevention message is unlikely to be effective without significant involvement of the health-care professional and explicit intervention designed to change behavior. As indicated in Figure 7.1, these factors in combination have the potential to make a significant impact on family health. This point is illustrated in Case Study 7.1.

Case Study 7.1
Providers as Change Agents

Consider a family of four (father, mother, 18-year-old daughter, and 12-year-old son) whose members enjoy optimal health. Optimal health does not necessarily mean the family members are disease free. In fact, the father suffers from heart disease and has had a mild heart attack. The school psychologist has diagnosed the son as having attention-deficit/hyperactivity disorder (ADHD). The daughter is away at college and is involved in a sexual relationship. This family is likely to have many different caregivers (a primary care physician, nurse practitioner, dentist, cardiologist, psychiatrist) and institutions (health-care providers' offices, a regional hospital with a cardiac center, the college health service, the local elementary school, a large national health insurer) functioning to ensure that their optimal health status is maintained. As indicated in Figure 7.1, these institutions and health-care providers are elements of a complex system that, at its best, functions to enhance health status.

It is clear that the family's health-care providers must adopt a preventive orientation to address the father's heart disease. Such a perspective also is essential to ensure that the son is successful in school and that the daughter deals with her sexual relationship in a responsible manner. Many health-care professionals will have the opportunity to provide care to these family members based on "caring principles." These same professionals are likely to be called upon to build relationships with family members and to teach optimal health-care practices. Professional organizations of physicians and nurses in the local community may be involved at a policy level in health-care issues that are sure to affect this family. Each of the providers in this system functions as a caregiver and, ultimately, as a change agent in the sense that much of the care that they provide is designed to change the attitudes and behaviors of family members and to bring about changes in social policies. Through such complex mechanisms, the optimal health status of this family can be maintained.

Perspectives

Perspectives provide a system of values that guide professional practice. The perspectives discussed below are essential to effective health-care practice with families. The value of prevention is obvious. Problems addressed early reduce health-care costs and needless suffering. Unfortunately, the U.S. health-care system is crises oriented (i.e., we wait until a health problem arises before intervening) rather than prevention oriented. However, through its *Healthy People* initiative, and more recently, *Steps to a Healthier US*, the U.S. Department of Health and Human Services has announced a bold shift in its approach from a disease-care system to a health-care system (U.S. Department of Health and Human Services, 2003). Thinking of families as systems embedded in larger ecological systems may yield critical intervention points and opportunities to reinforce and enhance clinical treatment. A caring orientation (Roach, 1987) involves a host of behaviors that ensures competent and compassionate practice.

Prevention

Historically, prevention was conceptualized in terms of (a) primary interventions practiced before an organism experienced biological disease; (b) secondary prevention practiced after a disease had developed but before significant suffering; and (c) tertiary prevention practiced after suffering or deterioration had occurred (Gordon, 1983). A more recent classification system for prevention (Institute of Medicine, 1994) included (a) universal interventions, targeted to entire populations identified as "at risk"; (b) selective interventions, targeted to subgroups of the population at higher than average risk of developing a disorder; and (c) indicated interventions, targeted to "high-risk" individuals with some detectable symptoms. For example, the National Center for Injury Prevention and Control (2002) suggested a number of potential strategies to reduce youth violence. Education of the general population concerning the role of society in promoting violence might be thought of as a universal intervention, training in conflict resolution for high school students as a selective intervention, and social skills training for children with behavioral problems as an indicated intervention.

Promising Strategies

Although the implementation of effective prevention programs is a complex undertaking, the literature suggests some promising prevention strategies to assist families in maintaining optimal health. Giving parents information and education about postoperative care appears to be related to less pain and postoperative vomiting in children (Kristensson-Hallstrom & Elander, 1997). This case demonstrates that an educational intervention helps to facilitate children's recovery time and to decrease the number of days in the hospital setting. Hovell et al. (1999) reported that counseling sessions with families are effective in preventing exposure to "environmental tobacco smoke" among asthmatic children. Heiberger (2004) described the key role nurse practitioners can play in empowering parents to prevent sudden infant death syndrome (SIDS). The National Center for Injury Prevention and Control (2002) suggested numerous strategies for preventing youth violence that range from adult mentoring to weaponless schools to prohibition of alcohol sales to recreational activities. Similarly, evaluators describe a host of programs that appears to be effective in preventing infectious disease, cardiovascular illnesses, drug abuse, and teen pregnancy. These examples provide evidence that well-conceived and evaluated prevention programs have the potential to reduce negative health outcomes. See box for an example of a strategy that addresses one of today's most alarming health challenges—obesity.

Implications for Work with Families

Health-care professionals must be proactive in providing preventive health care. Typically, the health-care professional will not have the opportunity to schedule appointments to discuss preventive strategies; such strategies must be communicated at opportune times. Consider a young boy or girl in the emergency department because of head trauma that might have been prevented by wearing a bicycle helmet. Appropriate counsel and education might prevent a brother or sister from suffering the same fate. Similarly, if the health-care professional encounters a teenage girl who is using alcohol or other drugs, it is probably prudent to counsel her on pregnancy prevention. These examples suggest that the health-care professional must continuously seek opportunities to provide effective prevention services.

In addition, research and theory suggest that health-care providers must intervene at the system and community levels to effectively prevent many negative health outcomes. Legislative and policy strategies are typically directed to higher levels of aggregation than individual clients. Table 7.1 provides several examples of interventions that focus on the individual in contrast to strategies that focus on the system or community level. Therapy for individual youths who have committed acts of violence and elective social skills training are aimed at changing the individual's attitudes and behavior. In the case of therapy, the intervention occurs after the disease or negative health outcome is present, whereas in the case of elective social

Promoting KidsWalk-to-School Day

In the United States, only about 1 of every 10 trips to school is made by walking or bicycling. Of school trips 1 mile or less, only 31% are made by walking, and within 2 miles of school, just 2% are made by bicycling. Research suggests that the decline in walking and bicycling may be contributing to the number of overweight children.

To increase opportunities for children to engage in physical activity, Washington State has promoted KidsWalk-to-School Day and the creation of safe walking routes for children to raise awareness about the importance of walking to school. The Washington Coalition for the Promotion of Physical Activity (WCPPA) and the Oregon Coalition for the Promotion of Physical Activity (OCPPA) collaborated to develop a KidsWalk-to-School Day packet of material that included the Walkability Checklist, the Neighborhood Walking

Table 7.1

283

Individual and System/Community-Level Interventions
Designed To Address Youth Violence

Level	Rehabilitation	Prevention
Individual	Therapy with individual youth who have committed acts of violence	Elective social skills training for youth with behavior problems
System/Community	Boot camps for juvenile offender	A policy requiring social skills training in all second-grade classrooms

skills training, the intervention occurs after symptoms have developed but before any major negative outcomes occur. Boot camps for juvenile offenders and required social skills training in all second-grade classrooms also are designed to change attitudes and behaviors. However, at the system or community level, entire groups of individuals are subjected to the intervention.

Family Systems

The family systems perspective is based on the notion that the person or patient is embedded in a family system that, in turn, is embedded in a larger ecological system. According to Foster-Fishman, Salem, Allen, and Fahrbach (1999), the ecological view has several important features. First, people and contexts are interdependent; that is, individual actions are influenced by the

Safety Guide, the Centers for Disease Control and Prevention's (CDC) KidsWalk-to-School Guide, a list of related educational Web sites, and a Safe and Active Routes to School presentation on CD-ROM. This packet was distributed to community leaders who are interested in promoting walk-to-school efforts.

The KidsWalk-to-School program encourages physical activity as an integral part of a child's daily routine. This program demonstrates the importance of promoting walking and bicycling to school to help increase the likelihood that children will engage in physical activity and carry this habit into adulthood. In addition, KidsWalk-to-School promotes the development of safe walking and bicycling routes and safe pedestrian practices to potentially reduce injury among children.

Note. Adapted from "Steps to a Healthier US: A Program and Policy Perspective—Prevention Programs in Action," by U.S. Department of Health and Human Services, 2003, Washington, DC: Author.

characteristics of the settings that people occupy. Second, individuals are subjected to multiple contextual influences. People usually inhabit many different settings simultaneously, and each setting may have specific influences on behavior. Third, beliefs, values, and norms define what is acceptable in the various settings people occupy.

Examples of the effects of system-level variables abound in the health-care literature. Jason, Anes, and Birkhead (1991) identified the importance of ecological factors in adolescent smoking prevention, and Jason et al. (1997) suggested that system-level variables must be addressed in treating chronic fatigue syndrome. Hobfoll (1998) stated that an ecological perspective has important ramifications for addressing human immunodeficiency virus (HIV) disease and prevention. For some individuals, personal and financial resources are more likely to be used to acquire a romantic partner than as a means of ensuring safer sex practices (Hobfoll, 1998). Thus, interventions designed to enhance access to resources at the individual level may not be sufficient to overcome cultural norms that place a high level of importance on having a romantic partner. A second example involves the adjustment of children with a sibling who is chronically ill. Family systems theory suggests that parental and family variables are likely to influence the successful adjustment of children to living at home with a sibling who is chronically ill. For example, Sargent et al. (1995) studied the responses of 254 siblings with a brother or sister who had cancer. Findings indicate that siblings are likely to feel distress about family separations and disruptions, lack of attention, focus of the family on ill children, negative feelings about themselves and family members, cancer treatments and effects, and fear of death.

Promising Strategies and Implications for Work with Families

Strategies that view the family as part of a larger ecological system hold great promise for effectively addressing health-care issues for families in a holistic manner. In the examples cited above, treatment of the individual or intervention at the individual level is conceptualized in terms of the influences of family and community variables. Thus, treatment of depression and antisocial behavior in children must address family issues, and effective interventions for HIV prevention must address community norms as well as individual behavior.

Theory and research suggest that the awareness of the illness of a brother or sister is important to the healthy development of siblings (Hughes & McCollum, 1994). Situations in which children who are critically ill are hospitalized for extended periods of time are likely to precipitate a number of family issues such as care for siblings, financial concerns, transportation to and from the hospital, as well as needs for support and stress management. In turn, these factors are likely to influence the success of treatment and the length of time required for recovery. It is clear that patients and their families are greatly influenced by their own individual qualities as well as qualities of other significant individuals and outside environmental forces. To provide the most effective health care in a holistic manner, health-care professionals must adopt a family systems perspective and consider a variety of ecological factors and forces.

Caring

Caring is a dynamic, multidimensional, and universal concept that enhances the preservation of human dignity. It is composed of nurturing activities, processes, and decisions that are essential for human birth, development, growth, and peaceful death. Caring behavior is manifested through attributes such as compassion, clinical competence and knowledge, confidence, conscience, and commitment (Roach, 1987). Caring professionals have control over their emotions and the clinical situation. They are self-reliant and they anticipate problems and provide the highest quality care. Roach suggested that professional caring involves self-donation and self-transcendence; that is, caring arises out of a concern for and response to the patient or family.

Implications for Work with Families

Neglect of caring skills is abundantly demonstrated in Marc Fisher's (1998) article, "The Doctor is Out." In this insightful article, the author described his son's rare, chronic condition and the impact this disorder and the realities of the current health-care system have on his family. Fisher's words, probably too familiar to many parents, demonstrate a health-care system that has relegated caring to a second or third level of priority. Fisher (1998) said his son's story is about

> what it means to be a patient, what it means to be adrift in the roiling sea of information that is medicine today, what it means to be searching for answers amid the warring faction of doctors, hospitals, managed care administrators, lawyers and fellow patients. (p. 8)

Fisher described a system in which physicians are protected from patients' "unremunerative questions" and one in which "HMOs and insurance companies want you to quit calling your doctor so often" (p. 8). The need for health-care professionals to develop caring skills cannot be overemphasized, particularly in the current environment. Such skills may, to some extent, serve as an antidote to large, impersonal, and uncaring bureaucracies.

Summary

Advocating for a prevention orientation in health-care delivery, viewing families as unique systems embedded in larger ecological systems, and incorporating principles of caring practice are critical perspectives that may serve to facilitate optimal health care for children and their families. Prevention may provide ample opportunity to define at-risk individuals and intervene before symptoms become severe. Adoption of a family systems perspective allows health-care providers to explore a wide variety of variables that are likely to influence the success of treatment. Finally, the incorporation of principles of caring into service delivery helps ensure competent and compassionate interactions with children and family members.

Skills

The second tier of Figure 7.1 describes several skills essential to the effective provision of health care for families. Whereas command of clinical skills is an obvious requirement for competent health-care practice, mastery of additional skills such as teaching, communication, and relationship building will often facilitate the health-care professional's work with families. Most health-care professionals develop these skills to some extent, and courses related to health teaching and communication are often part of curricula for many health-care professions. However, the skills described below may be neglected or relegated to a second or third level of importance given the demands of health-care practice. Teaching, communication, and relationship building are interdependent and should be viewed as adjuncts to clinical practice and complements to the essential perspectives outlined above. Finally, using these skills provides the opportunity to address family health-care concerns in a holistic manner.

Teaching Skills

Numerous teaching approaches are available to health-care professionals. Most teaching in health-care settings has as its goal the transfer of specific knowledge as a step in changing behavior. For example, teaching a family about proper dietary habits is an attempt to reinforce healthy behaviors and change unhealthy behaviors. Several principles may assist health-care professionals in developing more effective teaching techniques. Research findings indicate that if a desired behavior change seems overwhelming or impossible to implement, patients or learners will not be likely to attempt to change their behavior. This is true even if the patient is capable of performing the required skills. Breaking a large goal or behavior change into smaller goals or tasks that can be readily mastered is a simple strategy that may enhance chances of success. The health-care professional also may provide aids to ensure success, such as allowing the child or parent to practice while providing feedback concerning progress. Other principles of effective teaching include making the information relevant to the family's lifestyle and health problems, and providing rewards and feedback.

Table 7.2 287

Comparison of Traditional and Empowering Processes for Asthma Education

Variable	Traditional	Empowering
Setting	Classroom setting: Seats arranged in rows.	Classroom setting: Seats arranged in a semicircle
Role of the professional	Professional lectures from the front of the class. Professional educator is portrayed as the expert.	Professional educator sits within semicircle Professional acts as a facilitator and resource person with emphasis on parent–professional partnerships
Role of the parents	Passive learners	Active learners Emphasis on parent–professional partnerships Parents recognized as experts who know their child best, have personal experience with child's illness, and can suggest how to adapt asthma management to fit family lifestyle
Teaching strategies	Primarily lectures	Interactive (e.g., parents share impressions, concerns) Emphasis on behavior change (e.g., learning to assess, interpret, and respond appropriately to changes in child's asthma; practicing proper use of asthma devices) Individualization and application of theory about each topic to own situation through use of common scenarios Emphasis on shared problem solving and learning from each other Repetition and review Monthly follow-up phone calls to family

Note. From "Empowering Parents Through Asthma Education," by M. McCarthy, J. Hansen, R. Herbert, D. Wong, M. Brimacombe, and M. Zelman, 2002, *Pediatric Nursing, 28*(5), p. 468. Copyright 2002 by Jannetti. Reprinted with permission.

The concept of empowerment is now a well-established theoretical perspective in patient and parent education. Empowered families feel a sense of control and mastery over their situation as opposed to relying on professionals to meet their needs. For a comparison of traditional and empowering processes to asthma education, see Table 7.2. Although both traditional and empowering approaches to teaching parents can result in increased knowledge, McCarthy and colleagues (2002) reported significantly higher scores on measures of sense of control, ability to make decisions, and ability to provide care, for parents who participated in an empowerment approach to asthma education.

Implications of Using Effective Teaching Skills

Many critical implications of using teaching strategies exist in working with families. First, teaching is a primary prevention tool. The value of prevention is noted in the previous section. Second, health-care professionals who work with families during an illness have unique opportunities to implement effective teaching that may enhance healing and wellness. In such situations, the health-care professional can observe family coping and adaptation to a disease. In the case of children, such awareness may transcend various developmental stages and needs and may afford the health-care professional to act proactively to teach appropriate content and therapeutic strategies. For example, Eddy et al. (1998) found that preadolescent children with cystic fibrosis had greater stress and treatment problems when they had conflicts with parents. Eddy and colleagues (1998) suggested that, when developing interventions, health-care professionals should consider key developmental transition points, children's and family members' perspectives about their illnesses, and family relationship patterns. Milteer and Jonna (1996) indicated that providing high-risk, urban families with the appropriate information to address specific social issues is an important means of ensuring that their children are appropriately immunized. Providing relevant teaching content for families can serve as a powerful preventive intervention and, in other cases, as an effective strategy to address illness.

Communication Skills

It is commonly held that communication is the most important strategy in working with families in any health-care setting. Reviews of research suggest that communication is often identified as an area in which health-care professionals need to improve. Horn, Feldman, and Ploof's (1995) research described stressors for families who have children with chronic illnesses that require lengthy hospitalizations. These researchers suggested that personal emotions and communication problems with the health-care team are predominant stressors. Similarly, Evans (1996) reported that mothers of children who are hospitalized state that they often feel stressed and out of control because of the impact of disease and treatment. To help these mothers, it is essential that health-care professionals communicate with families by negotiating and clarifying (Evans, 1996).

Other researchers find that parental stress over the uncertainty of a child's prognosis may interfere with family coping and child management (Tomlinson, Kirschbaum, Harbaugh, & Anderson, 1996). Parental involvement in children's care can be stressful especially when children are required to undergo unpleasant procedures (Callery, 1997). Because having a parent present can reduce a child's anxiety (Blesch & Fisher, 1996), providing information about options parents have to help their children as well as creating a nonjudgmental atmosphere regarding their choices are critical elements of good communication in this regard.

In an interesting study by Melnyk, Alpert-Gillis, Hensel, Cable-Beiling, and Rubenstein (1997), opportunities were created for parents to feel empowered concerning the health outcomes of their critically ill children. The researchers used effective communication to educate parents about such topics as children's responses as they recover from critical illnesses and how parents might assist their children in coping with the stress experience. Participants in the intervention group felt empowered and provided more support to their children during intrusive procedures. These participants also reported less negative mood states, decreased parental stress related to their children's emotions and behaviors, and fewer posttraumatic stress symptoms 4 weeks following hospitalization. Similarly, Watson (1995) found that supplementing the spoken word with booklets, videos, tape-recorded interviews, and play helped support families of children with end-stage renal failure.

Experience and research indicate that empathetic, respectful, and genuine communication leads to trusting, empowering, therapeutic, and collaborative relationships (Northouse & Northouse, 1992). Carkhoff and Truax (1967) provided an important perspective regarding empathy, respect, and genuineness. Empathy involves active participation in and understanding of the individual's and family member's feelings or ideas. The health-care professional must sense, share, and accept the client's feelings. Three basic behaviors are associated with empathy: (1) awareness and acceptance of the self as a feeling person; (2) listening to messages and identifying the patient's or family members' feelings; and (3) responding to feelings exhibited in specific messages (e.g., use of paraphrasing techniques). By exhibiting empathetic behaviors, the health-care professional will become aware of the child's uniqueness and individuality. The child or family member, in turn, will perceive the health-care professional as caring and feeling, which ultimately will facilitate open communication and trust.

Feelings of being respected are important for the child or family member to experience her or his right to exist as a unique human being. The health-care professional must exhibit a receptive attitude that demonstrates value for feelings, opinions, individuality, and uniqueness. Also, the health-care professional must show a high level of commitment to understanding through a willingness to explore subjects that are important to the family. Finally, the health-care professional must convey acceptance and warmth by being nonjudgmental (free from prejudice) and must develop a high level of immunity to being embarrassed, shocked, dismayed, or overwhelmed by the child or family member's thoughts or behaviors. This requires appropriate verbal as well as nonverbal communication. Respect affirms the strengths and the problem-solving capabilities of the family.

Genuineness is synonymous with concepts such as authenticity, good faith, and sincerity. It is a sharing of self exhibited by behaving in a natural, spontaneous, and nondefensive manner. However, the health-care professional must be sensitive to the family's readiness for specific messages. For example, self-disclosure is appropriate, but only when the family is ready to respond positively to the disclosure. As trust is established, the health-care professional can become more open and spontaneous while adhering to the principles of empathy and respect. It is important to avoid using self-disclosure to manipulate, give advice, or influence a family to further the health-care professional's own goals. If empathy and respect are part of genuine communication, such personal motivations are not likely to occur (Carkhoff & Truax, 1967).

Implications of Using Effective Communication Skills

Whether labeled as inadequate information, paternalism, limited negotiation, or lack of clarification, troubled communication is at the root of many problematic family and professional partnerships (Evans, 1996; Horn, Feldman, & Ploof, 1995). Many problems in health-care settings can be traced to the way professionals talk to and otherwise interact with families. Most communication problems can be transcended if health-care professionals use empathy, respect, and genuineness along with basic therapeutic techniques (Carkhoff & Truax, 1967).

Good communication skills are not innate. Health-care professionals must learn appropriate techniques to effectively communicate with families. By incorporating communication skills into their repertoires, health-care professionals can accurately gather information and understand the inner worlds and thoughts of the families they serve. According to Sirkia, Saarinen, Ahlgren, and Hovi (1997), adequately tutored parents provide more cost-effective care because they avoid prolonged hospitalizations. It is clear that effective communication provides a variety of beneficial outcomes for children and their families.

Relationship Building

A critical skill in working with families involves the need to facilitate parental and professional collaboration at all levels of health care. Eddy and colleagues (1998) claimed that forming supportive collaborative relationships with parents of children with a chronic illness such as cystic fibrosis should be an early intervention. Such partnerships increase the chances that parents will be open in sharing the stresses and hassles experienced in the daily care of their children. Some important steps in building collaborative relationships include (a) good communication with clarity of vision and a foundation for active involvement of all in goal setting; (b) use of educational materials and strategies that account for the psychologic needs of the learner; and (c) development of relationships that build on the strengths of individuals and families (U.S. Department of Health and Human Services, 1996). In establishing collaborative relationships, it is important that common goals be developed and shared. The presence of a common goal that supersedes individual goals is a distinguishing characteristic of collaborative relationships (Julian, 1994).

Melnyk et al. (2004) reported exciting findings from a parent empowerment program on the coping outcomes of critically ill children and their mothers. Mothers in the experimental group received a three-phase educational–behavioral intervention program called Creating Opportunities for Parent Empowerment (COPE), which focused on increasing (a) parents' knowledge and understanding of the range of behaviors and emotions that young children typically display during and after hospitalization and (b) direct parent participation in their children's emotional and physical care. Control mothers received a structurally equivalent control program. COPE mothers reported significantly less parental stress and participated more in their children's physical and emotional care on the pediatric unit, compared with control mothers. Six months after discharge, COPE children exhibited significantly fewer withdrawal symptoms than did control children, as well as fewer negative behaviors and externalizing behaviors at 12 months. Study findings indicated that mothers who received the COPE program experienced improved maternal functional and emotional coping outcomes, which resulted in significantly fewer child adjustment problems, compared with the control group.

In a qualitative study by Woodgate and Kristjanson (1996) describing how parents and nurses responded to hospitalized young children experiencing pain from surgical interventions, nurses primarily provided technical care and used limited pain assessment approaches. These nurses were not able to adequately alleviate the children's pain. However, parents provided comfort measures and vigilant monitoring of their children's pain, suggesting a powerful, potential collaboration. Similarly, Pederson and Harbaugh's (1995) exploratory study found that nurses' lack of time and heavy workload impeded their use of nonpharmacologic pain management techniques. In this study, nurses perceived parents as helpful in implementing nonpharmacologic pain management techniques with children. Because of health-care changes, pain management has increasingly become the responsibility of the family in the home environment (Ferrell, Rhiner, & Ferrell, 1993). Researchers have found that optimal pain medication administration by the patient or family member does not always occur (Callahan, 1998; Ferrell, Rhiner, Cohen, & Grant, 1991). Collaborative relationships between health-care professionals and families may provide the opportunity to provide effective pain management treatment in the hospital and home setting.

Neill (1996) examined parents' views and experiences in participating in their children's (ages 2–5 years) hospital care, and found that parents clearly wished to participate at the level of their own choosing. Families preferred professionals to be responsible for their children's clinical care, while they continued to be responsible for their children's normal day-to-day care. Problems reported by parents centered on the paternalistic nature of the relationship with the health-care team and on communication. Interestingly, parents of children who experienced single, short hospital admissions found involvement in their children's care particularly difficult. Kawik (1996) found that nurses and parents had different perceptions of their individual roles. Parents were willing to be involved in caring for their hospitalized children yet experienced difficulties because of inadequate information and the nurses' reluctance to relinquish control of nursing care. Consequently, the nurse–parent relationship was not always conducive to a partnership approach. Researchers stressed the importance of developing guidelines to help educate professionals concerning the health-care needs of patients and families (Neill, 1996; Turner, 1997).

Implications of Using Relationship-Building Skills

To develop common goals, health-care professionals need to continually investigate the needs of caretakers of critically ill patients, especially children (Scott, 1998). Consistent identification, prioritization, and incorporation of parental needs into a plan of care are important steps in building collaborative relationships. Interestingly, Scott suggested that parental needs usually revolve around

- knowing the expected outcome of medical treatment,
- being given honest answers,
- being assured that the best care is given,
- seeing and visiting children frequently, and
- being notified of any changes in the condition of their children.

It appears as though collaborative relationships between family members and health-care professionals may serve as a valuable tool in providing optimal health care. Parental participation has now become an accepted feature in the care of children in hospitals. Collaborative relationships can maximize family members' confidence and competence in caring for their children. This is an important element in family-centered care (Johnson, 1990).

Summary

In summary, health-care professionals must strive to develop teaching skills, communication skills, and skills necessary to build collaborative relationships with parents and other family members. Teaching and communication provide avenues to new knowledge and represent the initial steps in behavior change. Skills related to relationship building provide a basis for intervention. All of these skills serve to facilitate treatment and may ultimately enhance the physical and psychosocial health of children and families. At a minimum, such skills are essential to developing trusting and therapeutic relationships. For more about relationships between health-care professionals and families, see Chapter 12.

Systemic Conditions

Systemic conditions represent social statuses, social states, or organizational practices and policies. Systemic conditions might be perceived as those key features of the environment that are likely to influence the character of health care in the United States in the next decade. This section identifies several features of the current environment, including (a) the adherence to scientific/biomedical beliefs about health care, (b) poverty and inadequate access to health-care resources, (c) the proliferation of technology and broad access to health-care information, and (d) home care and other alternative practice settings. In future years, these conditions are likely to have lasting implications for how health care is delivered in the United States, and to have a dramatic impact on families.

Adherence to Scientific/Biomedical Beliefs About Health Care

It is important for health-care professionals to realize that families have varied health beliefs (King, 1984). For the individual, beliefs are influenced by such things as (a) past experiences with the health-care system (e.g., degree of helpfulness, barriers to care), (b) family members' and influential others' experiences, (c) thoughts and cognition, (d) biochemical/structural strengths and weaknesses (e.g., level of wellness, perceptions related to disease), (e) culture, and (f) socioeconomic status. Although beliefs and experiences are varied, the scientific/biomedical health paradigm (Herberg, 1989) is the dominant health belief system for the majority of families in the United States.

The following are some of the values associated with the scientific/biomedical health paradigm:

- *Determinism*—Cause and effect relationships exist for all natural phenomena.
- *Mechanism*—Life is compared to the structure and function of machines.
- *Reductionism*—All life can be reduced or divided into smaller parts.
- *Dualism*—Mind and body are separated into two distinct entities.

In contemporary Western cultures, the scientific/biomedical health paradigm leads to an understanding of health in physical and chemical terms, and disease is viewed as the breakdown of the human machine. Thus, families and health-care professionals use terms such as wear and tear (e.g., stress), external trauma (e.g., injury, accident), external invasion (e.g., pathogens, infection), and internal changes (e.g., chemical imbalances or structural anomalies; Herberg, 1989).

Weaknesses of the Scientific/Biomedical Health Paradigm

All health belief systems, even the dominant value system in the United States, have strengths and weaknesses. Health-care professionals need to assess whether the scientific/biomedical health paradigm is leading to the best outcomes for children and families. Some serious weaknesses associated with the scientific/biomedical health paradigm include (a) the fragmentation of health-care services, (b) the lack of research and treatment that are holistic or preventive in nature, (c) the lack of health care that considers the mind–body connection, (d) the symptomatic treatment of diseases versus determining causation, and (e) "prescriptionism," or heavy reliance on pharmaceutical interventions. Some of the weaknesses of the scientific/biomedical paradigm are illustrated in Case Study 7.2.

Case Study 7.2
A Holistic Perspective

Throughout her life, a petite, undernourished 15-year-old had a chronic colon condition that resulted in inflammation and bleeding. Over time, surgeons removed most of the organ (the treatment of choice in our health-care paradigm). However, surgery produced little relief. As a last resort, the adolescent consulted a practitioner who used multiple health-care paradigms in her practice. During an initial interview, the health-care provider determined that physical growth was a primary concern for the adolescent.

The physician and her patient formed a collaborative relationship and a plan was developed. A very specific mind–body treatment regime was initiated. Over many months, the adolescent achieved her goals related to growth while keeping her chronic condition under control. In this case, the physician adopted a holistic perspective and focused on her client's major concerns. Treatment based on the scientific/biomedical health paradigm provided few answers for this patient.

Potential Responses

One role of the health-care professional is to reflect on the choices available to consumers. Most current treatment options are influenced by the scientific/biomedical health paradigm, and are developed and provided by private-sector enterprises. It is reasonable to ask if such treatments are always the best options for specific children and their families. Being aware of and understanding the strengths and weaknesses of the predominant health paradigm may lead to interventions based on alternative views of health and treatment for some children. Thus, health-care professionals might explore and incorporate practices from other health paradigms and cultures (e.g., holistic health, magic–religious health) into their interactions with families. Because some of these approaches may not be profitable, governmental entities and individual health-care providers must take a larger role in research and dissemination of alternative health-care treatments. In any case, health-care professionals can work together with families to strive to find the best approaches to treatment, even if those approaches deviate from the dominant health-care paradigm.

Poverty and Inadequate Access to Health-Care Resources

Many segments of the population struggle to acquire needed health-care services (e.g., homeless and low-income children and families, grandparents raising their children's children, foster children, the medically uninsured). Some of the reasons families are medically underserved involve individual factors, health-care professional factors, and system factors. When working with families, questions come to mind, such as the following:

- Is the individual or family in a state of readiness to comprehend information given to them?
- Are pain, fatigue, stress, and issues related to learning–teaching principles (e.g., varied learning styles, retention, comprehension differences) preventing optimal access to care?
- Are health-care professionals prepared to interact with children and families in a caring manner?
- Do system/organizational policies support a variety of approaches to education and teaching?

The answers to these and other such questions are important. In many cases, individual, professional, or system factors interfere with the provision of optimal health care.

Problems with the Current Situation

Many of the families experiencing difficulty in accessing health-care services also are the most in need. For example, in 2000, 5.6 million grandparents had grandchildren under 18 years of age living with them (U.S. Census Bureau, 2001). Approximately 7% of all grandparents provide extensive caregiving (30+ hours per week or 90+ nights per year) for their grandchildren (Fuller-Thompson & Minkler, 2001). Many grandparents are raising children with special needs, including HIV, child abuse and neglect, and neurologic deficits resulting from parental abuse of drugs. Research indicates that some of these grandparents are suffering from significant financial burdens, feelings of anger and resentment toward their own children, and mental health problems (Kelley, Yorker, & Whitley, 1997; Roe, Minkler, Saunders, & Thomson, 1996).

There is also concern that the impact of stressors on custodial grandparents and their responses to the stressors may ultimately be harmful to the psychosocial adjustment of their grandchildren. Roe et al. (1996) asserted that grandparents need to reclaim their own lives, learn how to take care of themselves, and find resources and support groups. Others state that custodial grandparents may be particularly in need of mental health services, especially if they are caring for grandchildren with behavioral problems (Emick, 1996; Kelly, Yorker, & Whitley, 1997). Unfortunately, inadequate access to health-care resources is a barrier for optimal health for the growing population of grandparent-headed households.

Garwick, Kohrman, Wolman, and Blum (1998) found that many families think that quality of health care and barriers to services and programs are major problems. Issues of access include lack of services, lack of insurance coverage or cooperation, and lack of sensitivity to diversity. Even access to needed services for foster children has been related to difficulties arising from community reactions to foster parenting (Barton, 1998). For a growing number of consumers, in general, dealing with billing departments or insurance companies is difficult and may result in failure to acquire needed care for their families. Garwick et al. (1998) concluded that health-care professionals and policy makers need to transform rhetoric about family-centered care into action.

Heck and Parker (2002) reported interesting results from a study they conducted to test the hypothesis that among children of lower socioeconomic status, children of single mothers would have relatively worse access to care than children in two-parent families. They found that although at high levels of maternal education, family structure did not influence physician visits or having a usual source of care, at low levels of maternal education, single mothers appeared to be *better* at accessing care for their children than those mothers with low levels of education in two-parent families. The investigators concluded that children in two-parent families whose mothers are less educated do not always have access to Medicaid, and that public health insurance is critical to ensure adequate health-care access and utilization among children of less educated mothers, regardless of family structure.

Regular contact with the health-care system is especially important for families of children with special health-care needs. The current U.S. health-care system is not designed to meet these needs: "At the heart of our system is the traditional physician–patient interaction. While effective, these interactions occur infrequently at best and typically last no longer than 30 minutes every several months" (U.S. Department of Health and Human Services, 2003, p. 6). Whether the child is sick or well, a family spends far more time making independent decisions—outside of the physician's office—that affect the child's health and does so with minimal training or information. This is particularly true for the uninsured, who have very limited access to health-care services.

Potential Responses

Various written materials and textbooks advocate intervention models designed to improve access to health-care resources. Usually these models involve case management strategies; family assessment models; and family advocacy, counseling, teaching, referral, and follow-up. These techniques and strategies prove to be effective in certain circumstances. Other strategies are continually being developed and deployed. Technology and the Internet may provide easy access to some types of health-care services. Advances in procedures, diagnostic tools, and innovations in how services are delivered may make health care more accessible to many consumers.

One innovative technique for improving access to health-care resources is the same-day surgery or satellite health-care site. Same-day surgery or satellite health-care sites for minor surgical procedures seem to offer win-win situations for families and health-care providers. In these settings, families become important partners with the health-care team in the provision of care. Parents often are with their children during the preoperative and the postoperative phases. Parental presence for anesthesia induction is important for reducing stress in children and enhancing recovery. However, for this system to work effectively, parents must be viewed as major collaborators and educated about their role in caring for their children. There must be opportunities for parents to ask questions and discuss fears and concerns. Same-day surgery sites also seem to be environmentally friendly (i.e., facilities are smaller, fewer parking difficulties, fewer personnel to get to know) and are frequently owned by small groups of physicians who have a vested interest in keeping their customers happy.

To provide optimal health care, it will become more important for health-care professionals to implement strategies that increase access and connect families to appropriate resources. Health-care professionals must find ways to help relieve the stress of inadequate access to health-care resources. An added burden concerns the maze of procedures created by current health insurance practices. Families without health insurance or those that receive minimal support from the government often are forced to make difficult decisions concerning the quality of care their family receives. Inadequate access to health-care resources exacerbates existing health-care problems. Health-care professionals must be aware of how issues of access, including limited financial resources, affect individualized plans of care for children and their families. They also need to be aware of resources that can help families, and disseminate this information to families in a timely and coherent manner. Finally, health-care professionals and policy makers should consider a variety of solutions to make health-care resources readily available to all community members. Many strategies discussed in this chapter will assist health-care professionals in decreasing the barriers that lead to inadequate access to health-care resources for families, especially for those individuals and families who are underserved, poor, and diverse.

The Proliferation of Technology and Widespread Access to Health-Care Information

Access to the Internet and technology has the potential to dramatically alter how health care is provided to families. There is little question that a vast amount of health-care information is currently available on the Internet. Web sites are devoted to specific diseases and conditions that provide families with access to expert medical opinions. In some cases, private companies will prepare reports about specific medical conditions and treatment options. Some hospital Web sites have extensive communications channels for patients and their parents (Rees, 2002). Fisher (1998) discussed his journey and experiences (positive and negative) through various online services to find information about his son's serious medical condition. He noted the value of access to Web-based information, but also identifies several challenges. His comments serve as a primer for online medical searches.

Changes Associated with Technology and Access

The Internet, access to information, and the current climate in health-care provision seem to have altered the traditional relationship between health-care professionals and families. Fisher (1998) cited Alan Rees, a professor emeritus at Case Western Reserve University, who summarizes the relationship as "adversarial." Rees concluded that information is the patient's best recourse, given the current health-care environment. Tom Ferguson, a Texas physician and consultant who is a leading advocate for online medicine, is quoted in Fisher's article:

> The line between patient and doctor is gone.... We're in the early stages of a great power shift from doctors to savvy patients. Doctors aren't the gatekeepers in health care anymore. When I was in med school, I was trained never to let the patient know you don't have a 100 percent answer to a question. We reduced medicine to oversimplified formulas. Now, consumers have access to the same information. They can go online and find the best doctors and the best treatments. (p. 8).

It is clear from this quote that technology may produce a number of changes in how care is provided in the future. Health-care professionals must develop new techniques and procedures that will allow families access to useful and accurate information.

Potential Responses

Appropriate use of the Internet and other technologic aids to information exchange appear to serve a useful function. Tetzlaff (1997) stated that consumers appear positively disposed toward online solutions. Online ser-

Information That Might Be Included on a Medical Web Site	• Dictionaries to help patients and families understand medical terminology • Health-care protocols to empower patients and families • Medication worksheets, including common and uncommon side-effects • Procedural worksheets detailing common medical treatments • Photographs and information about health-care professionals

vices can offer a broad range of information at great levels of detail in a timely fashion. Further, Internet communication with families via e-mail is one way to increase access to health-care resources. An e-mail delivery system might be used to confirm appointments, report information (e.g., "Your lab test is normal."), and answer questions. Some health-care agencies are already online and connect such interactions to electronic medical records. With many families online and many others having access through local schools and libraries, it is important that health-care professionals and policy makers adopt useful Internet strategies for sharing information and expanding access to health-care resources. It is also important that when strategies like those discussed above are implemented, health-care professionals develop and teach protocols for how to access the World Wide Web and pertinent Web-based resources. Clark (1997) recommended teaching families how to use browsers, search engines, and key word searches. The categories of information commonly found on medical Web sites are listed in the box.

The Boston Baby CareLink is an example of the use of computers, the Internet, and other communication technologies designed to provide access to medical resources to a wide rage of populations from newborns to the chronically ill to the elderly in frontier, rural, suburban, and inner city areas. For example, Boston Baby CareLink sponsors a videoconference focused on educational and emotional supports for families of high-risk newborns. This information can be accessed by Internet users across the globe. The National Library of Medicine funds this and other telemedicine projects that provide widespread access to information about health care (U.S. Department of Health and Human Services, 1998).

Aside from the use of computers and the Internet as illustrated by the Boston Baby CareLink, numerous other technologic strategies exist for increasing access to health-care information. Families might be encouraged to bring tape recorders to the health-care setting. If families do not own such devices, some might be acquired and made available for loan. Simply taping a conversation with a health-care professional might help families

- Important assessment tools that could be completed prior to office visits (ADHD behavioral assessments for parents, children, teachers)
- Answers to frequently asked questions
- References to resources that might help increase patient access to services (transportation passes, maps)
- Health-care handouts for patients, families, school personnel, and so on
- Reference lists of favorite helping and healing books

share information with loved ones. Teaching receptionists and scheduling personnel how to schedule appointments so that children and their families are not burdened by long waits to see health-care professionals represents a simple technology. Telephones also are an effective means of communication. In many cases, telephone calls provide a continuum of care to postsurgical patients. Making follow-up phone calls to patients and family members improves health-care outcomes (Chewitt, Fallis, & Suski, 1997).

Technologies including the Internet and a variety of other mechanical and electronic devices have the potential to make health-care information available to families and to increase access to health-care resources. The Internet is already a powerful communication tool that is readily available to many consumers. However, it will be necessary to educate consumers and to develop procedures to ensure that information obtained through the Internet and other technologic channels is accurate and "user friendly." Although the Internet is a potentially helpful tool for health-care professionals in their work with families, many challenges to responsible use must be addressed.

Home Care and Other Alternative Practice Settings

As the result of advances in scientific knowledge and technology, the number of patients—especially children—living with chronic illnesses is increasing. Some parents report that home care options provide them with greater freedom, more privacy, and less disruption to family life (Collins, Stevens, & Cousens, 1998). Collins and colleagues also stated that caring for children is a positive experience for most families. In addition, as morbidity increases and health-care cost-containment demands occur, the need for access to a variety of assisted living arrangements and home health-care services will increase. Health-care professionals will be called on more frequently in the next decade to provide assistance to families caring for critically ill loved ones and to provide a variety of services in nontraditional settings.

Impact on Families

Caretakers often express fears and concerns regarding symptomatic care of their children and other family members, and they need considerable support. For example, families may have insufficient knowledge of parenting skills and inadequate support systems, and they may be unable to help with vital childcare tasks (Jenkins, 1996). Managing the care of a medically fragile child at home often means finding unique solutions for the child's needs as well as providing emotional, educational, and financial support (Kilinski, 1997). For successful home care, parents need access to continuous supervision, help and support of well-trained personnel, and knowledge about respite care and quality day care services (Sirkia et al., 1997; Watson, 1995).

Potential Responses

Formal home visitation programs may provide the opportunity to assist families with the care of loved ones at home (Corbin & Strauss, 1991;

Watson, 1995). In the case of children, Watson (1995) recommended not only visiting the home but also visiting the nursery school and primary care physician. Home visitation offers an effective mechanism to ensure ongoing caretaker education and social support linkages with public and private community services. Health-care professionals can help families assess their ability to implement treatment regimens and to recognize signs of complications or symptoms in the child.

Health-care professionals must also help families address their ability to manage disabilities and come to terms with their own psychosocial responses (e.g., management of social isolation, financial hardships, constriction of time, identity insults, profound sense of loss). Formal home visitation programs need to include physical and emotional support, as well as tangible ways to relieve parents and other caretakers of the continuous 24-hour care of their children and other family members. Further, in cases of life-threatening conditions, emotional support must continue after the child's death.

Ozonoff and Cathcart (1998) described a unique home care program called TEACCH. This program was designed for families of autistic children. The home-based intervention was effective in positively enhancing the development of young children with autism. Parents were taught how to work with their preschool, autistic children in the home setting and how to focus on cognitive, academic, and prevocational skills for later school success (Ozonoff & Cathcart, 1998). Others have found that early home interventions during the first year of life can promote a nurturing home environment and can reduce the developmental delays often experienced by low-income, urban infants with nonorganic failure to thrive (Black, Dubowitz, Hutcheson, Berenson-Howard, & Starr, 1995). In these examples, home visitation programs provided many of the services necessary for sustained care of children with chronic conditions. These services included access to highly trained health-care professionals who provided advice and support.

Adopting the Role of Change Agent

To be a change agent means to facilitate or aid the process of change in a deliberate manner. Change can occur at a variety of levels. At the individual level, the health-care professional must assist the patient to define appropriate and healing behaviors, and take action to ensure such behaviors are adopted. Prochaska, Norcross, and DiClemente's (1994) transtheoretical model is a key tool for changing behavior at the individual level. Some strategies to effect change at the system level include (a) political action; (b) planning, needs analysis, and evaluation; and (c) grassroots movements. Each of these topics is addressed after a brief discussion of why the change agent role is so important.

The Importance of the Change Agent Role

Historically, teaching, communication, relationship building, and even medical treatment have represented significant health-care interventions. However, in the absence of deliberate action to change behavior, these strategies were insufficient to produce true health and wellness. For example, educational campaigns designed to promote the use of seat belts were only marginally successful. However, educational campaigns in combination with laws requiring seat belt use and enforcement garnered more support. Similarly, smoking cessation programs have not typically resulted in decreases in public expenditures for providing health care for cigarette smokers. However, class action suits against the tobacco industry have produced significant resources that may ultimately defray public expenditures and enhance the quality of life for individuals affected by smoking-related illnesses.

It is imperative that health-care professionals perceive themselves as change agents and work at both the individual and system levels. To truly address the psychosocial needs of children in health-care settings requires a long-range perspective focused on the change agent role. The list of potential changes in policies that could benefit families and children in health-care settings includes the following:

- universal health insurance
- expanded research and development of treatments for chronic illnesses such as HIV
- funding for and implementation of formal prevention programs that address family issues such as substance abuse and child neglect
- access to quality childcare services
- immunization programs
- guaranteed parental leave for mothers and fathers after the birth of a baby

The Role of Change Agent at the Individual Level

Several models are available to assist health-care professionals in advocating for change at the individual level. The transtheoretical model of behavior change (TTM) developed by James Prochaska and his colleagues is a particularly effective tool (Prochaska, Norcross, & DiClemente, 1994). In the TTM model, behavior change is conceptualized in terms of movement through a series of discrete stages:

1. Precontemplation
2. Contemplation
3. Preparation
4. Action
5. Maintenance

Individuals in the *precontemplation* stage are characterized by resistance to recognizing and modifying problem behaviors. They have no intention of changing their behavior in the next 6 months. *Contemplators* recognize a problem and are seriously considering changing their behavior. At the *preparation* stage, individuals intend to take action to change their behavior in the next 30 days. At the *action* stage, individuals are performing the desired behavior change at the designated criterion level. The *maintenance* stage represents continuous, long-term change wherein the person works to consolidate behavioral and cognitive/experiential gains made while transitioning through the previous stages to avoid relapse.

Smoking cessation is an example that illustrates the effectiveness of the TTM model. The negative impact of smoking on the smoker's health and secondhand smoke on other family members is well documented. Consider a family consisting of a father, mother, and preschooler with asthma. The father frequently smokes at home and in the presence of his son. According to the health-care provider's assessment, the father is at the precontemplative stage in the TTM model (he has no intention of changing his behavior). An effective intervention for the father might include education about the harmful relationship between smoking and asthma. As the father begins to consider changing his behavior (the contemplation and preparation stages), an effective intervention might focus on developing a plan to limit smoking to outside of the home. As the plan is put into place (action stage), the health-care provider might praise the father for his effort and point out the benefits for his son. In the maintenance stage, an effective intervention might involve periodic assessment of the extent to which the plan is working to reduce asthma symptoms in the son.

The Role of Change Agent at the System Level

At the system level, strategies to effect change are just as complex as those at the individual level. Situational factors such as goals, resources, and urgency help to determine an appropriate strategy to use for system-level change.

Political Action

Political action and policy development can be thought of in terms of "decision making through both private and public mechanisms occurring in city councils, hospitals, small businesses, community organizations, universities, courts and state legislatures" (Phillips, 2000). In a more comprehensive sense, political action and social policy might be also be thought to encompass neighborhood advocacy, media campaigns, and judicial policy making (Phillips, 2000). Political action and policy making are usually directed toward changing social conditions through a variety of tactics. Social planners and community organizers have developed a wide variety of strategies to effect social change that range from formal planning with community representatives to highly confrontational tactics designed to disrupt social activities. Children from hungry households are twice as likely to miss school as children from nonhungry households. Children who skip breakfast are less attentive, more likely to have discipline problems, and perform significantly less well in problem solving. Change related to such variables may require concerted political action.

Peters (1998) suggested several steps in effecting social change that include (a) being educated about various issues that influence the political agenda, (b) developing specific plans for change, (c) defining and prioritizing needs, and (d) developing a power base. Porter (1991) described several situations wherein political action and policy development resulted in significant changes in health-related issues. In one situation, an obstetrician organized members of a community and succeeded in placing adolescent health-care services in a local school. His motivation was based on high teen pregnancy rates and the inability of teens to access prenatal health care. In a second example, a minister's wife and public health nurse were successful in convincing the local medical community to open a free clinic in a migrant labor camp. The free clinic eventually became the basis for a formal arrangement at the county level to provide needed medical services to migrant workers.

A myriad of health-care issues calls for political action and social policy strategies. For example, the Tufts University Center on Hunger, Poverty, and Nutrition reports that low-income children depend on school lunches for one third to one half of their daily nutritional intake. The health-care implications of school lunch programs are numerous. When school is not in session, some children are not eating (Chern, 1997). Hungry children from low-income families are more likely to develop anemia and have higher rates of illness (Chern, 1997).

Planned Change, Needs Analysis, and Evaluation

A variety of theorists, including Julian and Lyons (1992) and Green and Kreuter (1991), have defined specific models that are applicable to health planning. The health planning enterprise usually consists of several distinct steps that lead to desired actions. Planning theorists divide planning models or approaches into a number of distinct categories. Two of the more prevalent approaches include rational and strategic planning. Rational planning is characterized by a comprehensive review of possible solutions and the selection of the best possible alternative. Strategic planning is more focused on defining two or three critical success factors and implementing strategies to achieve specific objectives.

In addition to defining a particular course of action, the planning function should address needs assessment and evaluation of progress toward desired outcomes. A needs analysis is a tool for decision making. A critical question addressed by needs analyses focuses on whether health-care services are available to a specific population and, if so, whether the services are adequate. If inadequate, it must be determined what specific actions are needed to correct the inadequacy.

For example, Schable et al. (1995) interviewed 541 women with HIV or acquired immunodeficiency syndrome. At the time of the interviews, 478 women were part of family units (mother and children) and 234 of those family units consisted of two or more children. The most common caretaker was the mother alone (46%). Grandparents were caretakers in 16% of the families; in 15% of the families, both mother and father were caretakers. Almost one quarter of the children of mothers who used injection drugs or lived alone, in a shelter, or with friends were cared for by their grandparents. Only 30% of the mothers knew about childcare assistance services, and only 8% had used these services. This information led planners to conclude that increased provisions for childcare assistance and planning for future permanent placement of orphaned children were urgently needed. These researchers identified the gaps in services and projected future needs of HIV-infected women.

Finally, health-care agencies must start evaluating their success in achieving desired outcomes as part of the effort to change conditions at the system level. This is an essential part of the planning process and in many cases leads to improved services for children and their families. For example, if health-care professionals conducted lead poisoning screenings at a public library or local shopping mall, several evaluation questions such as the following are particularly relevant:

- Did the intervention make a difference?
- Were children referred appropriately?
- Did families whose children had high levels of lead seek treatment for their children?
- Was the treatment effective?

Evaluation procedures provide a structured means to answer such questions, which provide a basis for changing interventions in ways that more effectively address identified needs.

Grassroots Movements

A grassroots movement represents an alternative approach to system-level change. One model for using grassroots strategies is Freire's train-the-trainer program (Hope & Timmel, 1990). It is an effective, culturally sensitive, health-care strategy that works well to empower diverse individuals, families, and local communities. The train-the-trainer program has been used in Third World countries to provide outreach and health care to underserved families.

In central Ohio, a team successfully implemented Freire's program to meet the needs of medically underserved families (Julian, Strayer, & Arnold, 1998). The train-the-trainer program presents practical methods for

- group process and team building to build a sense of community,
- breaking through apathy with empowerment strategies, and
- developing critical awareness of the causes of various problems and determining true needs.

An important philosophy of this model is having the participants themselves choose the content of their education rather than having experts develop curricula for them (i.e., development must rise from the community served). Besides providing care to those who have minimal access to health-care delivery systems, the train-the-trainer model helps families transcend themselves and their limitations by drawing from their internal capacities as well as referencing a reality that is greater, outside of, and beyond themselves (Farley, 1993).

Miller (1997) documented a successful grassroots program called the Birthing Project. The Birthing Project provides pregnant women with a role model who acts as an advocate to help them navigate the maze of health-care options and determine where to receive necessary prenatal care during their pregnancies. These advocates are with the pregnant women prenatally, for the birth of their child, and during the first year of the neonate's life. In the first 3 years of the program, there was a 30% decline in the African American infant mortality rate and a decline in drug-exposed babies in the Sacramento area (Miller, 1997).

Volunteers provide a critical resource for many grassroots initiatives. It is important to follow a policy of inclusion—not exclusion—and to enable all who wish to and are able to be volunteers. In such situations, health-care professionals or other responsible parties will need to train and retrain volunteers until they feel competent and confident. Health-care providers also will need to assist in the development of leadership to sustain participation and address issues related to power and barriers. Volunteer coalitions are a wonderful way to reach out to those who have difficulty accessing health care.

Summary

Adopting the role of change agent may lead to fundamental alterations in attitudes and behaviors. Such change often has the capacity to dramatically alter health-care practices and promote optimal family health. Prochaska, Norcross, and DiClemente's (1994) TTM model offers a particularly appropriate tool for facilitating change at the individual level. Political action; planning, needs analysis, and evaluation; and grassroots movements represent a variety of tools that might be used to produce change at the system or community level. Such change has the potential to dramatically benefit large numbers of people and to prevent suffering. Thus, the health-care professional should be acutely aware of the importance and value of the change agent role at the system/community level as well as at the individual level.

Self-Care

This chapter ends with some thoughts about self-care and personal fulfillment. This is a fitting end to a chapter devoted to how professionals might enhance health-care delivery for the families that they serve. The most effective health-care professionals have studied their own motivations and aspirations. They have clarified their own life missions and clearly understand how their personal strengths and weaknesses correspond to professional values and health-care goals at the individual and system levels. Such introspection is an important complement to the health professional's efforts to provide physical, social, and psychologic support to children and their families. Introspection and personal understanding also may lead health-care professionals to seek balance in their own lives. This means engaging in physical activity, healthy eating, stress management, relaxation, and other health-enhancing behaviors.

Conclusion

As time passes, the health-care professional will develop considerable expertise and may assume administrative and training roles. Such roles may include serving as mentors to novice professionals or acting to counter the societal and institutional forces that prevent caring, effective, and holistic health-care delivery. Advocacy for effective health care and action as change agents are also rewarding options for some health-care professionals. Our advice to novice health-care professionals is to view themselves as leaders and to practice leadership based on the perspectives and skills defined in this chapter. Effective health-care professionals must strive to (a) adopt preventive strategies and interventions when possible, (b) view families as systems embedded in larger ecological systems, and (c) provide service in a manner consistent with the principles of "caring." Skills related to teaching, communication, and relationship building also are likely to enhance service delivery. Finally, attention to features of the environment, such as technology and social norms, will provide a basis for the development of effective health-care interventions. When combined with the role of change agent, these activities are likely to significantly enhance well-being and quality of life. In the long run, such efforts will serve all children and families in their efforts to be healthy and happy.

Study Guide

1. Describe the four factors suggested as essential to effective family health care.

2. What is the role of the health-care professional as a change agent?

3. Define *prevention*—historically and presently.

4. List and discuss promising prevention and intervention strategies involving families.

5. Describe the levels of prevention and intervention that are essential to optimal health outcomes.

6. Define and contrast individual versus ecological perspectives on prevention and intervention.

7. How can "caring" be instilled and maintained in health-care professionals?

8. Describe effective and ineffective teaching with families.

9. What techniques can "empower" children and their families in health-care encounters?

10. Develop a plan for changing system practices and beliefs about children who are chronically ill.

11. How might computer technology enhance or decrease quality of health-care encounters for children and their families?

References

Barton, S. (1998). Foster parents of cocaine-exposed infants. *Journal of Pediatric Nursing, 13*(2), 104–112.

Black, M., Dubowitz, H., Hutcheson, J., Berenson-Howard, J., & Starr, R. (1995). A randomized clinical trial of home intervention for children with failure to thrive. *Pediatrics, 95*(6), 807–814.

Blesch, P., & Fisher, M. L. (1996). The impact of parental presence on parental anxiety and satisfaction. *AORN, 63*(4), 761–768.

Callahan, D. (1988). Families as caregivers: The limits of morality. *Archives of Physical Medicine and Rehabilitation, 69,* 323–328.

Callery, P. (1997). Caring for parents of hospitalized children: A hidden area of nursing work. *Journal of Advanced Nursing, 26*(5), 992–998.

Carkhoff, R., & Truax, C. (1967). *Toward effective counseling and psychotherapy.* Chicago: Aldine.

Chern, E. (1997). Healthy meals = healthy kids: Bringing subsidized breakfast and summer lunch programs to communities improves health. *Children's Advocate,* 1–12.

Chewitt, M. D., Fallis, W., & Suski, M. (1997). The surgical hotline. Bridging the gap between hospital and home. *Journal of Nursing Administration, 27*(12), 42–49.

Clark, T. A. (1997, May). *Utilizing the World Wide Web as an educational tool for chronic illness.* Paper presented at the 33rd Annual ACCH Conference, Washington, DC.

Collins, J., Stevens, M., & Cousens, P. (1998). Home care for the dying child. A parents' perception. *Australian Family Physician, 27*(10), 610–614.

Corbin, J., & Strauss, A. (1991). A nursing model for chronic illness management based upon the trajectory framework. *Scholarly Inquiry for Nursing, 5*(3), 155–174.

Eddy, M., Carter, B., Kronenberger, W., Conradsen, S., Eid, N., Bourland, S., & Adams, G. (1998). Parents relationships and compliance in cystic fibrosis. *Journal of Pediatric Health Care, 12*(4), 196–202.

Emick, M. A. (1996). Custodial grandparenting: New roles for middle-aged and older adults. *International Journal of Aging & Human Development, 43*(2), 135–154.

Evans, M. (1996). A pilot study to evaluate in-hospital care by mothers. *Journal of Pediatric Oncology Nursing, 13*(3), 138–145.

Farley, S. (1993). The community as partner in primary health care nursing and health care. *Nursing & Health Care, 14*(5), 224–229.

Ferrell, B. R., Rhiner, M., & Ferrell, B. A. (1993). Development and implementation of pain education program. *Cancer, 72,* 3426–3432.

Ferrell, B., Rhiner, M., Cohen, M., & Grant, M. (1991). Pain as a metaphor for illness. Part I: Impact of cancer pain on family caregivers. *Oncology Nursing Forum, 18,* 1303–1309.

Fisher, M. (1998, July 19). The doctor is out. *The Washington Post Magazine,* p. 8.

Foster-Fishman, P. G., Salem, D. A., Allen, N. E., & Fahrbach, K. (1999). Ecological factors impacting provider attitudes towards human service delivery reform. *American Journal of Community Psychology, 27*(6), 785–816.

Fuller-Thompson, E., & Minkler, M. (2001). American grandparents providing extensive child care to their grandchildren: Prevalence and profile. *Gerontologist, 41,* 201–209.

Garwick, A., Kohrman, C., Wolman, C., & Blum R. (1998). Families' recommendations for improving services for children with chronic conditions. *Archives of Pediatric Adolescent Medicine, 152*(5), 440–448.

Gordon, R. S. (1983). An operational classification of disease prevention. *Public Health Reports, 98*(2), 107–109.

Green, L. W., & Kreuter, M. W. (1991). *Health promotion planning: An educational and environmental approach.* Mountain View, CA: Mayfield.

Heck, K., & Parker, J. (2002). Family structure, socioeconomic status, and access to health care for children. *Health Service Research, 37*(1), 173–186.

Heiberger, G. (2004). Empowering parents for SIDS prevention: Nurse practitioners play a key role. *Advanced Nursing Practice, 12*(5), 57–58.

Herberg, P. (1989). Theoretical foundations of transcultural nursing. In J. S. Boyle & M. M. Andrews (Eds.), *Transcultural concepts in nursing care* (pp. 3–65). Glenview, IL: Scott, Foresman, & Co.

Hobfoll, S. E. (1998). Ecology, community, and AIDS prevention. *American Journal of Community Psychology, 26*(1), 133–144.

Hope, A., & Timmel, S. (1990). *Training for transformation*. Gwerw, Zimbabwe: Mambo Press.

Horn, J., Feldman, H., & Ploof, D. (1995). Parent and professional perceptions about stress and coping strategies during a child's lengthy hospitalization. *Social Work Health Care, 21*(1), 107–127.

Hovell, M. F., Meltzer, S. B., Zakarian, J. M., Wahlgren, D. R., Emerson, J. A., Hofstetter, C. R., Leaderer, B. P., Meltzer, E. O., Zeiger, R. S., O'Connor, R. D., Mulvihill, M. M., & Atkins, C. J. (1999). Reduction of environmental tobacco smoke exposure among asthmatic children: A controlled trial. *Chest, 106*(2), 440–446.

Hughes, M. A., & McCollum, J. (1994). Neonatal intensive care: Mothers' and fathers' perception of what is stressful. *Journal of Early Intervention, 18*(3), 258–268.

Institute of Medicine. (1994). *Reducing risks for mental disorders: Frontiers for prevention intervention research*. Washington, DC: National Academy Press.

Jason, L. A., Anes, M. D., & Birkhead, S. H. (1991). Active enforcement of cigarette control laws in the prevention of cigarette smoking. *Journal of the American Medical Association, 266*, 3159–3161.

Jason, L. A., Richman, J. A., Friedberg, F., Wagner, L., Taylor, R., & Jordan, K. M. (1997). Politics, science and the emergence of a new disease: The case of chronic fatigue syndrome. *American Psychologist, 52*, 973–983.

Jenkins, R. (1996). Grieving the loss of the fantasy child. *Home Health Care Nurse, 14*(9), 690–695.

Johnson, B. (1990). The changing role of families in health care. *Children's Health Care, 19*(4), 234–241.

Julian, D. (1994). Planning for collaborative neighborhood problem-solving: A review of the literature. *Journal of Planning Literature, 9*(1), 3–13.

Julian, D., & Lyons, T. (1992). A strategic planning model for human services: Problem solving at the local level. *Evaluation and program planning, 15*, 247–254.

Julian, T., Strayer, J., & Arnold, R. (1998). Project Community CARE: A neighborhood health intervention. *Community Psychologist, 31*, 18–20.

Kawik, L. (1996). Nurses' and parents' perception of participation and partnership in caring for a hospitalized child. *British Journal of Nursing, 5*(7), 430–437.

Kelley, S. J., Yorker, B. C., & Whitley, D. (1997). To grandmother's house we go ... and stay: Children raised in intergenerational families. *Journal of Gerontological Nursing, 23*(9), 13–20.

Kilinski, R. (1997, Spring). Redefining the meaning of home care: Caring for children outside the hospital environment requires special skill and a focus on family support. *Pediatric Homecare Journal*, 18–20.

King, J. (1984). The health belief model. *Nursing Times, 80*(43), 53–55.

Kristensson-Hallstrom, I., & Elander, G. (1997). Parents' experience of hospitalization: Different strategies for feeling secure. *Pediatric Nursing, 23*, 361–367.

McCarthy, M., Hansen, J., Herbert, R., Wong, D., Brimacombe, M., & Zelman, M. (2002). Empowering parents through asthma education. *Pediatric Nursing, 28*(5), 465–473, 504.

Melnyk, B., Alpert-Gillis, L., Feinstein, N., Crean, H., Johnson, J., Fairbanks, E., Small, L., Rubenstein, J., Slota, M., & Corbo-Richert, B. (2004). Creating opportunities for parent empowerment: Program effects on the mental health/coping outcomes of critically ill young children and their mothers. *Pediatrics, 113*, 597–607.

Melnyk, B., Alpert-Gillis, L., Hensel, P., Cable-Beiling, R., & Rubenstein, J. (1997). Helping mothers cope with a critically ill child: A pilot test for the COPE intervention. *Research Nurses Health, 20*(1), 3–14.

Miller, C. (1997, November/December). Sisterly support, healthy babies: With one-on-one mentoring for moms. The Birthing Project boosts babies' health. *Children's Advocate*, 1–12.

Milteer, R., & Jonna, S. (1996). Parental reasons for delayed immunizations in children hospitalized in a Washington, DC, public hospital. *Journal of the National Medical Association, 88*(7), 433–436.

National Center for Injury Prevention and Control. (2002). *Best practices of youth violence prevention: A sourcebook for community action*. Atlanta, GA: Centers for Disease Control and Prevention.

Neill, S. J. (1996). Parent participation. *British Journal of Nursing, 5*(2), 110–117.

Northouse, P. G., & Northouse, L. L. (1992). *Health communication*. Norwalk, CT: Appleton & Lange.

Ozonoff, S., & Cathcart, K. (1998). Effectiveness of a home program intervention for young children with autism. *Journal of Autism and Development Disorders, 28*(1), 25–32.

Pederson, C., & Harbaugh, B. (1995). Nurses' use of non-pharmacologic techniques with hospitalized children. *Issues in Comprehensive Pediatric Nursing, 18*(2), 91–109.

Peters, S. (1998). Grassroots glory: Organizing a campaign that works. *Advances for Nurse Practitioners, 6*(3), 51–54.

Phillips, D. A. (2000). Social policy and community psychology. In J. Rappaport & E. Seidman (Eds.), *Handbook of community psychology* (pp. 397–421). New York: Kluwer Academic/Plenum.

Porter, P. (1991). Ways and means of providing primary and preventive health services. *Journal of Health Care for the Poor and Underserved, 2*(1), 167–173.

Prochaska, J., Norcross, J., & DiClemente, C. (1994). *Changing for good*. New York: Morrow.

Rees, T. (2002). Web site helps families cope with childhood illnesses. Children's Hospital of Philadelphia undergoes Internet expansion. *Profiles in Healthcare Marketing, 18*(2), 37–41, 43.

Roach, M. (1987). *The human act of caring: A blueprint for the health profession*. Ottawa, Ontario, Canada: Canadian Hospital Association.

Roe, K., Minkler, M., Saunders, F., & Thomson, G. (1996). Health of grandmothers raising children of the crack cocaine epidemic. *Medical Care, 34*(11), 1072–1084.

Sargent, J., Sahler, O., Roghmann, K., Mulhern, R., Barbarian, O., Carpenter, P., Copeland, D., Dolgin, M., & Zeltzer, L. (1995). Sibling adaptation to childhood cancer collaborative study: Siblings' perceptions of the cancer experience. *Journal of Pediatric Psychology, 20*(2), 151–164.

Schable, B., Diaz, T., Chu, S., Caldwell, M., Conti, L., Alston, O. M., Sorvillo, F., Checko, P. J., Hermann, P., & Davidson, A. J. (1995). Who are the primary caretakers of children born to HIV infected mothers? Results from a multi-state surveillance project. *Pediatrics, 95*(4), 511–515.

Scott, L. D. (1998). Perceived needs of parents of critically ill children. *Journal for the Society of Pediatric Nursing, 3*(1), 4–12.

Sirkia, K., Saarinen, U., Ahlgren, B., & Hovi, L. (1997). Terminal care of the child with cancer at home. *Aceta Paediatrics, 86*(10), 1125–1230.

Tetzlaff, L. (1997). Consumer information in chronic illness. *Journal of American Medical Information Association*, *4*(4), 284–300.

Tomlinson, P., Kirschbaum, M., Harbaugh, B., & Anderson, K. (1996). The influence of illness severity and family resources on maternal uncertainty during critical pediatric hospitalization. *American Journal of Critical Care*, *5*(2), 140–146.

Turner, P. (1997). Establishing a protocol for parental presence in recovery. *British Journal of Nursing*, *6*(14), 797–799.

U.S. Census Bureau. (2001). *Census 2000 Supplementary Survey*. Washington, DC: Author.

U.S. Department of Health and Human Services. (1996). *Models that work: Compendium of innovative primary health-care programs for underserved and vulnerable populations*. Bethesda, MD: DHHHS/HRSA/BPHC.

U.S. Department of Health and Human Services. (1998, July/August). Can access to information enhance access to care in medically underserved areas? *Gratefully Yours*, 1–8.

U.S. Department of Health and Human Services. (2003). *Steps to a healthier US: A program and policy perspective—The power of prevention*. Washington, DC: Author.

Watson, A. (1995). Strategies to support families of children with end-stage renal failure. *Pediatric Nephrology*, *9*(5), 628–631.

Woodgate, R., & Kristjanson, L. (1996). A young child's pain: How parents and nurses take care. *International Journal of Nursing Studies*, *33*(3), 271–284.

The Health-Care Environment

Mardelle McCuskey Shepley

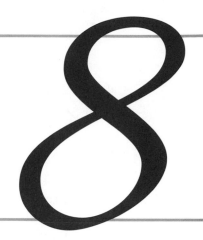

Objectives

At the conclusion of this chapter, the reader will be able to:

1. Define "environment" and summarize the general impact of the environment on functioning, development, and behavior.
2. Discuss the aspects of the environment in health-care settings that may affect behavior, development, and recovery, highlighting those that have research support.
3. Describe innovative approaches to designing children's health-care environments.
4. Determine changes in health-care delivery for children, and draw implications for relevant environmental design changes.

esign is a very broad-based discipline focused on issues of problem solving. Designers encompass a variety of professionals, including architects, interior designers, industrial designers, furniture and fabric designers, landscape architects, and urban designers. Although they are not primary caregivers, designers have an important role to play in health care.

The primary source of psychosocial support of children in the health-care continuum will always be caregivers and their programs. As a secondary source, conscientious designers attempt to provide spaces that will support the endeavors of these individuals. Excellent healing environments reinforce excellent clinical quality, and, conversely, inferior environments can detract from fine clinical care (Fottler, Ford, Roberts, & Ford, 2000). Designers also aspire to create environments that will directly support the well-being of children and their families. These environments are intended to be inherently healing by reducing stress and providing appropriate settings for normalized activity.

A recent analysis of more than 400 research studies by The Center for Health Design shows a direct link between patient health and quality of care and the way a hospital is designed (The Center for Health Design, 2004). Designers can have an impact on many health-care settings. In the traditional context, building types might range from home care settings to ambulatory care facilities, from day surgery to hospitals, and from skilled nursing facilities to hospices. Additionally, health care can be delivered in a variety of other environments, the primary purposes of which might focus on other services. Among these related building types are day care centers, halfway homes, schools, and community and recreational facilities. In addition to these specific spaces and buildings, designers that advocate a holistic healing process would argue that the health-care environment encompasses communities and regions. The healthy communities movement is a grassroots effort, which is gaining steam as we move into the 21st century. However, while supporting this compelling, holistic view of healthy environments, this chapter focuses on the spectrum of microenvironments.

The following discussion will address the health-care environment from five perspectives: first, a summary of terms and objectives of *psychosocial issues,* as defined by environmental psychologists; second, examples of *alternative design philosophies* that support family- and patient-centered care; third, general *design recommendations for pediatric hospitals;* fourth, *alternative caregiving environments;* and finally, more controversial (and frequently scientifically supported) *dimensions of healing environments.*

Psychosocial Issues

Environmental psychology, or "the study of transactions between individuals and their physical settings" (Gifford, 1987, p. 2), is a new science, the basic tenets of which are steadily being formulated. Gifford continued, "In these transactions, individuals change the environment and their behavior and experience are changed by the environment. Environmental psychology includes research and practice aimed at using and improving the process by which human settings are designed" (p. 2). Although the vast majority of design professionals are not trained as environmental psychologists, the more experienced are aware of some of the basic axioms and incorporate them into their design solutions. Many of these precepts are intuitively obvious, although, when not overtly identified, they are easily lost in the morass of objectives that must be accommodated in a design project.

The importance of the environment in health care was eloquently articulated in the form of a theory proposed by Lawton and Nahemow (1973). Their theory, the Press-Competence model, suggests that the more compromised patients are with regard to their physical or emotional health, the more susceptible they may be to negative aspects of the physical environment. Environments with a high level of *press* (very challenging) are appropriate when the competence level of an individual is high. When competence is low, an overtaxing environment is not suitable. In these two conditions, adaptive behavior is most successful. The difficulty takes place when the environment is inappropriately matched with the competence level of the individual. Hospitals, for example, which may be confusing or technologically overstimulating, can undermine a patient's self-confidence. Gerontologists developed the Press-Competence model, however, and the place of children within this theory must be considered. Are children more vulnerable to the physical environment than adults? If we assume that adults, having more experience in the world, are more callused to environmental stimulation, then we should expect children to be more sensitive to it.

In spite of its youth, the field of environmental psychology deals with very important psychosocial issues. These include (a) control, (b) privacy and social interaction, (c) personal space, (d) territoriality, and (e) comfort and safety. All of these terms are interrelated, and it is often difficult to speak of one without incorporating the others into the definition.

Control

The concept of *locus of control* originated in personality theory and generally refers to the perceived seat of social control. When an individual's health or the health of a family member is compromised, the resultant mindset is one of disempowerment or lack of control. A physical environment that prohibits individuals from managing their space can contribute to this disempowerment. Studies have shown that the negative aspects of environmental stress can be mitigated when individuals feel they can control their space (Evans, 1982). The well-known environmental psychologist Dr. Roger Ulrich (1999, 2000, 2001) included the provision of a sense of control as one of his four primary health facility design guidelines.

A health-care environment can undermine control in many ways. One of the classic examples is impeded *wayfinding*. Wayfinding is the behavior an individual exhibits when attempting to locate or arrive at a destination. When the design of a building results in poor wayfinding, that individual may become frustrated and lost. Adults who have been lost as children recount that experience as among the most frightening of childhood, and can find this experience very intimidating as adults, as well. With regard to health-care settings, an individual may enter into a frustrating wayfinding situation in an already distracted state because of poor health or concern about the poor health of a friend or family member. The unpleasantness of this disorientation is exacerbated by these stresses.

Various techniques can be employed to mitigate the potentially confounding aspects of a building's configuration, including the location of landmarks (e.g., plants or paintings) at critical intersections of the building; placement of windows along circulation paths to orient individuals relative to the outside of the building; clear designation of building entries; and massing of buildings to suggest their interior use. Buildings with massing that support wayfinding are buildings whose shape and size suggest the activity that takes place inside. For example, an auditorium might appear on the outside as a large windowless volume and a corridor might be articulated as a long linear element. The objective is to allow the viewer to guess how the interior is organized simply by looking at the exterior envelope. Surprisingly, signage is not the primary means of providing wayfinding, although it can be very useful as a redundant system. There are several excellent articles and books on this topic, including Carpman and Grant's *Design that Cares* (2001).

In addition to wayfinding, other examples of how an environment can deprive a patient or family member of control include the following:

- inability of patient or family to control room temperature
- inability of patient to control lighting from bed
- inability of patient to open or close window shades from bed
- inability to see out of a window because cubicle curtains, bed railings, or furniture block the view
- inability to open a door because of the strength required to overcome the door mechanism
- inability to turn a door knob to open a door because of weakness associated with illness or medications
- inability to pass a wheelchair through a narrow entry
- inability to use a toilet because of lack of adjacent space to make a transfer off a wheelchair
- inability to have privacy when needed

- inability to control noise
- absence of spaces that support the presence of family members

An additional source of frustration for a child can be an environment that is designed at adult scale. Ergonometrically correct pediatric furniture and plumbing fixtures and conveniently placed door hardware and light switches are small gestures that can increase the accessibility of a child's environment. Appropriate healing environments enhance feelings of efficacy rather than compromise them. The resultant sense of control helps reduce stress levels.

Privacy and Social Interaction

Health-care environments should provide opportunities for both privacy and social interaction. According to Altman (1975), privacy is directly related to control issues in that privacy can be defined as the selective control of social interactions. Patients and families may wish to control access not only to themselves, but also to groups with which they identify. The ability to control interactions is so important that these skills may be even more important than the interactions themselves.

In a health-care setting, privacy and social interaction can be accommodated through seating and furniture configuration, furniture and casework design, room configuration, and floor plan layout. Seating arrangements can directly support or undermine social interaction. Sociopetal seating, which orients chairs to enable conversation, has an effect opposite to that of sociofugal seating, which discourages interaction by orienting seats away from one another (see Figures 8.1 and 8.2).

Sociopetal seating is not necessarily preferred over sociofugal seating. In a study of adult ICU waiting rooms, Fournier (1994) found that families sought both kinds of seating, those that allowed family members to be alone and those that allowed them to commiserate with other families visiting the ICU. The sharing of information that can take place in a sociopetal environment can support parents in coping with their crisis (Hughes, McCollum, Sheftel, & Sanchez, 1994).

Furniture and casework (built-in counters and cabinets) also can be designed to encourage or discourage interaction. Highly elevated nurses' stations may be intimidating to children (and adults) who wish to interact with nursing staff. Similarly, room configuration can influence privacy. The placement of the restroom relative to the bed can be manipulated to allow nursing staff to observe activity once they enter the room, but protect patient visibility from general passersby. Finally, the floor plans of nursing units should be flexible enough to accommodate a variety of activities along the private-to-socially interactive spectrum.

In addition to spatial and visual privacy, auditory privacy is an equally significant concern. When patients share rooms, they are privy to one another's personal phone conversations as well as their discussions with medical

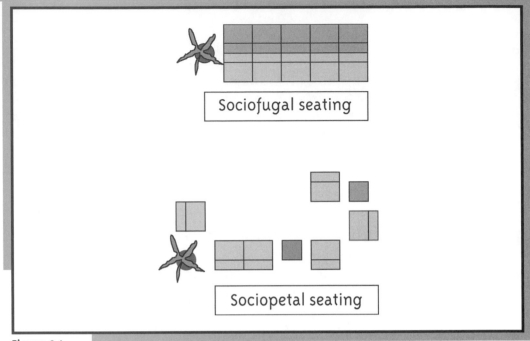

Figure 8.1.
Sociopetal seating supports conversation, and sociofugal seating discourages social interaction.

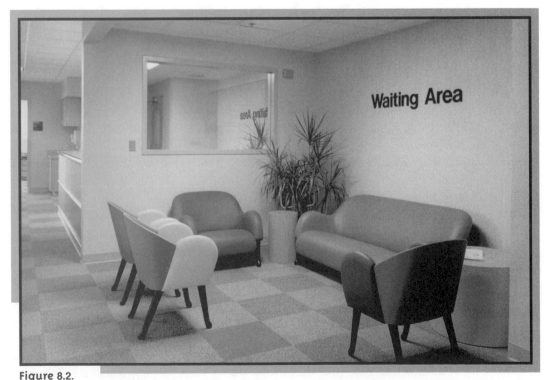

Figure 8.2.
Seating can be arranged to support conversation. *Note*. Photograph used with permission of Hackensack Medical Center.

staff, family members, and visitors. Private rooms are preferred by many to reduce this intrusion. If grieving rooms are not provided for parents who have experienced the loss of a child, then they must withhold their response or demonstrate their loss publicly. Interestingly, outdoor space is sometimes used to provide privacy. The introduction of a fountain into a public area, either indoor or outdoor, will generate enough "white noise" to allow individuals to have a private conversation without being overheard. Designers can also enhance auditory privacy by using acoustical, maintainable materials to control sound.

Personal Space

Robert Sommer (1969) defined personal space as "an area with invisible boundaries surrounding a person's body into which intruders may not come." More colloquially, personal space is thought of as the imaginary bubble around oneself that defines one's relationships with others. Sommer noted,

> Hospital patients complain not only that their personal space and their very bodies are continually violated by nurses, interns, and physicians who do not bother to introduce themselves or explain their activities, but that their territories are violated by well-meaning visitors who will ignore "No Visitors" signs. Frequently patients are too sick or too sensitive to repel intruders. (p. 28)

The literature on personal space behavior relevant to this chapter is of two kinds: general studies in settings other than health-care facilities, and studies in health-care facilities. In general studies on children's personal space, the methodology most frequently used involves asking the child to position a figure, such as a doll or silhouette cutout, relative to a figure of himself or herself in the context of a given situation. For example, Strayer and Roberts (1997) found that 5-, 9-, and 13-year-old boys place vignette characters closer to themselves when they felt greater empathy with the characters.

One of the interesting aspects of personal space behavior is that it may vary with age. This variation is particularly challenging in the design of pediatric units because the developmental age of the patients ranges dramatically. When recording the behavior of children ages 2 to 4 years old, Okano (1985) found that the higher the mental age of the children, the farther away from themselves they would place a silhouette of someone they disliked. Researchers also have noted that children demonstrate increased distancing of caretakers as they become older (Rheingold & Eckerman, 1970). In a related study, Burgess and McMurphy (1982) observed the behavior of children 6 months to 5 years old and found that distance from adults increased with age, but distance to playmates decreased. Although infants (age 6 to 18 months) stayed close to their adult caretakers, toddlers and preschoolers avoided the space around these adults.

Of the few studies examining the spatial behavior of children in health-care settings, one noted that hospitalized children participating in a program of planned play demonstrate more positive feelings in life-space drawings than those without a planned program (Gillis, 1989). In another study, Schoffstall (1984) examined the effect of the stress of hospitalization on the personal space of children by examining the distancing of stimulus figures by hospitalized and nonhospitalized children 7 to 13 years of age. The study measured stress levels and distancing patterns in response to figures representing mothers, fathers, nurses, doctors, strangers, and friends. The researcher predicted that hospitalized children would distance figures more than do nonhospitalized children, and although the overall trend supported this prediction, the data were not statistically significant. The study indicated, however, that the increased stress associated with hospitalization was correlated with increased distances from nurses, doctors, and male strangers. Schoffstall concluded that personal space serves as a buffer to protect individuals from a perceived threat.

In a related study, Sanfilippo (1994) focused on the personal space and coping behaviors of terminally and chronically ill children with HIV and cancer. Three groups of children—HIV symptomatic, those diagnosed with cancer, and healthy children—were compared. HIV-positive children perceived their parents to distance themselves farther away from them than did children with cancer. All sick children reported greater distancing of parents than that perceived by their mothers.

Proxemic behavior is integral to the concept of personal space. Hall (1969) described *proxemics* as "the interrelated observations and theories of man's use of space as a specialized elaboration of culture" (see Figure 8.3). Hall identified four types of psychologic distance: public, social, personal, and intimate. Public distance in a hospital setting might be observed when a medical resident makes a presentation to interns. In this situation, the speaker generally stands at least 12 feet from an audience. Social distance is expressed frequently in health-care settings. This proxemic characteristic is the distance at which informal business takes place, such as asking questions at the information counter or making purchases at the gift shop. Social distance is thought to be between 4 and 12 feet. Personal distance is kept between individuals who know one another, or when private information must be shared. Personal distance is often exercised in an exam room or inpatient room and, according to Hall, ranges from 18 inches to 4 feet. Intimate distance (less than 18 inches) is the distance at which caregiving might take place, particularly by friends or family members. Direct contact is not unusual. Natural conflicts, however, may take place when a caregiver who is unknown to the patient must trespass into the intimate space of a patient to provide treatment or assess health.

In a recent study (Edwards, 1998), adult patients and staff in a critical-care setting were evaluated regarding their perceptions of the use of space and touch. Using behavioral observation and interviews, the researcher found that normal spatial behavior was interrupted, and that "rules" differed for patients and staff. Both staff and patients defined the patient's personal

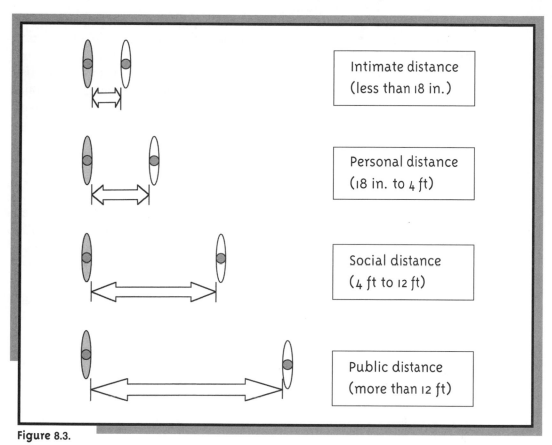

Intimate distance
(less than 18 in.)

Personal distance
(18 in. to 4 ft)

Social distance
(4 ft to 12 ft)

Public distance
(more than 12 ft)

Figure 8.3.
There are four types of psychologic distance: public, social, personal, and intimate.

space as containing the curtain, bed, and adjacent furniture. Although patients accepted the intrusion of staff into this space, they did not accept intrusions by other patients.

Proponents of proxemic theory suggest that different cultures have different spatial behaviors. Awareness of these cultural differences is critical in contemporary health settings. Caregivers are serving multicultural communities, so awareness of differences between groups will enable them to increase their effectiveness (see also Chapter 10: Cultural Influences in Children's Health Care). Researchers propose that one's sense of spatial distancing may vary depending on cultural or ethnic background. Certain groups may have smaller personal space requirements and be more comfortable with physical contact. Olson (1999) identified those groups as Arabs (from Iraq, Kuwait, Saudi Arabia, Syria, United Arab Republic); Latin Americans (from Bolivia, Cuba, El Salvador, Mexico, Ecuador, Paraguay, Peru, Puerto Rico, Venezuela); and Southern Europeans (from France, Italy, Turkey). Non-contact groups may include Asians (from China, Indonesia, Japan, Philippines, Thailand); Northern Europeans (from Australia, England, Germany, the Netherlands, Norway, Scotland); and Indians and Pakistanis. North

Americans have been described as falling into the noncontact group; however, our progressively multicultural composition may result in a behavioral shift.

What are the environmental implications of proxemic behavior for children and their families? Because of the diversity of needs, designers should be careful to provide a variety of furniture arrangements and room activity densities to correspond to differing spatial perspectives.

Territoriality

The third commonly used term in environmental psychology is territoriality. Gifford (1987) defined territoriality as a pattern of "behavior and attributes" based on perceived, attempted, or actual control of a quantifiable physical space. Territoriality can be differentiated from privacy in that it addresses domain and ownership rather than sense of personal separation. As with privacy, there are multiple realms of territory ranging from primary territory to public territory (Altman & Chemers, 1980). Primary territory in a hospital would be the patient's room. A hospital dining room is normally public territory. Lyman and Scott (1967) noted three ways in which a territory may be disturbed: (1) invasion (when a territory is physically entered by an outsider), (2) violation (when a territory is purposely modified by an outsider), and (3) contamination (in which something inappropriate is left behind in a territory). In the context of a hospital or clinic waiting room, territory would be invaded if a stranger sat between two family members having a conversation. The space would be violated if that stranger took a coat sitting on a chair in that conversational unit and moved it. It would be contaminated if the intruding individual spilled a cup of coffee and left it behind.

A single person may control a territory. In hospitals, territories controlled by individuals include patient rooms, nursing stations, and exam rooms. Groups can also control territories. A hospital billing office and the living room of a home are examples of territories under the control of several people. Subterritories can exist within the boundaries of public space: The corner of a waiting room that a family has been occupying for an extended period naturally evolves into its territory.

Spontaneous territorial gestures are evident throughout health-care environments. They include the following:

- photographs or drawings in a patients room (see Figure 8.4),
- relocation of furniture by families in waiting rooms to accommodate their needs,
- advertisements for activities in a nursing station,
- placement of coats and belongings on furniture in a waiting room, and
- decorations on a playroom wall.

Other more permanent territorial markers are signage, elevated nursing station counters, and locked doors (see Figure 8.5).

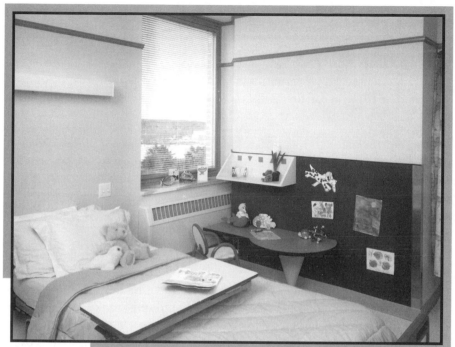

Figure 8.4.

Space should be provided at the bedside for personal belongings. *Note.* Photograph used with permission of Newton-Wellesley.

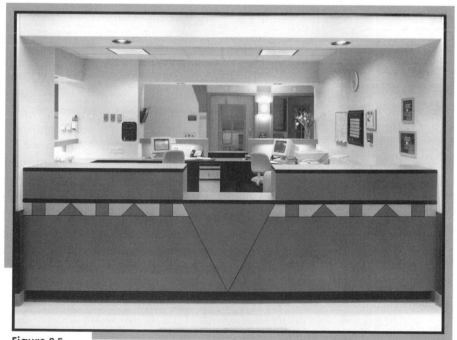

Figure 8.5.

Nurses' stations can be a barrier for children. Lowering the counter to child height will help to eliminate unnecessary territorial markers. *Note.* Photograph used with permission of Newton-Wellesley.

It is important to distinguish between personal space and territory. Personal space is "carried around" with an individual as he or she moves, whereas territory is associated with a particular physical environment. One of the few studies on territorial behavior in a health-care setting (Allekian, 1973) focused on adult patients and found that patients experienced anxiety when intrusions of territory took place, but when personal space was intruded upon, patients accepted the violation indifferently. It can be argued that "healthcare settings are effective socially when they have clear boundaries that create territories for people" (Shepley, Fournier, & McDougal, 1998). Clarity of ownership helps deflect potential conflict.

Comfort and Safety

Although comfort and safety do not represent traditional themes in environmental psychology, they are critical aspects of psychosocial well-being and are related to issues of control and privacy. The majority of the studies on comfort needs in pediatric health environments focus on family members (e.g., Kasper & Nyamathi, 1988; Kirschbaum, 1990). Meyer, Snelling, and Myren-Manbeck (1998) noted that parents may be intimidated by the "unfamiliar physical surrounds, and the equipment." Farrell and Frost (1992) identified the following personal needs of parents related to the physical environment:

- a place to rest,
- a place to take care of personal needs,
- a nearby telephone,
- a nearby bathroom,
- available refreshments, and
- solitude (a place to be alone).

In a modified Delphi study, Endacott (1998) cited the following other areas of family need: physiologic assessment, psychosocial needs, family-centered care, hygiene needs, nutrition needs, appropriate stimulation and rest, cultural needs, spiritual needs, specific interventions related to physiologic need, dependable equipment, safety needs, and collaboration with other professionals. Areas of need identified in the first round of the research were carried in the second round as "standard practices." For these items, 80% to 100% of the subjects agree that they should be routinely implemented. Of this group, those items relating to the physical environment included emergency equipment at bedside, accommodation for parents, and refreshment facilities for parents.

Studies of environmental comfort needs, other than those of parents, are limited. In a review of the literature on the needs of children (Price, 1994), the category of physical environmental needs was not included. In a review of research exploring parental experiences, Noyes (1998) noted that no studies have yet examined different ethnic and cultural groups, non-parental family members, or the family as a unit. Studies with regard to children are also limited. Oksala and Merenmies (1989) used nurse-administered questionnaires to determine child needs in an ICU during the first day, the middle day, and the last day in intensive care. The most clearly articulated need throughout all periods was the need for rest and leisure, both of which are dependent upon the physical environment. The need for "beauty and aesthetic experiences, and sensory integrity" became more prevalent toward the end of the stay. Unfortunately, this study represents the observations of the children's needs by nursing staff, rather than a direct articulation of need by children.

Design professionals who are aware of all these psychosocial issues—control, privacy and social interaction, personal space, territoriality, and comfort and safety—will be better able to support the efforts of caregivers and the well-being of patients and their families.

Alternative Design Philosophies

Philosophies on healing environments generally address social ambience rather than physical space. A handful of philosophies, however, have evolved with a clear focus on the physical environment. The best known of these are Planetree, The Eden Alternative, Easy Street, and Anthroposophy.

Planetree

Angela Thieriot founded Planetree in response to her own unpleasant hospital experiences. Reacting in part to what she recognized as the need of patients to become educated about their illness, she began by developing a health resource center where patients could access information. This concept eventually achieved its hospital incarnation in a 13-bed medical unit at a large San Francisco hospital (Orr, 1995).

According to Planetree's current brochure, the mission of Planetree is

> to serve as a catalyst in the development and implementation of new models of health care which cultivate the healing of mind, body and spirit; are patient-focused, value-based, and holistic; and integrate the best of western scientific medicine with complementary healing traditions, practices and approaches. (Planetree, 1999a)

The fact that Planetree is known for the physical environments that support its goals is unusual for a health-care philosophy, and therefore of particular interest to designers. Planetree environments are typically fully accessible and home-like, and include a variety of elements that support patients and their families, such as

- resource libraries,
- kitchenettes,
- art carts,
- patient-welcoming nursing stations,
- lounges,
- activity rooms,
- chapels,
- gardens,
- overnight family sleep spaces,
- fountains, and
- healing gardens. (Planetree, 1999a)

Spaces are available for patient privacy as well as social opportunities. Break areas are provided for staff to allow them to reenergize.

Planetree supports values that have been adopted by most children's health organizations, although there are few children's facilities that have fully incorporated its philosophies and blueprint. One exception is the Wendy Paine O'Brien Adolescent Treatment Center (Samaritan Hospital) in Phoenix, Arizona. A recent remodeling of this facility involved taking the glass barriers out of the nurses' station and increasing the family visiting areas. Proposed projects for the Treatment Center include a patient–family resource center, healing garden, gift shop, and chapel (Planetree, 1999b). Planetree currently has affiliates distributed around the United States (see Web site: www.planetree.org/affiliates.html), yet its philosophy remains on the health-care periphery (Romano, 2002).

The Eden Alternative

The Eden Alternative program, founded by Dr. W. H. Thomas, is similar to the Planetree program in that it focuses on the psychosocial needs of patients and addresses these needs through the physical environment (for publications by Thomas, see Appendix 8.1). The 10 beliefs of the Eden Alternative program are as follows (The Eden Alternative, 1999):

1. The psychologic conditions of "loneliness, helplessness, and boredom" are responsible for a huge component of human suffering.
2. Contact with children, plants, and animals is essential to the human community.
3. Loneliness can be mitigated by access to human or animal companionship.

4. Providing care and graciously receiving care are virtues in the human community.
5. Trust addresses the needs of the moment.
6. Meaning nourishes the human spirit.
7. Medical treatment is the servant rather than the master of human caring.
8. The wisdom of seniors grows in proportion to the respect accorded them.
9. Human growth and human life are integral.
10. Wise leadership is essential.

The Eden Alternative program considers a supportive physical environment to be essential to its success. Although the program is focused on seniors and adults, the general philosophy can be readily applied to children and their families. "Loneliness, helplessness, and boredom" are chronic problems for long-term care patients of all ages. Architecture that facilitates social interaction, empowers children to control their physical environment, and stimulates the imagination is highly desirable in long-term pediatric settings.

Easy Street

Easy Street is a rehabilitative environment designed to simulate real-life experiences. Developed by David Guynes in 1985, the environment is used by adults who are attempting to reintegrate themselves into the mainstream by practicing on environments that more closely proximate what they will encounter in the real world. These environments include portions of checkout stands, cars and buses, turnstiles, restaurants, and mailboxes. Although Easy Street was created for adults, Guynes also developed an alternative for children. This alternative, Rehab 1 2 3, was designed around a gameboard concept that, like Easy Street, used the environment to support rehabilitation (Moore & Jordan, 1997; see Figure 8.6).

Anthroposophy

Founded by Rudolph Steiner in 1924, the Anthroposophical Society supports a philosophy focusing on "opening up to the various spiritual realms connected with human life through our conscious understanding" (Anthroposophical Society, 1999). The world famous Vidarkliniken, in Jarna, Sweden, embodies these values in its architecture. The intent of this facility is to provide a "sense of living order" (Logsdon, 1995). Farms and a bakery provide activities on the site, in addition to a health facility for children and adults (Malkin, 1992). The philosophy reflected in the building assumes an evolution on the part of the healing patient from containment to exploration.

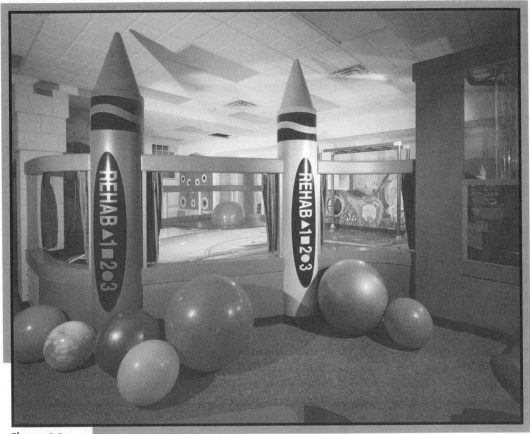

Figure 8.6.
Designed around the concept of the gameboard, Rehab 1 2 3 simulates a nonhospital environment to support rehabilitation. *Note.* Photograph used with permission of Guynes Design.

Most designers begin their projects seeking goals that will help guide the design process. Planetree, The Eden Alternative, Easy Street, and Anthroposophy provide philosophical approaches that can be readily embraced in the development of new facilities.

Design Recommendations for Hospital Environments

Much has been written about traditional hospital and ambulatory care environments, and the reader is advised to consult these references for more detailed information (see Appendix 8.1). With regard to some of the specific psychosocial factors described above, the design guidelines summarized in

Healthcare Environments for Children and their Families (Shepley et al., 1998) are particularly relevant. Regarding the hospital environment as a whole, the authors make the following recommendations.

Access

The entry and reception to the hospital should provide a supportive experience for children and their families by being welcoming, accessible, clearly designated, and of the appropriate scale. Consideration of such issues provides a "gentle" entry into an environment that may hold many unknowns for children and their families. The site of the facility should be designed to be psychologically supportive by clearly indicating destination locations, by supporting convenient access to buildings, and by being safe. Having a drop-off area near the entrance, for example, accommodates individuals carrying belongings and equipment. The exterior of the building must also support accessibility and wayfinding through the message it communicates in its exterior massing and circulation systems (corridors and elevators). For example, the organization of the building should be evident and well-marked, and separate corridors and elevators should be designated for the transport of critically ill patients.

Child Spaces

Spaces occupied by pediatric patients should be located near the services that hospital staff members are trying to provide. Psychologic support can be communicated by the inclusion of spaces that allow for social interaction (e.g., lounges, large patient rooms), privacy (e.g., areas or wall spaces dedicated specifically to a patient), and access to nature (e.g., appropriately located windows, gardens, outdoor play areas). The environment should reflect child-centered care by providing areas such as playrooms or teen rooms for age-appropriate activities, adequately-scaled furniture and light controls, and choices in types of space.

Family Spaces

If spaces are not provided for family members, conflicts can occur with staff and opportunities for parents to care for their children may be curtailed. Adequate space for guests within the patient room is essential, and the basic needs of a parent who might be confined to the hospital for an undetermined period of time must be taken into account. Such needs range from the basics (e.g., restrooms, showers, kitchenettes) to helping family members maintain their link to the outside world (e.g., computers, telephones, workspace).

Staff Spaces

The needs of staff are often overlooked in hospital design. When staff needs are not considered, staff morale may be low and existing patient spaces may have to be usurped for staff functions. Environments that support privacy (e.g., personal storage, staff lounges) and staff collaboration (e.g., conferences areas, large workstations) will indirectly benefit patients by supporting the psychologic state of caregivers.

Building Systems

Details such as lighting, acoustics, and ambience are important in hospital environments. If lighting is varied and flexible, then staff, patients, and families will have a greater sense of efficacy because a variety of tasks and activities will be supported. Natural light also should be considered because it clearly contributes to feelings of well-being. The negative impact of unwanted noise on sleep has been documented. Additionally, family and staff may wish to have private conversations and require spaces that are acoustically controlled. Sound-absorptive materials (e.g., carpet, acoustical ceiling tile) coupled with operational protocols involving noise control (e.g., beeper systems rather than public address systems) can go a long way toward eliminating noise problems. Lastly, aesthetics cannot be overlooked as an important factor in a supportive hospital stay. The application of "trendy" colors can be avoided if the designer seeks universal design solutions, such as the incorporation of nature elements and healing art.

Recent Trends in Hospital Design

Innovations in hospital design reflect a growing awareness of and attention to psychosocial needs of children and their families. Two trends include parent training spaces and single-room NICUs.

Parent Training Spaces

Training spaces are critical to the psychological comfort of parents. Such amenities are relatively common in NICUs and PICUs (see Figure 8.7). These spaces are provided with the equipment that the child will be using at home, most typically ventilators, oxygen, or infusion therapy (Dittbrenner, 1999). According to a government report (U.S. Congress, 1987), children who are ventilator-dependent may need two ventilators, in addition to an emergency battery, oxygen tank, suction machine, nebulizer, manual resus-

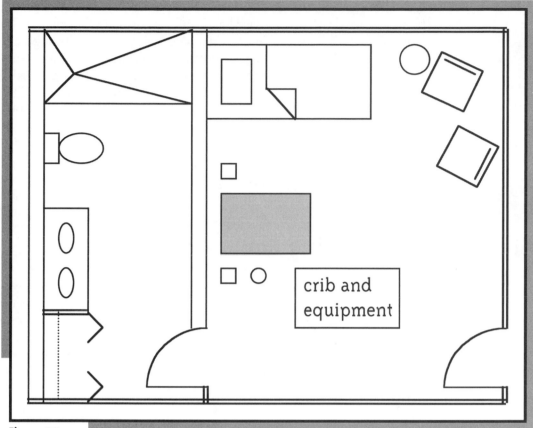

Figure 8.7.
NICU parent training room. Training spaces, common in neonatal intensive care units (NICUs) and pediatric intensive care units (PICUs), are critical to parents' psychological comfort.

citator, and infusion pump. Equipment and supplies should be in place at home prior to the child's arrival (Harris, 1988).

Single-Room NICUs

One of the recent trends in neonatal intensive care unit design has been the creation of private NICU rooms. Traditionally, neonates have been placed in large rooms with 10 to 50 isolettes or smaller bays with 4 to 6 patient stations. Regarding infants, private rooms will enable customized light levels and control noise. Both of these factors may positively influence a baby's ability to sleep and potentially promote healing. Regarding families, individual rooms will provide more privacy and the possibility of sleeping near one's child. Additionally, should a child die or an emergency (code) take place, all families would not have to be exposed to the incident. On the downside, separate rooms may reduce the opportunity for spontaneous communication between families. Additionally, some parents and staff may feel more confident when the babies are directly supervised and staff can respond quickly. Lastly, construction costs will increase due to expanded space needs. Although research suggests that window views have a positive impact on patients and families, windows are not required in these private rooms. If windows are mandated (which should be encouraged), this would be another cost factor. The provision of private-room NICUs may be a wonderful trend, or create serious challenges. Because several health organizations are constructing or have already built such facilities and many organizations are contemplating similar projects, it is important that results of current studies on these facilities be incorporated into the design decision-making process.

Alternative Caregiving Environments

The hospital room setting typically is the first to come to mind when considering pediatric health-care environments; however, there are other settings in the health-care continuum. Three of these settings—rooming in, cooperative care, and home care—are gaining importance in children's health care. Rooming in and health system–sanctioned home care have been in existence long enough to confirm their usefulness in the spectrum of healing environments. Cooperative care is newer and represents the step between rooming in and home care.

Rooming In

Although the majority of children's hospitals have adopted rooming in, it is useful to summarize the design implications of this operational policy. Johnson, Jeppson, and Redburn (1992) recommended that in addition to sufficient space for sleeping and caregiving activities of families, space should be provided for a parent lounge, food preparation area, laundry, library, and consultation and teaching space. White (1993) also recommended dedicated storage and telephones. Another element of support for rooming in with a child would be a communications outlet that can be linked via modem to a computer. While parents express a strong need to be near their child, parents should also have ready access to respite spaces such as outdoor seating areas, lounges, and cafeterias.

Cooperative Care

Cooperative care involves the participation of a nonmedical care partner, but unlike rooming in, the patient is not located in a full-fledged medical unit. The cooperative care center may be on another floor of the inpatient building, or in an adjacent building. To qualify for this program, the patient must require acute hospitalization, but not need continuous care. He or she must be capable, with the support of a care partner, of attending centralized eating facilities and clinical sessions (Grieco, Garnet, Glassman, Valoon, & McClure, 1990).

According to Douglass (1994), the unique characteristics of a cooperative care unit are the separation between residential and support spaces, the hospitality ambience of the design, and the absence of nursing stations. Cooperative care has been used most frequently with geriatric patients, although the concept could be appropriate for children and their families if used as the transition between acute and home settings.

Rhode Island Hospital, University of Nebraska Medical Center, and the Tisch Hospital (NYU Medical Center), among others, have cooperative programs, although the author was unable to identify a program spe cifically dedicated to pediatrics. Shepley and colleagues (1998) suggested that the rarity of existing cooperative care units for children may be the result of physician concern that children should be kept in acute care settings until they can go home. They also suggested that the benefits of remaining in an acute care setting may be outweighed by the stress of being in an institutional setting.

Home Care

The number of medically fragile children being cared for at home is increasing rapidly (Chapman, 1998; "Fulfilling a Responsibility to the Pediatric Patient," 1998; Gerbetz & Goulish, 1998). Reasons cited for the increase in children being treated at home are (a) the development of ventilators and other sophisticated equipment for home use, (b) the recognition that hospitalization is stressful for children, and (c) the reimbursement structure. Because the pediatric market is linked to managed care and Medicaid, rather than Medicare (as with geriatric patients), it stands on firmer financial ground (Dittbrenner, 1999). Pediatric care also is one of the better sources of private pay (Dittbrenner, 1999). Concern about the susceptibility of children to nosocomial infections while in the hospital may be another reason home care has grown (Dittbrenner, 1999). Essentially, "pediatric homecare services have increased to support a nurturing environment in which families' needs for medical assistance and normal lifestyles combine to meet the comprehensive care needs of the medically fragile child" (Chapman, 1998, p. 12).

Although the medical and familial aspects of pediatric home care have been addressed in the literature, very little has been said about the physical environment needed to support children in these settings. However, Shepley and colleagues (1998) have suggested design criteria for generic home care settings (see box).

Design Criteria for the Home Care Environment	• Accessibility for emergency personnel • Space for portable equipment • Family sleep space • Access to outdoors • Emergency call system • Patient-accessible communication systems • Bedside control of lighting, television, and temperature

Visual impairment and limited mobility bring additional design considerations. Lang and Sullivan (1986) have identified the following design guidelines to address the special needs of children who are visually impaired or blind:

■ The colors in the room of a child who is visually impaired should be highly contrasting.
■ Reflective materials and suspended objects can be used to attract the attention of a child who is visually impaired to the environment at large.
■ Sound-making objects can be used in the room of a child who is blind to expand the environment.
■ Floor textures can be used to define different spaces.
■ Furniture should be located around the perimeter of the room.

Leibrock (1993) offered the following suggestions for children of limited mobility:

■ Handrail heights should not exceed 26 inches.
■ Lever handles should be used in showers to avoid accidental bumping, or an integral temperature control should be used to avoid scalding.
■ Shower controls should be a maximum of 32 inches above the floor.
■ Adjustable tables should be provided with sufficient clearance below to accommodate a wheelchair.

Additional factors particularly pertinent to pediatric home care that might be considered are (a) accommodations for siblings, (b) location of child's room near the entry to accommodate visitors, (c) opportunities for stimulation, (d) access to nature, and (e) extension of home environment to school and day care.

Accommodations for Siblings

According to Chapman (1998), siblings "are the least prepared members of the family to accept a medically frail child as part of the family unit" (p. 13). How can the physical environment support their needs? To some siblings, the introduction of home care may feel like an invasion of their pri-

- Views outside
- Easy access to bathroom and snacks
- Sufficient space in family room for child in wheelchair or hospital bed
- Secure storage for medications

Note. Adapted from *Healthcare Environments for Children and Their Families,* by M. Shepley, M.-A. Fournier, and K. McDougal, 1998, Dubuque, IA: Kendall-Hunt.

vate space. Home size permitting, siblings should be given a space of their own, even if just a study nook or a wall where they can hang posters. These gestures support the innate need for personal space and are a healthy expression of territoriality.

Room Near Entry

The presence of visiting caregivers in the home can feel like an intrusion (Chapman, 1998), in spite of the beneficial contributions they make. One way of reducing this intrusiveness is to select the room nearest the entry for the child's bedroom. This will eliminate the need for caregivers to pass through any more of the house or apartment than necessary. This lack of penetration into the household may also make visitors of the child feel more comfortable.

Opportunities for Stimulation

As Dittbrenner (1999) pointed out with regard to children, "the patients are not just ill; they are growing. They need stimulation in addition to healthcare, medication and feeding" (p. 13). One source of stimulation will be proximity to the heart of family life, perhaps the kitchen or family room. Another source should be a connection to the outside world. In an apartment, the connection might be a view of the street; in a home, a view of the street or yard.

As always, however, a balance must be struck between stimulation and a restful environment. Oksala and Merenmies (1989) found that the need for "rest and relaxation" was strongly essential during the entire stay in a PICU, while the need for "beauty and aesthetic experiences" became more important during the latter portion of the stay. This latter need is probably similar to what might be appropriate for the home care experience.

Access to the Outdoors

The importance of nature in the life of a child was examined in a 1991 study by Sebba, which found that adults identify the most significant experiences of their childhood as being located in the outdoors. Educators argue that being outside fosters all aspects of a child's development (Davies, 1996). Lack of access to the outdoors may be the single most unpleasantly institutional dimension of a hospital environment. In addition to providing a normalized environment, researchers have associated access to nature with reduced stress and the resultant healing effects. Researchers at Johns Hopkins University found that 29% of patients who listened to nature sounds and viewed a nature mural during bronchoscopy found pain control to be good or excellent as opposed to 20.5% of patients in the control group (Diette, Lechtzin, Haponik, Devrotes, & Rubin, 2003). Additionally, views of the outdoors support orientation through diurnal and seasonal clues. A protected space where a child can be outdoors should be sought. This could be the stoop or roof of a multistory building or the yard or porch of a house.

Extensions of Home

According to an interview with Jay A. Perman of the Virginia Commonwealth University's Medical College of Virginia, it is important to stop thinking of home in the traditional sense. For most children, schools or day care centers have become an extension of home (Chapman, 1998). Ready accessibility to such facilities is necessary, and this need has been met more frequently since the passing of the Americans with Disabilities Act. Family-focused care incorporates "homecare, school and community-based resources that will encourage the family's autonomy..." (Chapman, 1998, p. 13).

Dimensions of Healing Environments

Caregiving environments, as discussed above, address specific settings. Dimensions of healing environments are not setting-specific. They can be applied to any health-care environment. Dimensions of healing environments can be defined as universal qualities of spatial experience that, when appropriately administered, contribute to the therapeutic process. Access to nature, the impact of light and color, and art, music, and sensory therapies are examples of healing dimensions about which studies have been conducted. Some cultures include geomancy as a cluster of therapeutic factors. The effectiveness of most of these proposed healing qualities has been scientifically substantiated, but some, such as geomancy, still require confirmation.

The notion that the physical environment influences healing is directly related to the concept of *psychoneuroimmunology*. Before describing the dimensions of geomancy, nature, light and color, and art, music, and sensory therapies, psychoneuroimmunology should be defined.

Psychoneuroimmunology

Psychoneuroimmunology (PNI) can be defined as "a transdisciplinary scientific field concerned with interactions among behavior, the immune system, and the nervous system" (Solomon, 1996, p. 79). Proponents of PNI suggest that stress can compromise the immune system, thereby interfering with healing. Since research indicates that the environment can create stress, this theory supports the need for stress reduction in health-care settings.

Studies involving psychoneuroimmunology are becoming more commonplace in traditional medical journals. Fueled by the contributions of psychologists interested in the mind–body paradigm, a variety of articles are available discussing the possibilities of PNI (e.g., Cerrato, 1998; Kiecolt-Glaser, 1998; Moore, 1998; Morgan, 1998). Recent articles tend to reinforce the more scientific aspects of PNI.

Geomancy

Geomancy, defined as divination by means of figures, lines, or geographic features, is prevalent in Asian cultures, and *Feng Shui*, Chinese geomancy, has experienced a rebirth in popularity in recent years. A variety of books are available on Feng Shui (see Appendix 8.1). The Feng Shui philosophy, which is still embraced by many Asians, means "wind, water" (Govert, 1993), and is used to evaluate the implications of certain spatial configurations and design. The purpose of Feng Shui is to "enhance energy flows" and create a positive space. Rossbach and Lin (1991) have applied the following Feng Shui guidelines to hospitals:

- Avoid long corridors leading directly from doors.
- Place bed so patient can see the door from a kitty-corner perspective.
- Avoid heavy furniture or furniture behind the bed projecting into the space.
- Provide good views.
- Avoid adjacent beds.
- Place no bed directly between the door and the window.

Although Feng Shui appears to be philosophic and abstract, many of its precepts are based on the practical experiences of observers. The author's experience with projects reviewed by professional Feng Shui experts is that many of their suggestions are compatible with the requirements of Western technology, particularly with regard to structure and safety.

Several other cultures have similar building philosophies, including the Indian *Vastu* described as "the art of correct setting in order to optimize the benefits of five basic elements of nature … and the influence of magnetic fields surrounding the earth" (Purush & Padam, 1998). There are five components of stable buildings: orientation, theory (*Vastu Purush Mandala* [see Appendix 8.1]), proportion, canons of Vedic (Hindu) architecture, and character. According to Vastu philosophy, hospitals fall into the category of public buildings—one of five categories of architecture established in ancient texts. An example of a typical design guideline for hospitals would be that an "L" or "U-shaped" building should be open to the northeast, and heavy in the southwest (Panditji, 1999).

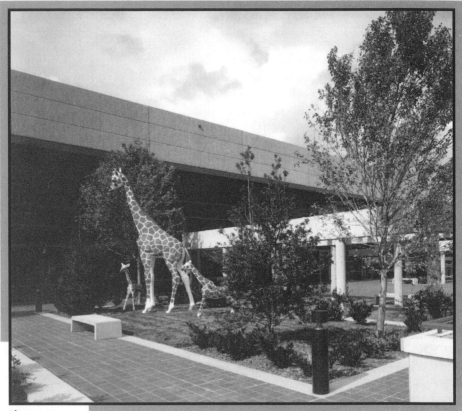

Figure 8.8.
Views of nature and access to outdoor spaces are essential to stress reduction.
Note. Photograph used with permission of Odell Associates.

Access to Nature

The affinity most children have for the outdoors is evident (see Figure 8.8). Dr. Edward O. Wilson (1986) used the word *biofilia* to describe the innate affiliation humans have with other living things. Steve and Rachel Kaplan (1989) suggested that our preference for the outdoors is the result of the critical contribution to our survival that is provided by an understanding of nature. According to their research, the nature scenes that have the most appeal are those that balance interest with understandability. Ulrich also has conducted studies demonstrating that views of nature may reduce stress and therefore support healing (Ulrich, 1984), as well as studies showing that driving through landscaped areas resulted in lower blood pressure and higher preference than billboarded, urban areas (Parsons, Tassinary, Ulrich, Hebl, & Grossman-Alexander, 1998). Unfortunately, there have been no studies examining the impact of views on children in health-care settings.

In a more quantitative study, Olds (1995) asked subjects to imagine where healing would take place. Participants, who included architects, designers, social workers, psychotherapists, nurses, parents, and students, responded with drawings. Seventy-five percent included the outdoors, nature elements, objects drawn with the suggestion of motion, and vistas. Light, animals, and beauty were also common components.

Studies and books on the impact of healing gardens have proliferated. Marcus and Barnes (1995) conducted research on the gardens in four hospitals. They found that people who used the gardens used them frequently and reported positive mood outcomes. Marcus and Barnes offered the following suggestions:

- Exterior and interior environments should contrast.
- Gardens should accommodate reduced patient mobility and provide protection.
- Extra security should compensate for the perceived insecurity suggested by outdoor spaces.
- Stimuli with an external focus should be provided.
- Physical and psychological journeys should be suggested in garden configurations.
- Gardens should provide options for both privacy and socialization.

Gardens are also an essential part of the Planetree philosophy. "Bringing nature inside through the use of plants, fountains, and skylights as well as encouraging patients, families and staff to go outside into garden areas whenever possible can help transform institutions into healing environments" (Planetree, 1999; see Figure 8.9). Several Planetree facilities incorporate significant nature components, including a three-story waterfall at MidColumbia Medical Center, a water sculpture in the ICU at Griffin Hospital, and a solarium in the rheumatology unit in Trondheim, Norway (Planetree, n.d./ 2004a; n.d./2004b).

Nature is important in the life of a child. As previously mentioned, Sebba (1991) found that adults identify the most significant experiences of their childhood as being located in the outdoors. Regarding selection of specific nature images, non–hospital-based studies on landscape preferences of children suggest that children prefer landscapes of the environments with which they are most familiar (Lyons, 1983) and that younger children (11-year-olds) demonstrate less preference for landscapes suggesting risk than older children (16-year-olds; Bernaldez, Gallardo, & Abello, 1987). This finding is sympathetic with the Press-Competence model discussed earlier, which suggested that the more competent the individual, the more adaptive the behavior in a challenging environment.

Light and Color

Literature relating to light and color includes three main topics: studies on chronobiology, studies on access to light, and studies on the impact of color.

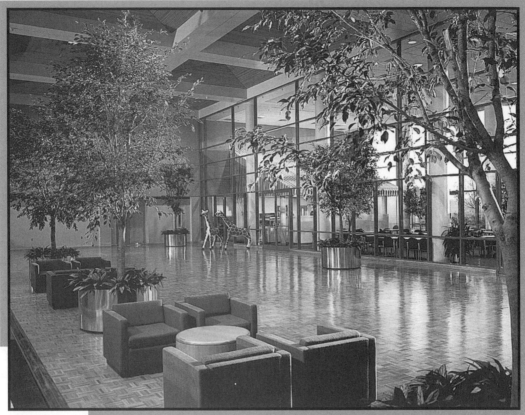

Figure 8.9.
Bringing nature inside can help transform institutions into healing environments. *Note.* Photograph used with permission of Odell Associates.

Chronobiology

The relationship of light to biologic and physical patterns of life is called chronobiology. Diurnal and season fluctuations are believed to affect the healing process, and a variety of studies confirm that adjusting light levels in nurseries to reflect diurnal variation has a positive effect on infants. As for seasonal variation, when the days are very short, some individuals are described as experiencing *seasonal affective disorder,* or SAD. Seasonal affective disorder can be defined as the negative psychologic state associated with the lack of exposure to daylight during winter months. Although there are studies that support this concept, there is insufficient evidence to fully substantiate its scientific base. Preliminary studies on children that support the argument for a causal relationship between winter and depression include Rosenthal (1995) and Carskadon and Acebo (1993). Milman and Bennett (1996), however, report that adolescent hospitalizations for suicide attempts are not related to time of year.

Access to Light

Studies on access to light generally focus on preferences expressed for daylight and window views. Previous efforts to eliminate windows in classrooms have been abandoned due to the resultant negative effects on academic performance and behavior. Research in work environments also demonstrates the preference of individuals for natural light in their workspace.

Impact of Color

Research on the physical or psychological impact of color is limited. It is generally believed that soft colors are less stimulating than bright, saturated colors (Kleeman, 1981). The intention of chromotherapy is to cure illness by exposure to specific colors or color palettes. Documented research on the effectiveness of this technique is not available.

There are several theories that may be useful in the development of health-care facilities, however, including theories about "lazure" painting, full-spectrum palettes, and neutral backgrounds. Lazure painting, which is the multilayered, semitransparent technique used at Vidarkliniken, varies in tint from blue to rose depending on the health status of the patient (Marberry & Zagon, 1995). Marberry and Zagon recommended full-spectrum color, "a balanced mix of various proportions of tints and shades" from the seven colors of the spectrum. The intent of this approach is to provide a range of coordinated colors, as would appear in a natural environment. Planetree advocates a neutral background palette.

Most designers feel that children have different color requirements than adults, and usually justify this position based on what are perceived to be developmental differences. Research indicates that strong colors may play a role in infant development and that toddlers express a preference for bright colors. However, the extension of this argument suggests that the palette must shift to accommodate children ages 2 to 18 years. Unless this population is separated spatially, it would be difficult to provide the implied universal palette.

Art, Music, and Sensory Therapies

Almost all health-care facilities now advocate the integration of art into health-care environments. Many facilities also incorporate music and aroma therapy in their programs. (See Chapter 4 for more details on the arts in children's health-care settings.)

Art

Several studies examining the art preferences of adult populations have been conducted in hospital environments and demonstrate that patients prefer realistic to abstract art images. Children's art preferences have not been studied in health-care environments; however, McGhee and Dziuban (1993, 1994) found similar preferences for realistic art among children in nonmedical settings. Other issues that have been examined regarding children and art include the impact of previous exposure to art (Bowker & Sawyers, 1988), verbal responses to art (Ramsey, 1990), the impact of cognitive style (Salkind, 1993), and aesthetic perception (Winner, 1986).

Music

Music has been used for two purposes in health-care settings: to cover up unwanted noise, and to act as a stress reducer. Parkin (1981) found that music reduced the stress of children prior to examination in a dental clinic. The majority of pediatric studies, however, have taken place in neonatal intensive care unit settings. Collins and Kuck (1991) found an increase in oxygen saturation in neonates when uterine sounds were played. Standley and Moore (1995) had similar findings when babies listened to lullabies; however, oxygen saturation fell when the music stimulus was removed.

Sensory Therapies

Aroma has been used as a distracting and soothing device in MRI rooms and as an orienting element in an Alzheimer's unit. In the former case, the smell of cookies has been piped into an MRI unit to help calm a patient undergoing a test. In the Alzheimer's unit, it is used for redundant spatial cueing to help a resident locate the kitchen by smell. There are no specific studies on the use of aroma therapy in children's environments, although it would be interesting to conduct a study on their preferences, as smell has been found to be effective in generating memories.

Conclusion

The field of environmental psychology is a new one, with discoveries being made every day. The range and exploratory nature of the material presented in this chapter lead us to conclude that more research is required on the relationship between the built environment and psychosocial factors influencing children and their families. The information contained herein should be applied judiciously until prototypes are fully tested and studies are corroborated. Regardless, consumers should demand that the designers who are developing projects base their decisions on the best information available. Designers should ask those who use or work in pediatric health-care environments—families, caregivers, and even the children themselves—to provide input to designers regarding their needs. The informed decision maker takes into account the role of environmental psychology, alternative design philosophies, alternative caregiving prototypes, and the potential healing contributions of specific environmental variables.

Study Guide

1. What types of (physical) environments best promote health and healing?

2. Describe the aspects of the environment that are particularly important to children's healing or continued developmental needs.

3. Compare and contrast psychosocial issues defined by environmental psychologists to those supportive of family- and patient-centered care.

4. List and discuss aspects of environmental design related to children's health care that are supported by research.

5. Discuss alternative design philosophies and draw implications for designing health-care environments for children.

6. Describe innovative environmental approaches in child health-care settings.

7. What are the dimensions of healing environments, and how can they be incorporated into child health-care settings?

8. Define *psychoneuroimmunology* and discuss its implications for children's health care.

9. Discuss various therapies as related to children's health care and cite supportive research.

10. List emerging health-care demands and treatments for children, and suggest environmental changes essential to healing and normalization.

© 2005 by PRO-ED, Inc.

APPENDIX 8.1

Resources for Health-Care Environments

Eden

Thomas, W. H. (1996). *Life worth living: How someone you love can still enjoy life in a nursing home*. Acton, MA: VanderWyk & Burnham.

Thomas, W. H. (1999). *Learning from Hannah*. Acton, MA: VanderWyk & Burnham.

Traditional Hospital and Ambulatory Care Environments

Johnson, B., Jeppson, E., & Redburn, L. (1992). *Caring for children and families: Guidelines for hospitals*. Bethesda, MD: Association for the Care of Children's Health.

Malkin, J. (1992). *Hospital interior architecture*. New York: Van Nostrand Reinhold.

Psychoneuroimmunology

Morgan, L. (1998). Psychoneuroimmunology, the placebo effect and chiropractic. *Journal of Manipulative and Physiological Therapeutics, 21*(7), 484–491.

Feng Shui

Craze, R. (1999). *Feng shui*. North Pomfret, VT: Trafalgar Square.

Edwards, J. (1999). *Asian elements: Natural balance in eastern design*. San Francisco: Soma Books.

Mandala

Brauen, M. (1998). *The mandala: Sacred circle in Tibetan Buddhism*. Boston: Shambhala Publications.

Leidy, D. P., & Thurman, R. A. (1997). *Mandala: The architecture of enlightenment*. Boston: Shambhala Publications.

Music

Hicks, F. (1995). The role of music therapy in the care of the newborn. *Nursing Times, 91*(38), 31–33.

Mazer, S., & Smith, D. (1991). The power of space. *Child Health Design, 4,* 13–15.

References

Allekian, C. (1973). Intrusions of territory and personal space. *Nursing Research, 22*(3), 236–241.

Allgemeine Anthroposophische Gesellshaft. (n.d./1999). *Anthroposophical Society.* Retrieved February 6, 2006, from www.goetheanum.org/aag.html?&L=1

Altman, I. (1975). *The environment and social behavior.* Monterey, CA: Brooks/Cole.

Altman, I., & Chemers, M. (1980). *Culture and environment.* Monterey, CA: Brooks/Cole.

Bernaldez, F. G., Gallardo, D., & Abello, R. P. (1987). Children's landscape preferences: From rejection to attraction. *Journal of Environmental Psychology, 7*(2), 169–176.

Bowker, J. E., & Sawyers, J. K. (1988). Influence of exposure on preschooler's art preferences. *Early Childhood Research Quarterly, 3*(1), 107–115.

Burgess, J. W., & McMurphy, D. (1982). The development of proxemic spacing behavior: Children's distances to surrounding playmates and adults change between 6 months and 5 years of age. *Developmental Psychobiology, 15*(6), 557–567.

Carpman, J., & Grant, M. (2001). *Design that cares* (2nd ed.). New York: Wiley.

Carskadon, M., & Acebo, C. (1993). Parental reports of seasonal mood and behavior changes in children. *Journal of the American Academy of Child and Adolescent Psychiatry, 32,* 264–269.

The Center for Health Design. (2004). *Evidence-based hospital design improves healthcare outcomes for patients, families, and staff.* Retrieved July 28, 2004, from www.healthdesign.org

Cerrato, P. L. (1998). Understanding the mind/body link. *RN, 61*(1), 28–31.

Chapman, D. J. S. (1998). Family-focused pediatric home care. *CARING Magazine, 17*(5), 12–15.

Collins, S., & Kuck, K. (1991). Music therapy in the neonatal intensive care unit. *Neonatal Network, 9*(6), 23–26.

Davies, M. (1996). Outdoors: An important context for young children's development. *Early Child Development and Care, 115,* 37–49.

Diette, G., Lechtzin, N., Haponik, E., Devrotes, A., & Rubin, H. (2003). Distraction therapy with nature sights and sounds reduces pain during flexible bronchoscopy: A complementary approach to routine analgesia-bronchoscopy. *Chest, 123,* 941–948.

Dittbrenner, H. (1999). Pediatric homecare as a viable service. *CARING Magazine, 18*(2), 12–13, 15.

Douglass, V. (1994). *Cooperative care study.* Unpublished manuscript, Texas A&M University, College of Architecture, College Station, TX.

Edwards, S. C. (1998). An anthropological interpretation of nurses' and patients' perceptions of the use of space and touch. *Journal of Advanced Nursing, 28*(4), 809–817.

Endacott, R. (1998). Needs of the critically ill child. *Intensive and Critical Care Nursing, 14*(2), 66–73.

Evans, G. (Ed.). (1982). *Environmental stress.* Cambridge, England: Cambridge University Press.

Farrell, M., & Frost, C. (1992). The most important needs of parents of critically ill children: Parents' perceptions. *Intensive and Critical Care Nursing, 8,* 130–139.

Fottler, M., Ford, R., Roberts, V., & Ford, E. (2000). Creating a healing environment: The importance of the service setting in the new consumer-oriented healthcare system. *Journal of Healthcare Management, 45,* 91–107.

Fournier, M.-A. (1994). *L'aménagement des aires d'attente dans les unités de soins intensifs pour adultes.* (The design of family waiting rooms in intensive care units for adults.) Unpublished master's thesis, Laval University, Quebec, Canada.

Fulfilling a responsibility to the pediatric patient. (1998). *CARING Magazine, 17*(5), 16–17.

Gerbetz, N. J., & Goulish, D. G. (1998). Improving continuing care for children: Collaboration between homecare and hospital social work. *Continuum, 18*(4), 1, 3–7.

Gifford, R. (1987). *Environmental psychology: Principles and practice.* Boston: Allyn & Bacon.

Gillis, A. J. (1989). The effect of play on immobilized children in hospital. *International Journal of Nursing Studies, 26*(3), 261–269.

Govert, J. (1993). *Feng Shui: Art and harmony of place.* Phoenix, AZ: Daikakuji.

Grieco, A., Garnett, S., Glassman, K., Valoon, P., & McClure, M. (1990). New York University Medical Center's cooperative care unit: Patient education and family participation during hospitalization—The first ten years. *Patient Education and Counseling, 15,* 3–15.

Hall, E. T. (1969). *The hidden dimension.* Garden City, NY: Doubleday.

Harris, P. (1988). Sometimes pediatric homecare doesn't work. *American Journal of Nursing, 88*(6), 851–854.

Hughes, M., McCollum, J., Sheftel, D., & Sanchez, D. (1994). How parents cope with the experience of neonatal intensive care. *Children's Health Care, 23*(1), 1–14.

Johnson, B. H., Jeppson, E. S., & Redburn, L. (1992). *Caring for children and families: Guidelines for hospitals.* Bethesda, MD: Association for the Care of Children's Health.

Kaplan, S., & Kaplan, R. (1989). *The experience of nature.* New York: Cambridge University Press.

Kasper, J. W., & Nyamathi, A. M. (1988). Parents of children in the pediatric intensive care unit: What are their needs? *Heart & Lung, 17,* 576–581.

Kiecolt-Glaser, J. K. (1998). Psychological influences on surgical recovery: Perspectives from psychoneuroimmunology. *American Psychologist, 53*(11), 1209–1218.

Kirschbaum, M. (1990). Needs of parents of critically ill children. *Dimensions of Critical Care Nursing, 9,* 341–352.

Kleeman, W. (1981). *The challenge of interior design.* Boston: CBI.

Lang, M. A., & Sullivan, C. (1986). Adapting home environments for visually impaired and blind children. *Children's Environments Quarterly, 3*(1), 50–54.

Lawton, M. P., & Nahemow, L. (1973). Ecology and the aging process. In C. Eisdorfer & M. Lawton (Eds.), *The psychology of adult development and aging* (pp. 619–674). Washington, DC: American Psychological Association.

Leibrock, C. (1993). *Beautiful barrier-free.* New York: Van Nostrand Reinhold.

Logsdon, R. (1995). Understanding the application of Lazure painting techniques. *Journal of Healthcare Design, 7,* 205–212.

Lyman, S. M., & Scott, M. B. (1967). Territoriality: A neglected sociological dimension. *Social Problems, 15,* 235–249.

Lyons, E. (1983). Demographic correlates of landscape preference. *Environment & Behavior, 15*(4), 487–511.

Malkin, J. (1992). *Hospital interior architecture.* New York: Van Nostrand Reinhold.

Marberry, S., & Zagon, L. (1995). *The power of color: Creating healthy interior spaces.* New York: Wiley.

Marcus, C. C., & Barnes, M. (1995). *Gardens in healthcare facilities: Uses, therapeutic benefits, and design recommendations.* Martinez, CA: The Center for Health Design.

McGhee, K., & Dziuban, C. D. (1993). Visual preferences of preschool children for abstract and realistic paintings. *Perceptual and Motor Skills, 76*(1), 155–158.

McGhee, K., & Dziuban, C. D. (1994). Visual preferences of Mexican preschool children for abstract and realistic paintings. *Perceptual and Motor Skills, 79*(1), 240–242.

Meyer, E. D., Snelling, L. K., & Myren-Manbeck, L. K. (1998). Pediatric intensive care: The parents' experience. *AACN Clinical Issues, 9*(1), 64–74.

Milman, D., & Bennett, A. (1996). School and seasonal affective disorder. *The American Journal of Psychiatry, 153*, 849–850.

Morgan, L. G. (1998). Psychoneuroimmunology, the placebo effect and chiropractic. *Journal of Manipulative and Physiological Therapeutics, 21*(7), 484–491.

Moore, N. G. (1998). The Getting Well Program: Digging deep to find healing. *Alternative Therapies in Health and Medicine, 4*(3), 29–30.

Moore, P., & Jordan, T. (1997). Children's health design: Improving child health outcomes with Rehab 1 2 3. *Journal of Healthcare Design, 9*, 137–140.

Noyes, J. (1998). A critique of studies exploring the experiences and needs of parents of children admitted to pediatric intensive care units. *Journal of Advanced Nursing, 28*(1), 134–141.

Okano, K. (1985). Development of personal space in 2- to 4-year old children. *Journal of Human Development, 21*, 30–37.

Oksala, R., & Merenmies, J. (1989). Children's human needs in intensive care. *Intensive Care Nursing, 5*, 155–158.

Olds, A. (1995). Nature: The essential healing environment. *Child Health Design, 9*, 3–5.

Olson, T. (1999, October 11). *Analysis of cultural communication and proxemics.* Retrieved January 12, 2000, from www.unl.edu/casestudy/456/traci.htm

Orr, R. (1995). The Planetree philosophy. In S. Marberry (Ed.), *Innovations in healthcare design.* New York: Van Nostrand Reinhold.

Parkin, S. (1981). The effect of ambient music upon the reactions of children undergoing dental treatment. *Journal of Dentistry for Children, 48*(6), 430–432.

Parsons, R., Tassinary, L., Ulrich, R., Hebl, M., & Grossman-Alexander, M. (1998). The view from the road: Implications for stress recovery and immunization. *Journal of Environmental Psychology, 18*, 113–140.

Planetree. (1999). *Components of Planetree.* Retrieved July 28, 2004, from www.planetree.org/components.html

Planetree. (n.d./2004a). *Planetree: Informational brochure.* Derby, CT: Griffin Hospital.

Planetree. (n.d./2004b). *Planetree affiliates.* Web site: http://www.planetree.org/pat_affiliates.htm

Price, S. (1994). The special needs of children. *Journal of Advanced Nursing, 20*, 227–232.

Purush, J., & Padam, A. (1998). *Vastu: Reinventing the architecture of fulfillment.* New Delhi, India: Vedams Books International.

Ramsey, I. L. (1990). An investigation of children's verbal responses to selected art styles. *Journal of Educational Research, 83*(1), 46–51.

Rheingold, H., & Eckerman, C. (1970). The infant separates himself from his mother. *Science, 168*, 78–90.

Romano, M. (2002). Slow growing: Planetree philosophy sprouts new branches of support but remains on the healthcare periphery. *Modern Healthcare, 32*(32), 30–33.

Rosenthal, N. (1995). Syndrome triad in children and adolescents. *The American Journal of Psychiatry, 152*(9), 1402.

Rossbach, S., & Lin, T. (1991). Feng Shui for healthcare design. *Journal of Health Care Interior Design, 3*, 17–25.

Salkind, L. W. (1993). The relationship of gender, age, and cognitive style to preference for works of art. *Dissertation Abstracts International, 53*(8-A), 2653.

Sanfilippo, M. D. (1994). Personal space and coping in terminal and chronically ill children. *Dissertation Abstracts International, 54*(8-B), 4406.

Schoffstall, M. C. (1984). The effect of the stress of hospitalization on the personal space of children. *Dissertation Abstracts International, 46*(5-B), 1717.

Sebba, R. (1991). The landscapes of childhood: The reflection of childhood's environment in adult memories and in children's attitudes. *Environment & Behavior, 23*(4), 395–422.

Shepley, M. M., Fournier, M.-A, & McDougal, K. (1998). *Healthcare environments for children and their families.* Dubuque, IA: Kendall-Hunt.

Solomon, G. (1996). Understanding psychoneuroimmunology (PNI) and its applications for healthcare. *Journal of Healthcare Design, 8,* 79–83.

Sommer, R. (1969). *Personal space: The behavioral basis of design.* Englewood Cliffs, NJ: Prentice Hall.

Standley, J., & Moore, R. (1995). Therapeutic effects of music and mother's voice on premature infants. *Pediatric Nursing, 21*(6), 509–512.

Strayer, J., & Roberts, W. (1997). Children's personal distance and their empathy: Indices of interpersonal closeness. *International Journal of Behavioral Development, 20*(3), 385–403.

The Eden Alternative. (1999, November 9). Our 10 principles. Retrieved July 29, 2004, from http://www.edenalt.com/10.htm

Ulrich, R. (1984). View through window may influence recovery from surgery. *Science, 224,* 420–421.

Ulrich, R. (1999). Effects of gardens on health outcomes: Theory and research. In C. Cooper Marcus & M. Barnes (Eds.), *Healing gardens: Therapeutic benefits and design recommendations* (pp. 27–86). New York: Wiley.

Ulrich, R. (2000). Environmental research and critical care. In D. Kirk Hamilton (Ed.), *ICU 2010.* Houston, TX: Center for Innovation in Health Facilities.

Ulrich, R. (2001). Effects of healthcare environmental design on medical outcomes. In A. Dilani (Ed.), *Design and health—The therapeutic benefits of design.* Proceedings of the Second International Conference on Design & Health, 2000, Stockholm, Sweden: Svenskbyggtjanst.

White, R. (1993). *Recommended standards for newborn design.* South Bend, IN: Memorial Hospital.

Wilson, E. (1986). *Biofilia.* Cambridge, MA: Harvard University Press. (Reprint)

Winner, E. (1986). Children's perception of "aesthetic" properties of the arts. *British Journal of Developmental Psychology, 4*(2), 149–160.

Spiritual Issues in Children's Health-Care Settings

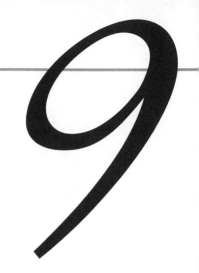

Lynn B. Clutter

Objectives

At the conclusion of this chapter, the reader will be able to:

1. Define "spirituality" and discuss children's development of and understanding of spirituality.
2. Discuss ways in which spirituality may influence children's reactions to illness and health-care experiences.
3. Determine theories of spirituality and draw implications for care of children in health-care settings.
4. Recommend various approaches to the use of spirituality with children in health care.

any aspects of health care proceed with little thought of spiritual care. The spiritual aspect of life is often dealt with much like politics, with the perspective that "the less said the better" is the best policy. Most people, however, believe that there is a spiritual aspect of life and that God does exist. Health care of children usually involves times of crisis, illness, injury, or at the least, change. Any of these times can bring spiritual aspects into focus for the child, parent, or family member (Kloosterhouse & Ames, 2002). Health-care professionals can provide spiritual care in a way that offers comfort, hope, encouragement, and respect, and can use spiritual strength to better the outcome of overall care.

The goal of this chapter is to equip professionals with information useful for providing spiritual care to children and their families. Although a knowledge base in religion is valuable, and having awareness of a religion in general can help with the care of specific children and families, this chapter will not include a discussion of this nature. Instead, an annotated bibliography of selected references regarding religions is provided in Appendix 9.1. An overview of spirituality is followed by theoretical and developmental aspects of spirituality. Spiritual care will be described. Because literature specific to children's spirituality is limited, it is hoped that the strategies given will demonstrate the variety of spiritual care options available to health-care providers. Barnes, Plotnikoff, Fox, and Pendleton (2000 suppl., p. 905) stated, "Spirituality and religion can serve as key organizing principles in the lives of children and their families, particularly in relation to children's illness, health, and healing."

The Importance of Spirituality

Spiritual issues are important for several reasons. Spirituality is regarded as a basic characteristic of humanness important in human health and well-being. Houskamp, Fisher, and Stuber (2004) reported that initial qualitative data suggest that even children experience themselves as spiritual beings, and that understanding and connecting with them around their spiritual lives can be an important adjunct to treatment. Spirituality affects people's worldview and meaning in life. Dunn and Dawes (1999) consider religious and spiritual orientations as significant as ethnicity, race, culture, social class, and gender because many fundamental beliefs are rooted in religion. People of all ages and circumstances have a spiritual dimension: "An individual is a spiritual person even when disoriented, confused, emotionally ill, cognitively impaired, or delirious" (Carpenito, 1997, p. 452). According to a U.S. national survey, nearly 80% of people believe in the power of God or prayer to improve the course of illness (Wallis, 1996). To ignore individuals' spiritual needs denies them a holistic approach to care (Espeland, 1999).

Physical Health Benefits

A mounting body of evidence points to the power of the "faith factor." For example, deeply spiritual or religiously committed individuals experience less stress—cope better with it—they have fewer drug and alcohol problems, less depression, and lower rates of suicide, and they enjoy their lives and marriages more than do the less religious in society (Gallup & Lindsay, 1999). Medical studies also have found measures of physical improvement with those having certain spiritual characteristics. Larson and Koenig (2000) reported that nearly every medical study that has considered religion has found it to be a positive factor; well-designed studies generally reveal a beneficial relationship between religious commitment, practices, and attitudes and patients' well-being.

People who report higher levels of strength of spirit tend to have higher measures of well-being in mind and body. Individuals with acute or chronic illness who report higher levels of spiritual health and religious commitment also report higher levels of physical and psychosocial well-being, more hope, less depression, less loneliness, greater compliance with health care, and improved coping and quality of life (Highfield, 2000).

In a study of the epidemiology of religion and health, Levin (1994) reviewed data on the effects of religion on outcomes of conditions including heart disease, cancer, tuberculosis, and suicide. He found that 22 out of 27 studies that included a religious variable (e.g., church affiliation, regular religious involvement) reported a significant positive effect, and 4 had a positive effect (although the studies were not large enough to be statistically significant). Marwick (1995) interpreted these findings as suggesting, although not proving, that "lack of religious involvement seems to be a risk factor [for poorer health]" (p. 1562).

Desire for Spiritual Care

Findings indicate that people want spiritual care, especially when hospitalized (Winseman, 2004). People seem to be seeing spirituality as something more than religion. The percentage of people who have thought a lot about "the basic meaning and value of their lives" rose to 69% in 1999 (Gallup & Lindsay, 1999). Some individuals do not find religion important and do not want spirituality addressed in medical care; however "for the more than 70% of the population for whom religion is central to life, treatment approaches that are not sensitive to spirituality may leave patients feeling disaffected" (Larson & Koenig, 2000, p. 84).

Desire for spiritual care among children has not been fully assessed, yet some studies show children need and value spiritual care (Carson, 1989; O'Brien, 1999; Pehler, 1997; Shelly, 1982; Silber & Reilly, 1985). Spiritual care may be especially important to children during times of illness or injury when health-care professionals can have valuable input (Davies, Brenner, Orloff, Sumner, & Worden, 2002). Smith and McSherry (2004) contended that if children are to be given the opportunity to develop to their full potential, fostering spiritual growth must be a part of the process of caring for them.

Unfortunately, in some cases health-care providers may base their impressions regarding children's and families' desire for spiritual care on their own value systems or on what they see in the health-care setting. These impressions can be significantly different from the reality of most people in general. Koenig, Bearon, Hover, and Travis (1991) examined religious beliefs and practices among physicians ($n = 130$), nurses ($n = 39$), patients ($n = 77$), and families ($n = 60$). Patients found religion to be the most important factor enabling them to cope 43.8% of the time, families rated it 56.1% of the time, nurses 25.6%, and physicians only 8.7%. This gap in orientation can hinder the recognition of and care for spiritual needs of patients in health-care settings.

The underemphasis of spiritual care in the nursing profession is well known (Narayanasamy & Owens, 2001; Piles, 1990). Physicians have also acknowledged a lack in the area of spiritual care (King & Bushwick, 1994). Reasons include lack of education regarding its significance, inability to recognize signs of spiritual need, or a belief that addressing spiritual needs is not within the profession's scope of practice. The trend of religious groups in the United States to unburden themselves of hospitals may further de-emphasize spiritual care in health-care settings. Until the early 20th century, almost all hospital development was the result of private donations motivated by Judeo-Christian ideals of "charity, love for one's neighbors, and dedication to a ministry of healing" (Bilchik, 1998, p. 38). Now, both Christian- and Jewish-owned centers are selling ownership and are merging with secular facilities. This trend is expected to continue. At the same time that U.S. consumers are wanting more humanity, touching, healing, and listening, health care is becoming less personal and more mechanized. Many people want to be helped to mobilize their personal faith to get well or stay well, but that resource may not be available (Bilchik, 1998).

Children's Spiritual Care in Health-Care Settings

If spirituality is one of the defining aspects of people, as many programs teach, and if spirituality affects the other aspects of people (e.g., physical, mental, social), then consideration of children's spirituality is an important part of children's health care (Alderson, 1996; Ratner, Johnson, & Jeffery, 1998). Further, when spirituality is viewed as a concept distinct from religion, it can be inclusive of all people—including children. Spiritual care too often is viewed as an optional extra, something that can be neglected without adverse effect for patient or family, yet often spiritual needs hold the key for appropriate intervention (Thurston & Ryan, 1996). Blockley (1998) provided an example of a 7-year-old boy, Cory, who sustained a fractured femur in a motor vehicle accident that killed his younger sister and left his mother in critical condition in the ICU. Cory was restless in a way that could not be accounted for by fear or pain. He could not get to sleep. His nurse closed the curtain and asked what he did at home before he went to sleep. Cory outlined the routine and added in a whisper, "and then I would sit on Mummy's knee and we would say the 'Our Father' together" (Blockley, 1998, p. 56). The nurse was able to provide pre-sleep spiritual and emotional care, having found the "key to his restlessness," and medication was never needed.

Until recently, very little has been written about children's spiritual lives because the 'normal' spiritual life was believed to be that of an adult. However, through the writings of persons such as Robert Coles (1990), adults are now much more aware that children do have their own spiritual lives and, when we are willing to listen, they will tell us about their spiritual ideas and experiences. This is especially true of children who are ill or grieving—sometimes their hurt makes them very willing to express themselves (Fosarelli, 2000).

Parents and health-care professionals frequently think that it is better to spare children from discussions of spirituality. This is not often in the child's best interest:

> Children do much better physically, emotionally and spiritually when their ideas are sought and they are included in important discussions.... Even though we may be uncomfortable with their questions and their emotions, we must not shy away from hearing them out and wondering with them. (Fosarelli, 2000, p. 7)

Children typically know when they need to talk. Because religion is part of the human experience in so many instances, it is definitely a part of the experience when we are ill, and children are often ready to talk about it. According to Coles (2000),

> We should give children the permission to share with us what is on their minds, and so, my advise is to ask directly about the role of spirituality and religion in their lives and listen for the enormous insight you will hear. (p. 6)

Definition of Terms

A foundation for providing spiritual care begins with an understanding of terms. For example, the *spiritual* aspect of an individual is not equivalent to the *religious* aspect. Many patients are excluded from spiritual care when spirituality is confined in that way (Brown-Saltzman, 1997; Dunn & Dawes, 1999; Emblen, 1992; Espeland, 1999). Spiritual has been described as "anything that preserves, supports, and/or develops the nature of man's relationship to God" (Espeland, 1999, p. 36). However, in the pediatric setting it may be difficult to separate religious affiliation from spiritual expression (Kenny, 1999). See box for definitions of terms related to spirituality.

Theoretical Underpinnings of Spirituality

Various writers have used developmental theories to deduce spiritual care strategies. For example, in her classic book, *The Spiritual Needs of Children* (1982), Judith Shelly took Erikson's Eight Ages of Man (Erikson, 1963) and explained spiritual care appropriate for each stage (Shelly, 1982, 2000). Others have used Erikson's information as well in spiritual care application (Barnum, 1996; Carson, 1989; Fulton & Moore, 1995; Hart & Schneider, 1997). Carson

Definitions of Terms Related to Spirituality

Belief—the holding of certain ideas; to hold dear, love, cherish (Fowler, 1981).

Faith—a confidence or trust in a person or thing (Hart & Schneider, 1997); an orientation of the whole person, giving purpose and goal to one's hopes and strivings, thoughts and actions (Fowler, 1981).

Faith communities or *religious communities*—congregations such as churches, synagogues, mosques, temples, or cathedrals where religion is practiced.

God—supreme presence, divine power, supernatural power, Divine, Ultimate Other, Great Mystery, Spring, Source, Spirit, and Divine Consciousness, supreme being, higher power, energy, force, power within, your personal definition of transcendence; a source of love, creativity, a social transformation.

Human spirit—the dimension of any individual that is distinct from physical, psychological, or social dimensions; the aspect of self that gives meaning and purpose to life (Espeland, 1999).

Religion—a set of cumulative traditions, symbols, rituals; service and worship of a god or supernatural power; a set of beliefs about God upon which practices are based (Fowler, 1981).

Spiritual care—activities that assist individuals to find meaning and purpose in life, to continue relationships, and to transcend beyond the self

(1989) provided an overview of three faith development theories including Aden's eight stages of faith, Westerhoff's four stages of faith, and Fowler's seven stages of faith. James Fowler's widely used work (Fowler, 1981, 1996; Fowler & Keen, 1978) is influenced by the theoretical work of Erik Erikson, Jean Piaget, and Lawrence Kohlberg. These stages of faith are shown to apply to people of any or no religion because faith is viewed as being universally present (see Table 9.1).

Other spiritual care authors have analyzed theoretical underpinnings of spirituality (Burkhardt, 1991; Nierenberg & Sheldon, 2001). Piaget's Stages of Cognitive Development have been related to spiritual development (Hart & Schneider, 1997; Pehler, 1997; Shelly, 1982). Discussions of Kohlberg's work on moral development (Fowler, 1981; Kohlberg, 1981, 1984; Shelly, 1982) and Maslow's theory of human motivation (Barnum, 1996; Carson, 1989) have shed light on spirituality in children.

Nursing theories are mixed in content and depth regarding spirituality (Barnum, 1996; Hancock, 2000; Martsolf & Mickley, 1998; O'Brien, 1999; Oldnall, 1996; Price, Stevens, & LaBarre, 1995). However, nursing has gained much ground in the area of addressing spiritual issues by developing nursing diagnoses concerning spiritual well-being and spiritual distress (Cavendish

(Fulton & Moore, 1995); may include activities such as holding, comforting, play therapy, providing pain control, and fostering of parental participation in the child's care (Hart & Schneider, 1997).

Spiritual development—a dynamic process that differs from physical, emotional, or social development, in which a person becomes increasingly aware of the meaning, purpose, and values in life (Carson, 1989).

Spiritual distress—the state in which the individual experiences or is at risk of experiencing a disturbance in his or her belief or value system that is a source of strength and hope (Carpenito, 1997).

Spiritual health or *well-being*—one's views and behaviors in the search for hope and meaning in life, which express a relationship with a higher power or some meaning to a transient dimension (Carpenito, 1997), and vary according to the child's age, religious tradition, and the severity of the illness (O'Brien,

1999); the integrating aspect of human wholeness characterized by meaning and hope (Clark, Cross, Deane, & Lowry, 1991); the center of a healthy lifestyle, which enables holistic integration of one's inner resources (Clark & Heidenreich, 1995).

Spiritual needs—meaning and purpose, love, trust, hope, forgiveness, and creativity (Carson, 1989).

Spiritual pain—the loss of or separation from God or institutionalized religion; the experience of evil or disillusionment; a sense of failing God; the recognition of one's own sinfulness; lack of reconciliation with God; a perceived loneliness of spirit (O'Brien, 1999).

Spirituality—dynamic principles developed throughout the lifespan that guide an individual's view of the world; influence his or her interpretation of a higher power, hope, morals, loss, faith, love, and trust; and provide structure and meaning to everyday activities (Hicks, 1999).

Table 9.1

Fowler's Seven Stages of Faith

Stage	Age	Characteristics
1. Primal faith	Infancy	A prelanguage disposition of trust forms the mutuality of one's relationships with parents and others to offset the anxiety that results from separations that occur during infancy.
2. Intuitive–projective faith	Early childhood	Imagination, stimulated by stories, gestures, and symbols and not yet controlled by logical thinking combines with perception and feelings to create long-lasting images that represent both the protective and threatening powers surrounding one's life.
3. Mythic–literal faith	Childhood and beyond	The developing ability to think logically helps one order the world with categories of causality, space, and time; to enter into the perspectives of others; and to capture life meaning in stories.
4. Synthetic–conventional faith	Adolescence and beyond	New cognitive abilities make mutual perspective-taking possible and require one to integrate diverse self-images into a coherent identity. A personal and largely unreflective synthesis of beliefs and values evolves to support identity and to unite one in emotional solidarity with others.
5. Individuative–reflective faith	Young adulthood and beyond	Critical reflection on one's beliefs and values, understanding of the self and others as part of a social system, and the assumption of responsibility for making choices of ideology and lifestyle open the way for commitments in relationships and vocation.
6. Conjunctive faith	Midlife and beyond	The embrace of polarities in one's life, alertness to paradox, and the need for multiple interpretations of reality mark this stage. Symbol and story, metaphor and myth (from one's own traditions and those of others), are newly appreciated as vehicles for grasping truth.
7. Universalizing faith	Midlife or beyond	Beyond paradox and polarities, persons in this stage are grounded in a oneness with the power of being. Their visions and commitments free them for a passionate yet detached spending of the self in love, devoted to overcoming division, oppression, and brutality.

Note. From *Spiritual Dimensions of Nursing Practice* (p. 29), by V. B. Carson, 1989, Philadelphia: Saunders. Copyright 1989 by Saunders. Reprinted with permission.

et al., 2001). Language that recognizes the importance of spiritual care is also in national and international codes of ethics.

Assessment of Spirituality

Health-care providers work diligently to anticipate care needs before they are crying out to be heard. The same should be true when it comes to spiritual needs of children. The way anticipation of needs happens is through building one's professional knowledge base and then adequately assessing the child and family. Highfield (1997, p. 238) asserted, "the first step in spiritual assessment is up to the caregiver. Leaving it to vulnerable patients to raise spiritual and religious questions risks ignoring some of their most devastating concerns and most powerful resources."

How the health-care provider views spirituality affects his or her own ability to assess spiritual needs and give care. If there is openness or even a welcoming viewpoint toward encounters of a spiritual nature, care will be strengthened. Providers should be theologically honest, speak the language of children, enter into the child's world, be sensitive to nonverbal and verbal information, respect privacy, and let the child take the lead (Sommer, 1989; O'Brien, 1999). Personal beliefs, feelings, perceptions, and experiences regarding spirituality are important. Basic questions to examine one's own beliefs include "How do I define the meaning of life?" "What is my relationship with a higher power?" and "How are my spiritual beliefs incorporated into my practice?" (Hicks, 1999). If we have struggled and come to a place of peace regarding spiritual aspects of life, we are free to help others and are not bound up in our own bewilderment. We have a base or core of spiritual belief.

Health-care professionals must avoid having damaging input into a child or family's spiritual life. One way to do this is to "avoid imposing one's own ideas on the patient while encouraging patients to voice their spiritual needs and questions" (Wright, 1998, p. 82). Aggressively passing on one's own beliefs without adequate assessment, or without a direct request from the client for our beliefs, can cause needless spiritual distress. Spiritual interactions should be about the child and family.

Assessment of Family Spirituality

A child comes to a health-care situation with the backdrop of family life and experiences that will radically affect the care experience. A child learns about health and illness, right and wrong, life and death, and faith in God within the context of a family (Anderson & Steen, 1995). After assessing the parents' spiritual needs, it is often easier to understand their child's needs.

During a crisis, children easily sense fear and anxiety in their parents. If parents are supported in their coping efforts, children are better able to handle the ups and downs of hospitalization. Parents are better able to support their child if health-care professionals provide adequate information and incorporate them into the child's care. Parents may well be experiencing spiritual distress with the hospitalization of a child, and may express this distress through anxiety, hostility, and blaming (Hart & Schneider, 1997). Parents are often at the bedside, but other family members may be in a waiting room. It may be helpful for the health-care professional to go to the waiting room or even on a break to the cafeteria to talk with family members. Once away from the child, a parent may have much to share. This type of break from the monotony-with-intensity can be a spiritual assessment opportunity. Parents may share valuable pieces of information about the child or family. On the other hand, they may say nothing but feel a burden lifted. They may let go of some grief.

Spiritual Assessment of Children

An assessment may be structured or unstructured, brief or comprehensive. Sound assessment is more important for children than for adults. Children have a limited ability to communicate, particularly about abstract concepts. Sources for data collection include direct observations, a patient's chart, doctors, referral sheets, and other health team members' observations (Still, 1984).

Much of spiritual assessment can be done through simple observation of people, interactions, and environment (see Figure 9.1). Look around the room for religious objects or materials. Sacred books, religiously based storybooks, cards or gifts, music or videotapes, or even the child's own artwork reflect spiritual beliefs. Observe the child's behavior, spiritual practices, those who provide spiritual support, and what support is provided.

Often children do not use religious words. Observe for anxiety, stalling, nightmares, regression, loneliness, parents' perceptions of the child's subtle behavior changes, hostility, blaming, or expressed spiritual needs (Anderson & Steen, 1995). Does the child mention God? If so, what is said? These sorts of observations make a significant difference in objectifying beliefs and differentiating those of child versus parent. These observations are noninvasive and useful.

In spiritual care literature, structured spiritual assessments have various categories. Several examples are provided. Stoll referred to four areas of spiritual assessment: concept of God, sources of hope and strength, religious practices, and relation between beliefs and health (Stoll, 1979). Anderson and Steen adapted Stoll's four areas of assessment for use with children and parents. Table 9.2 is the work of Anderson and Steen (1995). Its strength is in the questions that are directed toward the child or parent/adult caregiver and that are linked with particular aspects of spiritual concern.

With children, categorizing spiritual assessment questions according to developmental stage can be useful. Clutter (1991) offered an extensive list of age-appropriate questions categorized for use with children who are preschool, school-age, or adolescent, as well as questions for adults/parents.

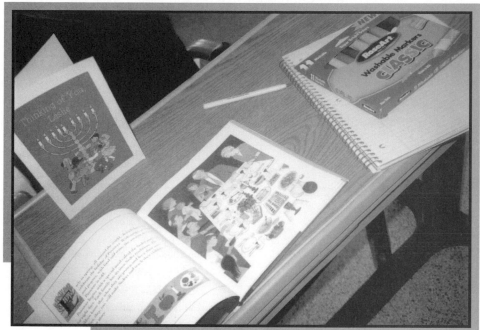

Figure 9.1.

Presence of spiritual materials can indicate the importance of spiritual aspects to a particular child and family. *Note.* Photograph by Lynn Clutter. Used with permission.

Taking a child's spiritual or faith history is another way to categorize spiritual assessment information. The purpose of this type of history is to gather baseline, background information; make careful observations; listen carefully; and inquire about and note any cues that are spiritual in nature. The faith history enhances knowledge of sources of strength, identifies spiritual challenges for child and parent, and identifies major life or faith change points.

A spiritual history does not have to be lengthy. Puchalski (2000a) developed a simple spiritual history tool that uses the acronym FICA. An explanation and questions suitable for children include the following:

- F—Faith or beliefs; what the individual believes; "Do you believe in God?"
- I—Importance and influence; how important spiritual issues are in the person's health and life; "Do you think about God a lot or a little?"
- C—Community; the religious community involvement of the person; "Do you worship God somewhere with other people?"
- A—Address; how the person would like their health-care provider to address these issues in their care; "Do you want to talk about this kind of thing with me?"

The strengths of a tool such as the FICA are its simplicity and speed of use, yet breadth of application and depth of information received from patients. Phrasing questions with "Tell me about your ..." may yield longer

Table 9.2

Spiritual Assessment Questions for Parents and Children

Area of Spiritual Concern	Person to Answer Question	Faith Assessment Question
Concept of God	Parent/Adult caregiver	Is faith or God important to you? How? How is God involved in your life? How is God involved in the life of your child? How would you describe God? Does your child have an interest in faith or God? How do you answer your child's questions about God? Does your child have a favorite Bible story? What is it? Why does he (or she) like it?
Concept of God	Child	Have you thought about God during this time? What is God like? How does God work? Does God make everything happen? Do you believe God causes ___? How do you see God acting or not acting now? Do you have a favorite Bible story or character? What do you like about this story?
Sources of strength and hope	Parent/Adult caregiver	Who do you turn to when you need help? How do they help? Is your faith important to you now? How is it important right now? What helps you when you feel afraid or alone? What gives you strength during difficult times? Are your beliefs a source of strength and support during hard times?
Sources of strength and hope	Child	How do you feel when you are in trouble? Who do you tell when you feel afraid (or sad, scared, alone, happy)? Who do you like to talk to when you feel that way? Who else? What makes you feel afraid (or sad, scared, lonely)? What helps you feel better?
Faith practices	Parent/Adult caregiver	Is your faith important to you now? How is it important? Are there faith practices that are important to you or your child now? What practices are important? Has having a sick child made a difference in your faith practices? Is prayer important to you? In what ways? Is the Bible or another book or symbol helpful to you? How? Are there any other helpful faith practices that we should be aware of?
Faith practices	Child	Have you thought about God? Are there things that you do that help you feel closer to God? What are they? Do you ever pray or talk to God?

Note. From "Spiritual Care: Reflecting God's Love to Children," by B. Anderson and S. Steen, 1995, *Journal of Christian Nursing, 12*(2), p. 15. Copyright 1995 by *Journal of Christian Nursing*. Reprinted with permission.

answers to the FICA. Children are often very willing to give honest answers to these types of questions.

The mnemonic "B-E-L-I-E-F" is the basis of McEvoy's (2000) spiritual history. The pediatric health maintenance visit is a time when this history can be incorporated. Categories are B—belief systems, E—ethics, L—lifestyle, I—involvement in a spiritual community, E—education, and F—future events. McEvoy provides specific spiritual history questions and summaries of categories.

Dunn and Dawes (1999) encouraged the use of a spirituality-focused genogram to explore this dimension of the child and family. Untapped spiritual or religious resources for care or client coping may be seen. Sample questions to consider when constructing spirituality-focused genograms include

- What are the first religious or spiritual experiences you can remember?
- What role does religion or spirituality have in your everyday life or times of crisis?
- What defining experiences or individuals have influenced the development of your sense of spirituality or religion?
- What were significant transitions and/or critical life events in the history of your family?
- What impact, if any, did religion or spirituality have in making sense of or coping with those life events? (p. 254)

Highfield (2000) pointed to the importance of focusing the assessment on strengths. The child and family can rely on these strengths through illness and crisis. They will buoy the child and allow others to provide support by encouraging the use of his or her own strengths. Therefore, strengths should be identified and documented for further use. For example, if a child listens to a spiritual tape, later sings one of the songs and has a brighter outlook, and the mother states, "She really loves that song," the notation, "Gains strength from use of spiritual music tapes" could be charted for future intervention.

Sometimes the use of known tools can bring a formality that yields valuable data but is less threatening for both client and health-care provider. Many formal spiritual assessment tools are available for adults; some apply to children. Some tools can be completed by patient or parent alone then discussed later. Some tools are formatted as spiritual interviews with questions. Appendix 9.1 is an annotated bibliography of spiritual care tools for use with children, adults, research, practice, and chart documentation.

Spiritual Distress

Sometimes people are "cut off from their spiritual roots in facing the crisis of illness, dying, and death. Even people who are religious may lack the spiritual energy to cope with crisis situations" (Bailey, 1997, p. 242). Though spiritual distress may not be discernable biologically, it is accepted in society as real and must be dealt with by health professionals (Piles, 1990). Learning to identify spiritual distress is the first step (Smucker, 1996; Sumner, 1998).

Indicators of spiritual distress include loss of meaning and purpose in life, a diminished sense of love and relatedness, and a lack of forgiveness (Georgesen & Dungan, 1996; Shelly & Fish, 1988; Stoll, 1989). McHolm (1991) listed 13 indicators of spiritual distress:

1. unable to accept self
2. description of somatic complaints
3. cues about relationships with others
4. cues about guilt and forgiveness
5. cues about religious or spiritual needs
6. inadequate coping
7. despair or hopelessness
8. fear
9. depression
10. helplessness
11. anorexia
12. silence
13. bitterness

Another validation study (Twibell, Wieseke, Marine, & Schoger, 1996) identified the following as defining characteristics of spiritual distress:

- spiritual emptiness
- disturbance in beliefs
- no reason for living
- request for spiritual assist
- concern over meaning in life
- questions beliefs
- doubts beliefs
- unable to practice rituals
- detached from self or others

Sometimes spiritual distress in children is expressed as anger, resentment, exaggerated fear, self-blame, questioning the meaning of one's own existence, or questioning the moral and ethical implications of the therapeutic regime (Fina, 1995). Additional cues for children may include crying, nightmares, asking numerous questions, and regressive behavior. Often this distress is expressed at nighttime or bedtime hours (Fulton & Moore, 1995). Repeated questions or resistant behavior can occur as well (Treloar, 1999).

When Children Are Dying

According to Taylor, Amenta, and Highfield (1995), dying is a spiritual event. Cox (2000) pointed out that grief, loss, and death can be powerful times for children to experience spiritual growth, wholeness, and holiness. Palliative spiritual care has become a topic of current focus (Field & Behrman, 2003) as health-care provider skill is especially important during this stage of care. Those who are dying can have quite a different spiritual reality, especially if they are suffering. Suffering is defined as "a loss of wholeness and the distress and anguish that accompany it." It is also the "experience of brokenness" (Attig, 1996, p. 20). Table 9.3 identifies care of children with spiritual anguish.

Attig (1996) explained that "terminal illness interrupts the ongoing stories of children's lives ... it truncates their future and changes utterly both the shape and content of the remaining pages and chapters of their lives and the character of their biographies as wholes" (p. 20). Similarly, but stated about cancer, the terminal illness "intrudes on patients' lives, pulling the rug out from under them, and handing them a new script for life" (p. 20).

Illness seems to set children apart, and they often find it difficult to participate in or to feel "at home" in their families, friendships, and communities. They can also lose their sense of spiritual place or have fears of what lies beyond the boundaries of this life. Feeling disconnected from that which once brought value, hope, and meaning, and distant from what brings consolation and comfort leaves children or adolescents with "soul pain" (Attig, 1996). There is a longing for the embrace of those who share life with them and a yearning to feel at home in the world. Listening is so vital: "Careful and sensitive listening to patients who have spiritual beliefs, regardless of our own personal beliefs, can ease the pain of dying" (Lyon, Townsend-Akpan, & Thompson, 2001, p. 559). Many children are filled with questions that cry for honesty. Health-care providers can present clear, honest answers that orient children to present realities and what lies ahead of them (Sommer, 1989).

It is not always easy to give honesty in the face of death. In the following example, Dr. Christina Puchalski discovered how hard honesty seems and yet how amazing children are.

> Sara was a nine-year old girl dying of metastatic cancer with an estimated few months to live. Both the doctor and mother wondered how (or if or when) they should tell Sara that she was dying. "Sara's mother and I were so caught up in the tragedy of a young child's shortened life that we could not see that Sara was at peace with herself." One evening after drawing another blood sample, Sara looked up at her doctor and asked if she ever knew anyone close to her who died. The doctor shared that her fiancé, Eric, had died two years before. Sara teased her with an impish grin and the childhood rhyme: "Eric and Christina sitting in a tree, K-I-S-S-I-N-G." With many giggles, then very seriously said, "a tree in heaven and when you die you'll see him again. Since I am going to die soon, I'll give him a hug for you." Sara turned to her mother and said, "I'll be okay, Mommy." (Puchalski, 2000b, p. 3)

Table 9.3

Characteristics and Care of Children with Spiritual Anguish

Characteristics

Young Children

- uninhibited
- persistent in questioning
- open about what frightens them
- read well the anxieties of caregivers
- sense caregiver anguish
- express anguish nonverbally in play, through images in drawing or painting, or in behaviors that signal distress, such as tears, agitation, outbursts of anger or hostility, refusal to eat or to cooperate with treatment
- lethargic, withdrawn, have prolonged silences, turn toward the wall, hold themselves in fetal position, have clinging behaviors

6–12-Year-Olds

- candid in revealing concerns when they feel safe
- reluctant to ask questions or show fright for fear of discouraging response
- read well the anxieties of caregivers
- sense caregiver anguish
- hold concerns inward to please, protect, or hold close their anxious caregiver
- focus on present with hopes focused on immediate future

Adolescents

- fear exposure and rejection
- hold questions back for fear of embarrassment
- shield their privacy
- find more comfort in communication with peers
- express themselves (share with those they select) through poetry, diaries, journals, art, music
- focus on future (that their meaningful lives lie ahead) so they feel deep deprivation, resent unfairness of their condition, anguish over unrealized potential
- long for but realize they will not fully have adult experiences
- struggle with hopelessness
- dread the return to greater dependence

Puchalski (2000b) pointed out that adults can complicate things with intellectual and rational thinking: "In many ways, children are more in touch with their spirituality because of their innate sense of wonder and imagination. They can often 'see' a reality beyond the everyday, physical world most people live in" (p. 3). Their perceptions are unfettered and unencumbered.

Puchalski's sharing opened the door for the child to share. Traditionally, the "therapeutic relationship" has been described as only including talk of the *patient's* life. However, in times of crisis or critical need, adults and children are looking for authentic communication that can be readily supported by personal examples. Maugans (1996) wrote,

At times, revealing one's own personal spirituality may be appropriate if it helps in building the patient–physician relationship [or that of patient

Table 9.3 *Continued.*

367

Characteristics and Care of Children with Spiritual Anguish

How To Help
1. Create a safe, secure place permeated with trust.
2. Allow and welcome expression of anguish.
3. Recognize the need for comfort.
4. Overcome own fears of being overwhelmed by the pain and anguish that might be expressed.
5. Avoid signaling in word or deed lack of receptivity to expressions of anguish.
6. Remember that symptom control cannot replace intimacy with child or mute expression of suffering.
7. Offer presence free of agenda (be companion as they suffer).
8. Learn the power of special interventions such as image or dream work, art or music therapy.
9. Support prayer or meditation to express and process spiritual anguish.
10. Minister to fears (e.g., separation, abandonment).
11. Assure that they need not be alone unless they choose to be so.
12. Believe and state that they will always be worthy of caring attention.
13. Address helplessness and powerlessness by including children in decision making for treatment, symptom control, where they live, choices in shaping their daily lives.
14. Remind them that they had no choice about their condition but can choose how they live in response to its intrusion and death's shadow.
15. Encourage them that their life remaining can be precious; then focus on opportunities for meaningful experiences, achievements, and expressions.
16. Help them face the spiritual challenges of leaving this life.
17. Assure them that they will always be in the hearts of those who love them, that we won't forget them.
18. Be honest.
19. Invite them to tell what they believe and hope about life beyond.

Note. Adapted from "Beyond Pain: The Existential Suffering of Children," by T. Attig, 1996, *Journal of Palliative Care, 12*(3), pp. 20–23. Copyright 1996 by T. Attig. Adapted with permission.

with other health care provider] or in breaking down barriers that have developed over conflictual belief systems. Generally this is done at the request of the patient and only if the physician [or other health care provider] feels capable. (p. 15)

Immanent Justice

One common type of spiritual distress that occurs with children is termed *immanent justice*. This is the belief that illness is a punishment for wrongdoing. Children can think that misdeeds have caused the illness. These beliefs are primarily, but not exclusively, found in children under 7 years of age (Pehler, 1997). Children may voice these perceptions, or perceptions may remain as internal concerns. Keeping these beliefs or fears inside can be spiritually damaging. When voiced, however, misperceptions can be corrected. Measures can be taken by health-care providers to offer different viewpoints.

Distorted Images of God

Individuals, including children and adolescents, can have distorted images of God (Ryan, 1996). Due to developmental-level differences, children may have unexplored feelings that cause negative reactions to God or others. These images may be of an angry, demanding, "scowl on his face" God rather than a kind, comforter, counselor, healer image of God. The child may think one way but feel another; that is, images of God are not the same as ideas of God. Parents, early caretakers, or spiritual community members can affect these images. The distortions of God, such as one who is abusive, a bully, unreliable, weak, or one who abandons can sometimes be changed through new examples of caring others, prayer, or through talk. Providing a competing image (such as God with a loving smile looking at and holding the child) can push away the painful image (Ryan, 1996).

Sommer (1989), a chaplain, spoke of the dying child and stated,

> It is helpful to share with children that God loves all people—especially little children—so they will not fear the prospect of going to be with an angry or mean God after they have died. Second, children need to be given a positive image of what lies beyond death. Because children have vivid imaginations, unless we fill the void of afterlife with positive images they may fill it with monsters and images of separation and darkness. (p. 232)

Intense Spiritual Experiences

Sometimes, religious beliefs, particularly of ultra-religious sects, or various spiritual experiences can be very intense. When are these normal and when are they psychotic episodes? The following criteria are helpful for identifying when referral is needed. According to Greenberg and Witztum (1991), psychotic episodes

- are more intense than normative religious experiences in their religious community;
- are often terrifying for the individual;
- are often preoccupying and the individual can think of little else;
- are associated with deterioration of social skills and personal hygiene; and
- often involve special messages from religious figures. (p. 554)

While intense but not distorted, some spiritual experiences may be awesome and preoccupying. The difference is that these experiences are strengthening in nature. It can be difficult for mental health therapists who lack knowledge of the basic tenets of a particular religion to differentiate religious beliefs and rituals from delusions and compulsions (Greenberg & Witztum, 1991). Nontherapists should document any signs of mental instability, seek out interdisciplinary communication, and refer to clergy or mental health specialists when applicable. Preepisode functioning, stressful precipitants, onset of any new symptoms, and postepisode functioning should be noted if a child has an intense religious experience (Lukoff, Lu, & Turner, 1995).

Perceived Lack of Spiritual Support

Another facet of spiritual distress can be within the spiritual support system itself. Parents—especially those of children with disabilities—have sometimes experienced the church's support being limited and fragile or not comprehensive enough to meet the many strains of long-term disability. "Many people with disabling conditions are angry at their church for what feels like a lack of caring support, a feeling that carries over to their relationship with God" (Webb-Mitchell, 1993, p. 42). While the health-care team cannot resolve this dilemma, members can assist parents and children in realizing that a local church may not have enough resources to meet the multiple spiritual needs that are present. Encourage parents to explore widening their support systems so they can avoid cutting off valuable, though limited, support from those usual spiritual communities.

A Developmental Approach

Interventions with children differ, depending on the age of the child. Health-care professionals should know some basic developmental-stage aspects of care prior to any care of children. Major illness or injury can alter spiritual development with the possibility of regression; however, an understanding of developmental concepts enhances spiritual care of children.

Below are developmental concepts associated with each general developmental stage of childhood. This information is summarized and linked with age-specific interventions for infants, toddlers and preschoolers, school-age children, and adolescents in Table 9.4.

Newborns and Infants

Loss can affect trust, and thus can affect the spiritual support for a baby. Children under the age of 2 years do not understand the concept of death

Table 9.4

Developmentally Specific Spiritual Care Interventions

Developmental Staging	Interventions
Infants **Erikson:** *Trust versus mistrust* Requires sensitivity and consistency in meeting needs. Basis of self-identity and hope established. **Piaget:** *Sensorimotor* Uses senses, motor skills, reflexes to explore. Trial and error and "insight" problem solving. **Fowler:** Stage 0: *Undifferentiated* No concept of right or wrong; no apparent religious beliefs or convictions to guide behavior. However, beginnings of faith are established with the development of basic trust through developing a relationship with their primary caregiver.	1. Actively listen to parental concerns. Be alert to the possibility that they may perceive their child's illness as some kind of religious omen or punishment. 2. Build self-worth by reassuring parents about the adequacy of their parenting skills. 3. Attend to emotional and physical needs of infants. Encourage parental presence. Provide safe, consistent care that is loving and accepting. 4. Encourage and facilitate the continued use of a religious support system for the family. Suggest to caregivers the possibility of using a religious-based support system. If desired, assist them in finding an appropriate support system.
Toddlers and Preschoolers **Erikson:** *Autonomy versus shame* (1–3 years) Limits (firm and consistent) lead to security. Acquires "will," feeling of self-control basis for self-esteem. *Initiative versus guilt* (3–5 years) Energy used in problem solving. "Conscience" develops. Begins cooperation. Beginning of purpose. **Piaget:** *Preoperational* Self-centered; perception from own point of view; literal interpretation of works and actions; judges things for outcome, consequence to self. **Fowler:** Stage 1: *Intuitive–projective* Imitates the behavior of others; imitates religious gestures and behaviors of others with very limited comprehension of any meaning or significance of activity. Follows parental beliefs as part of daily life, but without an understanding of their basic concepts.	1. Teach and coach the parents to assist the child in positive coping behaviors. 2. Reassure the child that she or he is not being punished (by God or other authority figures) for the disease or hospitalization. 3. Using the information gained in the assessment, continue with routines from home, such as daily activities, limit setting, and religious rituals. 4. Appropriately initiate discussion of love and caring from a Higher Power, using developmentally correct language to relieve anxiety and loneliness. 5. Show the child behavioral qualities of love, acceptance, trust, respect, caring, setting of firm limits, and disciplining without anger. 6. Don't underestimate the child's level of comprehension. Respond to questions in an understandable, concrete manner. Give logical reasons for religious behavior.
School-Age Children **Erikson:** *Industry versus inferiority* Wins recognition by producing things, solving problems, and finishing tasks. **Piaget:** *Concrete operations* Interpersonal collaboration and competition. Social reciprocity and sense of fairness. Uses	1. Be alert to anxiety about being punished by a deity. 2. Provide appropriate, concrete explanations in response to questions regarding spiritual beliefs. 3. Continue with religious rituals. When appropriate, promote the use of prayer.

(continues)

Table 9.4 *Continued.*

371

Developmentally Specific Spiritual Care Interventions

Developmental Staging	Interventions
School-Age Children (*continued*) elementary logic and manipulation of actual objects and experiences. **Fowler:** Stage 2: *Mythical–literal* Spiritual development closely related to experiences and social interactions. Usually has a strong interest in religion and is able to articulate his or her faith. Conscience is developing.	4. Encourage the child's personal relationship with his or her God. 5. Model behaviors that show forgiveness and acceptance. 6. Promote continued contact with school or church peers.
Adolescents **Erikson:** *Identity versus role confusion* Searches for self-identity. Begins socially responsible behavior and coping with emotions. Develops ideology and philosophy of life. Looks for powers and limits. **Piaget:** *Formal operations* Sees world from many and different perspectives. Thought is independent of concrete reality; is flexible; and manipulates symbols, forms hypotheses, and theories. **Fowler:** Stage 3: *Synthetic–conventional (preadolescent)* Becomes increasingly aware of spiritual disappointments. Begins to reason and question some of established parental religious standards. May drop or modify some religious practices. Stage 4: *Individuative–reflective (adolescent)* Becomes more skeptical and begins to compare religious standards of family with standards of others. A time of asking questions and searching for answers.	1. Provide an open, accepting attitude. Provide an atmosphere for the adolescent to discuss the implications of this illness in terms of philosophical and religious beliefs. 2. Encourage continued contact with friends and classmates. Use support groups with which the youth feels comfortable. Some may seek religious support groups from members of their peer groups. 3. Encourage the use of religious rituals if the adolescent desires to continue using them. 4. Provide answers to questions in an unbiased manner that encourages participation and stimulates his or her personal thinking. 5. Take the time to develop an honest, trusting relationship with the teen. 6. Assess and document verbalizations of the teen's values and beliefs.

Note. Adapted from "Spiritual Care of Children with Cancer," by D. Hart and D. Schneider, 1997, *Seminars in Oncology Nursing, 13*(4), pp. 266, 268, 269. Copyright 1997 by Aspen. Adapted with permission.

but do respond to the loss of a significant person. They sense changes in daily routines and perceive sadness and anxiety. They demonstrate awareness of the absence of a significant person by exhibiting altered feeding patterns, crankiness, and altered sleeping patterns (Mangini, Confessore, Girard, & Spadola, 1995).

Anything that promotes trust between caretaker and a baby is valuable for the baby's spiritual development (Leduc, 2001). "Through consistent, loving care of their needs, infants develop a sense of trust, belonging, and self-worth. These are all prerequisites for the development of a relationship with a Higher Being." (Hart & Schneider, 1997, p. 266). Infants need predictable routines, normalcy, and a consistent nurturing caregiver. Parental comfort such as holding, rocking, singing, and talking to the infant develops trust (Hart & Schneider, 1997).

Mangini, Confessore, Girard, and Spadola (1995) described 6-month-old-Jason, a previously healthy infant, who was admitted for failure to thrive. Jason's father had died in a plane crash 2 months earlier. His mother was exhausted and tearful. She reported that the baby had been vomiting, was disinterested in feeding, and needed to be held constantly. Interventions included physical care for Jason (allowing his mother to rest), supportive listening by staff to Jason's mother, an opportunity for her to attend an in-hospital parent coffee hour, and an outside referral to a support group for grieving spouses. Jason and his mother responded well. Consistency of schedule and meeting Jason's basic needs diminished the negative effects of loss. The supportive listening allowed for spiritual and emotional support of his mother, helped increase her coping skills, and thus made her better able to help her baby.

Toddlers and Preschoolers

Any concrete approach that builds comfort is helpful for toddlers, such as (a) the thought that God is their protector, (b) simple prayers, (c) having religious stories read to them, (d) having picture discussions with comforting picture or images such as those in picture Bibles, (e) participating in their activities of normal living such as mealtime grace or bedtime prayers, and (f) activities of religious holidays or rituals (see Figure 9.2).

Toddlers are beginning to develop a conscience and perceptions of right and wrong (Erikson, 1963). "Concrete cognitive thinking with beginning conscience can lead preschoolers to believing that an illness is a punishment for a 'bad' thought or action" (Hart & Schneider, 1997, p. 267). This concrete thinking can also lead to literal spiritual interpretations. For example, 3-year-old Amy asked her mother to sing "Turn Your Eyes Upon Jesus" at bedtime. Amy kept lifting her head and looking around to "turn her eyes on Jesus" instead of being lulled to sleep (Steen & Anderson, 1995). Toddlers need predictability in the daily schedule, clear expectations from consistent caregivers, clear structure yet the ability to explore within the structure, and opportunities to exert their independence and to develop their self-worth (Hart & Schneider, 1997).

Preschoolers require both self-assertion and self-discipline, consistent expectations, and appropriate discipline. They need to feel loved and secure, maintain a regular schedule and religious practices or rituals, and be surrounded by familiar objects, even in health-care settings (Hart & Schneider, 1997).

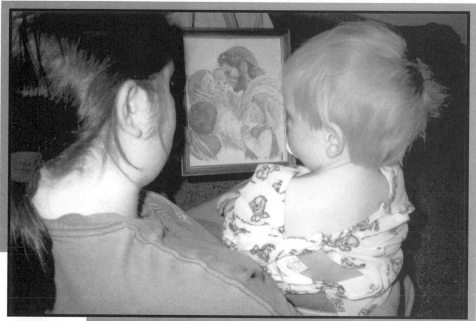

Figure 9.2.
Spiritual pictures that portray caring or comfort can evoke pleasure, even with very young children. *Note.* Photograph by Lynn Clutter. Used with permission.

School-Age Children

Young school-age children have a limited ability to communicate needs or feelings. They may give no verbal hints about spiritual needs yet may give cues about their own religious beliefs. However, inner pain or distress is most often inferred by behaviors.

School-age children lack abstract thinking, so concrete interventions are appropriate. Reading spiritual passages or prayer books, saying learned or spontaneous prayers, and discussing meaning of prayers, sacraments, or family worship rituals may be parts of their lives. However, they may just as easily indicate needs by what they do not say or do. For example, they may avoid eye contact, display anger, frustration, or manipulative behaviors, or resist the plan of care (Fulton & Moore, 1995).

Providing a supportive environment, trusting relationship, time and opportunity to unlock spirituality will enhance spiritual well-being and help to identify any distress (Ebmeier, Lough, Huth, & Autio, 1991). Care will offer a developmentally appropriate means to gain control over their situation (Fulton & Moore, 1995). Active involvement in spiritual intervention choices (e.g., drawing, listening to music) can help as the decision making gives control.

School-age children are "learning and growing through producing and accomplishing things. They begin to feel competent and successful through mastery of knowledge and skills" (Hart & Schneider, 1997, p. 266). They may ponder the cause and require assurance of causes—not their own—for their illness, and may require explanations for their illness. They are exploring new awareness of forgiveness, acceptance, guilt, and the differences between supernatural and natural.

Religious concepts are still concrete. Talking with their God in prayer can nurture their spiritual relationship (Hart & Schneider, 1997). School-age children may think about what God does and how He does it. They may believe in good and evil, which can lead to feelings of fear and guilt (Steen & Anderson, 1995). Because they have a limited tolerance for acute sadness, they may be upset one moment and asking to go out to play the next (Mangini et al., 1995).

Pre-Adolescents

Pre-adolescent children, ages 9 to 12 years, are developing their sense of right and wrong behavior on a moral level. They understand time, space, quality, and causality. They are growing in their understanding of life and death. They have interest in biological details and need to have their questions answered accurately and honestly (Mangini et al., 1995). A broad question about spirituality and availability to hear their responses may focus the pre-adolescent enough to promote growth.

Adolescents

Spirituality among adolescents involves ideological concerns more than rituals or religious customs. This change is largely due to the development of abstract thinking. Their focus is more on internal aspects of religious commitment and of developing a strong personal relationship with a Higher Power. The search for identity may involve exploring spiritual belief systems to discover meaning, purpose, and hope in life (Hodge, Cardenas, & Montoya, 2001; Holder et al., 2000; Pullen, Modrein-Talbott, West, & Muenchen, 1999; Stewart, 2001). They need to find meaning in suffering and illness (Hart & Schneider, 1997).

Teens are open to spiritual counsel at times. They are sometimes willing to talk with health-care providers about how the current health issue affects beliefs or meaning in life, and to deal with questions such as, "Why me?" Teenagers may participate in spiritual activities, receive visits from peers, cherish some privacy, talk on the phone about spiritual matters, or worship privately in their room (Hockenberry, Wilson, Winkelstein, & Kline, 2003). Adolescents may find strength by creating new religious rituals in the sickroom. They want a sense of normalcy, and desire some sense of control over decision making in their plan of care.

Adolescents may demonstrate spiritual strength in the midst of crisis or challenges (Cavendish et al., 2001). O'Brien cites the "win-win" words of Anna, a 13-year-old diagnosed with escalating Ewing's sarcoma with metastasis who said, "If God heals my body, then it will be wonderful and I can be a missionary and tell people about Him, but if He doesn't then I will die and be with Jesus, so there's no way I can lose" (O'Brien, 1999, p. 218).

Open and accepting attitudes help adolescents to discuss spiritual beliefs. Providing answers to questions and encouraging their involvement is appreciated. Having visits from peers can provide youth support. However, teens may be very concerned with their image and not want peers or others to see them weak.

General Concepts of Spiritual Intervention

In general, health-care providers should support children's existing faith. Inner resources or individualized spiritual expression can be supported in ways that continue their meaningful influence in the life of the child. Sometimes, especially during pivotal life events such as the diagnosis of cancer, completion of treatment, or return of disease progression, children and adults experience severe spiritual disequilibrium. Supporting their existing faith and helping them clarify or identify what is meaningful in their lives can be helpful.

Health-care providers can also support the faith of the family (Wilson & Miles, 2001). While cultural and religious awareness is valuable for care, one does not need to be an expert on religion to support existing faith. In many care situations, sensitive support is key in the presence of suffering. Some children and family members will simply want to discuss their religious beliefs. Health challenges can bring spiritual questions or conflicts to the forefront of one's thinking. It may be much easier to discuss problems with health-care providers who are not in a person's spiritual sphere of involvement. In this case, listening skills are primary. Beyond listening and once a health-care provider identifies the patient's or family member's formal religious belief system, it is possible to locate very significant resources. For example, the teachings of spiritual leaders can be very health promoting. Written resources or suggestions of compatible spiritual practices that will help the client's physical and emotional situation may then be offered.

Religions have rituals, various spiritual practices, sacraments such as communion or anointing with oil, baptism, circumcision, or various traditions surrounding care of the sick. Because religion holds pervasive life value to the patient, and health-care intervention is superimposed on that life, health-care providers have a responsibility to make room for the beliefs and practices that the patient holds dear. Children who are involved with a church or spiritual group may benefit from ongoing involvement with members while they are receiving health care. Regular participation in healthy religious activities (e.g., prayer, scripture reading, worship attendance, healing ceremonies, community service, referral to and collaboration with clergy) have been shown to have health benefits (Matthews, 2000).

"Spiritual care of children should reflect the fact that 'children want to have fun'" (Thayer, 2001, p. 180). Having fun linked with spiritual life often is powerfully effective. For example, "the making of 'spiritual bracelets' (akin to friendship bracelets, except that the colors of threads represent different spiritual values) can both prompt discussions about faith and other values and allow the child to create a gift."

Fostering spiritual growth is another important principle. Illness "can be viewed as an opportunity—as an occasion to redefine values, to encounter uncertainty, and to seek out greater purpose and connectedness" (Waldfogel, 1997, p. 965). The child may have ability greater than adults to express spiritual concerns when facing physical or emotional challenges. The health-care provider can maintain a readiness to hear and truly be with a child during this time. Spiritual growth is fostered through comfort, companionship, conversation, and consolation measures. Accepting, reassuring, caring, visiting, listening, concrete communications being "real" (not contrived), and sharing "straight" answers are valuable in care. The health-care provider can intervene in these measures or link others with the child (Kenny, 1999). Spiritual or religious coping strategies are nearly always associated with adaptive health outcomes (Pendleton, Cavalli, Pargament, & Nasr, 2002).

Health-care providers can also promote the use of spiritual strength. Many people with life-threatening illnesses—including children—have "phenomenal courage that is grounded in their spirituality, empowering them to life with deepened faith, hope, love, peace, and joy" (Bailey, 1997, p. 242). The ability to transcend the crisis with this strength is exactly what health-care providers need to support (Batten & Oltjenbruns, 1999; Marshall, Mandleco, Olsen, & Dyches, 2001).

Additionally, Clark, Cross, Deane, and Lowry (1991, p. 68) mentioned the notion of "spirit-to-spirit encounter between caregiver and patient that includes the patient's acknowledgment of trust in the caregiver." Quality care, in their view, must include this spirit-to-spirit encounter.

Direct Spiritual Practices or Interventions

The following section outlines spiritual care interventions that demonstrate the myriad of options available to the health-care provider in spiritual work with children. Familiarity with strategies gives professionals an internal "toolbox" that will be useful at the moment of planned or spontaneous spiritual care.

The Ministry of Presence

Authors refer to this quality in various ways. Authentic human presence, being there, being with, and caring presence all refer to the same aspect

(Gallia, 1996). Presence has been described as foundational for compassion. Kendall (1999) indicated that aspects of bedside nursing such as "hands on" care, "accompanying," and "watching" give "presence" to the vulnerable patient. Zerwekh (1997, p. 260) uniquely described this quality as "presencing." Presencing converts the word presence, a noun describing a quality, into a verb expressing action. Kenny (1999) stated,

> The ability to be with children in this way confirms their uniqueness and offers acceptance of them and their experience. Out of this trusting contact, avenues of communication can open that are unique to the child and his/her developmental stage. (p. 32)

Within the concept of the ministry of presence, the professional must be committed and devoted to the child's growth. Just our authentic presence can bring a measure of settling or healing to the child and family, we must be able to be truly present in the face of suffering, pain, sorrow and grief. By doing this, we offer strength that may be desperately needed. Shelly and Fish (1988) and Fulton and Moore (1995) called it the therapeutic use of self with empathy, vulnerability, humility, and commitment.

Relational contacts decrease as people come to the end of their lives (Bowers, 1974). Yet, nurses and others who are present at these and other critical times can share warmth, caring, and compassion. When one is authentically present with a patient, alertness and sensitivity to the spiritual needs of that patient and of the self are enhanced.

So very often, talk is not needed—especially with children. Being there makes the difference. Nurses are at the bedside around the clock in many health-care situations. This is a wonderful advantage because presence alone can build trust and strengthen relationships. Sterling-Fisher shared some gracious wording that a health-care provider may use that sets a time limit but conveys authentic presence: "I need to be leaving in about 20 minutes but I'm not in a hurry. I'm here to be with you" (Sterling-Fisher, 1998, p. 247).

Conveying Acceptance

Having true regard and respect for a person conveys acceptance and invites children to open their lives to us. Judith Shelly described the importance of "unconditionally welcoming a child." Having unconditional acceptance and love allows the child to feel safe, secure, and able to express his or her real self (Shelly, 1995). *Empathetic regard* is another descriptive phrase that implies acceptance.

Active Listening

Active listening has been cited as a means to assure caring (Clark & Heidenreich, 1995; Sellers & Haag, 1998), confirm a child's uniqueness (Kenny,

1999), confirm acceptance, and tell the child that the listener is open or trustworthy when it comes to listening to their history and spiritual stories. Active listening can allow children—who are egocentric by developmental stage—to be the center of our attention for the time we are with them. This forum is powerful in touching the being of a child and allowing the child to lead us to the areas of greatest spiritual need.

It takes caring, with a true desire to know the child—to truly share yourself with a child. O'Brien talked about listening with a loving heart (O'Brien, 1999). Listen to what is shared. Listen to what is not said. Children will usually not express their needs in spiritual terms. It is up to us to listen for the needs or to listen for the strengths. Comments such as, "It isn't fair to have asthma" (example from Fulton & Moore, 1995) may be a lead to broad opening questions. However, before any questions, listening is necessary. Listening may lead to discovery of the "gift" to be affirmed or the needs to be met (Hungelmann, Kenkel-Ross, Klassen, & Stollenwerk, 1996).

In his culminating work of research, *The Spiritual Life of Children*, Robert Coles (1990) shared a marvelous insight gleaned from William Carlos Williams:

> I am with a child, and I want some information—and he'll clam up, or she'll stare at me stonily. I'll get impatient. I'll get angry. On a good day, though, I'll remember what I shouldn't have forgotten—what I've learned after hundreds and hundreds of house calls: When a kid falls silent I should keep my eyes open.... Pay attention to the wordless narration that can take place as a child uses his or her face, arms, or legs, or, as child psychiatrists have learned, a paintbrush, [or] some crayons. (p. 167)

Crisis situations warrant private listening without interruption. Mangini and colleagues (1995) explained,

> You can create the sense of a timeless space in which you are fully present and focused on the situation. The other person should sense that you are fully there for them and have all the time they need for you to be with them. (p. 562)

Listening cannot be overemphasized.

Therapeutic Spiritual Communication

Talking with a child or family member about spiritual matters is, in itself, an intervention that can bring strength. Sometimes therapeutic listening will give way to spiritual discussions. During these discussions, health-care providers can employ communication methods such as facilitating, clarifying, validating feelings and thoughts, or identifying sources of strength and hope (Sellers & Haag, 1998). No matter what spiritual counseling skills a health-care provider feels he or she has, therapeutic spiritual communication can take place. Simply by using the content of the person's own words and adding therapeutic, supportive communication skills, much can be accomplished.

Reflective Communications or Further Questions

A question such as, "To whom do you turn when you need help?" lets clients clarify spiritual values, resources, and experiences (Sellers & Haag,1998). "What are some of the lessons you've learned from this experience?" is an example of a question that can be fairly easy to ask but can yield meaningful spiritual answers. Other helpful questions are, "What aspects of spirituality would you like me to keep in mind as I care for you?" and "How has your spiritual history been helpful in coping with your illness?" (McBride, Arthur, Brooks, & Pilkington, 1998).

Prayer

Prayer is the main spiritual tool for seeking God's help. It is reaching out beyond ourselves for some and looking inward for others (Harmon & Myers, 1999). Patients use prayer for themselves in times of crisis. Parents commonly pray for their children who face a crisis. Health is a primary focus of prayer (Magaletta, Duckro, & Staten, 1997).

Prayer seems to benefit the doer and the receiver. Those who pray may feel less burdened because they have been able to do something about the problem. It seems to be a way of "mastering a seemingly uncontrollable situation" (Cerrato, 1998). There may be a feeling of relaxation, release of endorphins, and release of other natural "tranquilizers" (Hughes, 1997). Physical, emotional, social, and spiritual strengths have been described as being associated with noncontact intercessory prayer, personal private prayer, or face-to-face joint prayer (Matthews, 2000; Roberts, Ahmed, & Hall, 2002). Meaning in suffering, coping, and perceptions of well-being for patients are recurrent results of prayer.

Prayer can be a petition, request, adoration, reparation, meditation, or contemplation; it can be thanksgiving, vocal, mental, discursive, affective, centering, mystical, private, or communal (O'Brien, 1999; see Figure 9.3). Harmon and Myers (1999) identified petition, intercession, confession, lamentation, adoration, invocation, and thanksgiving as forms of prayer. In short, there are many types of prayer. Levin (1996) reviewed four dimensions of prayer, which are listed in Table 9.5 with examples.

Being aware of different dimensions or types of prayer is valuable for the health-care provider. Different types of prayer may bring different results for children. Variety in prayer may prove helpful. O'Hara (2002)

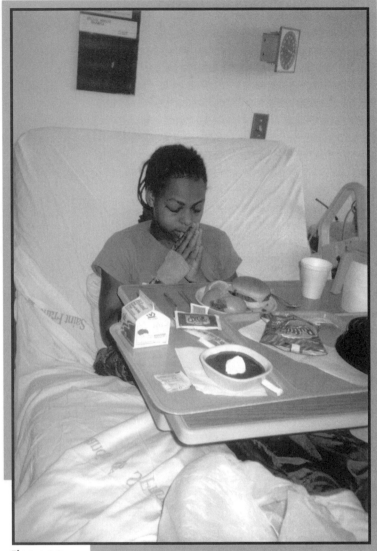

Figure 9.3.
Spiritual routines such as saying grace before meals can be maintained in various health-care settings. *Note.* Photograph by Lynn Clutter. Used with permission.

pointed out that how a person prays and what happens when he or she prays is more important information than frequency of prayer. The following example demonstrates prayer situations with children.

Sharon was a patient in critical condition after a cardiac arrest. Gail (11 years old) and Karen (8 years old) were wide-awake at night. Gail suddenly said to the nurse, "I wish Sister Marie was here. She was my primary schoolteacher, and she really meant a lot to me. She would understand!" Karen said, "I don't know what I'm going to do if Sharon [a

Table 9.5 381

Four Dimensions of Prayer

Dimensions of Prayer	Examples of Prayer
Ritual/recitational	Readings, reciting of prayers
Conversational/colloquial	Conversing with God in a less formal way
Petitionery/intercessory	Requesting something specific from God
Meditative	Reflective, listening, experiencing, and worshipping God

Note. From "Replenishing the Spirit by Meditative Prayer and Guided Imagery," by K. Brown-Saltzman, 1997, *Seminars in Oncology Nursing, 13*(4), pp. 255–259. Copyright 1997 by Saunders. Reprinted with permission.

third child in the same hospital] dies!" Gail responded, "I can't believe that this hospital doesn't even have a place to pray! I mean, isn't that what hospitals are all about?" The nurse responded, "Even though we don't have a special place, we could pray right here. Would you like that?" The girls eagerly agreed, sat on the bed, held hands and prayed. This prayer opened the way for discussion of death. (Still, 1984, p. 4)

Hart and Schneider (1997, p. 269) offered the following guidelines for initiating and intervening through prayer if prayer seems suitable:

- Be prepared to offer the prayer—"Would you appreciate prayer at this time?"
- Allow the child or family to make the choice—"Yes, it couldn't hurt!"
- Pray … blessing, petition, formal prayer, and so on. If the nurse is praying, the prayer should be kept short and simple, endeavoring to reflect the child's feelings, fears, and concerns.

Wording must be comfortable for the health-care provider. Often, however, the point when initiation of prayer is appropriate, the health-care provider may not come up with ready words. The box presents 10 ways to word the same offer for prayer and demonstrates that there are many ways to word things well.

Prayers can be short and simple, reflecting the child's feelings, fears and concerns, and "opening the lines of communication between the child and God" (Anderson & Steen, 1995, p. 16). Prayers may change with developmental stage. Earliest prayers of young children are vague because children have an indistinct understanding of prayer. In the next stage, children view prayer as a routine, external activity. In the third stage, children view prayer as a private conversation with God with less egocentricism (Steen & Anderson, 1995).

As a cautionary word, it is important to distinguish prayer as an adjunct to care and not an alternative. Post, Puchalski, and Larson (2000) discussed

Ten Different Wording Styles for Initiating the Offer of Prayer	1. "Would you like me or a spiritual advisor to pray with you now?" 2. "Would you appreciate prayer at this time?" or "...about the things we've discussed?" 3. "Would saying a prayer be helpful for you?" 4. "I would be happy (honored, able to, most willing to) say a prayer with you if that would help." 5. "Some people find prayer valuable at times like this. Would that be the case with you?"

this very thought about physicians and analyzed the ethics of physicians offering prayer. Citing a national poll (Yankelovich Partners, Inc., 1996), they show that 48% of patients in the United States want prayer with their physicians and 64% of Americans think that physicians should join their patients in prayer if the patients ask. Their viewpoint is that the client should initiate prayer; that if a religious leader is present, that person should lead; and physician-led prayer is acceptable only when pastoral care is not readily available. Further, "A physician who initiates prayer without first being asked presents an ethical concern in that patients might easily feel coerced" (p. 581).

The medical literature has mixed viewpoints on initiation of prayer, as does the nursing literature. While physicians—responsible for diagnosing and treating illness—may have a greater concern over any hint of religious coercion than other health-care providers, some degree of their caution is true for others as well. Patients should have the choice of having verbal prayer or not.

Proclaiming a Blessing

In many ways, people rely on the strength, hope, belief, and faith of others to get through difficult times. We have an ability to bestow a blessing upon an individual as an "intentional act of speaking God's favor and power into someone's life" (Anderson & Steen, 1995, p. 16). The Book of Psalms and various other sacred writings have many written blessings. Even for those living in death's shadow, health-care providers can foster strength where there was helplessness and powerlessness:

> Our confidence and affirmation that the life remaining can be precious can encourage the same appreciation in them and counter feelings that they are burdens upon others or failures. We can help them to focus upon remaining opportunities for meaningful experiences, achievements, and expressions. (Attig, 1996, p. 23)

6. "Do you ever say prayers at times like this?"
7. "I know a couple of children who have had a special prayer written on a paper or index card and it has helped them. Do you think something like that would be good for you?"
8. "Did you know you could write (or make a song out of) a special prayer that is your very own to God? I'd pray it with you if you ever did that."
9. "I like to pray about things like that. Do you?"
10. "This card of yours says 'God meets us when we pray.' What do you think about that? Would that help now?"

Meditation

A wide variety of meditation practices are used throughout the world. Both eastern and western religions include meditation, as do American Indians. Physiologic changes associated with meditation identified in studies with adults include a decrease in heart rate, decrease in respiration rate and oxygen consumption, altered skin conductance, EEG changes, and biochemical changes (Harmon & Myers, 1999). In addition to physiologic findings, studies on individuals with psychologic disorders and those coping with stress, anxiety, insomnia, or pending surgery report benefits with the use of meditation (Harmon & Myers, 1999). On the other hand, several studies have shown adverse effects in certain population groups with "over-meditation" (Harmon & Myers, 1999).

Attig (1996, p. 23) recommended encouraging children to use prayer and meditation to express and process spiritual anguish. Of course, if children indicate that meditation is part of their lives, health-care providers should facilitate its practice in the health-care setting through means such as assisting in providing privacy.

Touch

Human touch can convey spiritual compassion in a way that words cannot. Children are especially responsive to touch. Referred to in religious literature (Mark 10:13, the *Bible*), human touch is important from birth to death, and is a powerful means of uniting people.

Many types of touch are suitable for spiritual intervention with children. Patting, stroking, tussling of the hair, touching or holding a hand, patting or gently grasping a forearm or shoulder, patting a back, putting an arm around, rocking, soothing, holding, or even nestling can have their place with babies or children (see Figure 9.4). Anderson and Steen (1995) described John, an 18-year-old boy who was hospitalized and in the terminal stages of leukemia. He was depressed and hopeless. His nurse offered a backrub, which was

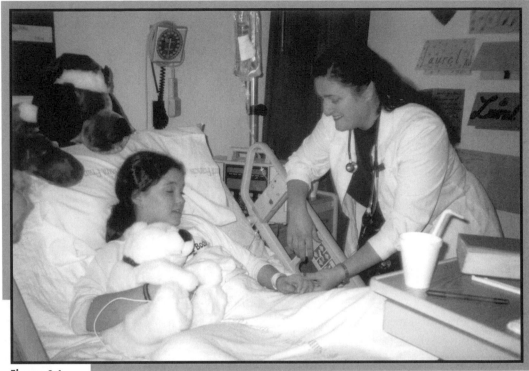

Figure 9.4.

Empathy, vulnerability, humility, and commitment to being present can all be conveyed through touch. *Note.* Photograph by Lynn Clutter. Used with permission.

readily accepted. John said that she was the first person who had touched him during the month he had been hospitalized. Claassen (1998) demonstrated the value and communication benefit of touch toward children with multiple disabilities. Empathy, being vulnerable, humility, and commitment to being present through the time of support are important elements in therapeutic use of self (Anderson & Steen, 1995; Carson, 1989; Shelly & Fish, 1995). These qualities can be expressed through touch. Spiritual communication often comes with close proximity and healthy types of compassionate touch.

Therapies of Non-Western Origin

A variety of philosophical beliefs or cultural principles give way to alternative or complementary therapies. Holism, as described by the Holistic Nurses Association in England, indicates that health proceeds from a balance of physical, spiritual, psychological, and social needs (Patterson, 1998). Holistic nursing, which emphasizes self-organizing, self-renewal, and self-transcendence with the ability to be self-assertive, does not infer complementary therapies, but may use them.

Ancient Eastern philosophy, quantum theory, and the interconnectedness of all energies seem to have a strong link (Patterson, 1998). An array of lesser known spiritually linked therapies or practices are derived largely from Chinese medicine, Aborigines of Australia, Native North American Indians, ancient Eastern or ancient Indian spiritual traditions, many of which involve the flow of energy. Spiritual healing is connected with energy fields or centers and is not linked with religion or God or a Higher Power. Spiritual healers work with universal energy fields, human energy fields, laws of energy, energy systems, and the interconnectedness of energy or the flow of energy that happens when people become "well balanced" (Patterson, 1998).

Therapies that have New Age origins (Barnum, 1996; Sellers & Haag, 1998) may be herbal, aroma, chanting, and prayer rituals with tefillins, chakras, or dantians. Healing through various therapies or channeling energies from one to another are aspects of New Age, American Indian, Aboriginal, or Chinese beliefs.

Guided Imagery

Brown-Saltzman (1997) described the use of imagination, thoughts, senses, position, and internal images that create positive messages. The new images create new patterns or ways of seeing things. Imagery is used to reframe experiences and perceptions, facilitate problem solving, and increase a client's sense of control.

Children are very able to use imagery. Computer programs have been developed to help children have positive health images (e.g., a computer game that has Pac-Man-type "body cells" that "eat" cancer cells). One can use spiritual images as well (e.g., Psalms 91:4: "He will cover you with his feathers, and under his wings you will find refuge" [New International Version, the *Bible*]). This evokes an image of a comforting, protecting God that children understand and can mentally picture.

Spiritual References, Bibliotherapy

Bibliotherapy tools can be sacred scriptures, devotional materials, written reflections on beliefs, poems, spiritual teaching tapes (audio, video), or sacred stories. The possibilities are vast. With children and adolescents, the written word can draw on the imagination of hearts and minds. Certain materials such as a Bible storybook, may be beloved and much read. Books can provide support and motivation because readers can identify emotionally with characters to gain understanding.

Health-care providers can observe a child's belief system then identify books that may be useful. Timing and appropriateness of the book are important in acceptability to the child and parent. Often spiritual books will be brought from home to the health-care setting.

Cress-Ingebo and Chrisagis (1998) described two types of bibliotherapy: (a) finding the right fit of literature for readers to use by themselves, and (b) having an interactive, discussion approach. With the latter approach, the health-care provider must be prepared to discuss the material when the patient is ready to process content. Reading to the child allows opportunity for a private or discussive approach. Often with an interactive processing, the child may benefit from emotion clarification as emotions emerge.

Anderson and Steen (1995) provided an example of bibliotherapy with a parent. The nurse preparing a 4-year-old child for surgery observed the child's mother reading the Bible. The nurse offered to share one of her favorite passages. The child's mother not only accepted the offer, she also asked the nurse to pray with them for strength. Later, at a time of fear and apprehension for the family, the nurse was able to share a scripture—a welcomed encouragement.

Autobiographical scrapbooks and literature are very comforting and reassuring, they promote insight and reflection, and improve communication. These, in turn, empower the spirit of the child to find meaning and purpose in life (Fulton & Moore, 1995).

Adults read sacred scriptures to feel closer to God, find peace, have meaning in life, stand against wrongs in society, be open and honest with self, and gain love toward others (Gallup & Lindsay, 1999). Children may or may not read for the same reasons. Piles (1990) pointed out that before initiating the sharing of scripture with patients, the health-care provider should have some sense of when this would be an appropriate intervention.

Reassurance or Encouragement

Spiritual encouragement can take many forms. Support of the belief in God's caring presence, care notes, prayers that are written, and visits by trusted friends are examples of reassurance (Clark et al., 1991). Sellers and Haag (1998) described the ministry of caring that takes many forms. Even a visit from a pet can convey acceptance and encourage a child. A comment such as, "Blackie loves you in bed or outside … just like God," can offer a concrete symbol of reassurance. The Bible teaches Christians to encourage one another every day (Hebrews 3:13). Some children who are in health-care facilities may go days without encouraging words. With keen assessment and descriptive skills, nurses can regularly share specific encouragement with children and their families. Seeing the day-to-day progress gives nurses a position to share the parameters that demonstrate growth, which can be reassuring and foster hope.

Adapting the Physical Environment

Health-care providers can create spiritually supportive environments. Advocating for spiritual comfort or modifying the physical surroundings are two avenues of intervention. Employing the use of a family waiting room or a private area, and posting notes on doors to maintain privacy at times, can allow for spirituality. Providing a private area is a valuable intervention, especially with pastoral visits or meditations. Having a hospital chapel with beepers available for parents to use allows a parent of a child in surgery some freedom of space. Fina (1995) stated,

> Orthodox Jewish parents may wish to chant, pray, or use tefillins (i.e., leather thongs used in prayer rituals) or prayer shawls. Islamic families may need a private place in which to wash and lay out their prayer rugs. Christian families may desire a private area in which to hold hands and pray aloud or to say a rosary. Prayer rituals and meditations may last for many hours. It is not unusual for family members to tell me that their prayers are for physicians and staff members caring for their child. (pp. 558, 560)

Instilling Hope

Hope can be a curative element or a preventive intervention. Health-care providers can have hope themselves, foster hope in others, or discourage feelings of hopelessness. The role of influence is one that cannot be taken for granted. In fact, some believe nurses should take ownership of their key role in enabling patients to have hope (Clark et al., 1991). Reed (1992) stated, "Hope which in part represents a connectedness to possibilities and powers beyond the current situation, is frequently cited [in the literature] as the factor that can make a critical difference in the healing process" (p. 354).

Hope can be for life, recovery, and well-being. Hope can also exist for death and the hereafter. Health-care providers can assess the hope level of patients and families then support or influence accordingly. Hopelessness, the lack of hope, can hinder well-being. When the family places trust in their higher power, hope can rekindle. Hope in the capacity of the health-care team can be reassuring as well.

Maintaining hope of life in the face of death is an aspect that can affect those around. Porter (1995) described one parent's hope of life for her baby in the midst of staff having given up on the possibility. After the newborn survived her birth defect of gastroschesis, subsequent multiple complications and surgeries, and went on to live to adulthood, her nurse reflectively commented, "Perhaps the most valuable lesson I've learned is to listen to parents, get a feel for their instincts, show them how much I care and, most of all, never to say 'never'" (p. 26).

Children Giving Back

An example of someone who has given back may be the best way to share the value of this intervention. Fina (1995) described Matthew, who at 12 years of age had a near-total amputation of his hand with seven surgeries and a month of hospitalization. The experience pushed the family's coping strategies to the limit. Matthew received spiritual care from the chaplaincy department and often from the family's Rabbi. Later, at the time of Matthew's bar mitzvah, part of Matthew's right of passage was to donate the silk flower table centerpieces from the celebration to the surgical family waiting area where "they often had prayed together" (Fina, 1995, p. 564). This act of giving took the experiences at the children's hospital and placed a positive, lasting memory of a gift with them. This probably served as a healing act related to this chapter of Matthew's life.

Children who are chronically ill, hospitalized, or who have experienced critical illness or injuries are very able—at some point in time—to help other children. They can have very meaningful messages that benefit adults and children. One question for a child is "Do you spread love to others?" (Sterling-Fisher, 1998).

Nearly every religion encourages love and giving, both as actions and as noble character qualities. Health-care providers may facilitate "giving back" or simply allow it to happen in the health-care setting. Health-care providers who value the belief that giving back helps children spiritually will be attuned to opportunities such as identifying a child who is struggling, a child who may be strong, and a means of connecting the two. They will foster outlets for individual children, and will encourage family members to find outlets for giving. We foster spiritual growth when we foster giving in children.

Journaling and the Use of Diaries

Writing can be useful for children, particularly those with spiritual issues surrounding chronic or terminal illness. Journals are especially helpful for adolescents. "Some adolescents are as verbally articulate or as sophisticated in their thinking as adults. Yet adolescents tend to fear exposure and rejection more, hold questions back for fear of embarrassment, shield their privacy, and find more comfort in communications with peers" (Attig, 1996, p. 22). Journaling allows youths to explain themselves privately and without time or interactive pressure. For example, an individual experiencing a crisis of faith went to the ocean, discussed the crisis, then wrote an essay illustrating water-related images. This process helped her move through spiritual pain to deepened faith, hope, and courage (Bailey, 1997).

Picture Therapy

Coles (1990) used this tool in work with school-age children in a classroom setting to encourage them to talk about topics that would evoke inner spiritual beliefs. Having a picture such as a sick child in someone's arms or care can simply be shown to a child. Usually they will offer comments or questions. The health-care provider can guide the comments once a child's voluntary comments fall silent. Questions such as, "What do you think this child is wondering?" can give way to comments that reflect the child's inner concerns. Answers can also be followed by more self-reflective comments such as, "He's lucky. His mom holds him." Even simple pictures of children out of magazines can be useful for particular aspects of spiritual care. Some children respond more readily to pictures than words. Adolescents can be prompted with questions such as, "If you were this person, what would you be thinking?"

Use of Memory, Reminiscence

Remembering important life events can be quite important for children. For young children, remembering fun, special, close to family, or close to God memories can be enjoyable, encouraging, and healing. Health-care providers can use reminiscence for assessment and trust-building. A concrete and creative approach is creating a "memory island." This involves having the child or family bring pictures and memorabilia to "create their own island." The island could be a poster board, scrapbook, or basket. This strategy allows "others to join in the celebration of the person's life in a visual manner and assist in the acceptance of life" (study participant in Sellers & Haag, 1998, p. 345). Memories can bring to the forefront meaning, purpose, and satisfaction of life. Another approach is having the child, or the child and family members, share memories of "I remember when..." Spiritual themes are often present.

Forgiving Self or Others

Forgiveness can be an act, a process, and an attitude. Giving and receiving forgiveness brings healing and peace. Children can have powerful experiences of forgiveness. One young child said he "felt lighter or something" after he had forgiven his father for leaving him. A 6 year-old girl reported that she does not get that "tight neck where I can't swallow when I think of her" after she forgave the person. An adolescent athlete was furious at the "guy who gave me this broken foot that makes me be out of basketball the whole season." Once he chose to forgive, he was able to say, "It wasn't really his fault anyway." His affect changed and he felt he could better handle the problem.

One helpful method of assisting children to forgive is the use of poetry. The poem "Wild Geese" (Oliver, 1992) begins with, "You do not have to be good. You do not have to walk on your knees for a hundred miles through the desert, repenting." Gustavson (2000, p. 329) stated, "You can easily see that this poem might be used in sessions with persons who are struggling to forgive themselves, or who may be having a hard time forgiving another person." The poem can spark a conversation on a topic that the child may have been reluctant to talk about.

Much of the 12-step materials first developed by Alcoholics Anonymous include information on forgiveness. Children can experience the same freeing from bitterness and hostility that adults experience once they decide to let go of the pain and forgive the offender. On the other hand, when a child has experienced abuse, too much willingness to forgive can be a red flag for psychosocial distress (McCullough, 2000).

Humor

"Joy is one of the spiritual strengths that enable people to survive—including the capacity to see the funny side of life" (Bailey, 1997, p. 245). Humor can relieve emotional tension and grief, bring health-care providers and families closer together, and allow people to stand back from the difficult situations and see other sides (Sterling-Fisher, 1998). According to McFadden (1990), authentic humor is an expression of spiritual maturity because, although it cannot eliminate suffering, it can momentarily relieve the pain. Children with spiritual resilience often exhibit humor or a "lighter" perspective. Humor and pleasure can be important parts of a child's spiritual experience.

Play

The health-care provider can observe what gives a child pleasure, find favorite types of play, then let the child have ample opportunities to have fun without the thought of illness. For example, the father of a girl with multiple disabilities and multiple hospitalizations was in the room with his daughter. A nurse brought three finger puppets and said, "Would you like to see these? Here is the dad; here are the other two puppets." Her dad put one on and the daughter had the others. They started playing and soon were lost in play, talking with "puppet voices" to each other for about 10 minutes. Their voices were animated and they laughed. They were unaware of anything else. What a wonderful connecting experience this was, with a rarely present dad. Health-care providers can enter the child's world rather than forcing the child to enter theirs. "The child's world is characterized by play" (Sweeney & Landreth, 1993, p. 351). Spiritual care can occur in the context of that play.

Spiritual play helps for gaining insight into the child but is especially therapeutic because it opens the spiritual dimension indirectly using the natural mode of communication. It also allows mastery, free expression, and fun. Points of pleasure can give way to trust and spontaneous comments. Child-centered play therapy allows the child to "talk" through the process of play, and does not require the child to be cognitive and verbal (Sweeney & Landreth, 1993).

Children's anxiety may be so great as to paralyze their imaginations and inhibit their capacity to play (Piers & Landau, 1980). What helps these children are opportunities to play, the safety of symbolic play, and play therapy. Play therapy provides the environmental situation to, as Sweeney says, "grow, to change, and to heal. It is a spiritual process." Our role is to communicate four messages: "I'm here, I hear you, I understand, and I care" (Landreth, 1991, p. 182).

Using stuffed dolls or animals, puppets, or simple finger puppets (easy to keep in the pocket) is perfect. Talking with transitional objects like this is appropriate, especially with young children who can easily give these toys human qualities and will sometimes open up more readily than with a person they do not know well. Using a third-person technique (e.g., "Some children tell me that they worry when they have to go for tests. I wonder how it is for you.") and identifying a change that would facilitate spiritual well-being can be helpful.

The Arts and Imagination

Music, visual arts, storytelling, poetry, and other expressive arts can be used to address spiritual issues. For example,

> John was a fiercely angry six-year-old boy with leukemia. He hated the hospital, fought against the needles and nurses, and understood well the toughness of life. The only things I knew about John before I visited him in his hospital room were that he had a brother named Rory and that he often threw things at people who came to visit him. When I arrived, I was greeted with a shower of liquid. At the same time, I heard something hit the floor beside me—John's bedpan.
>
> I tried to appear undaunted, as if the stains on my blouse might be tears or punch or rain from the parking lot. "John, tell me three things about your brother, Rory, and I will get out of here fast," I began. John proceeded to relay three of the most disgusting facts that he could think of.
>
> Still trying my best to appear unshaken, I asked him if he knew the song "Pop Goes the Weasel." When he seemed hesitant, I handed him a musical instrument that made loud noises when you slapped it hard. John was the type of child that loved to make loud noises. "I want you to slap this as hard as you can at the part that goes pop," I said. I improvised a song: "Passes gas and picks his nose, and then he tries to hug me. He gets the mail, he bit my dog's tail. That's [pop] my brother, Rory."
>
> As it turned out, John was so taken by the song that he asked if we could call his brother and sing the song over the phone to him and then record it on tape for his parents. I gladly agreed. It was the beginning of a great relationship. (Lane, 1994, p. 118)

Not only did Lane break the anger, she reached John on his terms. This silly and shocking "music" touched the boy and broke away from the disease and clinical procedures. Music has been shown to have so many physiological, psychological, and spiritual benefits (see Chapter 4). When a child's spirituality and music are combined in care, powerfully effective changes can happen. Not only is music therapeutic in general, but it can spiritually reach children and provide a medium for children to communicate.

Lorrie's story is another example of the strength of spirituality and music. Lorrie had cancer. Her favorite song was "Jesus Loves Me." While in the hospital, she was asked to compose another verse to the song, the singing of which was very meaningful. Later, while in a coma, her music therapist visited and sang the song with Lorrie's verse, then said, "Isn't that beautiful, Lorrie?" Lorrie aroused from her coma and nodded. She soon returned home, and before her death, was calmed regularly through her mother's singing of her verse (Lane, 1994, p. 28).

Children may be receptive to **music therapy,** such as hearing spiritually based or sacred songs, and active singing or playing instruments (O'Brien, 1999; Sellers & Haag, 1998). Music is a part of all cultures and religions in some way, and especially in association with worship. Music has been incorporated into care in various ways, including during the postoperative recovery period (Heiser, Chiles, Fudge, & Gray, 1997), general spiritual care (O'Brien, 1999), pain management (Zimmerman, Pozehl, Duncan, & Schmitz, 1989), and distraction from procedures (O'Brien, 1999).

Art therapy is valuable as a tool with children having spiritually linked issues (Koepfer, 2000). The work with issues somehow happens as a by-product of working with media. Feelings can be expressed during the process or in the created outcome. For example, "the construction and decoration of a 'prayer or meditation pillow' not only offers opportunities for activity, creativity, and discussion but also leaves the child with a physical object that may later be helpful in meditation or prayer" (Field & Behrman, 2003, p. 166). Drawing and painting are discussed in general terms in Chapter 4. However, in a spiritually directed art session, requests for certain pictures can be given such as, "Will you please draw a picture of…"

- Anything at this time [note: sometimes this brings to paper and discussion what is foremost on the child's mind]
- How you feel now
- God or specific spiritual leader, such as Jesus, Moses, Mohammed, Higher Power [note: Allah is not to be pictured in the Islamic belief system]
- A story from a sacred book
- A place of worship, such as synagogue, mosque, Mecca, temple, church, home
- A place where you feel close to God
- A time when you felt close to God
- You with people who help you be close to God

Spiritually related developmental changes in children's drawings have been noted. Anderson and Steen (1995) cited a study from 1944 that found that (a) children ages 3 to 6 years drew God as king living in clouds, (b) children ages 7 to 12 years drew faith symbols (Jewish Star of David or Christian cross), and (c) youth ages 13 to 18 years drew diverse things from conventional views of God to abstract things such as rainbows or sunrises (Pendleton et al., 2002).

Robert Coles used the **viewing of works of art** to inspire spiritual discussions among school-age children (Coles, 1990). For example, when showing the portrait "The Doctor," by French artist Luke S. Fildes, that depicts a sick girl with a doctor, Coles wrote, "I have learned to ask nothing, to say nothing. Eventually the questions always come—inquiries that, of course, make their own statements" (Coles, 1990, p. 110). This approach of letting the artwork evoke the thoughts is fairly nonthreatening, can be directed by the choice of picture offered, and can reveal aspects of children's perceptions that may not otherwise emerge.

Telling stories that are spiritual in nature, or those that encourage positive spiritual qualities such as courage can be excellent in use with children (Taylor, 1997). The stories need to be consistent with the child's beliefs. "What makes one a Christian, a Jew, a Hindu, or a Muslim, is the sacred, master story of the religious community that shapes and nurtures each person's identity" (Webb Mitchell, 1993, p. 148). These are the Old and New Testaments, the Hebrew Bible, and the Qur'an. Parts of the child's master story can be comforting to hear. The narrative approach can be a valuable tool for distraction and for incorporating spiritual content that can make a difference in health-care situations. Stories shape children's understanding of life, who they are, their faith, family, and the world around them. The telling or hearing of a story can be an act of care. A concept embedded in a story can bring lasting meaning for a child.

Sometimes **writing poetry** is of great value in health-care settings for children, adults, and for health-care providers as well. A child may capture and identify a spiritual, emotional, physical, or social need they are having, in their poem. This is valuable because professionals seek to locate areas of needed healing and offer interventions accordingly. Merely the process of writing the poetry is therapeutic. The sharing with others can strengthen, as well.

In her book, *In-Versing Your Life: A Poetry Workbook for Self-Discovery and Healing*, Cynthia Gustavson (1995) used a procedure of pairing poems with exercises for personal growth. This process can be exemplified by having people write, "I used to be…but now I am…." Once, an adolescent who recently gave birth filled in the metaphor with, "I used to be a beautiful flower, but now I am a stem, because I am broken" (Gustavson, 2000, p. 329). Though the girl had returned to her support group and her baby was 2 weeks old, this was the first time she had spoken to anyone.

Another example of a verse is, "I am…but I will be…." Sometimes filling in the blanks can pull inner feelings out into the open in a way that talking never can. It is important that the poem match the person's developmental level, but poetry therapy can be used with children as young as 4 years of age. There are four stages in the process of using poetry for therapy. The individual

- identifies with the poem and feels it has something to say to him or her,
- examines the poem and discusses its meaning,

- thinks about other meanings to compare and contrast under-standings (not necessarily what the author intended but what the client feels), and
- integrates own perceptions of meaning into his or her own self-understanding (Gustavson, 2000).

Much could be said about children's wonderful **capacity to imagine,** and the use of this tool for spiritual care. Books and all media "capture children's imagination." Health care is only scratching the surface of use of this marvelous resource of children. Even very young children can abandon themselves to positive imaginations. For example, children who know they are dying find strength in imagining what heaven is like. Some caregivers use a "magic carpet" to help children imagine trips to heaven or a land of no pain so that children may then talk about their hopes, wants, or worries (Field & Behrman, 2003). Parents of dying children find security in the belief that they will see their child again. Sometimes parents imagine, with pleasure, that reunion in heaven. Imagination can be used as a distraction, as when having a painful procedure. Imagination can soften a willful perspective or change a mood. Imagining the great stories of sacred books can bring a role model to one's recollection or can be applied to the current situation.

Horticultural or Pet Therapy

The media of plants, or "horticultural therapy" has value in work with children. "Gardening combines physical, mental, and emotional involvement and stimulates an interest in the future" (Gough, 1986, p. 165). It uses a living medium and requires someone with responsibility, time, energy, and care. Plants are responsive to care and do not discriminate (Gough, 1986). Spiritual growth can happen tangentially.

The unconditional love of a pet can touch souls of any age. An increasing number of hospitals have pet therapy programs where specially trained dogs and other animals visit children in a group or at the bedside. Proximity, caretaking, and nurturing are valuable and can help to "reach the core" of a child. After playing with a pet, children are noticeably calmed and often more receptive to spiritual care.

Critical Moments for Spiritual Interventions

Often in life there are vulnerable times when spiritual care—that otherwise would not be possible—is welcomed with open arms. Health-care professionals can be sensitive to cues and structure time or interventions accordingly when possible. Making use of these "open windows" can dramatically change the course of care.

A clinical nurse specialist (CNS) and parents who had experienced the sudden infant death of their third child while overseas shared such a moment. The parents scheduled an appointment with the CNS to learn how to deal with the grief of their other children. Knowing that this family had many issues of grief, and being willing to take additional personal time if necessary, the CNS arranged an appointment at the end of a work day. Her broad opening comment to the parents was, "I never really heard how everything happened that day. Will you share that with me?" This comment alone gave way to 5 hours of the spilling of grief. The intensity of sharing was so great that there was not a thought of stopping. The CNS spoke very little and engaged in active listening to the talk and grief of each parent. At the end, the parents were exhausted but settled in a way that was lasting. There was prayer and the provision of literature on children's grief. Every "critical moment" experience is certainly not this long. Some can be very brief but with equally lasting results.

Often children open up just before bedtime. This is a valuable time to unlock spiritual and emotional issues for children. The wise health-care provider will set aside time at the child's bedtime to use for this purpose. Nighttime can also be that settling time when the provider can provide extra physical touch and special care such as combing hair or giving extra pillows. These special ministrations open doors for critical moments and allow the provider to demonstrate value of the child, unconditional acceptance, and love without words.

Baptism

Baptism is a Christian practice. Infant baptism is important for Roman, Byzantine, Coptic branches of Catholicism, Greek Orthodox, Episcopal, Lutheran, Methodist, and Presbyterian churches. For members of these denominations, additional grief can occur if the newborn has not been baptized. Baptist, Assembly of God, Charismatic, Disciples of Christ, Church of Christ, Mennonite, and Pentecostal denominations do not practice baptism in infancy, but do at older ages (Reeb & McFarland, 1995).

When a baby is critically ill, those of certain religions may desire infant baptism. The box describes procedures for emergency infant baptism.

Referrals to Providers of Spiritual Care

The question may arise as to who should provide spiritual care. In general life, the range is broad; in health-care settings, the same is true. Sometimes a formal clergy member or chaplain is appropriate; other times, family members

Emergency Baptism

If death seems inevitable and imminent:

1. Take the initiative and identify parental wishes.
2. Notify chaplain or social service department of parents' desire with the name and phone number of desired minister or priest.
3. If spiritual care provider is not available at time of imminent death, perform the baptismal rite:
   - Call infant by name (or "child of God" if not named)
   - Pour less than 30 cc. tap or sterile water, or even D5W on baby's head and say, "(name), I baptize you in the name of the Father and of the Son and of the Holy Spirit." (Note that the Methodist rite is to put hands in water and place wet hands on baby's head. The Lutheran rite has the water poured on the head three times.)

do a fine job with children, and sometimes friends offer welcomed care. However, a multidisciplinary team approach is valuable for spiritual care. First, using a team approach, more people can assess for spiritual distress or well-being. Second, the most appropriate person on the team can plan and intervene. Third, a coordinated effort of care for the whole person can happen. Barnes and colleagues (2000, p. 903) offered some excellent general guidelines for integrating spiritual and religious resources into pediatric practice. Additionally, the book *Health Care and Spirituality: Listening, Assessing, Caring* (Gilbert, 2002) uses a multiprofessional authorship to describe various patient experiences with multidisciplinary spiritual care. Certain members of the health-care team or community have specific expertise that other members can call upon in times of need. These members include chaplains, pastoral caregivers, community ministers, spiritual advisors, parish nurses, and other community resources.

Chaplains and Pastoral Caregivers

Many hospitals and hospices have a pastoral care or chaplains department (see Figure 9.5). Some have excellent skill with children. Chaplains frequently rely on referrals from health-care providers concerning patient emergencies and whom they should visit (VandeCreek, 1997). With changes in health care, these departments are feeling the impact of dwindling resources and are focusing on coordination with other disciplines. Before or

4. Give the parents or family members documentation of
   - name of the nurse who baptized (with permission)
   - date
   - time
   - place
   - name given to the infant
5. If the parents wish, notify their church or a local church (of the family's denomination) and request that the baptism be recorded in that church's registry. Give the same documentation as in Item 4 above.

Note. From "Emergency Baptism," by R. M. Reeb and S. T. McFarland, 1995, *Journal of Christian Nursing, 12*(2), pp. 26–27. Copyright 1995 by *Journal of Christian Nursing.* Reprinted with permission.

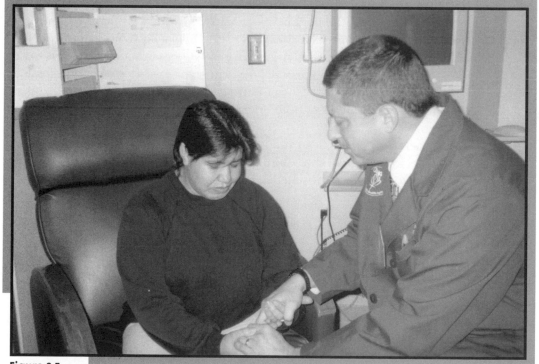

Figure 9.5.
Visits and prayer from a hospital chaplain can bring support in the midst of suffering and bring hope and encouragement to a weary parent. *Note.* Photograph by Lynn Clutter. Used with permission.

after surgery is a time children commonly wish to talk with clergy members or participate in a religious ritual such as prayer or blessing. Often they will see their minister or cleric before coming to the hospital but they may have last-minute "crises of confidence or faith." During these times, it is important for health-care providers to arrange for a quiet, private space suitable for the visit (Fina, 1995).

Chaplains are formally designated pastoral caregivers (O'Brien, 1999). According to Burke and Matsumoto (1999), a chaplain functions with patients, families, or others by creating meaning or theological reflection and serving as

- a trustworthy listener,
- a pastor away from home,
- a calming presence,
- a fellow sojourner among the bereaved,
- a generator of ethical concerns, and
- an educator in using spiritual resources to cope.

In making the decision to call for a chaplain, children or family members will often give cues indicating need. Also, health-care providers may ask directly (e.g., "Susie, would a visit from the hospital chaplain be helpful for you at this time?"). The chaplain can also be alerted that a family is having a particularly difficult time or has a child with a difficult diagnosis. A visit by the chaplain early in the child's hospital stay can open doors of communication and lay groundwork for future support that can be vital to the family (Fina, 1995). Chaplains can participate in confidential discussions about assisting the patient if the patient gives permission and the consent is written in the "progress note" section of the medical record (Wagner & Higdon, 1996).

Often it is the nurse at the bedside who is able to give ample spiritual comfort. However, as with all interventions, individuals need to recognize limitations and determine when referral is needed. For example,

> A youth has sustained a gunshot wound to the head and is in surgery. Family members are in the waiting room sobbing with uncontrolled grief. The nurse's words are helpful but do not change the situation. The nurse offers to call someone from the family's church. The Pastor comes and enters the situation with physical presence during the crisis, with touch, spiritual care, words of counsel, words of comfort, prayers, scriptures, and love. The time factor alone is more than the nurse can offer. The depth of past relationship allows the Pastor to uniquely know what will make a difference. The spiritual care—specific to the family's belief system—brings a settled calm to those who are waiting. The Pastor is available to help after the surgery and to offer ministry to family and to the youth. The nurse is able to observe and assess the changes while the Pastor does the work of ministry.

Pastoral Counselors

These counselors are clergy and others who have received graduate training in both religion and behavioral science for a clinical practice that integrates psychological and theological disciplines (Jordan & Danielsen, 1997). Many pastoral counselors are certified by the American Association of Pastoral Counselors (Woodruff, 1995), which also accredits pastoral counseling centers and training programs. Pastoral counselors combine counseling and spiritual values using resources of prayer, scripture, and participation in congregations. They often pay special attention to the religious history of a child and family, which is used for identifying pathology or resources for coping. Because of the emphasis on historical information, childhood images and experiences are important.

Parish Nurses

Parish nursing is a specialized area of professional nursing that focuses on health promotion within the context of the beliefs, values, and practices of a faith community (Practice and Education Committee, 1997). A Lutheran minister named Granger Westberg introduced the concept in the United States in 1982. As a hospital chaplain, Reverend Westberg realized that health care was more than diagnosing and treating illness. Parish nurses focus on health as wholeness to prevent or minimize illness and emphasize the role of faith in health, illness, and healing (Bay, 1997).

With access to health care becoming increasingly complex and many people having inadequate health insurance coverage, parish nursing fills a need. The church is the best "health place" in the community for several reasons. It is the only agency that interacts with people from beginning of life to end. It has structure for education, encourages volunteerism, and offers opportunity for community involvement. The church's mission is one of health for the whole person. Also, new community members use it as a resource for services, and in rural areas, it may be the only "health place" available (Solari-Twadell & Westberg, 1991).

Individuals and families that do not use regular health care may have the church as their primary social link from week to week. A parish nurse may see and know families that have not received health care for reasons such as difficulties with time and transportation, fear, distrust, or lack of finances. The types of offerings to the congregation include screenings, health fairs, workshops, classes, individual and family appointments, referrals, and visits to home, extended care facility, or hospital (Biddix & Brown, 1999). Roles of the parish nurse include being health educator, personal health counselor, coordinator of volunteers, advocate and community liaison, and integrator of relationships between faith and health (Bay, 1997). In a study of 40 parish nurses with 1,800 client interactions, Rydholm (1997) found that half of the parish nurses' activities dealt with physical problems while the other half were spiritual or psychosocial concerns. Another study identified spiritual care as the fourth most common intervention used by parish nurses (Weis, Matheus, & Schank, 1997).

Parish nurses are not in competition with public health or community health services. They do not provide home health-care services or perform invasive nursing procedures. They do work in collegial relationships with these agencies to enhance health-care delivery (Shank, Weis, & Matheus, 1996). Parish nurses, functioning in faith communities, are "advocates, educators, gatekeepers to community resources, informal counselors for life transitions, motivators for healthy living, spiritual nurturers and coordinators of faith community volunteers" (Abbott, 1998, p. 265). The focus is on healing, nurturing, "being," rather than curing or "doing" (O'Brien, 1999). For example, for a family that is financially limited or without transportation, a parish nurse may conduct home visits for developmental issues, health concerns, parent education, and explanations of doctors' comments. If the child is hospitalized, the parish nurse may visit and work in coordination with the hospital nurse, providing an important and trusted resource for the child, family, and hospital staff.

Simington, Olson, and Douglass (1996) estimated that there were at least 3,000 parish nurses employed in parishes across the United States in the mid-1990s. The Carter Center says that about 3% of the U.S. congregations have some kind of health promoter—many under the parish nurse title—and foresees the number growing by nearly 50% a year (Bilchik, 1998). According to the International Parish Nurse Resource Center (2004), there is a standardized core curriculum to prepare nurses in parish nursing. However, many more nurses are using this title in practice. Parish nurses usually have a bachelor of science degree in nursing (BSN); however, nurse practitioners and those with PhDs function in the role as well. Plans for a distinct certification have been considered (Martin, 1996). The American Nurses Association recognized parish nursing as a specialty practice in 1997, and published "The Standards and Scope of Parish Nursing" in 1998. Basic preparation courses and coordinators of preparation courses are available in many U.S. locations. Further information on parish nursing can be obtained through the resource centers listed in Appendix 9.2.

Other Community or Health-Care Team Resources

The use of referral can broaden the usual support system to include unique aspects of assistance. Health-care providers can benefit from "thinking outside the box" when it comes to gathering support through community resources. When health-care providers consider spiritual care of children as well as physical care, a completely different set of referral possibilities exist. For example, after initial assessment at one trauma center, in addition to chaplains, nursing staff usually initiate referrals to other support team members such as physicians, child psychiatrists, child life specialists, hospital trauma support teams, specialty nurses, social workers, and translators (Mangini et al., 1995).

In a community setting, health-care providers may suggest referral to a parent or patient, or make a referral with the family's permission. This referral could be a spiritually strong friend for a specific aspect of support, a spiritual official (i.e., a minister, shaman, guru, spiritual advisor), a support group, a librarian for books on specific subjects, or even a webliography (directory with hot links) to identify helpful spiritual sites.

Spiritual Experiences

Children sometimes have experiences that relate to their spirituality. One example might be in a specific experience of finding meaning in illness or injury. Parents often report that their child has a different attitude or perspective about life or toward them than they had before hospitalization. Sometimes children report experiences—such as dreams—or events that cause them to stop resenting their illness or being mad at God. Listening is usually an important way of encouraging children. While they may not have the language capacity to fully explain the experience, being there to care and listen can foster growth.

Spiritual Healing

Many patients participate in religious healing activities and find them to be helpful. Studies of religious practices among patients with arthritis found that minorities and lower socioeconomic groups commonly use religious healing activities to complement traditional medical care (Matthews, 2000). Waldfogel (1997) identified various studies indicating not only belief in faith healing, but attendance at services, and large percentages of people saying they had been cured.

A study of the trends in alternative medicine use in the United States from 1990 to 1997 revealed significant increases in spiritually linked types of therapy (Eisenberg et al., 1998). Therapies of "spiritual healing by others," "energy healing," and "self-prayer" were significantly increased in use from 1990 to 1997. Another study of 207 patients in a rural family practice demonstrated that 58% believed faith healers to be "quacks," 29% believed they could help some people whose physicians could not help, 21% had attended a faith-healing service, and 6% reported actually being healed (King, Sobal, & DeForge, 1988).

Thirty percent of people in the United States report that they have had "at some point in their lives a 'remarkable healing' related to a physical, emotional, or psychological problem" (Gallup & Lindsay, 1999, p. 2). Seventy percent of these people attributed the healing to supernatural forces, with 42% naming Jesus Christ, God, or a Higher Power, and 30% more stating their or other's prayers. Further, of these people who received the remarkable healing, 89% felt that it made them more aware of the importance of their spiritual life, and 84% said that it deepened their religious faith.

In a broad and spiritually sensitive understanding of healing, Carson (www.ihpnet/nrs4.htm, p. 9, accessed 5/6/01) identified various sources of healing:

- sacraments and religious rituals
- prayer—especially intercessory prayer
- medical technology, skills, and research
- persons gifted with healing abilities and powers
- faith in a Higher Power or Supreme Being
- persons who care, listen, counsel, and love us
- the source of life, energy, and healing power within ourselves

Health-care providers who are aware of these trends, attitudes, and experiences will be more inclined to assess the use of spiritual means of healing. Combining the strength of a patient's belief in spiritual healing with the commonly used health-care strategies can be beneficial for those who believe. For example, a child who believes that the laying on of hands and prayer can bring healing may want church elders or peers to visit the health-care setting to pray while holding one or both hands on the child. Facilitating an uninterrupted visit could yield positive results.

Mystical Experiences

A dramatic rise has occurred in the percentages of those who report mystical and near-death experiences, visions, and other unusual experiences (Lukoff, Provenzano, Lu, & Turner, 1999). Many believe in angels or angelic beings (see Case Study 9.1). There have been many positive aftereffects

Case Study 9.1
Angels

According to Blanton (2004), 78% of adults in the United States believe in angels. Children do as well. Some children in hospital settings have claimed to "encounter an angel" (Hudson, 1996, p. 26) or to have "seen Jesus." For example,

> A 3-year-old child graphically told his mother and nurse that Jesus came and showed him how to take out the tube in his mouth. He had successfully extubated the endotracheal tube and, when found, did not require reintubation because his condition had improved. He was soon released from the hospital.

This type of experience by a child usually brings comfort, but is also a critical moment for parents or health-care providers to listen and care. The physical care given must reflect the physical findings; however, often emotional settling and spiritual peace are evident. Anticipatory care is needed should the critical moment give rise to any difficulty or anxiety of the child or parent.

As many as 50% of individuals who have had near-death experiences have reported the presence of angels (Kennard, 1998). For example,

> Mallory was nine years old and had been diagnosed with terminal cancer. She knew she was dying and she was very afraid. One morning, she told her mother that three angels had come to her during the night. The angels had white wings and were very beautiful. They'd taken her on a trip to heaven. Mallory wasn't sick in the presence of the angels and even danced with them.
>
> Nine days before she died, Mallory made a videotape for other terminally ill children. She described the angels and heaven so that the children would not be afraid of death. She told them, "Believe what I say because it's true. It really is." (Kennard, 1998, p. 50)

Angels are seen in Judaism, the Talmud, the Kabbalah, the Bible, Muslim beliefs, Mormons, Buddhism, Hinduism, and Zoroastrianism (Kennard, 1998). Among other things, health-care providers should show spiritual respect by listening, remaining sensitive to the patient's interpretation, encouraging the patient to share with others, and documenting the event and any behavioral changes (i.e., from restlessness to calm alertness; Kennard, 1998).

from people who have experienced near-death or other mystical experiences. Mystical experiences are generally characterized as transient, extraordinary experiences marked by feelings of unity and harmonious relationship to the divine and everything in existence. "In several studies, people reporting mystical experiences scored lower on psychopathology scales and higher on measures of psychological well-being than did controls" (Lukoff et al., 1995, p. 468).

Near-death experiences (NDEs) have been estimated to occur in about one third of individuals having had close encounters with death. Further, numerous studies on the aftereffects of NDEs provide strong evidence of its nonpathologic nature. There can, however, be difficulties or adjustments afterward (Lukoff et al., 1995, p. 476). Children report vivid experiences. One hospitalized patient stated, "I tried to tell my nurses what had happened when I woke up, but they told me not to talk about it, that I was just imagining things" (Lukoff et al., 1995, p. 477). This should not be the case. Health-care providers can encourage children to share with parents and others, as well as explaining that this type of experience is not unusual. The child and supportive parent can focus on how it changes feelings, outlook, attitudes, and spiritual growth.

Miracles

Although Gladys had no family or friends, she had her cherished faith throughout life. When her doctor recommended amputation of her foot due to a purulent ulcer and poorly controlled diabetes, Gladys stated, "Dr. Jesus gonna heal me!" Four months later she went home with ulcer healed and foot intact. Is this "a miracle" or health care? Some say both. Gladys put her faith in God and believed He would heal her (Silva & DeLashmutt, 1998).

Gardner (1983) chronicled historical accounts of "miraculous" healings from the early 1900s with medical descriptions. Independent historical corroboration was cited for some of the cases of "almost inexplicable healing." While no attempt was made to prove that miracles occurred, historical written accounts were described.

Children can easily believe in miracles. They also can consider things to be "miracles" that are comprehensible or realistic to adults. Usually, children's beliefs and hopes are qualities of strength. Regarding miracles, it is important to ask, "What are you asking for?" It may be something simple such as, "another day together." Clarifying the language of miracles can allow for hope, as well as respectful and mutual accommodations between children, parents, and professionals (Rushton & Russell, 1996).

Religion-Motivated Medical-Care Avoidance

Religion and spirituality "can have both constructive and destructive influences on individual and family development" (Dunn & Dawes, 1999, p. 243). In some religious sects, some core values seek to avoid traditional means of health care. This can cause the most damaging aspects for children. Just as some cultures have their own healers and healing methods, some religious sects have a view of healing, and perhaps even value of human life, that differs significantly from the norm. Several of these sects will avoid medical services even to the point of death. Sects differ in reasons for what most would call medical neglect.

Grievously, children can be the victims. In an overview of deaths of children between 1975 and 1995, Asser and Swan (1998) identified and studied 172 deaths of children from families that practiced faith healing *in lieu* of medical care. Of this group, 145 of the children died of conditions for which expected survival rates with medical care would have exceeded 90%. Eighteen more had survival rates greater than 50%, and all but 3 of the children would have had some benefit from clinical help. Their conclusions point to the strong danger of faith healing to the exclusion of medical treatment.

Existing protection laws for children are different from state to state, especially in regard to religious exemptions. These laws may be inadequate to protect children from this form of medical neglect (Asser & Swan, 1998).

In Florida, for example, laws grant exemption from prosecution to parents who choose spiritual healing rather than conventional medical therapy for their children (Hartog, Freeman, Kubilis, & Jankowski, 1999).

Health-care providers are encouraged to work with children and families to intervene when religious values clash with traditional medical care. Wagner and Higdon (1996) offered an example of an effective and supportive team approach: The father, a minister, was refusing treatment on "religious grounds" for his 13-year-old daughter, newly diagnosed with diabetes. The physician consulted the chaplain, who talked with the father. The chaplain was able to ask the minister if his daughter's illness might be an opportunity for his faith to grow, and also result in his providing a better model for his parishioners. The physician explained that medicine could not cure but that the treatment would only manage symptoms. If she was cured, the chaplain and the physician promised the father attendance at one of his church's Sunday services to support the testimony that God had healed his daughter. The father felt his basic faith had been affirmed and was willing to embrace a new perspective and accept treatment for his daughter.

In many—perhaps most—of the religious groups that believe in faith healing, medical care is not neglected or avoided at all. In fact, many of the leaders strongly encourage medical review even with healing results that are dramatically visible or evident to the "healed" person. The follow-up medical care is considered "confirmation" or "documentation" of the healing that occurs in a manner different from those medically treated. People believing in divine healing commonly feel that medical follow-up is a responsible action and not at all threatening to their faith or an act of doubt toward their healing. One study in North Carolina revealed that 13% of patients attended faith-healing services regularly, and 6% reported having been healed by faith healers (King et al., 1988).

Documentation

Documentation of spiritual care is rarely found on patient records. Without documentation, an important aspect of patient care will not be communicated to other care providers to guide them in planning for holistic care (Broten, 1997). There can be avoidance of documentation of religious-sounding information and action due to the fear of censure from superiors. Highfield recommended that nurses use accepted standards, "such as the diagnoses of spiritual distress and potential for enhanced spiritual well-being (Carpenito, 1997) and keep documentation focused on what patients find helpful or unhelpful" (Highfield, 2000, p. 119). Additionally, chaplains or clergy can be involved to enhance care, collaboration, and agency acceptance of care.

Professionals can identify actions and documentation strategies that help the agency meet the Joint Commission for Accreditation of Healthcare Organizations (JCAHO) requirements for spiritual care (Highfield, 2000).

JCAHO requires that spiritual care be provided to all patients. Showing how spiritual care relates to the philosophy or mission statement of a facility aligns health-care provider–patient care with overall standards or values. Meeting JCAHO requirements does the same aligning, only with a strong benefit to the facility that may not have been considered.

Conclusion

Carson pointed out that there is a difference between providing care that is spiritual and spiritual care. Care that is spiritual "may contain no direct references to God, scripture, or anything religious, but the care is performed as part of a ministry of service and as such the nurse is reflecting God's presence and love to the patient in need" (Carson, n.d., p. 10). Carson listed the personal qualities necessary to become "a ministering person" (see box).

A Ministering Person	A ministering person is willing to do the following: 1. Enter into a relationship with another and share that individual's pain, need or crisis. 2. Listen, even when it causes some personal inconvenience. Raise necessary questions after listening. Say little or nothing, as the circumstance demands. 3. Be a companion to another's journey, especially when the journey becomes long and difficult. 4. Love the unlovable, the ungrateful, the uncooperative, the aggressive, and the unreachable.

Health-care providers are encouraged to first provide care that is spiritual. It is true that there are limits on time spent with patients. Also, there is a "difference between people who need just a little more and people who seem to never get enough" (Lane, 1994, p. 86). However, greater wholeness for children is marvelously possible when we provide whole person care that includes spiritual care.

Additionally, we have heard children and adults say things such as, "This illness has brought me closer to God;" or "Knowing that people are praying for me really helps;" and "Having this disease has made me a better person." These types of statements reflect the resources that come from spiritual strength and connectedness (Taylor & Mickley, 1997). Health-care providers have the opportunity to assist with spiritual coping strategies and, in so doing, buoy the spirit of each child and family we serve.

5. Accept one's brokenness, humanness, and mortality so as to better enter into relationships with those who are burdened by the difficulties of life.
6. Allow others to make their own decisions, supporting them through that process. Accept the reality that others may choose not to change.
7. Accept the reality that one cannot put an end to all the pain and suffering others face.
8. Encourage others to discover or rediscover their own values, goals, and dreams.

Note. From "Spirituality in Nursing Practice," by V. Carson, n.d. Accessed January 3, 2004, from www.ihpnet.org/nrs4.htm, pp. 8–9. Copyright 1989 by Saunders. Reprinted with permission.

Study Guide

1. What are the aspects of children's health-care encounters that may bring spiritual issues into focus?

2. In what ways might spirituality affect children's responses to illness and health-care experiences?

3. Are children likely to express spirituality in the same manner as adults? What differences are there, and why?

4. How can health-care providers' spiritual beliefs have a positive or negative effect on the care of children and their families?

5. What are some of the current changes in health care that influence the spirituality of care?

6. Describe three theories of spirituality and draw implications from each for spiritual care of children and their families.

7. List five things that health-care providers can do or say to assess children's spirituality.

8. How does spiritual distress differ from other forms of distress? What are the implications for intervention?

9. For each stage of children's development, discuss the critical issues of spirituality and cite appropriate interventions.

10. Outline direct spiritual practices and interventions that are useful in health-care settings.

APPENDIX 9.1

Resources for Religion

Annotated Bibliography of Selected References Regarding Religions

Carson, V. B. (1989). *Spiritual dimensions of nursing practice.* Philadelphia: W. B. Saunders.

Carson's text devotes an entire section on spirituality, religion, and health care. Chapter 4, contributed by Ruth Gerardi, examines Western Spirituality and Health Care. Tables of the beliefs and practices of many religious groups are present. Chapter 5, contributed by J. Patricia Martin, describes Eastern Spirituality and Health Care. Attitudes, beliefs, types of medicine, and various spiritual practices are covered. Chapter 6, contributed by Patricia C. McMullen, is on Religious Belief, Legal Issues, and Health Care. This chapter illustrates situations in which an individual's religious beliefs and medical treatment are in conflict— where there is spiritual distress. Appropriate interventions are described.

Coles, R. (1990). *The spiritual life of children.* Boston: Houghton Mifflin.

This text is the culmination of Dr. Robert Coles' career in studying children all over the world. Coles conducted thousands of home and school visits with school-age children. He has written over 40 books about children. This 358-page book is insightful with its numerous examples of children from Christian, Jewish, and Islamic families. Pictures drawn by children and profound insights on children's spirituality are included. One learns communicative techniques simply by reading the fascinating dialogues between Coles and the children.

Emblen, J. D. (1998). Suffering dialogues with five faiths. *Journal of Christian Nursing,* *15*(2), 27–29.

This creative article uses a nursing, emergency room case example with the death of a young man. The nursing care approach is divided into care for those who are of different religious beliefs. Humanism, Christianity, Buddhism, Hinduism, and Judaism are the religions covered. Sensitive client care is encouraged.

Engebretson, J. (1996). Considerations in diagnosing in the spiritual domain. *Nursing Diagnosis,* *7*(3), 100–107.

This article describes the traditions of Western and Eastern belief systems with the identification of common Western Judeo-Christian thought compared with other perspectives. Monotheism is contrasted with pantheism and polytheism. Transcendence, dualism, humanism, and atheism are described. Trends in postmodern synthesis of beliefs are explained. The final pages overview patient, health care, and caregiver tendencies with an encouragement to foster active participation of the patient with either spiritual distress or spiritual growth.

Halstead, M. T., & Mickley, R. (1997). Attempting to fathom the unfathomable: Descriptive views of spirituality. *Seminars in Oncology Nursing, 13*(4), 225–230.

This article explores a brief history of human thought as it relates to truth, self, meaning, and purpose. Eastern philosophic traditions including Hinduism, Buddhism, Confucianism, and Taoism are clearly described. Eastern philosophies and attitudes are covered as well. Muhammad, Allah, and God as Creator are described. Early Greek, German, and French philosophers such as Plato, Aristotle, Descartes, and Hegel are linked to current underpinnings of thinking. New Age philosophy is well described. Finally, definitions of religion and spirituality with nursing's view of spirituality are identified, along with research instruments for spirituality and spiritual well-being.

Hockenberry-Eaton, M., Wilson, D., Winkelstein, M. L., & Kline, N. (2003). *Wong's nursing care of infants and children* (7th ed.). St. Louis, MO: Mosby.

This text includes a discussion about the spiritual development of toddlers, preschoolers, school-age children, and adolescents. It also has segments on religion. The table on pages 58 through 62 is of religious beliefs that affect nursing care. The table has categories of beliefs about birth and death, beliefs about diet and food practices, beliefs regarding medical care, and comments. Twenty-six religions are discussed. This is a clinically useful table.

O'Brien, M. E. (1999). *Spirituality in nursing.* Boston: Jones and Bartlett Publishers.

The section entitled Spiritual Care and Religious Tradition (pp. 120–125) is an excellent, concise overview of world religions. Religions are categorized into Western spiritual philosophy and religions (Judaism, Christianity, and Islam) and Eastern spirituality (Buddhism, Hinduism, and Confucianism).

Web sites:

www.adherents.com/
www.barna.org/
www.beliefnet.com/
www.religioustolerance.org/
www.ciolek.com/wwwvlpages/buddhpages/otherrelig.html

Annotated Bibliography of Spiritual Care Tools

Barnes, L. L., Plotnikoff, G. A., Fox, K., & Pendleton, S. (2000, October). Spirituality, religion, and pediatrics: Intersecting worlds of healing. *Pediatrics, 106*(4 Suppl.), 899–908.

Table 2, on Page 904, is "Seven questions for learning about connections families and children make among spirituality, religion, sickness, and healing." These questions are valuable for clinical, religious, spiritual, or cross-cultural encounters. This excellent article has 162 references.

Cavendish, R., Luise, B. K., Bauer, M., Gallo, M. A., Horne, K., Medefindt, J., & Russo, D. (2001, July/September). Recognizing opportunities for spiritual enhancement in young adults. *Nursing Diagnosis, 12*(3), 77–91.

Page 85 has an excellent tool of 14 open-ended questions or "interview probes" for assessing spiritual needs of young adults.

Clutter, L. B. (1991). Fostering spiritual care for the child and family. In D. Smith (Ed.), *Comprehensive child and family nursing skills* (pp. 263–270). St. Louis, MO: Mosby-Year Book.

This includes a developmentally appropriate list of spiritual care assessment questions. Nursing process is reviewed with rationale for each step. Information is specific to children and parents.

Dudley, J. R., Smith, C., & Millison, M. B. (1995). Unfinished business: Assessing the spiritual needs of hospice clients. *The American Journal of Hospice & Palliative Care, 12*(2), 30–37.

This article contains lists of spiritual assessment topics, and includes an extensive list of open-ended spiritual questions.

Georgensen, J., & Dungan, J. M. (1996). Managing spiritual distress in patients with advanced cancer pain. *Cancer Nursing, 19*(5), 376–383.

This article describes the Dungan model of dynamic integration along with means to manage spiritual distress. Includes a table with six categories of nursing modalities of care.

Halstead, M. T., & Mickley, R. (1997). Attempting to fathom the unfathomable: Descriptive views of spirituality. *Seminars in Oncology Nursing, 13*(4), 225–230.

This article has a table of research instrumentation for spirituality and spiritual well-being.

Hart, D. & Schneider, D. (1997). Spiritual care for children with cancer. *Seminars in Oncology Nursing, 13*(4), 263–270.

This article includes child- and parent-specific assessment questions of religious preferences, activities, and use of support groups. Age- and stage-specific interventions are also included.

Hatch, R. L., Burg, M. A., Naberhaus, D. S., & Hellmich, L. K. (1998). The spiritual involvement and beliefs scale. *The Journal of Family Practice, 46*(6), 476–486.

This instrument is presented in full. It has 26 Likert-type format items. Validity and reliability information is presented along with comparison to other tools.

Hungelmann, J., Kenkel-Ross, E., Klassen, L., & Stollenwerk, R. (1996). Focus on spiritual well-being: Harmonious interconnectedness of mind-body-spirit—Use of the JAREL spiritual well-being scale. *Geriatric Nursing, 17*(6), 262–266.

This tool was developed as an assessment tool to establish a nursing diagnosis of spirituality. It has 21 Likert-type questions. Use of the instrument is demonstrated.

Kendall, M. L. (1999). A holistic nursing model for spiritual care of the terminally ill. *American Journal of Hospice & Palliative Care, 16*(2), 473–476.

Ten open-ended spiritual questions are presented in a table. The questions are designed for personal spiritual reflection.

Kerrigan, R., & Harkulich, J. T. (1993, May). A spiritual tool. *Health Progress, 74*(4), 46–49.

Chart documentation is the intent for the two tools presented. One is a checklist useful for quickly listing religious and spiritual care given. Another tool gathers spiritual belief and practice information about the patient. Each item has a detailed list of options to read and check.

Maugans, T. A. (1996). The SPIRITual history. *Archives of Family Medicine, 5*(1), 11–16.

This tool uses the pneumonic "SPIRIT" to list categories of questions. Details of the tool's use are presented.

McEvoy, M. (2000, September/October). An added dimension to the pediatric health maintenance visit: The spiritual history. *Journal of Pediatric Health Care, 14*(5), 216–220.

This tool uses the mnemonic "BELIEF" to categorize spiritual history, information for nurse practitioners constructing initial pediatric health maintenance visits.

O'Brien, M. E. (1999). *Spirituality in nursing.* Boston: Jones and Bartlett Publishers.

The Spiritual Assessment Scale is presented along with validity and reliability. The 21-item tool has a Likert scale and is included in its entirety.

Piedmont, R. L. (2001, January–March) Spiritual transcendence and the scientific study of spirituality. *Journal of Rehabilitation, 67*(1), 4–14.

The psychometrical strength of the Spiritual Transcendence Scale is evaluated and compared with other scales. An overview of spirituality measurement is presented. Use of spiritual constructs is encouraged as part of a multidimensional assessment battery.

Puchalski, C. M. (n.d.). A spiritual history. *Supportive Voice.* Web site: http://www .careofdying.org/SV/PUBSART.ASP?ISSUE-SV99SU&ARTICLE=J

A brief, four-area method of spiritual assessment is provided. Use and results with various people is demonstrated.

Soeken, J. (1989). Perspectives on research in the spiritual dimension of nursing care. In V. B. Carson (Ed.), *Spiritual dimensions of nursing practice* (pp. 354–378). Philadelphia: Saunders.

An overview of the research process, tools, and measurement scales in spiritually related topics is given.

Stoll, R. I. (1979). Guidelines for spiritual assessment. *American Journal of Nursing, 79*(8), 1574–1577.

This classic spiritual assessment article lists sections of: concept of God or Deity, sources of hope and strength, religious practices, relation between spiritual beliefs and health. Each section has a series of questions.

Swinton, J. (2001) *Spirituality and mental health care: Rediscovering a "forgotten" dimension.* Philadelphia: Kingsley.

The appendix (pp. 179–190) of this book compiles various spiritual models for assessment and intervention.

APPENDIX 9.2

Resources for Parish Nursing

The International Parish Nurse Resource Center at Deaconess Parish Nurse Ministries
475 East Lockwood Ave.
St. Louis, MO 63119
Phone: 314/918-2559
Toll-Free: 800/556-5368
www.ipnrc.parishnurses.org/index.phtml

Health Ministries Association, Inc.
295 W. Crossville Road, Suite 130
Roswell, GA 30075
Toll-Free: 800/280-9919
www.hmassoc.org/

Marquette University Parish Nurse Institute
Marquette University College of Nursing
PO Box 1881
Milwaukee, WI 53201-1881
Phone: 414/288-3809

References

Abbott, B. (1998). Ask home healthcare nurse: Parish nursing. *Home Healthcare Nurse, 16*(4), 265–267.

Alderson, P. (1996). Body language…decision-making, care of children, spiritual care. *Nursing Times, 1*(36), 31–33.

Anderson, B., & Steen, S. (1995). Spiritual care: Reflecting God's love to children. *Journal of Christian Nursing, 12*(2), 12–17.

Asser, S. M., & Swan, R. (1998). Child fatalities from religion-motivated medical neglect. *Pediatrics, 101*(4), 625–629.

Attig, T. J. (1996). Beyond pain: The existential suffering of children. *Journal of Palliative Care, 12*(3), 20–23.

Bailey, S. S. (1997). The arts in spiritual care. *Seminars in Oncology Nursing, 13*(4), 242–247.

Barnes, L. L., Plotnikoff, G. A., Fox, K., & Pendleton, S. (2000). Spirituality, religion, and pediatrics: Intersecting worlds of healing. *Pediatrics, 106*(4 Suppl.), 899–908.

Barnum, B. S. (1996). *Spirituality in nursing from traditional to new age.* New York: Springer Publishing Company.

Batten, M., & Oltjenbruns, K. A. (1999). Adolescent sibling bereavement as a catalyst for spiritual development: A model for understanding. *Death Studies, 23*(6), 529–546.

Bay, M. J. (1997). Healing partners: The oncology nurse and the parish nurse. *Seminars in Oncology Nursing, 13*(4), 275–278.

Biddix, V., & Brown, H. N. (1999). Establishing a parish nursing program. *Nursing & Health Care Perspectives, 20*(2), 72–75.

Bilchik, G. S. (1998, May 20). When the saints go marching out. *Hospitals & Health Networks, 72*(10), 36–42.

Blanton, D. (2004). *More believe in God than heaven.* Retrieved July 28, 2004, from http://www.foxnews.com/story/0,2933,99945,00.html

Blockley, C. (1998). Children, too, have spiritual needs. *Nursing Praxis in New Zealand, 13*(3), 56–57.

Bowers, M. K. (1974). *Counseling the dying.* New York: Aronson.

Broten, P. B. (1997). Spiritual care documentation: Where is it? *Journal of Christian Nursing, 14*(2), 29–31.

Brown-Saltzman, K. (1997). Replenishing the spirit by meditative prayer and guided imagery. *Seminars in Oncology Nursing, 13*(4), 255–259.

Burke, S. S., & Matsumoto, A. R. (1999). Pastoral care for perinatal and neonatal health care providers. *Journal of Gynecological and Neonatal Nursing, 28*(2), 137–141.

Burkhardt, M. A. (1991). Spirituality and children: Nursing considerations. *Journal of Holistic Nursing, 9*(2), 31–40.

Carpenito, L. J. (1997). *Nursing diagnosis: Application to clinical practice* (7th ed.). Philadelphia: Lippincott.

Carson, V. B. (1989). *Spiritual dimensions of nursing practice.* Philadelphia: Saunders.

Carson, V. B. (n.d.). *Course Title: Spirituality in nursing practice.* Retrieved January 3, 2004, from www.ihpnet.org/nrs4.htm

Cavendish, R., Luise, B. K., Bauer, M., Gallo, M. A., Horne, K., Medefindt, J., & Russo, D. (2001). Recognizing opportunities for spiritual enhancement in young adults. *Nursing Diagnosis, 12*(3), 77–91.

Cerrato, P. L. (1998). Spirituality and healing. *RN, 61*(2), 49–50.

Claassen, E. (1998). God's special children. *Journal of Christian Nursing, 15*(2), 21–23.

Clark, C., & Heidenreich, T. (1995). Spiritual care for the critically ill. *American Journal of Critical Care, 4*(1), 77–81.

Clark, C. C., Cross, J. R., Deane, D. M., & Lowry, L. W. (1991). Spirituality: Integral to quality care. *Holistic Nursing Practice, 5*(3), 67–76.

Clutter L. B. (1991). Fostering spiritual care for the child and family. In D. Smith (Ed.), *Comprehensive child and family nursing skills* (pp. 263–270). St. Louis, MO: Mosby-Year Book.

Coles, R. (1990). *The spiritual life of children.* Boston: Houghton Mifflin.

Coles, R. (2000). Face to face: Interview with Robert Coles, M.D. *Spirituality & Medicine Connection, 3*(4), 6–7.

Cox, G. (2000). Children, spirituality, and loss. *Illness, Crisis & Loss, 8*(1), 60–70.

Cress-Ingebo, R., & Chrisagis, X. (1998). Try a good book: Bibliotherapy as spiritual care. *Journal of Christian Nursing, 15*(2), 14–17.

Davies, B., Brenner, P., Orloff, S., Sumner, L., & Worden, W. (2002). Addressing spirituality in pediatric hospice and palliative care. *Journal of Palliative Care, 18*(1), 59–67.

Dunn, A. B., & Dawes, S. J. (1999). Spirituality-focused genograms: Keys to uncovering spiritual resources in African American families. *Journal of Multicultural Counseling and Development, 27*(4), 240–254.

Ebmeier, C., Lough, M. A., Huth, M. M., & Autio, L. (1991). Hospitalized school-age children express ideas, feelings, and behaviors toward God. *Journal of Pediatric Nursing, 6*(5), 337–349.

Eisenberg, D. M., Davis, R. B., Ettner, S. L., Appel, S., Wilkey, S., Van Rompay, M., & Kessier, R. C. (1998). Trends in alternative medicine use in the United States, 1990–1997. *Journal of the American Medical Association, 280*(18), 1569–1575.

Emblen, J. D. (1992). Religion and spirituality defined according to current use in nursing literature. *Journal of Professional Nursing, 8*(1), 41–47.

Erikson, E. K. (1963). *Childhood and society* (2nd ed.). New York: Norton.

Espeland, K. (1999). Achieving spiritual wellness: Using reflective questions. *Journal of Psychosocial Nursing, 37*(7), 36–40.

Field, M. J., & Behrman, R. E. (Eds.). (2003). *When children die: Improving palliative and end-of-life care for children and their families.* Washington, DC: The National Academies Press.

Fina, D. K. (1995). The spiritual needs of pediatric patients and their families. *AORN Journal, 62*(4), 556–564.

Fosarelli, P. (2000). The spiritual development of children. *Spirituality & Medicine Connection, 3*(4), 1, 7.

Fowler, J. W. (1981). *Stages of faith.* New York: HarperCollins.

Fowler, J. W. (1996). *Faithful changes.* Nashville, TN: Abingdon.

Fowler, J. W., & Keen, S. (1978). *Life maps: Conversations on the journey of faith.* Waco, TX: Word Books.

Fulton, R. A., & Moore, C. M. (1995). Spiritual care of the school-age child with a chronic condition. *Journal of Pediatric Nursing, 10*(4), 224–231.

Gallia, K. S. (1996). Teaching spiritual care: Beyond content. *NursingConnections, 9*(3), 29–35.

Gallup Jr., G., & Lindsay, D. M. (1999). *Surveying the religious landscape.* Harrisburg, PA: Morehouse.

Gardner, R. (1983). Miracles of healing in Anglo-Celtic Northumbria as recorded by the venerable Bede and his contemporaries: A reappraisal in the light of twentieth century experience. *British Medical Journal, 287*(6409), 1927–1933.

Georgesen, J., & Dungan, J. M. (1996). Managing spiritual distress in patients with advanced cancer pain. *Cancer Nursing, 19*(5), 376–383.

Gilbert, R. B. (Ed.). (2002). *Health care & spirituality: Listening, assessing, caring.* Amityville, NY: Baywood.

Gough, W. C. (February, 1986). A growing interest. *American Journal of Nursing, 86*(2), 165–166.

Greenberg, D., & Witztum, E. (1991). Problems in the treatment of religious patients. *American Journal of Psychotherapy, 45*(4), 554.

Gustavson, C. B. (1995). *In-versing your life: A poetry workbook for self-discovery and healing.* Lewiston, NY: Manticore.

Gustavson, C. B. (2000). In-versing your life: Using poetry as therapy. *Families in Society: The Journal of Contemporary Human Services, 81*(4), 328–331.

Hancock, B. (2000). Are nursing theories holistic? *Nursing Standard, 14*(17), 37–41.

Harmon, R. L., & Myers, M. A. (1999). Prayer and meditation as medical therapies. *Physical Medicine and Rehabilitation Clinics of North America, 10*(3), 651–662.

Hart, D., & Schneider, D. (1997). Spiritual care for children with cancer. *Seminars in Oncology Nursing, 13*(4), 263–270.

Hartog, M. A., Freeman, M., Kubilis, P. S., & Jankowski, R. A. (1999). Pediatricians' and social workers' knowledge and opinions of Florida's religious immunity laws. *Southern Medical Journal, 92*(4), 362–368.

Heiser, R., Chiles, K., Fudge, M., & Gray, S. (1997). The use of music during the immediate postoperative recovery period. *Association of Operating Room Nurses Journal, 65*(4), 777–778.

Hicks Jr., T. J. (1999). Spirituality and the elderly: Nursing implications with nursing home residents. *Geriatric Nursing, 20*(3), 144–146.

Highfield, M. F. (1997). Spiritual assessment across the cancer trajectory: Methods and reflections. *Seminars in Oncology Nursing, 13*(4), 252–254.

Highfield, M. F. (2000). Providing spiritual care to patients with cancer. *Clinical Journal of Oncology Nursing, 4*(3), 115–120.

Hockenberry, M., Wilson, D., Winkelstein, M. L., & Kline, N. (2003). *Wong's nursing care of infants and children* (7th ed.). St. Louis, MO: Mosby.

Hodge, D. R., Cardenas, P., & Montoya, H. (2001). Substance use: Spirituality and religious participation as protective factors among rural youths. *Social Work Research, 25*(3), 153–161.

Holder, D. W., Durant, R. H., Harris, T. L., Daniel, J. H., Obeidallah, D., & Goodman, E. (2000). The association between adolescent spirituality and voluntary sexual activity. *Journal of Adolescent Health, 26*(4), 295–302.

Housekamp, B., Fisher, L., & Stuber, M. (2004). Spirituality in children and adolescents: Research findings and implications for clinicians and researchers. *Child and Adolescent Psychiatric Clinics of North America, 13*, 221–230.

Hudson, T. (1996). Measuring the resuls of faith. *Hospitals and Health Networks, 70*(9), 22–28.

Hughes, C. E. (1997). Prayer and healing: A case study. *Journal of Holistic Nursing, 15*(3), 318–324, 325–326.

Hungelmann, J., Kenkel-Ross, E., Klassen, L., & Stollenwerk, R. (1996). Focus on spiritual well-being: Harmonious interconnectedness of mind-body-spirit—Use of the JAREL spiritual well-being scale. *Geriatric Nursing, 17*(6), 262–266.

International Parish Nurse Resource Center. (2004). *Information for parish nurses: The basic preparation course in parish nursing.* Retrieved July 22, 2004, from www.ipnrc.parishnurses.org/course/phtml

Jordan, M. R., & Danielsen, A. V. (1997, May). What is pastoral counseling? *The Harvard Mental Health Letter, 13*(11), 8.

Kendall, M. L. (1999). A holistic nursing model for spiritual care of the terminally ill. *American Journal of Hospice & Palliative Care, 16*(2), 473–476.

Kennard, M. (1998). A visit from an angel. *American Journal of Nursing, 98*(3), 48–51.

Kenny, G. (1999). Assessing children's spirituality: What is the way forward? *British Journal of Nursing, 8*(1), 28, 30–32.

King, D. E., & Bushwick, B. (1994). Beliefs and attitudes of hospital inpatients about faith healing and prayer. *The Journal of Family Practice, 39*(4), 349–352.

King, D. E., Sobal, J., & DeForge, B. R. (1988). Family practice patients' experiences and beliefs in faith healing. *Journal of Family Practice, 27*(4), 505–508.

Kloosterhouse, V., & Ames, B. D. (2002). Families' use of religion/spirituality as a psychosocial resource. *Holistic Nursing Practice, 16*(5), 61–76.

Koenig, H. G., Bearon, L. B., Hover, M., & Travis III, J. L. (1991). Religious perspectives of doctors, nurses, patients, and families. *The Journal of Pastoral Care, 45*(3), 254–267.

Koepfer, S. R. (2000). Drawing on the spirit: Embracing spirituality in pediatrics and pediatric art therapy. *Art Therapy, 17*(3), 188–194.

Kohlberg, L. (1981). *The philosophy of moral development: Essays on moral development* (Vol. 1). San Francisco: Harper & Row.

Kohlberg, L. (1984). *The philosophy of moral development: Essays on moral development* (Vol. 2). San Francisco: Harper & Row.

Landreth, G. (1991). *Play therapy: The art of the relationship.* Muncie, IN: Accelerated Development Press.

Lane, D. (1994). *Music as medicine.* Grand Rapids, MI: Zondervan.

Larson, D. B., & Koenig, K. G. (2000). Is God good for your health? The role of spirituality in medical care. *Cleveland Clinic Journal of Medicine, 67*(2), 80–84.

Leduc, E. (2001). Connecting with your infant's spirit. *Midwifery Today, 58,* 20.

Levin, J. S. (1994). Religion and health: Is there an association, is it valid, and is it causal? *Social Science Medicine, 38*(11), 1475–1482.

Levin, J. S. (1996). How prayer heals: A theoretical model. *Alternative Therapies, 2*(1), 66–73.

Lukoff, D., Provenzano, R., Lu, F., & Turner R. (1999). Religious and spiritual case reports on Medline: A systematic analysis of records from 1980–1996. *Alternative Therapies, 5*(1), 64–70.

Lukoff, D., Lu, F. G., & Turner, R. (1995). Cultural considerations in the assessment and treatment of religious and spiritual problems. *The Psychiatric Clinics of North America, 18*(3), 467–484.

Lyon, M. E., Townsend-Akpan, C., Thompson, A. (2001). Spirituality and end-of-life care for an adolescent with AIDS. *AIDS Patient Care and Standards, 15*(11), 555–560.

Magaletta, P. R., Duckro, P. N., & Staten, S. F. (1997). Prayer in office practice: On the threshold of integration. *Journal of Family Practice, 44*(3), 254–256.

Mangini, L., Confessore, M. T., Girard, P., & Spadola, T. (1995). Pediatric trauma support program: Supporting children and families in emotional crisis. *Critical Care Nursing Clinics of North America, 7*(3), 557–567.

Marshall, E. S., Mandleco, B. L., Olsen, S. F., & Dyches, T. T. (2001). Families of children with disabilities: Themes of religious support. 34th Annual Communicating Nursing Research Conference/15th Annual WIN Assembly, "Health Care Challenges Beyond 2001: Mapping the Journey for Research and Practice," held April 19–21, 2001, in Seattle, Washington. *Communicating Nursing Research, 34*(9), 333.

Martin, L. B. (1996). Parish nursing: Keeping body and soul together. *The Canadian Nurse, 92*(1), 25–28.

Martsolf, D. S., & Mickley, J. R. (1998). The concept of spirituality in nursing theories: Differing world-views and extent of focus. *Journal of Advanced Nursing, 27*(2), 294–303.

Marwick, C. (1995). Should physicians prescribe prayer for health? Spiritual aspects of well-being considered. *Journal of the American Medical Association, 273*(20), 1561–1562.

Matthews, D. A. (2000). Prayer and spirituality. *Rheumatic Disease Clinics of North America, 26*(1), 177–186.

Maugans, T. A. (1996). The SPIRITual history. *Archives of Family Medicine, 5*(1), 11–16.

McBride, J. L., Arthur, G., Brooks, R., & Pilkington, L. (1998). The relationship between a patient's spirituality and health experiences. *Family Medicine, 30,* 122–126.

McCullough, M. E. (2000). Forgiveness as human strength: Theory, measurement, and links to well-being. *Journal of Social and Clinical Psychology, 19*(1), 43–55.

McEvoy, M. (2000). An added dimension to the pediatric health maintenance visit: The spiritual history. *Journal of Pediatric Health Care, 14*(5), 216–220.

McFadden, S. H. (1990). Authentic humor as an expression of spiritual maturity. *Journal of Religious Gerontology, 7,* 131–141.

McHolm, F. A. (1991). A nursing diagnosis validation study: Defining characteristics of spiritual distress. In R. M. Carroll-Johnson (Ed.), *Classification of nursing diagnoses: Proceedings of the ninth conference* (pp. 112–119). Philadelphia: Lippincott.

Narayanasamy, A., & Owens J. (2001). A critical incident study of nurses' responses to the spiritual needs of their patients. *Journal of Advanced Nursing, 33*(4), 446–455.

Nierenberg, B., & Sheldon, A. (2001). Psychospirituality and pediatric rehabilitation. *Journal of Rehabilitation, 67*(1), 15–19.

O'Brien, M. E. (1999). *Spirituality in nursing.* Boston: Jones & Bartlett.

O'Hara, D. P. (2002). Is there a role for prayer and spirituality in health care? *Medical Clinics of North America, 86*(1), 33–46.

Oldnall, A. (1996). A critical analysis of nursing: Meeting the spiritual needs of patients. *Journal of Advanced Nursing, 23*(1), 138–144.

Oliver, M. (1992). *New and selected poems.* Boston: Beacon Press.

Patterson, E. F. (1998). The philosophy and physics of holistic health care: Spiritual healing as a workable interpretation. *Journal of Advanced Nursing, 27*(2), 287–293.

Pehler, S. R. (1997). Children's spiritual response: Validation of the nursing diagnosis spiritual distress. *Nursing Diagnosis, 8*(2), 55–66.

Pendleton, S. M., Cavalli, K. S., Pargament, K. I., & Nasr, S. Z. (2002). Religious/spiritual coping in childhood cystic fibrosis: A qualitative study. *Pediatrics, 109*(1), E8.

Piers, M., & Landau, G. (1980). *The gift of play.* New York: Walker & Company.

Piles, C. L. (1990). Providing spiritual care. *Nurse Educator, 15*(1), 36–41.

Porter, B. (1995). Joy comes in the morning: A newborn fights for life. *Journal of Christian Nursing, 12*(2), 23–26.

Post, S. G., Puchalski, C. M., & Larson, D. B. (2000). Physicians and patient spirituality: Professional boundaries, competency, and ethics. *Annals of Internal Medicine, 132*(7), 578–583.

Practice and Education Committee. (1997). *Scope and standards of parish nursing practice.* Huntington Beach, CA: Health Ministries Association.

Price, J. L., Stevens, H. O., & LaBarre, M. C. (1995). Spiritual caregiving in nursing practice. *Journal of Psychosocial Nursing, 33*(12), 5–9.

Puchalski, C. M., (2000a). Taking a spiritual history allows clinicians to understand patients more fully. *Journal of Palliative Medicine, 3*(1), 129–137.

Puchalski, C. M., (2000b). The gift of the child. *Spirituality & Medicine Connection, 3*(4), 3.

Pullen, L., Modrcin-Talbott, M. A., West, W. R., & Muenchen, R. (1999). Spiritual high vs high on spirits: Is religiosity related to adolescent alcohol and drug abuse? *Journal of Psychiatric & Mental Health Nursing, 6*(1), 3–8.

Ratner, P. A., Johnson, J. L., & Jeffery, B. (1998). Examining emotional, physical, social, and spiritual health as determinants of self-rated health status. *American Journal of Health Promotion, 12*(4), 275–282.

Reeb, R. M., & McFarland, S. T. (1995). Emergency baptism. *Journal of Christian Nursing, 12*(2), 26–27.

Reed, P. G. (1992). An emerging paradigm for the investigation of spirituality in nursing. *Research in Nursing & Health, 15*, 349–357.

Roberts, L., Ahmed, I., & Hall, S. (2002). Intercessory prayer for the alleviation of ill health. *The Cochrane Library, 3*, Article CD000368. Available from The Cochrane Library Web site, http://www.update-software.com

Rushton, C. H., & Russell, K. (1996). The language of miracles: Ethical challenges. *Pediatric Nursing, 22*(1), 64–67.

Ryan, J. R. (1996). Seeing God more clearly: Healing distorted images of God. *Journal of Christian Nursing, 13*(2), 23–28.

Rydholm, L. (1997). Patient-focused care in parish nursing. *Holistic Nursing Practice, 11*(3), 47–60.

Sellers, S. C., & Haag, B. A. (1998). Spiritual nursing interventions. *Journal of Holistic Nursing, 16*(3), 338–354.

Shank, M. J., Weis, D., & Matheus, R. (1996). Parish nursing: Ministry of healing. *Geriatric Nursing, 17*(1), 11–13.

Shelly, J. A. (1982). *The spiritual needs of children: A guide for nurses, parents and teachers.* Downers Grove, IL: InterVarsity Press.

Shelly, J. A. (1995). Welcoming children. *Journal of Christian Nursing, 12*(2), 3.

Shelly, J. A. (2000). *Spiritual care: A guide for caregivers.* Downers Grove, IL: InterVarsity Press.

Shelly, J. A., & Fish, S. (1988). *Spiritual care: The nurse's role* (3rd ed.). Downers Grove, IL: InterVarsity Press.

Shelly, J. A., & Fish, S. (1995). Praying with patients: Why, when and how. *Journal of Christian Nursing, 12*(1), 9–13.

Silber, T. J., & Reilly, M. (1985). Spiritual and religious concerns of the hospitalized adolescent. *Adolescence, 10*(77), 217–224.

Silva, M. C., & DeLashmutt, M. (1998). Spirituality and prayer: A new age paradigm for ethics. *NursingConnections, 11*(2), 13–17.

Simington, J., Olson, J., & Douglass, L. (1996). Promoting well-being within a parish. *The Canadian Nurse, 92*(1), 20–24.

Smith, J., & McSherry, W. (2004). Spirituality and child development: A concept analysis. *Journal of Advanced Nursing, 45*, 307–315.

Smucker, C. (1996). A phenomenological description of the experience of spiritual distress. *Nursing Diagnosis, 7*(2), 81–91.

Solari-Twadell, P. A., & Westberg, G. (1991). Body, mind, and soul. *Health Progress, 72*(7), 24–28.

Sommer, D. R. (1989). The spiritual needs of dying children. *Issues in Comprehensive Pediatric Nursing, 12*(2/3), 225–233.

Steen, S., & Anderson, B. (1995). Ages & stages of spiritual development. *Journal of Christian Nursing, 12*(2), 6–11.

Sterling-Fisher, C. E. (1998). Spiritual care and chronically ill clients. *Home Healthcare Nurse, 16*(4), 242–250.

Stewart, C. (2001). The influence of spirituality on substance use of college students. *Journal of Drug Education, 31*(4), 343–351.

Still, J. V. (1984). How to assess spiritual needs of children and their families. *Journal of Christian Nursing, 1*(2), 4–6.

Stoll, R. I. (1979). Guidelines for spiritual assessment. *American Journal of Nursing, 79*(8), 1574–1577.

Stoll, R. I. (1989). The essence of spirituality. In V. B. Carson (Ed.), *Spiritual dimensions of nursing practice* (pp. 4–23). Philadelphia: Saunders.

Sumner, C. H. (1998). Recognizing and responding to spiritual distress. *American Journal of Nursing, 98*(1), 26–31.

Sweeney, D. S., & Landreth, G. (1993). Healing a child's spirit through play therapy: A scriptural approach to treating children. *Journal of Psychology and Christianity, 12*(4), 351–356.

Taylor, E. J. (1997). The story behind the story: The use of storytelling in spiritual caregiving. *Seminars in Oncology Nursing, 13*(4), 252–254.

Taylor, E. J., & Mickley, J. R. (1997). Introduction. *Seminars in Oncology Nursing, 13*(4), 223–224.

Taylor, E. J., Amenta, M., & Highfield, M. (1995). Spiritual care practices of oncology nurses. *Oncology Nursing Forum, 22*(1), 37–39.

Thayer, P. (2001). Spiritual care of children and parents. In A. Armstrong-Daley & S. Zarbock (Eds.), *Hospice care for children* (2nd ed.; pp. 172–189). Oxford, England: Oxford University Press.

Thurston, C., & Ryan, J. (1996). Faces of God: Illness, healing, and children's spirituality. *ACCH Advocate, 2*(2), 13–15.

Treloar, L. L. (1999). Spiritual care assessment and intervention. *Journal of Christian Nursing, 16*(2), 15–18.

Twibell, R. S., Wieseke, A. W., Marine, M., & Schoger, J. (1996). Spiritual and coping needs of critically ill patients: Validation of nursing diagnoses. *Dimensions of Critical Care Nursing, 15*(5), 245–253.

VandeCreek, L. (1997). Collaboration between nurses and chaplains for spiritual caregiving. *Seminars in Oncology Nursing, 13*(4), 279–280.

Wagner, J. T., & Higdon, T. L. (1996). Spiritual issues and bioethics in the intensive care unit: The role of the chaplain. *Critical Care Clinics, 12*(1), 15–27.

Waldfogel, S. (1997). Spirituality in medicine. *Complementary and Alternative Therapies in Primary Care, 24*(4), 963–976.

Wallis, C. (1996, June 24). Faith and healing. *Time*, 58–63.

Webb-Mitchell, B. (1993). *God plays piano, too: The spiritual lives of disabled children.* New York: Crossroad.

Weis, D., Matheus, R., & Schank, M. J. (1997). Health care delivery in faith communities: The parish nurse model. *Public Health Nursing, 14*(6), 368–372.

Wilson, S. M., & Miles, M. S. (2001). Spirituality in African-American mothers coping with a seriously ill infant. *Journal of the Society of Pediatric Nurses, 6*(3), 116–122.

Winseman, A. (2004, April 27). Spiritual care crucial to healing the whole patient. *The Gallup Poll Tuesday Briefing.* Retrieved July 21, 2004, from www.gallup.com/content/login.aspx?ci=11500

Woodruff, C. R. (1995, Spring). Pastoral counselors and healthcare reform. *Treatment Today*, 31–32.

Wright, K. B. (1998). Professional, ethical, and legal implications for spiritual care in nursing. *Image: Journal of Nursing Scholarship, 30*(1), 81–83.

Yankelovich Partners, Inc. Telephone Poll for TIME/CNN. June 12–13, 1996.

Zerwekh, J. V. (1997). The practice of presencing. *Seminars in Oncology Nursing, 13*(4), 260–262.

Zimmerman, L., Pozehl, B., Duncan, K., & Schmitz, R. (1989). Effects of music in patients who had chronic cancer pain. *Western Journal of Nursing Research, 11*(3), 298–309.

Cultural Influences in Children's Health Care

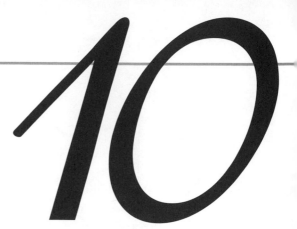

Lacretia Johnson

Objectives

At the conclusion of this chapter, the reader will be able to:

1. Discuss culture and cultural identity and the implications for understanding the reactions of children and their families to health-care experiences.

2. Determine the barriers to understanding and communication among health-care professionals and parents and children of different cultures, and outline approaches to improve understanding.

3. Delineate factors that have contributed to an increased awareness and concern for "cross-cultural competence" in health-care settings.

4. Outline "culturally competent" approaches to supporting children in health-care settings and encounters.

$\mathcal{E}$ ach decade, our evolving society continues to grow more demographically complex. In the United States, the representation of people from diverse racial, ethnic, and cultural backgrounds continues to grow (Hedayat & Pirzadeh, 2001). Data from the U.S. Bureau of Census (2001) indicate that the racial and ethnic composition of the United States is continuing to diversify, particularly with increases in those who come from non–White and non–Anglo backgrounds. It is estimated that by 2020 approximately 40% of school-age children in the United States will be from non–White ethnic groups (American Academy of Pediatrics [AAP] Committee on Pediatric Workforce, 1999). Conversely, the racial and ethnic composition of individuals in programs to train health-care practitioners to work with this diverse population does not mirror this racial and ethnic diversity found in the child and family (Lynch & Hanson, 1992). Moreover, according to the U.S. Bureau of Labor Statistics (1998), among the largest health-care profession—nursing—90% of registered nurses in the United States are White (see Table 10.1). Lack of diversity in language, socioeconomic status, and ethnicity may influence the provision of health services (AAP Committee on Pediatric Workforce, 1999).

This discrepancy between the diversity of the populations seeking health-care services and the diversity of the populations providing the services demonstrates the need for remedy on several levels. On one level, this disparity signals a greater need for organizational, systematic, and institutional solutions. A solution on this level may encompass having recruiting and hiring strategies that create a talented and diverse workforce to better serve a diverse family, which a recent policy statement issued by the AAP was developed to address (AAP Committee on Pediatric Workforce, 2000). However, Culley (1997) cautioned that the employment of minority ethnic workers, although desirable for many reasons, is not in itself a guarantee of improved service delivery. Citing Gerrish, Husband, and Mackenzie (1996), Culley (2001, p. 133) explained that "it cannot be assumed that minority ethnic health professionals who have undergone traditional training will necessarily practice in less Eurocentric ways or have the necessary skills to work in a culturally competent way with all minority groups."

On another level, there is a need to focus on the individual and thus to train and develop health-care practitioners to interact effectively and compassionately with people who may be culturally different from themselves. McEvoy (2003) recommended that rather than attempting to understand categories of culture, spirituality, and religion, perhaps more can be gained by

Table 10.1 423

Racial and Ethnic Demographics Among Registered Nurses

Demographic	Percentage
White (non-Hispanic)	86.6
African American (non-Hispanic)	4.9
Hispanic	2.0
American Indian/Alaskan Native/Hawaiian/Pacific Islander	0.7
Asian	3.5
Two or more races	1.2

Note. From 2000 Sample Survey of RNs, Health Resources and Services Administration, 2001, Washington, DC: Author.

focusing instead on understanding the individual child's or family's traditions, values, and beliefs and how these dimensions have an impact on the health of the child.

We each possess a cultural identity, and thus the situations in which a family and a practitioner of different cultures come together provide rich opportunities for challenge, growth, and personal and professional development for practitioners in the health-related professions. This chapter addresses several issues, including (a) how we define ourselves as cultural beings, (b) how we demonstrate and live our culture, (c) how others of similar and different cultural backgrounds view and react to us, and (d) how we view and react to others of similar and different cultures.

Many lenses exist by which we may view culture. Some of us may see ourselves as belonging to one distinct culture, whereas others may identify with two or more cultures. Simultaneously, some of us may identify strongly with the dominant culture found in the United States or identify primarily with another culture. Understanding culture is as much about understanding ourselves as cultural beings as it is about learning how to function effectively with those from other cultures. As people engaged in professions aimed at helping others in the context of meeting health-care needs, practitioners are sharing and cultivating more than just technical expertise about health-related issues. The practitioner is also engaging in interpersonal interactions and participating in highly personal and physically challenging experiences with children and their families.

Every interaction among humans is a cultural interaction. When we interact with those who come from similar racial or ethnic backgrounds, social and economic classes, educational experiences, values, traditions, and dress, often these interactions are embedded with common reference points, meanings, and assumptions. Because we share common reference points, the likelihood increases that we will understand each other. When common reference points are absent or few, either or both parties involved may not fully understand the perspectives and experiences of the other person, and thus interactions can result in dynamic tensions and discomfort.

Although many ways exist in which to frame a discussion about culture, presenting conceptual material about what is culture and the various dimensions of culture provides a context for the more practical concepts, such as how to engage in a process of becoming more cross-culturally competent and effective. First, we explore the definition and dimensions of culture. Terms such as culture, race, and ethnicity often may be used interchangeably, yet they are not interchangeable. Whereas on one level, providing a working definition of culture offers one way to present and anchor a concept that is sometimes misunderstood, presenting the various dimensions of culture adds several layers of complexity. Examples of the elements of culture relevant to interactions in a health-care context include communication styles, interactions in and uses of physical space, concepts of time, and assumptions about healing and health.

Second, we look at a *process* for developing cross-cultural competence. Because we each experience culture and possess a cultural identity and history, this section begins with helping one develop an awareness of the culture we each possess. In thinking about culture, it is tempting to look at the "other" as exotic and interesting, without realizing that the reason why the other appears exotic is most likely because we are judging the other against our cultural norm. Coincidentally, the "other" may perceive us as being just as exotic or idiosyncratic as we may perceive them. Because we each possess a culture and come from a worldview informed by numerous experiences, values, and traditions, which may or may not be shared by others with whom we come into contact, cross-cultural interactions contain a mixture of possibility and uncertainty for all who are involved.

Our worldview influences how we interact with others and how we construct meaning from events; therefore, it is important to think intentionally about how we construct meaning by working toward greater self-awareness rather than acting from unconscious biases or assumptions. Actively cultivating greater self-awareness regarding culture while simultaneously developing a repertoire of skills and competencies to function better in a cross-cultural situation is essential in developing cross-cultural competence.

This chapter presents the dimensions of culture, the within-group complexity found among members of any given culture, and information about developing cross-cultural competence. By providing information about terms and concepts related to culture, this chapter provides practitioners with a basic vocabulary for framing and discussing issues related to culture, as well as exposing practitioners to some of the complexity that is present in culture and is manifested in language and through experience. The section on developing cross-cultural competence begins with building self-awareness, followed by knowledge of other cultures, and it concludes with skills and knowledge in cross-cultural communication.

Culture

Culture is a powerful mechanism that guides our conscious and unconscious thoughts and activities; thus, culture influences the interactions between the practitioner, the family, and others who are a part of the support system and decision-making team for the child (Geissler, 1993). We each belong to a culture and operate within one or more cultural frameworks. Culture is dynamic and evolving, rather than static. All societies have cultural mores and practices that "guide human behavior and provide a socialization framework that shapes interaction" (Lynch & Hanson, 1992, p. 3). It is difficult—if not impossible—to be knowledgeable about *all* aspects of many cultures or even one culture. However, if one is to effectively interact with those from a different culture, it is important to be aware and knowledgeable of—as well as sensitive to—the many aspects and dimensions of one's culture and the cultures of one's family members.

Culture refers to the values, traditions, norms, customs, history, folklore, arts, and institutions shared by a group of people (Orlandi, 1992). Culture can exist on several levels. For example, consider how one's workplace or school encompasses several of the aforementioned components of culture. One may also identify with a particular racial group or nationality. Although the concepts of race and ethnicity are linked, they are not synonymous terms. Race is a way of *socially* defining individuals or a group of people based on "distinguishable physical characteristics," whereas ethnicity refers to one's membership in a group that is often "linked by race, nationality, and language with a common cultural heritage and/or derivation" (Orlandi, 1992, p. vi).

Culture involves the entire environment in which interactions among humans occur and is learned through instruction and imitation (Smith, 1995). Culture is more than just an abstract concept. Culture helps shape how one experiences and functions in different environments. Smith (1995), citing the work of Ali Mazrui, presents several functions of culture, including:

- how people view the world and construct reality through lenses of perception and cognition;
- how motivations for human behaviors are shaped, which may involve identical behaviors for two people, but because of different motivations, the behaviors hold different meanings;
- a basis for individual and group identity within a historical context encoded and described by oral, written, and social constructs;
- how value systems (e.g., beauty, morality, and justice) are defined and described; and
- the modes of communication expressed through language, art, music, dance, cuisine, and other means.

As one begins to develop a greater understanding of the multiple functions of culture, one also may realize that in cross-cultural situations, there is an increased probability that conflicts may occur based on differences in perceptions, values, communication styles, and motivations. Health-care practitioners may encounter families who speak a different language, cherish and operate from a different set of beliefs, or hold a different attitude about health and illness (Geissler, 1993). For example, the family may see illness as being connected to fate and thus feel that accepting the medical situation and providing comfort to manage the symptoms is more important than using an aggressive intervention to "cure" the body. When these differences are present, practitioners will need to work *with* the family to understand *their* desired outcome. This will enable the practitioner to develop an appropriate intervention and process.

The term *cross-cultural competence* appears throughout this chapter. Developing cultural competence is a multifaceted process. It requires us to cultivate an awareness of how culture shapes and influences our lives, how it plays a role in the lives of others who belong to a different culture, and how the interaction among people of different cultures has an impact on all who are involved. In addition to cultivating a greater awareness of culture in relation to oneself and others, cultural competence also means cultivating a set of skills to help individuals manage cross-cultural interactions effectively and appropriately. Although being cross-culturally competent is an asset for individuals in all professions, it is a particularly important asset for those working in health-care settings in which practitioners often work directly with families in situations that are highly personal and emotionally intense. (See box for definitions of cultural terms.)

Culture of the Family

Human experience is contextual. We thus operate from and function as individuals within contexts that contain other people, rules, and norms for behavior. In these systems, we affect others and are affected by others. In the

---

Definitions of Cultural Terms

Cultural competence—a compilation of academic and interpersonal skills that allow individuals to increase their understanding and appreciation of cultural differences and similarities within, among, and between groups.

Cultural imposition—the tendency of individuals to impose their beliefs, values, and patterns of behavior on other cultures.

Culture—the shared values, norms, traditions, customs, arts, history, and institutions shared by a group of people.

Ethnic—belonging to a common group—often linked by race, nationality, and language—with a common cultural heritage or derivation.

health-care setting, at least two types of culture are intertwined. The first is culture as it pertains to racial and ethnic groups; the second is the culture of the family. As we work with children, not only are we communicating and interacting with the child, but also we are interacting with family members, friends, and perhaps even clergy. These other people may be viewed as very important people in the child's and family's "world."

Because children are members of a larger system, such as a family, it is important to acknowledge the role of this system and its members in the life of the child (see Chapter 7, Families in Children's Health-Care Settings). Practitioners also need to work closely with the parents or other designated decision makers. Part of effective work with families requires understanding the family's concerns, priorities, needs, strengths, and resources, which are shaped in part by their cultural background. The racial and ethnic group in which the family most strongly identifies significantly shapes the family's rituals, behaviors, dynamics, and approaches. Understanding how the family system works, in addition to how culture plays a role in shaping the family system, may present multiple challenges for the practitioner who strives not only to be knowledgeable in the technical aspects of the profession, but also to be interpersonally effective.

Understanding the importance and centrality of the family is important in the health-care context and healing process. In addition to the child being affected by his or her health-care and healing experience, the family system is also affected by this experience. Parents, siblings, and others whom the family deems important are included in the process as participants and as witnesses. Much of what influences how the child and family experience the various aspects of the healing process and the health-care system is shaped by the assumptions and beliefs embedded in their cultural identity: "The health care provider must be aware of the meaning that families assign to the use of surgery and drugs for medical treatments, just as educators must be knowledgeable as to family beliefs about childrearing and developmental expectations" (Lynch & Hanson, 1992). In addition to needing to be mindful of a

---

Language—the form or pattern of speech—spoken or written—used by residents or descendents of a particular nation or geographic area or by any large body of people; can be formal or informal and include dialect, idiomatic speech, and slang.

Mainstream—usually refers to a broad population that is primarily White and middle class.

Nationality—the country where a person lives or identifies as a homeland.

Race—a socially defined population that is derived from distinguishable physical characteristics that are genetically transmitted.

Note. Adapted from *Cultural Competence for Evaluators: A Guide for Alcohol and Other Drug Abuse Prevention Practitioners Working with Ethnic/Racial Communities* (DHHS Publication No. 92-60067), by M. A. Orlandi (Ed.), 1992, Rockville, MD: U.S. Department of Health and Human Services.

family's perspective on various medical interventions (e.g., taking medications, surgery, diagnostic procedures), the practitioner needs to be aware of the differences in the ways in which people communicate, make decisions, and think about seeking outside assistance (Lynch & Hanson, 1992). McEvoy (2003) suggested three areas that can be used to broach culturally sensitive issues within the context of pediatric health care: (a) family beliefs and values, (b) family daily practices; and (c) community involvement. However, perhaps more basic than understanding the rituals and practices of families is first understanding how families define their concept of family (e.g., immediate family, extended family, close family friends), the roles of the members of the family, how the family makes decisions, and the family's view of illness or the health condition (Danielson, Hamel-Bissell, & Winstead-Fry, 1991).

It may be tempting for a practitioner to want to help families *change* so that the family functions more like those in the mainstream culture. In a more cross-culturally appropriate approach, the practitioner assists families in functioning in a new environment by helping them navigate through the mainstream culture, rather than encouraging them to strip their cultural identity. A practitioner can help families by (a) serving as an interpreter of mainstream culture; (b) learning about the family's approach to childrearing, health care, and socialization; and (c) helping to design a set of interventions that complement the family's preferences (Lynch & Hanson, 1992). Thus, "it may be the interventionist's role to provide information about the new culture that will help the family adapt to new demands and beliefs, while helping the family maintain the elements of their traditional culture of origin that they wish to preserve" (Lynch & Hanson, 1992, p. 12).

Cultural Assumptions, Bias, and Values

Culture is complex and "without a clear view of the full cultural process, we are led down the path of ineffectiveness, frustration, and conflict in our attempts to offer meaningful services and programs" (Smith, 1995, p. 15). In addition to realizing the complexity and richness of culture, we also must realize that we not only emerge from and are products of a culture, but also that we hold biases and make assumptions about those who have membership in a culture that is different from our own. Likewise, if a family is from a culture different from the practitioner's culture, the family may be cautious, anxious, or wonder whether the practitioner understands and respects their concerns, needs, and perspectives.

We each have biases as a product of living in a world that is rich with multiple perspectives, beliefs, and approaches. The world is complex and multifaceted and thus it may be easier to manage this complexity by comparing other people, events, and phenomena to *our* reference points, ideas, and experiences, which serve as our anchors. Theorists as well as health professionals "sometimes show bias toward families who do not share their own personal values and view of effective family functioning" or other practices

(Danielson et al., 1991, p. 143). Although bias is a reality in human existence, our biases may challenge our ability to function effectively in situations that bring into our lives cultures in which we are less familiar.

Although it is unrealistic to eliminate all traces of bias in our lives, we can strive to work effectively with families who have a cultural perspective that is different from ours. We each come from a culture and thus bring to and operate from a set of values and beliefs with every interaction and experience. This is true for a Latino practitioner working with an African American family, an African American practitioner working with a White family, a White practitioner working with a Native American family, and so on. Given the salience and presence of culture, we do not operate as a neutral party with a neutral perspective. However, if one happens to be a member of the dominant culture, this cultural perspective is likely to be reinforced by media images and political and educational institutions. Because of this multiple reinforcement of the dominant culture, people who hold membership in this culture may not notice the absence of other perspectives and approaches. As a consequence, the practitioner may assume that his or her culture's perspective and approach is the most "normal," efficient, and appropriate.

Along with belonging to a culture, individuals hold a set of values and assumptions that are connected with a particular culture. Our values are indicative of the importance, desirability, worth, or usefulness we place on an object, behavior, or belief. Our assumptions are the ideas and actions that we hold as true without demanding proof or evidence.

Some may consider themselves members of the dominant culture of the United States in which certain values and assumptions permeate many aspects of mainstream life (e.g., television, film, music, and political, educational, and social institutions). Others consider themselves outside of the mainstream or dominant culture. Whether considering ourselves to be members of the dominant culture or not, it is valuable at least to be aware of the values, assumptions, and beliefs typically associated with the dominant culture in the United States and some of the ways these are reflected in cultural courtesies and customs:

- *The notion that all people are more or less equal.* Women and men are treated with equal respect. People providing daily services (cab drivers, waitresses, secretaries, sales clerks) are treated courteously.
- *People freely express their opinions.* Freedom of speech is a major characteristic of the culture. However, some topics (sex, politics, religion, personal characteristics such as body odors) typically are not openly discussed, particularly with strangers.
- *Persons are greeted openly, directly, and warmly.* Not many rituals are associated with greetings; maybe a handshake, particularly among men.
- *People usually greet each other and get to the point of the interaction.* Eye contact is maintained throughout the interaction. It is considered impolite to not look at the person to whom you are talking.

- *Social distance of about an arm's length is typically maintained in interactions.* People (men, in particular) do not expect to be touched except for greetings such as shaking hands. People walking down the street together typically do not hold hands or put their arms around one another unless they are involved in an intimate relationship.
- *Punctuality and responsibility in keeping appointments are valued.* Time is valued and most people expect punctuality. It is considered rude to accept an invitation to someone's home and not go, or to make an appointment with someone and not keep it.

These values and assumptions of the dominant U.S. culture are also those inherent in the U.S. health-care system and are reflected in ways institutions and the employees within them operate and interact with families. An awareness of some of the ways in which other cultures' values may contrast with dominant U.S. values can provide a helpful starting point for health-care providers (see Table 10.2). For example, a family from a culture in which human interaction holds a higher value than time may arrive late for a scheduled clinic appointment. This would likely cause friction in a system that is structured by and places a high value on time.

Because many cultures exist in the United States, our attempts to learn from and interact effectively with those who have different values and assumptions may be enriching yet challenging. One starting point, however, is to be aware of the values and assumptions from which we are operating.

Values and assumptions have a role in constructing our ideas and beliefs about health care and how to interact with children. For example, mainstream culture in the United States may place a high value on preventing disease and the use of the latest technologic advances in medical practice. In dominant U.S. culture, it is not unusual to see the use of the latest diagnostic techniques and aggressive approaches to managing illness (Lynch & Hanson, 1992). In the dominant culture of the United States, there may also be an assumption that good health is a right and "that medical science should be able to cure everything" (Lynch & Hanson, 1992, p. 10–11).

One should not assume, however, that certain cultures considered "less modern" would routinely reject these technologic advances. Banks and Benchot (2001) reported that Amish people—who live in large multigenerational families on farms where hard work is valued and worldly conveniences such as electricity, telephones, and automobiles are usually shunned—are willing to accept and participate in modern health care if its value is clearly understood.

In terms of interacting with children, two central values in the mainstream U.S. culture are independence and privacy; thus, children are encouraged to be independent from an early age. An example of how this value is manifested is through a parent having separate rooms for each child and infant so that they may sleep alone. In contrast, many families from cultures such as those from Mexico, Central America, South America, and Asia may view isolating young children in a dark room and having them sleep alone in a crib or bed as inappropriate (Lynch & Hanson, 1992).

Table 10.2

431

Contrasting Beliefs, Values, and Practices

Anglo-American Values	Some Other Cultures' Values
Personal control over environment	Fate
Change	Tradition
Time dominates	Human interaction dominates
Human equality	Hierarchy/rank/status
Individualism/privacy	Group welfare
Self-help	Birthright inheritance
Competition	Cooperation
Future orientation	Past or present orientation
Action/goal/work orientation	"Being" orientation
Informality	Formality
Directness/openness/honesty	Indirectness/ritual/"face"
Practicality/efficiency	Idealism/theory
Materialism	Spiritualism/detachment

Note. Adapted from *Cross-Cultural Counseling: A Guide for Nutrition and Health Counselors,* by U.S. Department of Agriculture and U.S. Department of Health and Human Services, 1986, Washington, DC: Author.

Dimensions of Culture

In addition to functions of culture, several dimensions of culture exist (see Table 10.3). Rather than presenting a list of what aspects of the dimensions "typically" may be found in a given culture, the table outlines the ways in which cultural groups and families can vary, thus presenting information about the dimensions without overgeneralizing.

The dimensions listed reflect many aspects of culture and pay particular attention to the dimensions that are relevant to health-care issues and contexts. For example, just as approaches to independence manifested through approaches to sleeping can vary, so do approaches to feeding practices. For some cultural groups, mealtimes may be highly structured and for others, it is less defined. In some families, meals are served at the same time every day. In other families, a meal is prepared and then kept out so that the family members can take what they want when they want it (Lynch & Hanson, 1992). It is apparent that confusion can arise when a health-care professional instructs parents to give their child medication with meals without understanding what "mealtime" means to that family.

(*text continues on p. 434*)

Table 10.3

Dimensions of Culture

Dimension	Selected Considerations
Approaches to family planning, pregnancy, and birth	• contraception use • attitudes toward abortion • place of delivery (i.e., home, hospital, or birthing center) • use of midwife or physician for delivery • presence of the father and others (e.g., children, friends, and other family) during delivery • rituals after delivery
Beliefs about and attitudes toward death	• acceptability of organ and tissue donation • views on autopsy • views on cremation • preparation of the body after death • time between death and funeral rites • expression of grief
Childrearing practices	• response to a crying infant • attitudes toward independence of children • perspectives on and approaches to discipline • use of cloth, disposable, or no diapers • methods and timing of toilet training • attitudes toward child labor
Communication	• volume of voice • acceptability of interruptions • use of gestures • body movements (e.g., bowing) • touching (e.g., handshaking, hand holding, hugging, kissing) • cursing • repetition • boastfulness • style (e.g., indirect, tactful, blunt) • eye contact (e.g., direct, sustained, brief, looking away) • comfort in discussing feelings
Food practices	• fasting • frequency of meals • vegetarianism/veganism • food preparation (e.g., Kosher diet)
Gender and family roles	• decision-making processes • appropriate dress • expectations for participation and involvement of family and others during hospitalization • restrictions • views toward elders
Infant feeding practices	• breast or bottle feeding • weaning (e.g., abrupt, gradual)
Language issues	• oral and written proficiency in one's primary languages and in other languages • number of languages spoken

Table 10.3 *Continued.*

433

Dimensions of Culture

Dimension	Selected Considerations
Language issues (*continued*)	• whether the language of the dominant culture is primary or secondary
Perceptions of time	• attitudes toward punctuality (i.e., relaxed or strict observance) • focus (i.e., present, past, immediate future, long-term future) • taking medication (i.e., at scheduled times versus when one feels sick)
Reactions to pain	• private or expressive reactions • denial or acknowledgment of pain • expectations for medical intervention
Religious and spiritual beliefs and practices	• often intertwined with other dimensions of culture, such as beliefs about and attitudes toward death • private or public uses of prayer and meditation • presence of religious symbols and objects in room or on clothing • observances of the Sabbath
Sick care, healing practices, and interventions	• biomedical • holistic • magico-religious • use of spiritual healers • traditional
Views toward health-care professionals	• attitudes toward doctors, nurses, and other members of the health-care team • level of respect given and expected • questioning and challenging diagnosis versus not questioning diagnosis • views toward client being examined by a professional of a different sex • level of formality expected in interactions
Other dimensions	• attitudes toward transfusions and transplants • attitudes toward surgery • frequency of handwashing • expectations for privacy • discussion of outcomes (e.g., hope, optimism, fatalism) • support systems (e.g., immediate family, extended family, friends, church) • practice of regular physical examinations • attitudes toward health, healing, disability, and help seeking/intervention • practice of male and female circumcision • sleeping practices

Note. Adapted from "Home-Based Early Childhood Services: Cultural Sensitivity in a Family Systems Approach," by K. Wayman, E. Lynch, and M. Hanson, 1990, *Topics in Early Childhood Special Education, 10,* pp. 65–66. Copyright 1990 by PRO-ED, Inc. Adapted with permission.

Cultural differences sometimes involve ethical issues. For example, some cultures consider it cruel to inform adults as well as children about life-threatening diagnoses or risks involved in procedures. An understanding of different approaches to truth-telling when seeking informed consent is critical. Crow, Matheson, and Steed (2000) presented a excellent illustration of approaches to truth-telling through Korean, Southeast Asian, and American Indian case studies.

Complexity in Culture

Although the dimensions of culture presented in Table 10.3 are not exhaustive, they do illustrate some of the complexity contained within culture. Additionally, it is essential to remember that although patterns of beliefs and practices are found among members of a culture, individual differences also exist within cultural groups (Geissler, 1993). For example, two different families may be traced to a similar cultural background, but one child may be a visitor from another country and the other child may belong to a family who has been in the United States for several generations. Thus, the two different children may experience hospitalization and other health-care experiences in the United States differently. Both children come from a similar background, but may express themselves and their culture differently, for example, through dress and food choices. Culturally effective practitioners are aware not only of differences among cultures, but also are open and curious about complexity *within* a cultural group (see Figure 10.1). Culturally aware practitioners realize that just because two children come from a similar cultural background does not mean that their experiences, values, and beliefs are identical (Danielson et al., 1991).

Culture is an important factor in understanding human behavior, yet some other factors contribute to behavior and mediate the impact of culture. Some common factors include socioeconomic status, sex, age, education, and length of residence in a locale (Lynch & Hanson, 1992). Additionally, individuals vary in how strongly they choose to adhere to cultural patterns and practices. Some individuals may identify strongly with one particular group, whereas others may embrace the practices of several groups simultaneously (Lynch & Hanson, 1992).

Like other phenomena, the degree of cultural identity falls along a continuum. Although individuals may identify with a given cultural group by way of birthplace, skin color, language, or religious practices, these factors will not determine the *degree* to which individuals see themselves as members of a group (Lynch & Hanson, 1992). On one end of the continuum, a person may try to assimilate or adopt fully the values accepted by the mainstream or dominant culture. In contrast, a person may choose to participate in both the dominant culture and their culture of origin. On the other end of the continuum, some individuals may choose to identify more closely with their culture of origin, rather than with the dominant culture (Lynch & Hanson, 1992).

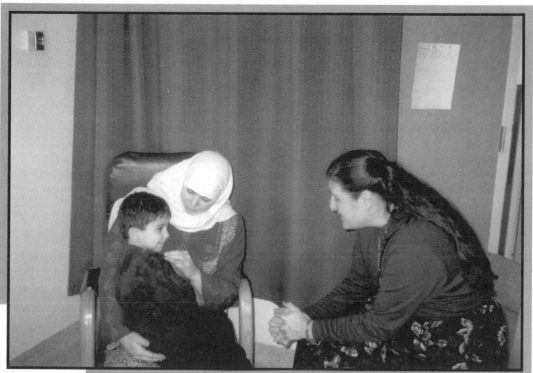

Figure 10.1.
Culturally effective practitioners are open and curious about complexity within a cultural group.
Note. Photograph by Lynn Clutter. Used with permission.

Cross-Cultural Competence

Becoming more cross-culturally competent is a process, rather than a destination, that involves developing awareness, behaving with intention, and possessing a desire to grow and continually evaluate one's progress. Cultural competence encompasses acquiring knowledge and developing a set of interpersonal skills, which allows "individuals to increase their understanding and appreciation of cultural differences and similarities" (Orlandi, 1992, p. vi).

Children learn and grow through this process. Although no human being is born with racist, sexist, or other oppressive attitudes, the very way that children learn to make sense of their world demands a focus on "differences." For example, early on, children notice differences and mentally organize these observations into categories. Attitudes about "us" and "them" are learned and reinforced in the home, school, church, and through the media. By age 3 years, children have learned to categorize people into "good" or "bad" based on superficial traits such as race or gender (Derman-Sparks & A. B. C. Task Force, 1989). As they learn the names of colors, they apply these names to skin color. Even before the age of 3, children may show signs of being

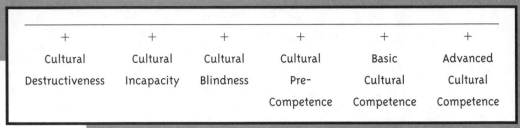

Figure 10.2.

Cultural competence continuum. *Note.* From "Services to Minority Populations: Cultural Competence Continuum," by T. Cross, 1989, *Focal Point, 3*(2), pp. 1–5. Copyright 1989 by The Research and Training Center on Family Support and Children's Mental Health. Reprinted with permission.

influenced by what they see and hear around them. By 4 or 5 years of age, children may use racial reasons for refusing to interact with others who are different from themselves, or they may exhibit discomfort around or even reject people with disabilities. By the time they enter elementary school, some children have developed prejudices built on stereotypes that remain until personal experience or someone attempts to correct them.

Regarding this process, Cross (1988) presented a 6-point continuum for cross-cultural competence ranging from cultural destructiveness to advanced cultural competence (see Figure 10.2). The points on the continuum can be described as follows:

1. *Cultural destructiveness*—actively carries out activities that destroy or disrupt cultural beliefs or practices.
2. *Cultural incapacity*—represents cross-cultural ignorance; often characterized by support of the status quo.
3. *Cultural blindness*—well-meaning but misguided "liberal" policies and practices based on the belief that if only the dominant cultural practices were working properly, they would be universally applicable and effective for everyone.
4. *Cultural precompetence*—reflects a movement toward the recognition that differences exist in individuals, families, and communities, and a willingness to begin to try different approaches to improve service delivery.
5. *Basic cultural competence*—acceptance and respect for difference, continuing self-assessment regarding culture, careful attention to the dynamics of difference, continuous expansion of cultural knowledge and resources, and a variety of adaptations to service models to better meet the needs of nondominant populations.
6. *Advanced cultural competence*—at the most positive end of the scale, characterized by actively seeking to add to the knowledge base of culturally competent practice by conducting research, developing new therapeutic approaches based on culture, publishing and disseminating the results of demonstration projects, and so on. In other

words, advocates for cultural competence throughout the system and for improved relations between cultures throughout society.

In developing cross-cultural competence, the goal for practitioners should not be perfection. Rather, the goal could be to cultivate a greater understanding, empathy, and sensitivity to those who have membership in cultures other than the practitioner's culture, as well as cultivating a set of skills to enable effective and productive interactions.

Cross-cultural competence is a multifaceted process. Lynch and Hanson (1992) outlined four aspects of cross-cultural competence:

1. The awareness of one's culture and limitations
2. An openness to and respect for cultural differences
3. A willingness to learn from intercultural interactions
4. An ability to use cultural resources during interventions

In contrast, cross-cultural competence does not mean adopting the values, beliefs, or behaviors of another culture, shedding one's cultural identity, or knowing everything about another culture. A culturally sensitive person recognizes that both differences and similarities exist between cultures. The culturally sensitive person strives to acquire knowledge about the cultural groups that live in one's region or state and thus knows the general parameters of those cultures. The culturally sensitive person also understands that cultural diversity has an impact on families' participation in intervention programs (e.g., health, education, social services; Lynch & Hanson, 1992).

Although cultural sensitivity is an aspect of cross-cultural competence, merely being culturally sensitive does not make one cross-culturally competent. With cross-cultural competence, we must have an ongoing commitment to understanding ourselves, our culture, our biases and assumptions, as well as to actively cultivate a set of *skills* to help us function effectively in cross-cultural situations. Cross-culturally competent individuals are aware of how they are affected by, and how they affect, others of different cultures. Further, they possess a repertoire of skills to aid in effective cross-cultural interactions.

When working with those from cultures different from our own, it is important to consider both the process of, the goals for, and the outcomes of the healing process. The process refers to the approaches, strategies, and techniques used in working with others and can be either appropriate or antagonistic for the child and family. The goals, however, refer to the desired outcomes from the process (Sue & Sue, 1990).

Benefits of and Challenges in Developing Cross-Cultural Competence

Anticipating the dynamics of and tension in cross-cultural interactions may hold a mixture of excitement about the possibilities for growth and learning for the practitioner, and anxiety in anticipating potential conflicts and miscommunication between the practitioner and the family. Sometimes interactions between practitioners and the family from different cultures may feel awkward for both parties. Nevertheless, such interactions can facilitate learning about a different culture and developing a greater understanding of ourselves, how we respond to those who are culturally different, and give us greater sensitivity to the tension that can be a product of interpersonal interactions.

We cannot easily discard the lenses created by culture in which we view the world, but we can cultivate a greater awareness of our culture and other cultures, and develop a set of skills to help us navigate more easily through culture's complex tapestry. A high level of awareness of, and sensitivity and openness to, the richness and variety of cultural identity requires intentional thought and action. Although acting with intent in regard to cultural differences requires energy and effort, the benefits for the practitioner include (a) personal and professional enrichment, (b) the acquisition of new knowledge, (c) the development of a repertoire of skills and competencies enabling one to function in a variety of circumstances, and (d) a better understanding of self.

Lynch and Hanson (1992) reported that for practitioners working with culturally diverse families, being cross-culturally competent enables one

- to feel comfortable and be effective in interactions with families;
- to interact in ways that help families from different cultures feel positively about the interactions and practitioner; and
- to accomplish the goals established by the family and practitioner.

In addition to the many benefits of being a more culturally aware and competent practitioner, one may encounter challenges that are a product of this journey. Perhaps one of the greatest challenges is developing a tolerance for ambiguity and contradiction.

Cultures evolve and contain a myriad of within-group variations. One culture can also be radically different from another, and even within a given culture, two people can vary in how strictly they adhere to the norms of that culture. In developing cultural competence, it is important to recognize and respect cultural differences, rather than minimize the salience of cultural identification or avoid those who come from diverse cultural backgrounds. It is essential to recognize the common humanity of individuals without negating or trying to strip away the distinct cultural identity of oneself or a child and family. Walking along a fine line of embracing common humanity and recognizing cultural distinction can be cognitively challenging. Lynch and Hanson (1992) outlined several reasons why it is challenging for people to understand or function in a culture that is different from their own:

1. One's understanding of his or her primary culture is generally established by age 5 years. The elements of cultural learning are numerous and include every interaction, odor, sound, and touch one experi-

ences. Such material is learned at an early age and becomes integral in one's thinking and behavior, and thus persists into adulthood.

2. Adults experience more difficulties in learning new cultural patterns than children for possibly two reasons: (a) adult patterns of behavior tend to be more established, and (b) adults have more information to manage than children.

3. One's values are often determined by one's first culture and when these values are used to function in a second culture, conflicts may result from contradictory values. Additionally, one's deepest values are expressed through long-standing behavior patterns.

4. People tend to look at other cultures through the lens of their first culture. One may therefore make errors in attempts to interpret the meaning of behaviors from another culture.

The challenges for a practitioner or child and family to function in or with another culture may manifest themselves through the experience of *culture shock*. "Every culture has subtle, if not unconscious, signs by which people evaluate what they say and do. Losing these cues produces strain, uneasiness, and even emotional maladjustment if the person is received badly" (Igoa, 1995, p. 39). Culture shock results when a series of disorienting encounters occur in which an individual's basic values, beliefs, and patterns of behavior are challenged by a different set of values, beliefs, and behaviors. When one is confronted with something that is unfamiliar (e.g., sounds, odors, sights, behaviors), one may experience interest, excitement, confusion, frustration, fear, anger, or disgust. Culture shock is particularly pronounced when individuals discover dramatic differences between their values and beliefs and the values and beliefs of the people around them. Although both the practitioner and the family can experience culture shock during interactions, the practitioner must remain effective and professional when working with the family. Developing cross-cultural competence is one way to manage culture shock.

Developing Cross-Cultural Competence

The rewards of becoming more cross-culturally competent are plentiful. With cross-cultural competence, one can function as a bridge between two or more cultures, possess a high degree of self-knowledge, and function more effectively during interpersonal interactions. The process of developing cross-cultural competence, however, is not necessarily easy. Becoming cross-culturally competent requires that we lower our defenses, take risks, and practice behaviors that may be unfamiliar and uncomfortable. We must be open, flexible, and willing to respect alternate perspectives. In other words, becoming more cross-culturally competent requires hard and diligent work. Lynch and Hanson (1992) listed three essential elements of cross-cultural competence that include possessing (a) self-awareness of one's values and assumptions, (b) knowledge of other cultures, and (c) skills in engaging successfully in cross-cultural interactions. To develop these elements of cross-cultural competence, practitioners need to

- have an awareness of the sociopolitical forces that affect the lives of the children and families they serve;
- understand that some of the barriers to effectively working with those who are culturally different are language, culture, and class;
- recognize the importance of worldviews and cultural identity in the healing process;
- understand differences in communication styles among different cultural groups; and
- be aware of one's own biases and attitudes. (Sue & Sue, 1990)

Self-Awareness

Gaining self-awareness is an important element for those who are striving to become more cross-culturally competent. Although we each have a culture, we are often unaware of how our behaviors, habits, and customs are grounded in our cultural backgrounds (Lynch & Hanson, 1992). Lacking self-awareness, we may look at other cultures as exotic or strange in comparison to our culture, particularly if we identify strongly with the dominant or mainstream culture.

As we consider becoming cross-culturally competent, it is not uncommon to want to try to eliminate all negative biases or attitudes from our thinking or to try to avoid making mistakes. The reality is that these are impossible tasks that deny the complexity of the self.

We have both conscious and unconscious thoughts, and we can experience a range of emotions and responses that may be triggered by cross-

---

Exploring Your Cultural Heritage

1. What ethnic group, socioeconomic class, religion, age group, and community do you belong to?
   - What about these groups do you find embarrassing or would like to change? Why?
   - What sociocultural factors in your background might be rejected by members of other cultures?
   - What did your parents and significant others say about people who were different from your family?
2. What do you believe or value?
   - How do you define health, disease, illness?
   - Are you usually on time? Early? Late?
   - How do you feel when others are late? Frustrated? Angry? Not respected? Fine? Philosophical?

cultural situations that range from curiosity, interest, and excitement to confusion, anxiety, frustration, and defensiveness. Perhaps it is unrealistic to completely eliminate bias from our lives. Instead we can strive to understand how bias operates in our lives on a deeper level by first developing an awareness of our biases, identifying the sources and functions of our biases, and thinking about whether and how to dismantle biases. Mistakes are a natural process and to avoid all mistakes is impossible; openness to learning from them is more important in developing cross-cultural competence.

As mentioned previously, developing cross-cultural competence is a process in which developing self-awareness is a fundamental component. One important piece related to this journey is thinking about how we can learn about our cultural heritage. Lynch and Hanson (1992) suggested that we ask ourselves the following questions:

- What is your family's place(s) of origin?
- When did your ancestors immigrate or come to the United States?
- Under what circumstances, or for what reasons, did your ancestors to come to the United States?
- What were your ancestors' political leanings?
- What jobs and status did your ancestors hold?
- What were your ancestors' beliefs and values?

Rollins and Riccio (2001) also offered questions to assist in exploring cultural heritage (see box). These questions are designed to help clarify beliefs and attitudes, and how these beliefs and attitudes affect how we work with people from different cultural backgrounds.

Knowing your own cultural heritage serves two functions: (a) to help gain a better understanding of the economic, social, and vocational changes

- What are your views on children's education?
- Are you comfortable with physical contact (e.g., touching, embracing)? How much and with whom?
- What are your religious views and biases? Do you adhere to religious rituals?
- What are your feelings on childrearing practices (including nutrition, discipline, play, roles)?
3. What experiences have you had with people from ethnic groups, socioeconomic classes, religions, age groups, or communities different from your own?
- What were those experiences like?
- How did you feel about them?
4. What personal qualities do you have that will help you establish interpersonal relationships with persons from other cultural groups?
5. What personal qualities may be detrimental?

Note. From "Strategies for Working with Culturally Diverse Communities and Clients," by E. Randall-David, 1989, Washington, DC: Association for the Care of Children's Health; and "Health Care of Immigrant Children: Incorporating Culture into Practice," by V. Niederhauser, 1989, *Pediatric Nursing, 15*(6), 569–574. Adapted with permission.

Suggestions for Gathering Information About Your Cultural Heritage	1. Ask about and listen to the stories of your oldest family members. 2. Look at family photographs, videotapes, and albums. 3. With permission, read the journals and letters of family members. 4. Look at notes of important events in places such as the family Bible or other important family texts.

our family and ancestors experienced; and (b) to provide a tool by which we can think about how our culture is similar to and different from others in tangible ways. It is also helpful to consider how our families and others who share our culture celebrate certain holidays, engage in religious practices, exhibit norms for behavior, etiquette, and interactions, and hold beliefs and values that guide our actions and behaviors (see box).

When we work and interact with others, we do so through a lens created by our values and thus we may make incorrect assumptions about those with whom we come into contact. These assumptions and biases may be "conscious or unconscious, active or passive, overt or covert, and intentional or unintentional," and a practitioner who acts from these biases may work inappropriately or ineffectively with a family (Churchill, 1995, p. 42). For example, a practitioner working with an Asian American family may assume that the members of this family will have difficulty in speaking and understanding English. As a result, the practitioner may speak to the family slowly and loudly. The reality may be that this family has been living in the United States for generations and has a firm command of the English language.

Knowledge of Other Cultures

Several strategies can be used to minimize unconscious cultural biases (Churchill, 1995; Lynch & Hanson, 1992):

1. *Engage in an assessment of feelings and attitudes about those from other cultures.* This complements the element of self-awareness.
2. *Learn about other cultures.* A starting point in this process is to ask yourself, and perhaps even make a list describing what you have learned about cultural groups other than your own. After you have made this list, consider what and who were your sources of information and whether the list presents other cultures as generally having positive or negative characteristics.
3. *Learn about the population with whom you have had little experience or prior contact.* Having culture-specific information about the people

5. Investigate forums (e.g., electronic genealogy) on the Internet.
6. Visit county courthouses for marriage records, birth and death records, and titles of land bought, sold, or occupied.
7. Explore church or parish records.
8. Visit public libraries for resources on genealogy.

Note. From "Developing Cross-Cultural Competence: A Guide for Working with Young Children and Their Families," by E. W. Lynch and M. J. Hanson (Eds.), 1992, Baltimore, MD: Brookes. Copyright 1992 by Brookes. Adapted with permission.

you encounter may help explain and illuminate the cultural values, beliefs, and behaviors you experience in cross-cultural situations. A variety of ways exist in which one can learn about other cultures (see box).

4. *Read about and expose yourself to current literature on the topics of diversity, inclusiveness, and racial and cultural awareness.* This will assist you in being informed about the critical inquiry and discussion on the topics, as well as provide you with new tools and approaches in your work with those from various cultures.

5. *Get to know and interact with people and professionals who come from varied academic, racial, and cultural backgrounds.* This contact will give you valuable experience in interacting with many groups of people and demonstrate the vast diversity that is found within any group of people.

6. *Challenge yourself and others by initiating discussions and posing questions about culture and cultural bias in courses, seminars, workshops, and other situations.* This step allows you to demonstrate your commitment to becoming more cross-culturally competent, but often involves some degree of intellectual and psychologic risk.

Cross-Cultural Communication

Beyond merely having conceptual information and discussing the saliency and functions of culture, it is important to understand how to function effectively in cross-cultural situations, particularly in terms of issues related to cross-cultural communication. In addition to remembering that individual differences and subgroup differences exist in all cultures, the practitioner should be sensitive to how a family defines themselves, what a family values, the needs the family articulates, and the way the family describes their race, ethnicity, and culture. It is also valuable to be mindful of differences in styles of communication. For example, some people from a particular cultural group may use a louder volume when talking, whereas others may tend to speak softly. A practitioner may mistakenly interpret a person who speaks more loudly as being angry, when actually they are not.

Approaches to Learning About Other Cultures	**E**ngaging in the following activities will help you to accumulate more *accurate* information about cultures different from your own: 1. Study and read about other cultures through poetry, history, biography, and fiction. 2. Work and talk with members of other cultures (e.g., friends, colleagues, neighbors) who are willing to be cultural mediators or guides for you.

Conversely, one may misinterpret a person who speaks in a softer voice as timid, indecisive, or incompetent, which is also an inappropriate assumption (Davidhizar, Dowd, & Bowen, 1998).

A practitioner should also be mindful of the use of personal space and touching. Touching another person may be acceptable in some groups and taboo in others. For example, touching can convey caring and empathy, or in the case of touching someone of a different gender, it may be seen as extremely inappropriate (Davidhizar et al., 1998).

In recent years, increasing numbers of educators of health-care professionals have addressed the need for their students to develop cross-cultural communication skills. In the case of medical schools, however, most programs relegate attending to the development of cross-cultural communication skills to nonclinical years, hindering skills development (Rosen et al., 2004). The Department of Family and Community Medicine at the University of New Mexico has taken a new approach and provides a cross-cultural training workshop designed to teach cross-cultural communication skills to third-year medical students. The workshop teaches cross-cultural awareness, interviewing skills, working with an interpreter, attention to complementary treatments, and consideration of culture in treatment and prevention. Surveys before and after the workshop demonstrated improvement in students' abilities to assess the culture and health beliefs of patients and negotiated issues regarding treatment (Rosen et al., 2004).

Culturally Sensitive Language and Terminology

Although a discussion of terminology may cause some to think about the debate over political correctness, it is important to be sensitive to language. "Amidst the battles over purported 'political correctness' lies one unmistakable reality—respect for the preferences of individuals in groups will enhance communication and the process of learning" (The National Conference for Community and Justice [NCCJ], 1999, p. 100).

3. Participate in aspects (e.g., community projects, holidays) of another culture.
4. Learn the language of another culture.
5. Attend seminars or take courses that focus on the experiences, histories, and issues of other cultures.

Note. From "Developing Cross-Cultural Competence: A Guide for Working with Young Children and Their Families," by E. W. Lynch and M. J. Hanson (Eds.), 1992, Baltimore, MD: Brookes; and "Cultural Countertransference," by M. Churchill, 1995, *Treatment Today, 7*(1), pp. 42–43. Adapted with permission.

Language is a powerful tool by which thoughts are conveyed and meaning is constructed. A culturally sensitive practitioner is intentional in and careful with how he or she uses language to reflect an understanding and desire to accurately communicate thoughts, as well as to respectfully address members of communities that are culturally diverse, complex, and rich.

Just as sensitivity to language is an important component to cross-cultural competency, so is making a special effort to pronounce someone's name correctly. It may be tempting to try to reduce discomfort that sometimes accompanies cross-cultural interactions by avoiding contact with someone of a different cultural background or trying to avoid saying the name of a person who has a less familiar name to the practitioner. For many people, names are an important piece of how they identify themselves and are reflective of their culture. If in doubt on how to pronounce a name, one can ask for the correct pronunciation and make a note of it.

On one level, verbal communication consists of the terminology used to describe the people with whom we interact. People may have a preference for certain terms when referring to themselves as people with a racial, ethnic, and cultural identity. When practitioners are unaware of or lack precision with the language and terminology they use, they risk alienating the people they are charged with assisting.

The following information, compiled by the National Conference for Community and Justice (NCCJ, 1999), discusses terminology commonly used to describe people who share membership in groups such as African American, Asian Pacific American, Caucasian, White, Latino American, and Native American. This list presents suggestions for minimizing the use of insensitive and alienating language and terminology, and it also presents areas of sensitivity for members of different racial and ethnic groups. These suggestions are merely a guide and should be used with caution. Within any group of people, individuals may have preferences for terminology they use to refer to their racial and ethnic group; therefore, a practitioner needs to be careful not only in thinking about what terms to use, but also about how and why to use these terms to make a racial or ethnic distinction. Complicating this process is that many people are bicultural or biracial and thus do not fit easily into one particular category. The following is terminology commonly used to refer to racial and ethnic groups:

- *African Americans.* The terms *African* and *African American* are not synonymous. African refers to the people or language of the continent of Africa, not a country. Some African Americans may prefer the term *black* (with a lowercase "b") or *Black* (with an uppercase "B") to the term *African American.* Do not refer to African Americans as colored, Negro, or minorities.

- *Asian Pacific Americans.* Recent immigrants may have their names written in the style of their homeland. For example, most Chinese names have two parts, family name followed by a personal name. These names may be hyphenated or may run together. It is generally good practice to double check individual preferences for listing their names. The term *Asian* refers to someone of Asian ancestry, but the term *Asian American* or *Asian Pacific American* refers to an American citizen with Asian ancestry. Do not refer to Asians or Asian Pacific Americans as Orientals. Oriental is an adjective that is used to describe an object (e.g., Oriental rug). Refer to people by their national origins (e.g., Chinese, Filipino, Japanese, Korean, Burmese, Vietnamese) if you are aware of their background.

- *Caucasians or Whites.* Americans of European descent may be recent immigrants who prefer to be identified by their national origin (e.g., Irish, Polish). Do not refer to Caucasians or White people as Anglos or WASPs (White Anglo Saxon Protestants). Other terms for Caucasian people are *white* (with a lowercase "w"), *White* (with an uppercase "W"), and *European Americans.*

- *Latino Americans.* Although Latino Americans are often portrayed as undocumented immigrants, many Latino American families have been American citizens for hundreds of years. The terms *Latino* and *Latina* refer to people of Latin American ancestry. Latino and Latina are generally the preferred terms by those in the community and by activists. Latino refers to men and Latina refers to women. The term *Hispanic*, which refers in general to those with Latin American or Spanish roots, is rarely used by these members of the community. When possible, replace the terms Latino and Latina with a specific designation (e.g., Puerto Rican, Cuban, Mexican).

- *Native Americans.* Native Americans usually identify with a particular tribal nation (e.g., Cherokee). It is good practice to ask them their preferred tribal identification. Recognize that the terms *American Indian* and *Native American Indian* are used interchangeably; however, some individuals may have a preference. Do not refer to American Indians as Redskins, Indians, or minorities.

Communication Styles

The first element of communication styles is nonverbal communication. Nonverbal communication encompasses such things as eye contact and facial expressions. Although a set of behaviors or gestures may look identical between two cultures, in different cultures these gestures can hold different meanings. For example, brief glances versus prolonged eye contact may be interpreted as sincerity, trustworthiness, and directness, or as disrespect and shame. Cultures also vary in the display of affect. Some cultures may demonstrate emotions through facial expressions, whereas others do not.

Another element is proximity and touching. Some cultures prefer communicating at an arm's length (approximately 3 feet) or closer, whereas people from other cultures prefer communicating from a greater distance. One way to tell a person's comfort with social distance is whether they back up during conversation (indicating discomfort with how close the other person is standing) or move closer. Interpreting touching is more complex because some of the factors that influence what is appropriate include gender, age, religion, and personal preference. For example, in some cultures, patting someone on the head or using the left hand to touch another is inappropriate and is associated with bodily waste (Lynch & Hanson, 1992).

A final element of communication style is body language, which refers to various body positions and posture. Gestures are encompassed in body language and are used to supplement or substitute for verbal communication. Gestures include the speed and range of arm movements, presence of head nodding, and pointing.

Effective Cross-Cultural Communication

Because cross-cultural interactions and communication are so complex and varied, it may be tempting to want to avoid engaging in such interactions. However, cultivating competence in cross-cultural situations requires a willingness to engage in such interactions and a willingness to explore differences with openness and respect, as well as using these interactions as opportunities to dispel myths and gain greater understanding (see Case Study 10.1). According to Lynch and Hanson (1992), some examples of effective cross-cultural communication include

- showing respect to individuals from other cultures;
- making multiple and sincere attempts to understand others' points of view;
- being open to learning new things;
- being flexible;
- having a sense of humor;
- possessing the ability to tolerate ambiguity;
- having an appreciation of other cultures; and
- having a desire to learn about those from other cultures.

Case Study 10.1
Creative Communication

While a Latino family was on a trip in the United States, their adolescent daughter, Maria, was diagnosed with cancer. The family decided to prolong their stay in the United States while their daughter received treatment at a U.S. hospital. The family's primary language was Spanish.

At the hospital where Maria was receiving treatment, the pediatric unit's child life program frequently used the services of an artist-in-residency program. In this program, artists are trained to use the arts in hospital settings, thus providing a form of support and a creative outlet for children facing the hospital experience.

The child life coordinator requested that an artist work with Maria and her sister. The artist was provided with written information about Maria's age, date of admission, diagnosis, and a note indicating that the family spoke little English. Because the artist spoke no Spanish, she was concerned about how she would communicate with Maria and her family.

When the artist went to Maria's room, she found that Maria, her parents, and her younger sister were present, as well as several members of the extended family. When the artist entered the room, the family was speaking in Spanish. Because of the artist's lack of Spanish-speaking skills, the artist used gestures and pointed to the supplies to indicate the purpose of her visit. The family briefly spoke some Spanish among themselves and then by using gestures, the family welcomed the artist into the room and expressed interest in doing the activity.

As the artist assembled her supplies, Maria and her younger sister expressed their excitement and curiosity about the project. The children had a Spanish/English primer, which had Spanish words and their English equivalents listed together. Along with the use of gestures, this primer served as the primary means for communication between the artist and the children during the session. To communicate, the children would use the primer to say words in English and the artist would use the primer to say words in Spanish. The children often smiled and giggled as the artist tried to pronounce words in Spanish, and the children often repeated the correct pronunciation and encouraged the artist to repeat mispronounced words. When the artist would say a word correctly, the children would say "good" or "very good." The children also used this as a time to practice their English.

The session ended with the children having an assortment of colorful beads that they made using polymer clay. In this session, the children also had an opportunity to interact with a member of the health-care team in a way that allowed them to have a sense of power and mastery through language. Working with these children also allowed the artist to develop her language and communication skills, and have the experience of being taught and helped by the people she was assigned to help.

This experience illustrates that while verbal language is an important mechanism for communication, there are many ways, including nonverbal, to express thoughts. Although the lack of language skills of the artist was anxiety-producing, her openness to *trying* to speak Spanish and allowing the children to teach her helped them feel a sense of mastery in the hospital.

Techniques for Effective Cross-Cultural Communication	1. Speak slowly and clearly. 2. Pause more frequently. 3. Use simple sentences. 4. Use active verbs. 5. Repeat each important idea. 6. Use visual measurements such as graphs or pictures. 7. Act out and demonstrate. 8. Focus on nonverbal behavior. 9. Remember that silence is communication. Listen. 10. Check comprehension.

Communication can take on increased importance in health-care settings in which comprehension may be critical to the health and welfare of a child or may have ethical implications. The box offers some techniques to facilitate effective cross-cultural communication. However, hospitals and other health-care institutions and agencies that are committed to providing culturally competent care offer written materials and signage translated into the languages most common in the populations they serve, have interpreters available to families within a reasonable period of time, and keep resource lists of agencies and individuals who can help when serving families from cultures less common to the area.

Conclusion

Throughout this chapter, the saliency and complexity of culture are mentioned in terms of how humans perceive the world and behave in it. For a child, the role of culture may manifest itself in a number of ways. For example, depending on a child's culture and other factors such as age and gender, children may exhibit different responses to pain or ways of relating to authorities. Some children may be very vocal when experiencing pain while others may be more stoic. Some children may desire comfort from physical contact through hugs while others may be less comfortable with initiating or receiving hugs. Some children may feel comfortable in having direct eye contact with those in authority positions, while other children may look away from an adult. By observing how the family interacts with the child, the practitioner can gain useful clues about what is culturally appropriate.

This chapter mainly focused on issues of cross-cultural competence on an individual level. One can argue that this is an appropriate focus for several reasons, particularly because we each possess the capacity to become more informed about ourselves and others and behave in a way that can help us work effectively and compassionately with others, especially if they come from a culture that is different from our primary cultural orientation.

Practitioners working in multicultural contexts should actively cultivate an awareness of self and others, and develop the skills to help to interact effectively with a variety of people. Research indicates that although nurses and other practitioners have identified a need for further education in meeting the cultural needs of their patients (Narayanasamy, 2003), much work is needed in this area. Regarding medical education, for example, a recent survey by the AAP revealed that despite the importance of culture in health care and the rapid growth of ethnic diversity in the United States and Canada, most medical schools in these countries provide inadequate instruction about cultural issues (Flores, Gee, & Kastner, 2000). Fisher, Bowman, and Thomas (2003) believe that teaching cultural issues in medical schools is not enough; content should be included at all levels—undergraduate, graduate, and continuing medical education.

Essential to the development of cross-cultural competence is the integration of education and training in the process of lifelong learning (AAP Committee on Pediatric Workforce, 1999). To complement individual efforts, it is also valuable to consider ways that the health-care industry or a particular organization can help create an environment that reflects the demographics of the child and family, and employs professionals that come from diverse backgrounds, therefore reflecting a rich array of cultures, perspectives, experiences, and styles.

Three possibilities for developing cross-culturally competent organizations include (a) encouraging and recruiting people of color into the human service professions, (b) providing staff development sessions covering the topic of intercultural competence, and (c) actively working to change practices that discriminate against people of color (Lynch & Hanson, 1992). Some may think that these changes can only be instituted by those administrators at the uppermost ranks in the organization, but each person has the power and responsibility to raise questions or concerns about discriminatory practices. Speaking on behalf of cultural fairness takes courage, much in the same way becoming a member of the health-care field takes courage to confront issues of illness, injury, and death.

Study Guide

1. Define *culture* and *cultural identity*.

2. What purpose does culture serve?

3. How does culture influence children's perceptions of and reactions to health care?

4. How can lack of common cultural reference affect the health care of children and their families?

5. Discuss factors that mediate culture's effects and list two to three ways in which these factors may affect children's health care.

6. Describe "cross-cultural competence."

7. List several aspects of cultural sensitivity and competence that are particularly essential to the effective coping of children.

8. Does lack of diversity among health-care providers, such as nurses, affect quality of children's health care? In what ways?

9. How can practitioners' cross-cultural competence enhance children's health care?

10. Discuss methods for improving cultural sensitivity and competence among health-care providers.

References

American Academy of Pediatrics, Committee on Pediatric Workforce. (1999). Culturally effective pediatric care: Education and training issues. *Pediatrics, 103*(1), 167–170.

American Academy of Pediatrics, Committee on Pediatric Workforce. (2000). Enhancing the racial and ethnic diversity of the pediatric workforce. *Pediatrics, 105*(1) (Pt. 1), 120–131.

Banks, M., & Benchot, R. (2001). Unique aspects of nursing care for Amish children. *American Journal of Maternal and Child Nursing, 26*(4), 192–196.

Churchill, M. (1995). Cultural countertransference. *Treatment Today, 7*(1), 42–43.

Cross, T. (1988). Services to minority populations: Cultural competence continuum. *Focal Point, 3*(2), 1–5.

Crow, K., Matheson, L., & Steed, A. (2000). Informed consent and truth-telling: Cultural directions for healthcare providers. *Journal of Nursing Administration, 30*(3), 148–152.

Culley, L. (1997). Ethnicity, health and sociology in the nursing curriculum. *Social Sciences in Health, 3*, 28–40.

Culley, L. (2001). Equal opportunities policies and nursing employment within the British National Health Service. *Journal of Advanced Nursing, 33*(1), 130–137.

Danielson, C. B., Hamel-Bissell, B., & Winstead-Fry, P. (Eds.). (1991). *Families, health, and illness: Perspectives on coping and intervention.* Boston: Mosby.

Davidhizar, R., Dowd, S. B., & Bowen, M. (1998). The educational role of the surgical nurse with the multicultural patient and family. *Today's Surgical Nurse, 20*(4), 20–24.

Derman-Sparks, L., & A. B. C. Task Force. (1989). *Anti-bias curriculum: Tools for empowering young children.* Washington, DC: National Association for the Education of Young Children.

Fisher, J. A., Bowman, M., & Thomas, T. (2003). Issues for South Asian Indian patients surrounding sexuality, fertility, and childbirth in the U.S. health care system. *Journal of the American Board of Family Practice, 16*, 151–155.

Flores, G., Gee, D., & Kastner, B. (2000). The teaching of cultural issues in U.S. and Canadian medical schools. *Academic Medicine, 75*(5), 451–455.

Geissler, E. M. (1993). *Pocket guide to cultural assessment.* St. Louis, MO: Mosby.

Gerrish, K., Husband, C., & Mackenzie, J. (1996). *Nursing for a multi-ethnic society.* Buckingham, England: Open University Press.

Health Resources and Services Administration. (2001). *2000 Sample Survey of RNs.* Washington, DC: Author.

Hedayat, K., & Pirzadeh, R. (2001). Issues in Islamic biomedical ethics: A primer for the pediatrician. *Pediatrics, 108*(4), 965–971.

Igoa, C. (1995). *The inner world of the immigrant child.* Mahwah, NJ: Erlbaum.

Lynch, E. W., & Hanson, M. J. (Eds.). (1992). *Developing cross-cultural competence: A guide for working with young children and their families.* Baltimore: Brookes.

McEvoy, M. (2003). Culture and spirituality as an integrated concept in pediatric care. *American Journal of Maternal and Child Nursing, 28*(1), 39–43.

Narayanasamy, A. (2003). Transcultural nursing: How do nurses respond to cultural needs? *British Journal of Nursing, 12*(3), 185–194.

Orlandi, M. A. (Ed.). (1992). *Cultural competence for evaluators: A guide for alcohol and other drug abuse prevention practitioners working with ethnic/racial communities* (DHHS Publication No. 92–60067). Rockville, MD: U.S. Department of Health and Human Services.

Randall-David, E. (1989). *Strategies for working with culturally diverse communities and clients.* Washington, DC: Association for the Care of Children's Health.

Rollins, J., & Riccio, L. (2001). *ART is the heART: An arts in healthcare program for children and families in home and hospice care.* Washington, DC: WVSA Arts Connection.

Rosen, J., Spatz, E., Gaaserud, A., Abramovitch, H., Weinreb, B., Wenger, N., & Margolis, C. (2004). *Medical Teaching, 26,* 126–132.

Smith, D. (1995). The dynamics of culture. *Treatment Today,* 7(1), 15.

Sue, D. W., & Sue, D. (1990). The culturally skilled counselor. In D. W. Sue & S. Sue (Eds.), *Counseling the culturally different: Theory and practice* (2nd ed., pp. 159–172). New York: Wiley.

The National Conference for Community and Justice. (1999). *Building bridges with reliable information: A quick guide about our community's people.* Washington, DC: Author.

United States Bureau of Census. (2001). *Overview of race and Hispanic origin: Census 2000 brief.* Retrieved July 22, 2004, from www.census.gov/prod/2001pubs/c2kbr01-1.pdf

United States Department of Agriculture. (1986). *Cross cultural counseling: A guide for nutrition and health counselors.* Washington, DC: U.S. Deparment of Health and Human Services.

Wayman, K., Lynch, E., & Hanson, M. (1990). Home-based early childhood services: Cultural sensitivity in a family systems approach. *Topics in Early Childhood Special Education,* 10(4), 56–75.

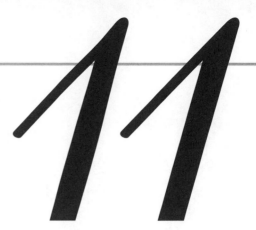

Ethical, Moral, and Legal Issues in Children's Health Care

Teresa A. Savage

Objectives

At the conclusion of this chapter, the reader will be able to:

1. Discuss the history of concern for, and identification of, ethical and legal issues in child health care.

2. Outline current legal, moral, and ethical issues in child health care, and draw implications for working with children in those settings.

3. Analyze the legal, moral, and ethical aspects of children making their own health-care decisions, versus parents, versus health-care professionals.

4. Discuss the emerging issues in children's health care and hypothesize future ethical, moral, and legal issues.

*A*s we entered the new millennium, some ethical issues in children's health care persisted, and some new ones have appeared. In the last 3 decades, health care for children has changed. Examples of changes include (a) improved neonatal and pediatric intensive care; (b) improved management for chronic illnesses; (c) recognition for improved communication during the dying process; (d) improvements in transplantation care; and (e) the emphasis on outpatient, home, and school settings, rather than the hospital, for delivery of health care. There has been, and continues to be, discussion of the child's rights, including the right to consent and the right to be included in clinical research. Violence perpetrated by children has been increasing, and some of society's response has been to hold children more responsible by treating them like adults in the criminal justice system. The burgeoning economy of the past decade stimulated much discussion of the need for better health-care coverage, but today more children remain without health-care insurance than ever before. This chapter will review some of the familiar issues, such as treatment decisions for the very small or very sick newborns, allocation issues, and research on children, but will also challenge conventional thinking on these issues and raise new issues to be faced.

Ethics and Ethical Decision Making in Health Care

Since the birth of bioethics in the 1970s, a great deal has been written about ethics and ethical decision making in health care. How to decide and who should decide are the central questions. For children, parents are the surrogate decision makers. Many of the ethical issues posed by various clinical situations revolve around the parents' responsibility to make treatment decisions for their children. The settings may be different, such as the neonatal intensive care unit, the outpatient clinic, the school, the research office, or the juvenile justice system, but parents or a legal guardian must decide what is in the child's best interests.

A number of approaches have been used for identifying and analyzing ethical issues in health care. The most popular approach is principlism, or the application of ethical principles. Autonomy, beneficence, nonmaleficence, and justice are the four primary principles most often mentioned in health-care ethics. In children's health care, autonomy would be exercised by parents, but the child's developing autonomy is important, especially in light of chronic or terminal illness. Beneficence (doing good) and nonmaleficence (preventing harm) undergird decisions for children, such as mandatory immunizations programs or the inclusion of children in clinical drug trials. Justice—how society allocates benefits and burdens—is seen in decisions regarding access to scarce resources, equitable selection in research, and supportive services for children with chronic illnesses or disabilities and their families. Application of principles sometimes falls short in facilitating decision making, but may help clarify the priorities and values of the parents and health-care providers.

Another approach is the ethic of care, which goes beyond applying principles to viewing the issue in its context. Gilligan (1982) first described this approach when studying women who were contemplating abortion. She found that the women considered the context of their situations, strove to preserve relationships, and made choices to relieve burdens, even if it meant self-sacrifice. The use of principles as a framework to unravel the complexities in clinical situations is helpful. Applying a principlism approach with an ethics of care approach, health-care providers can appreciate the values of the parents' and their own values in the context of a particular case. Combining both methods of analyzing a case is helpful in resolving the immediate clinical problems. Using the case as a way to learn and teach ethical decision making in the clinical setting is called *casuistry*.

Health-care providers see similar scenarios in their specialties—the preterm newborn, the child who needs an organ transplant, the adolescent who refuses treatment, the parents who want extraordinary treatment for their child. How these cases are approached guides future decisions in a heuristic manner. Health-care providers learn from casuistry, the application of ethical principles to specific cases, which then become instructive for future cases. This chapter follows a casuist format, using cases to illustrate ethical issues and ways to address those issues.

Decision Making for Children

Parents are responsible for making decisions, including health-care decisions, for their minor children. It is presumed that the parents have their children's best interests at heart. Parents' decisions are rarely challenged, and only if the decision appears to be against the child's interests. A common example in the health-care setting is the use of blood in treating children whose parents are Jehovah's Witnesses. When a life-threatening condition exists, and a blood transfusion is determined to be medically necessary to save the life of the child, parents are fully informed and asked for their consent. Parents who are Jehovah's Witnesses may refuse their consent because blood transfusions are forbidden by their religion. The physician has the option of seeking temporary custody for the purposes of consenting to the blood transfusion, and often this route is quickly accomplished through administrative channels in hospitals. The courts grant this shift of custody based on the belief that children should not forfeit their lives on the chance that they would choose their parents' religion upon reaching adulthood. Further discussion of conflict between parents and health-care providers will be discussed later.

Parents, as surrogate decision makers for their children, make health-care decisions based on the family's beliefs, values, and wishes. As children grow and mature, parents inculcate their beliefs and values. Although children may have specific preferences and wishes, parents are empowered to make the decisions regardless of a child's agreement or dissent. Not only is this paternalism acceptable, it is expected. In the case of an adult patient who is unable to make a health-care decision (lacks decisional capacity), a surrogate decision maker is expected to make decisions using the substituted judgment standard. The surrogate knows the wishes of the patient and, acting as the patient's substitute, relays those wishes as the patient would. The patient, having reached adulthood, had the capacity to make decisions and share beliefs, preferences, and wishes with the surrogate over time. Substituted judgment does not work with children because children are thought to lack decisional capacity until they reach adulthood. The age of majority, determined by state statute, is an arbitrary age, usually 18 or 21 years of age. Recognizing the arbitrariness of the age, health-care providers may wish to include the child in the decision-making process.

When a child requires a medical intervention, informed consent is sought from the parent or guardian. Additionally, the physician or nurse will discuss the proposed intervention in terms understandable to the child. Depending upon the intervention and its degree of necessity, the child's cooperation is sought, but the intervention may be performed without cooperation. Infants are given immunizations despite their crying and older children are restrained to have blood drawn when they are unable to cooperate. Nurses and other pediatric health-care providers demonstrate respect for the child through various methods of soliciting cooperation, but at times realize that it may be necessary to "force" a child to accept an intervention.

In 1995, the American Academy of Pediatrics (AAP) Committee on Bioethics issued a position statement on informed consent, parental permission and assent in pediatric practice. The Committee recognizes that consent involves making judgments for oneself and one's "unique personal beliefs, values, and goals" (AAP Committee on Bioethics, 1995, p. 315). Therefore, parents do not give "consent" but do give their informed permission. Three categories of consent were recommended. The first category relates to a child who lacks decisional capacity, and for whom parents make the decision unless there is evidence of parental abuse or neglect. The second category refers to the child whose capacity for decision making is developing but not yet sufficient, and in these cases the parents give permission but assent must be obtained from the child. The third category is for the child who has decisional capacity; he or she should be approached for consent. Parents would be consultants to the child, but the child's consent or refusal would be honored. No age level is assigned to the categories, nor is a method of assessment of decisional capacity presented. The assessment of decisional capacity is left to the health-care provider seeking consent.

It is generally accepted that capacity to consent is made by clinical assessment relative to the decision to be made. For example, assessing a child's capacity to decide which college to attend is different than assessing a child's capacity to decide whether to undergo an amputation for treatment of osteogenic sarcoma. Both decisions have long-ranging implications for the child's future. While both decisions are very important, the decision regarding the amputation is irreversible and potentially lifesaving. Some children at age 10 or 11 years may make either decision; some children at age 17 years may not have the capacity. Grisso and Appelbaum (1998) have identified the following four elements as necessary for the capacity to consent:

1. Understanding of the treatment-related information
2. Appreciation of the significance of the information for the patient's situation
3. Reasoning, which involves comparing alternatives and projecting what the impact could be on the patient's life
4. Expressing a choice

The physician or health-care provider assesses the patient for these elements for informed consent in relation to the decision facing the patient. A formal assessment, however, is done only when the patient's capacity to consent is questioned. For children, because they are presumed to lack capacity and legally are considered incompetent before the age of majority, little attention has been given to assessing their capacity to consent.

Grisso and Vierling (1978) delineated the following abilities children should have to reason:

- the ability to sustain attention to the important issues under discussion
- the ability to deliberate the issues
- the ability to weigh the pros and cons of the options
- the ability to consider the possible risks and the alternatives
- the ability to use both inductive and deductive reasoning

Some children may possess these abilities; some may not. Flavell (1985) found that there was not much difference between early, middle, and late childhood in having cognitive functions to make decisions. The AAP's position statement reflects an attitude shift toward children as autonomous persons. Strongly influenced by Bartholome's work in the "experience, perspective and power of children" (AAP, Committee on Bioethics, 1995, p. 314), the statement pushes the issues of a child's capacity to consent. Some opponents see the statement as going too far.

Ross (1997), a pediatrician and bioethicist, believes that competency is not sufficient for a change in practice. She believes the decisions children make are based on limited experience and subject to impetuosity. In those cases where the child is capable of making the decision, and he or she disagrees with the parents' decision, mechanisms already exist to emancipate the child (if appropriate and by a court order) and honor the child's wishes. Any further government involvement in family decision making is seen as inappropriate and unwanted. Ross challenges the movement to grant decision-making rights to children in the health-care context only. "Why," she asks, "can't a child buy cigarettes or elect to participate in school sports without parental consent?" (1997, p. 43). Child liberationists, by abandoning traditional paternalism, would allow children to make bad decisions. To only honor decisions with which the parents or health-care providers agree is not honoring the child's autonomy. Ross also disagrees with the recommendation that a third party become involved in the decision-making process. Parents' should have the final decision-making authority. Again, mechanisms exist to challenge parents if health-care providers believe that parents are not making decisions in the child's best interests. The AAP recommendations and Ross's critique offer the health-care provider thoughtful arguments for approaching decision making by children.

Both the AAP position and Ross's position use the best interest standard. How does one decide what is in a child's best interests? Kopelman (1997) described the standard in terms of identifying a *threshold*, the *ideal*, and as a *standard of reasonableness*. The issue of "best interests" is raised when parents decide against medical advice, when policymakers strive to improve laws to protect children, and in various court decisions bearing on a child's welfare. Threshold is a point in the process when a decision does not rise to the level of best interests. The level is usually a judgment call by the professionals involved. For example, a child who requires anticonvulsant medication does not bring the medication to school. When reached, the mother tells the school nurse that she has not had time to get the prescription refilled. Is this mother acting in the child's best interests? The threshold for best interests is that the child receives the medication without interruption. The ideal is the course of care that would be followed if there were no barriers (e.g., cost, time, distance). In another example, a child with cystic fibrosis has frequent visits to the emergency room. Parents are advised to put the child on a waiting list for a heart–lung transplant at a center several states away. The child is gravely ill and the only hope for survival is a transplant. The ideal would be that the child would get the transplant and recover to a healthy state. Using that same example, the standard of reasonableness hinges on *if* the child qualifies for the transplant and *if* the family can move to the distant state and afford to live there until the transplant and recovery period is over. How reasonable is it to assume that all parents could or should do this? Most parents may be willing, but do they have the means and is it reasonable to expect parents to do the ideal? The standard of reasonableness allows the best interests standard to be interpreted as what is reasonable in the specific situation with the specific players. Buchanan and Brock (1990) extended the discussion of best interests and reasonableness to this conclusion:

> Not only should the best interest principle as a guidance principle for parents' decision not be understood as requiring literal *optimization* of the child's interests in all cases, but also suitable *intervention* principles will allow parents considerable leeway—tolerating departures from what would be best for the child—in order to protect the family from intrusions that would violate the privacy which it requires if it is to thrive as an intimate union whose value to those who participate in it depends in great part upon its intimacy. (p. 237)

Although parents are the legal decision makers for children, there are some conditions for which parental consent is not needed. Emergency treatment can be provided without parental consent if delay in seeking consent could result in loss of life or greater injury to the child. Each state has non-emergency conditions for which children can be treated without parental consent. State statutes delineate the condition, the age of the child, and in some cases, the duration of the treatment. Conditions may be pregnancy, sexually transmitted diseases, substance abuse, or mental health disorders.

In 1993, the American Academy of Pediatrics issued a policy statement "Consent for Medical Services of Children and Adolescents" (AAP, 1993). The policy was recently revised in response to the development of a number of social, legal, and medical ethics considerations that have a direct impact on the policy (AAP, 2003). For example, the revised policy points out that financial reimbursement for emergency treatment of the unaccompanied minor may affect access to appropriate medical care and patient confidentiality. Although adolescents usually are covered by their family's insurance or by Medicaid, they may not have coverage for unaccompanied care, and they may not have the resources to pay for care themselves. The Emergency Medical Treatment and Active Labor Act (EMTALA) requires that treatment must be provided without consideration of reimbursement issues; however, uncompensated charges may result from the EMTALA requirement of treatment for all without regard to payment. Health-care providers must ensure that the financial issues surrounding a patient's treatment do not result in a breach of patient confidentiality, especially if an unintended parental notification may result for the receipt of an itemized medical bill. The policy statement has been endorsed by the American College of Surgeons, the Society of Pediatric Nurses, the Society of Critical Care Medicine, the American College of Emergency Physicians, the Emergency Nurses Association, and the National Association of EMS Physicians.

Although confidentiality is critical in treating adolescents without parental consent, it is not absolute. When an adolescent's condition may lead to suicide (such as in depression) or death, or if a teenage girl refuses surgery for an ectopic pregnancy, confidentiality may be breached. In ambulatory settings, procedures can be established to inform both parents and adolescents of the parameters for treatment, confidentiality, and when confidentiality could be breached. Strasburger and Brown (1991) suggested a form letter be sent to parents upon a child's 12th birthday notifying the child and parents that the child now qualifies for confidential adolescent health care. In addition, the office will have procedures for alternative billing and dual record keeping to ensure privacy of the encounters when teens desire to see the provider for conditions covered in the state's statutes. Health-care providers for children should be aware of their state's statutes relating to mature and emancipated minors—a designation that means a child under the age of majority can be treated without parental consent—and those statutes that cover specific conditions for which underage children can consent to treatment.

Increasingly, consumer groups are demanding quality health care and are more knowledgeable regarding health-care practices (Williams, 2002). O'Neill (2002) proposed that in such an environment, children need information to enable them to participate in the medical decision-making process. Thus, health-care professions need the ability to establish rapport and trust not only with the parents, but also with the child, through effective communication techniques.

Children with Chronic or Terminal Conditions

With chronic and terminal illness, children gain experience and a certain level of medical sophistication. If the condition is not addressed within the state statute, parental consent must be obtained for health-care decisions, and usually this does not pose a problem. Occasionally, there may be a disagreement, either between health-care providers and parents, or between parents and the child, about what the best course of care should be. For example, an adolescent who was treated for leukemia at a young age has now developed a secondary cancer. Recalling his experience, he refuses treatment and states he prefers to die than to accept surgery, chemotherapy, and radiation. His parents disagree and want him treated with maximal therapies. Health-care providers assess the teen's decisional capacity and are convinced that the teen is making an informed decision. Does it matter if the teen is 13 or 17 years old? According to the AAP position, the decision of the teen should be respected. Ross would say the parents should have final authority. Should the teen be treated against his will? Are there control issues aside from the cancer treatment that are undercurrents in the family relationships? In difficult situations like this, family mediation through a family therapist and ethics consultation to the family and health-care team may help in resolving the conflict.

Adolescence is a time for rebellion and testing limits. Children with chronic conditions who have followed health maintenance practices may be less attentive to these practices, and may suffer complications as a result. Feeling different from peers, the adolescent may wish to deny the chronic condition exists, or may neglect certain habits, such as checking blood glucose or performing self-catheterization. Should adolescents have the freedom to abandon health-preserving, and sometimes lifesaving, practices? Are parents who do not "force" their children to take their medicine, test their blood, or self-catheterize being neglectful? While respecting the developing autonomy of the adolescent, parents are still considered responsible for their children's health care. The degree to which parents should intervene is related to the likely severity of the consequences of noncompliance. Renal failure from hydronephrosis and urinary tract infections may result from forgoing inter-mittent catheterization, but it may take several years before the damage re-sults. Much like cigarette smoking, the results are not immediate and there-fore seem too remote to imagine. Forgoing insulin may result in immediate and unpleasant consequences, serving to reinforce the wisdom of compli-ance. Allowing the teen to test the limits risks the teen befalling harm. The concept of "dignity of risk" applies to the decision to allow the teen to make choices, even potentially harmful choices, in an effort to develop and exercise decision-making abilities. Oberman (1996) would reject this analysis. She finds chronic illness an impedance to developing autonomy, and that it is not surprising to find that adolescents with repeated hospitalizations regress developmentally. She urged an increased skepticism regarding adolescents' abilities to make health-care decisions, especially regarding forgoing life-sustaining treatment.

In conclusion, parents are responsible for health-care decision making for their children. How much to involve the child in the decision-making process is at the discretion of the parents. Health-care providers can help parents understand the capabilities to reason that their children possess, and should work with the parents in effectively communicating with their children, especially around sensitive topics such as sexual activity and termi-nal illness. Throughout the chapter, parental decision making will be revis-ited in the context of treatment decisions for selected conditions affecting children's health.

Ethical Issues Involving Newborns

Some specific ethical issues may be encountered at the time of birth. Three—mandatory newborn screening, circumcision, and imperiled newborns—are explored here.

Mandatory Newborn Screening

Every state and the District of Columbia have mandatory newborn screening for phenylketonuria (PKU) and congenital hypothyroidism (Hiller, Landen-burger, & Natowicz, 1997; Pass et al., 2000). (The reader is referred to Pass et al. for details of newborn screening programs, lists of screened disorders, and consent requirements.) Only two states, Maryland and Wyoming, require informed consent from parents prior to the screening. In the other states, parents are informed that the test will be done unless they have a religious objection. It is presumed that "no reasonable person" would refuse the screening to detect a condition that is treatable, although not curable. Some states have other tests that are part of the newborn screening, such as galactosemia, biotinidase deficiency, maple syrup urine disease, and HIV, to name a few. For example, New York tests for seroprevalence of HIV; however, mothers can indicate if they do not want to be informed of the test results (Kunk, 1998). Although many parents may desire that their newborn be screened for various conditions for which early intervention can eliminate the complications, they may not want screening for untreatable conditions. Since the mapping of the human genome, there is the possibility of screening for genetic conditions that may or may not ever manifest phenotypically. The selection of tests in the newborn screening depends upon each state's legislature and the effective lobbying of interest groups. The addition of screening for certain other conditions (e.g., cystic fibrosis, adult-onset conditions such as familial hypercholesterolemia, hypertrophic cardiomyopathy, long QT) has raised controversy. There is very little discussion in the literature about mandatory newborn screening. Annas (1982) predicted that more screening tests would be added to the newborn screening profile since informed consent was waived, and this has occurred. There has not been a public outcry against mandatory newborn screening without informed consent, but in light of the Human Genome Project, there may be some concern.

Initially, screening for PKU involved testing a wet diaper of a baby who had ingested a protein-based formula or breast milk for 72 hours or more. A positive result meant further testing; a diagnosis of PKU meant a lifetime of special diet without phenylalanine. Best of all, it meant that mental retardation from a metabolic malfunction could be avoided. For other tests that were added to the screening profile, a therapy was available to ameliorate the condition, such as thyroid supplementation for hypothyroidism. One condition being touted for inclusion in the newborn screening is cystic fibrosis. In cystic fibrosis, numerous mutations exist, and no single test can identify all mutations. Only one study has supported early treatment of screened children leading to improved survival rates (Dankert-Roelse, terMeerman, Martijin, tenKate, & Knol, 1989). However, although the pulmonary benefits of early diagnosis have been less well demonstrated (Wang, O'Leary, Fitzsimmons, & Khoury, 2002), newborn screening for cystic fibrosis has been found beneficial for improving nutritional status and early childhood growth (Merell et al., 2003).

Although cystic fibrosis treatment has improved over the last few decades, it is still considered a terminal disease. Does mass mandatory screening, on balance, provide a benefit to the newborn, parents, or public at large? Is the outcome of the newborn's condition improved by the screening? Do the benefits justify waiving parental consent? For adult-onset disorders, there are additional ethical concerns. Four tests for adult-onset cardiovascular disorders, hemachromatosis, familial hypercholesterolemia, hypertrophic cardiomyopathy, and long QT, are being considered for screening in the new-born period (Lashley, 1999). It is hoped that early intervention in these disorders may either prevent their phenotypic expression, or limit their detrimental effect on the body, but as yet no data support this. Like cystic fibrosis, there are many mutations for familial hypercholesterolemia, so a single test may produce a false negative. Because the technology is, or will be, available for screening more and more conditions in a newborn, is it a benefit to do this? The American Academy of Pediatrics issued a position statement limiting the use of genetic testing in children of late-onset conditions (2001), as has the American Society of Human Genetics and American College of Medical Genetics Report (1995). Informed consent involves the weighing of the benefits or potential benefits against the harms or possible harms. Can the harms be known? There is a fear of discrimination and stigma should an abnormal condition, or risk of an abnormal condition, be identified and the results placed in a medical record. This knowledge of the abnormal finding can affect the newborn who was tested, the parents, and possibly extended family who may be carriers of the abnormality. Will this knowledge affect the family relationships, the parent–infant attachment, and later, the child's self-image? Legislation prohibiting discrimination based on genetic test results has not been adopted in all states and there currently is no federal legislation. Many ethical issues must be considered, and if these tests are added to the newborn screening as it is currently performed in 48 states, parental consent is presumed. The implications of genetic testing are far-reaching, and although inclusion in the newborn screening may not cause a public uproar, the lack of informed parental consent is bothersome. Much more needs to be known about the presence of genetic markers and the effect on the child, family, and society by learning of these markers in the newborn period.

Questions also arise about genetic testing in children after the newborn period. The American Society of Clinical Oncology (ASCO) recently revisited this issue and updated its 1996 ASCO Statement on Genetic Testing for Cancer Susceptibility (American Society of Clinical Oncology, 2003). Regarding testing of children for cancer susceptibility, ASCO recommended that the decision to offer testing to potentially affected children should consider the availability of evidence-based risk-reduction strategies and the probability of developing a malignancy during childhood. When risk-reduction strategies exist or the cancer predominantly develops in childhood, ASCO believes that the parents have the right to choose or reject testing. In situations where increased risk of a childhood malignancy is absent, ASCO recommended delaying genetic testing until the individual is of a sufficient age to make an informed decision regarding such tests.

Circumcision

The American Academy of Pediatrics estimates that 1.2 million male infants are circumcised each year, despite past position papers that did not support routine neonatal circumcision (AAP Task Force on Circumcision, 1999). In

1989, after reviewing research on the relationship between circumcision and sexually transmitted diseases and urinary tract infection, the AAP modified its position paper to acknowledge that there may be a medical benefit for some infants, but that there are also risks, so the parents should be fully informed before consent is obtained. Revisiting the position statement in 1999, the AAP reiterated the position against *routine* neonatal circumcision; however, the decision is ultimately left to parents. Parents may consider their values, culture, ethnicity, and religious practices when making the decision. The AAP's position statement on female circumcision (AAP, Committee on Bioethics, 1998), referred to as *female genital mutilation* (FGM), does not acknowledge the family's values, culture, ethnicity, and religious practices. The Council on Scientific Affairs (1995) of the American Medical Association recommended all U.S. physicians oppose female genital mutilation. The United States has outlawed performing FGM on girls under 18 years of age. As abhorrent as FGM seems to be, the inconsistency between the tolerance for male circumcision and the prohibition against female circumcision bears further discussion.

Neonatal circumcision on males is a common procedure, done at the parents' request. In the past, no anesthesia or analgesia was used, and there is reason to believe that the procedure is still performed without attention to pain relief in many places (Maxwell & Yaster, 1999). In a "dispassionate analysis," Learman (1999) waded through the research of the proposed advantages and risks, both physical and psychological. He concluded that neonatal circumcision is a "health-neutral, cost-neutral intervention, especially when effective anesthesia is used" (Learman, 1999, p. 849), and it will probably continue as routine because of parents' health beliefs or religious practices and the desire for father–son concordance. In the United States, approximately 60% of male newborns are circumcised for nonreligious reasons (Goldman, 1999), although more than 80% of the men in the rest of the world are uncircumcised. Although male circumcision is not also called "genital mutilation," Goldman argued that circumcision is a cosmetic surgery done electively at the request of the parents, surrogate decision makers for the infant. He further argues that by the *Diagnostic and Statistical Manual of Mental Disorders* (*DSM–IV*; American Psychiatric Association, 1994) criteria, the psychologic parameters of assault, torture, and a threat to physical integrity are present; therefore, circumcision qualifies as trauma. The infant is physically restrained and his body is cut, often without benefit of anesthesia or analgesia. Goldman noted that parents make the decision about circumcision regardless of the discussion of risks and benefits, but based on their beliefs, religious practices, and whether the father, brother, or other male relatives have been circumcised. To this, Goldman responded that if uncircumcised men desired to look like other men, the rate of adult circumcision would be higher than 3 in 1,000. In the rest of the vast pro and con literature on neonatal circumcision, the conclusion is that parents should make the decision in their infant's best interests. If the decision to circumcise is left to the parents, what about the parents who seek circumcision for their daughter? Why is there such strong opposition to female circumcision, or FGM?

The procedures for FGM vary more than those for male circumcision. The AAP (AAP, Committee on Bioethics, 1998) described three types of female circumcision, although these types may vary within their categories as well. The first type involves the removal of the clitoral hood, the entire clitoris, or a puncture through the clitoris. The second type is the removal of the clitoris and labia minora. The third, called *infibulation*, is the same as the second, only the labia majora are cut and the raw edges sewn together covering the urethra and most of the vaginal opening. On the wedding night, the husband may need to cut this band of skin for the penis to penetrate the vagina for intercourse. Not restricted to a geographic area, the practices of FGM follow more ethnic and cultural lines. In the cultures that perform FGM, it is accepted as a rite of passage, necessary for the integration of the girl into her culture and to ensure eligibility for marriage. It permits mother–daughter concordance. Parents, deciding for their newborn daughter, may wish to integrate her into their society by having the procedure done in the newborn period, or they may wait until the child is older, even at the onset of menses. The reasons for the procedure are usually the same as reasons for male circumcision. One main difference is that FGM is usually performed by barbers (Toubia, 1994), older female relatives, or other untrained laypeople. A sharp, nonsterile object, such as a glass, razor, or sharp stone is used to cut. As with neonatal male circumcision, the girl is physically restrained, her body cut, and no anesthesia or analgesia is given. Although complications can arise from male circumcision, the likelihood of complications arising from FGM is great. There may be hemorrhage and shock, septicemia, gangrene, tetanus, keloid formation, urinary tract infection, pelvic inflammatory disease, and infertility. Performing FGM has been illegal in the United States since 1997 (Gibeau, 1998). Because FGM has been outlawed for children under 18 years of age in many countries, parents who want their daughters circumcised find nonprofessionals, usually within their own group, to perform the procedure. Toubia (1994) estimated that 6,000 girls are circumcised every day somewhere in the world.

Suppose that female circumcision were available as male circumcision, to be performed at the parents' request, under sterile conditions, and with attention to pain relief. What would be the objections then? It is an unnecessary procedure, but so is breast augmentation, which is done for a woman to meet her perception of the cultural norms of beauty and attractiveness. It offers no health benefit and, even if performed under aseptic conditions, can result in decreased sexual sensation, difficult and painful intercourse, and dangerous childbirth. Because it is also illegal for a health-care provider to reinfibulate the woman after childbirth, the circumcised woman may be distressed after childbirth with the appearance of her genitalia. Some women believe that intercourse is more pleasurable for the husband when his wife has been circumcised. Does the woman's desire to sexually satisfy her husband qualify as a "health benefit" to the woman? Our society permits cosmetic surgery to satisfy patients' perceptions of what is acceptable appearance (e.g., rhinoplasty, breast augmentation or reduction, liposuction, blepharoplasty, hair transplants, hair removal). Cosmetic surgery decisions are usually made by adults, but young girls may wish to have plastic surgery, such as rhinoplasty, while they are still under 18 years of age. A rhinoplasty may not have a physical health benefit, but may have a huge psychological benefit to the child and her parents. Why should parents be permitted to consent to other cosmetic surgeries but not to FGM?

There has to be a "middle ground" in respecting the cultural beliefs and practices of others and protecting children. U.S. society, even though it is becoming more pluralistic, rejects female circumcision as a barbaric, repressive practice without any merit. The reasons for its origin (to ensure and protect women's chastity from warring tribes and to prove a bride's virginity) are, arguably, no longer relevant, and the practice is perpetuated as a custom. As with male circumcision, the customs are deeply rooted and hard to abolish. It is useful to think about the arguments in favor of FGM (traditional practice, concordance between mother and daughter), which are *rejected* as being inherently coercive and oppressive, and how those arguments are used to *defend* routine neonatal male circumcision. Both male and female circumcisions are performed because they are traditional practices and they provide concordance between parents and their children of the same sex. Parents, as surrogate decision makers, usually have wide latitude in making decisions for their children. Approaches endorsing informed consent for routine male circumcision perpetuates the practice. If both female and male circumcision decisions are seen as a matter for parental informed consent, and the U.S. public may see the parallel arguments and their weaknesses, perhaps there will be a more careful consideration of the real benefits of the procedure to the child. Applying the informed consent approach to decisions on female circumcision, however, would mean that FGM could continue. Until society sees the arguments against routine male circumcision as morally compelling as against FGM, routine male circumcision will be viewed as another childrearing option.

Imperiled Newborns

Neonates who require intensive care treatment following birth are often referred to as *imperiled newborns*. They are imperiled—in danger of dying or suffering injury—because they are not able to live without specialized care. Such infants may have been born prematurely, experienced perinatal complications, or have problems with organs or organ systems interfering with normal functioning. Since the advent of neonatal care in the 1950s, infant mortality and morbidity have improved for imperiled newborns. Infants weighing less than 1 pound (450 grams) have survived; infants with previously lethal conditions, such as hypoplastic left ventricle, can be treated; and infants who are profoundly compromised at birth with Apgar scores of "0" can be successfully resuscitated. Some conditions remain untreatable. An infant born with anencephaly cannot survive an extended period without technologic assistance; however, infants with anencephaly pose a unique ethical problem that will be addressed later in this chapter.

Neonatal care has improved survival for preterm infants. In the early 1970s, the threshold of viability was around 28 weeks gestation. Today, infants born at 24 weeks gestation are considered viable, although not much progress has been made in lowering this threshold in the last 10 years. Neonatal care has become more sophisticated with the regionalization of neonatal care into perinatal centers; the proliferation of neonatal nurse practitioners; and research on neonatal medical treatment, nursing care, and the effect on the family. Widespread use of ventilators was just beginning in the 1970s, with all the concomitant care of pulmonary toileting, blood testing, X-raying, and nasogastric feedings. Iatrogenic problems such as pneumothoraces, pulmonary hemorrhages, and Mikity–Wilson disease (later called bronchopulmonary dysplasia) soon became apparent. Necrotizing enterocolitis was common, as was intraventricular hemorrhage. Parents could visit 24 hours, but could only touch their infants.

Also in the 1970s, Duff and Campbell (1973) published an article in which they acknowledged that 14% of the deaths in their Yale-New Haven Hospital nursery was the result of withholding or withdrawing treatment. The previously taboo subject of "letting babies die" was brought to public attention. The infants whose treatment was withheld or withdrawn were usually considered too small to save. The equipment and the skill of the staff limited the number of infants who could get a trial of neonatal intensive care. As the equipment became available, and the skills of the physicians and nurses improved, smaller and sicker babies were treated in the neonatal intensive care unit (NICU). Infants who in the past were given oxygen via hood and were kept warm were now being aggressively treated with ventilators and medications such as epinephrine and sodium bicarbonate. Some would still die despite aggressive treatment, but others would survive. Those survivors might experience complications of ventilator dependency, malnutrition and rickets, necrotizing enterocolitis necessitating surgery (and resulting in short gut syndrome), and intraventricular hemorrhage resulting in seizures and hydrocephalus. Withdrawal of treatment was considered for infants who suffered short gut syndrome or intraventricular hemorrhage. Withholding of additional lifesaving measures was also discussed with the parents.

Because of Duff and Campbell's article, there was concern that the deliberate withdrawing of life-sustaining treatment, usually in terms of discontinuing intermittent mandatory ventilation or extubation, would be seen as euthanasia. Many hospitals did not have "Do Not Resuscitate" policies; however, there were unit practices of "no codes" or "slow codes" in which resuscitative measures would be withheld or not effectively performed with the intent of resuscitating. Although outcomes could not be predicted, the fear was that infants who experienced a brain hemorrhage, short gut, or ventilator dependency would have a poor quality of life and their parents were informed of the possibility. With parents' agreement, treatment (i.e., the ventilator or cardiopulmonary resuscitation) would be withdrawn or withheld.

Infants who were born full term but experienced complications such as asphyxiation, or had congenital problems such as diaphragmatic hernia also were treated, but might have treatment withdrawn if the outcome looked poor. Criteria were published on selective treatment of infants with spina bifida, which recommended maximal treatment for low-level lesions and non-treatment for high-level lesions (Lorber, 1972). An infant with prolonged hypoglycemia who became flaccid and unresponsive, or an infant with Down syndrome could be left unfed at parents' request. Fost (1999) referred to this period as the era of serious undertreatment of infants who may have survived. It was an infant with Down syndrome who provoked the end of the undertreatment period.

The Baby Doe regulations (1984) came about in response to the death of an infant with Down syndrome. Baby Doe was born in Bloomington, Indiana, in 1982. He had esophageal atresia preventing anything from passing from the esophagus into the stomach. A common complication of Down syndrome, the atresia could be repaired surgically. The parents opted not to treat; they worked in special education and they were familiar with Down syndrome. A pediatrician thought the infant should be transferred to a neonatal intensive care unit where surgery could be performed, but the parents refused. The Indiana Supreme Court upheld the parents' right to make the decision when faced with two diverse medical opinions. The hospital and the state child welfare agency planned to appeal the Indiana Supreme Court decision to the U.S. Supreme Court, but the infant died at 6 days of age.

Margaret Heckler, the Secretary of (then) Health, Education, and Welfare in the Reagan administration, orchestrated the Baby Doe regulations. Section 504 of the Rehabilitation Act of 1973 was invoked, and hospitals that discriminated against infants on the basis of their disabilities were in danger of losing federal funds. Signs in both English and Spanish urged anyone who suspected discrimination to call a toll-free number. After a court challenge, the signs were reduced in size and placed in staff areas only, but the message was clear. The regulations became the Child Abuse Prevention and Treatment Act. The AAP (1984) urged the use of pediatric review committees to avoid judicial intervention. Ethics committees proliferated in hospitals across the nation. Decisions to withhold or withdraw treatment were no longer simply between parents and physicians, but were considered in terms of whether they would hold up to public scrutiny. Very preterm infants, infants with severe asphyxiation, and infants with other trisomies, such as Trisomy 18, were aggressively treated. Some authors argued that the regulations changed practices related to spina bifida or Down syndrome (Carter, 1993), and others maintained that the regulations did not give enough consideration to parents' rights or to infant suffering (Kopelman, Irons, & Kopelman, 1988). Fost (1999) described this time as the era of serious overtreatment. There was probably some overlap between the eras of undertreatment and overtreatment, as evidenced by the publication of a book by parents of a preterm infant whose treatment was continued despite their requests for discontinuation (Stinson & Stinson, 1979).

Since the early 1980s, aggressive treatment became standard. A "wait until certainty" approach before discontinuing treatment was adopted, supplanting a statistical prognostic approach. In the latter approach, the decision to forgo treatment was made if there was a possibility that the child could be disabled. Follow-up data showed reduced mortality, but did not always reflect the morbidity. Survivors had cerebral palsy, mental retardation, seizures, hydrocephalus requiring shunting, and a myriad of sensory deficits. For those who were less affected, attention problems and learning difficulties were reported. Early intervention programs flourished and targeted NICU graduates who were displaying developmental problems or were at risk for those problems. Legislation for integration and inclusion of children with disabilities was passed so that children could attend local schools and receive education as well as speech, occupational, and physical therapies if needed.

Another historical movement that has an impact on neonatal decision making is managed care. Survivors who were technology dependent had no place to go because nursing homes were not equipped to care for them, so some children remained in NICU for years. At a cost of $1,000 to $2,000 per day, upon their discharge or death their bills exceeded $1 million. Parents' insurance would sometimes be adequate, but some policies had caps and parents were expected to pay the bill when their insurance was exhausted. Discontinuing treatment because of parents' inability to pay was unimaginable. Parents were counseled to declare bankruptcy. Health-care reimbursement was changing. The federal government had started to reimburse according to diagnosis-related groups (DRG), although pediatric care was not included initially. Soon to follow, hospitalizations were paid according to diagnosis and complications. Companies purchased insurance plans that provided an incentive for employees to enroll in health maintenance organizations (HMO). For-profit groups began to purchase hospitals and health-care systems and to reorganize delivery of services to reduce costs and maximize profits to shareholders. The state of Oregon developed a system for prioritizing payment of health care for people covered by public aid funds. At the cusp of the cutoff for covered conditions were the extremely low birth weight infants. From a utilitarian perspective, there was little use in covering health-care costs for infants under 500 grams, 23 weeks gestation, or those born with anencephaly (Hadorn, 1991).

What impact does this history have on decision making today? There is still a tension between parental rights to consent or refuse treatment as surrogates for their children and the rights of children to be treated. Although many NICUs will treat the smallest infants, those under 500 grams or 23 weeks gestation, guidelines have been proposed for determining when treatment is obligatory and when its benefits may be ambiguous (Wisconsin Association of Perinatal Care, 1997), and the AAP (2002) issued a clinical report regarding decision making for infants born between 22 and 25 weeks gestation. Even with breakthroughs such as surfactant replacement therapy, jet ventilation, nitrous oxide, and other cutting-edge treatments, mortality has not significantly changed in a decade. Because of the inability to predict disability with certainty, treatment is expected to continue. Some activists in the disability community believe that withholding treatment for a child with disabilities (or probable disabilities) demonstrates a lack of respect and devalues the lives of people with disabilities (Brennan, 1995; Charlton, 1998; Gallagher, 1995; Shapiro, 1994). Others suggest that we are overdue for a specific process-based public policy approach to futility determinations on a case-by-case basis (Clark, 2002).

Parents of children in NICUs need to know the likely course of their child's hospitalization. The "window of opportunity," a point in the course of a child's treatment in which withholding or withdrawal of treatment will result in death, is more difficult to defend. Quality of life determinations are subjective; no one can know the quality of life of another person. Saigal et al. (1999) found that health-care providers underestimate the quality of the lives of children with disabilities, and it is possible that they impart their bias to the parents (Asch, 1998). Catlin (1999) found that most physicians would not choose for their own children the very treatment they are providing. She found that physicians experienced much angst over their duty to treat and their belief that treatment was not always in the infant's and family's best interests. The physicians believed that they were treating at the request of the parents and because if a good outcome was possible, they *had* to treat. Framing it in a moral sense versus a legal sense, most of the physicians felt compelled to treat because that is what they were trained to do. They stated they were eager to have guidelines drafted by their peers, not imposed by the government, so that they could make individual decisions about the appropriateness of treatment (Catlin, 1999). The ethical question has been, Should extremely low birth weight infants who are at risk for disabilities be treated? Since Baby Doe, the question has become, At what point, if ever, is it ethically justifiable to discontinue treatment of infants at risk for disabilities? Is the decision exclusively the parents'?

Of interest are the results of a comparative study of ethical dilemmas in French and American NICUs regarding parental role (Orfali, 2004). France and the United States have opposed models of decision making: parental autonomy in the United States (as described above) and medical paternalism in France. Findings revealed that French physicians do not ask parents for permission to withdraw care (as expected in a paternalistic context); but symmetrically, American neonatologists (despite the prevailing autonomy model) tend not to ask permission to continue. Orfali concluded that the ongoing medical authority on ethics remains the key issue.

Wilder (2000) reviewed outcome literature for extremely preterm infants and drew these conclusions: Resuscitation is not reasonable and not likely to be successful in infants born between 20 and 22 weeks gestation, but should be attempted in infants over 22 weeks gestation. After a trial of therapy, the infant's condition should be reassessed and decisions made regarding continuation of life-sustaining treatment.

Ethics committees provide a forum for discussion, and ethics consultants can be a sounding board for health-care providers and parents. Often an ethics consultant can help focus the questions if communication between parents and the NICU staff breaks down. What are the goals of treatment? What are the expectations of the parents? What is the treatment plan? See Case Study 11.1 for an illustration of a typical case in a NICU.

Case Study 11.1
Matthew and Virgil

Matthew and Virgil were born at 25 weeks gestation to a 38-year-old primipara who conceived on her third in vitro fertilization (IVF) attempt. Mrs. F. delivered despite bedrest and continuous tocolytic infusion. Matthew, the first twin, weighed 600 grams at birth and had Apgars of 1^1, 3^5, and 5^{10}. Virgil weighed 490 grams and had Apgars of 0^1, 1^5, and 3^{10}. The twins were immediately resuscitated at birth and transferred to NICU. They were placed on protocol for infants under 1,000 grams, which included surfactant therapy, oscillator ventilation, hyperalimentation and lipids, and minimal handling. By 72 hours of age, Virgil showed a Grade IV intraventricular hemorrhage (IVH) by ultrasound, seizures, hypotension, and sepsis. Matthew showed a Grade II or III intraventricular hemorrhage, but was hemodynamically stable. Parents were given daily updates, and on Day 3, the attending neonatologist, Dr. M., met with parents and explained how each twin was doing. As he discussed Virgil's IVH, Mr. and Mrs. F. requested that treatment be discontinued. They stated that they had an agreement with their perinatologist that they could "call the shots" and Virgil's "brain damage" was unacceptable. They did not want a child who "drooled and couldn't walk or talk," and if the neonatologist couldn't guarantee that Virgil would be normal, they wanted all treatment to stop. Dr. M. discussed Virgil's possible developmental outcomes and the uncertainty of predicting. He also shared the suggested guidelines for decision making for infants at this gestational age. The parents again reiterated that if there was a chance Virgil would not be normal, they would rather he died. The neonatologist stated that he could not discontinue treatment, but he would place a "Do Not Resuscitate" (DNR) order in the infant's chart. He wrote the order and called the ethics consultant.

The ethics consultant reviewed the twins' charts, spoke with the nurses and residents involved in their care, and met with Dr. M. The parents told the nurses and residents that the preterm labor was unexpected. They scrupulously followed the perinatologist's instruction, so they did not expect any complications. They both were successful in their careers and attributed that success to careful planning and determination. They were elated when this cycle of IVF resulted in twins, but they would be happy if only one survived. The perinatologist had explained to them that if they had a multiple gestation, they could choose to have a fetal selection procedure where "excess fertilized embryos" could be "terminated" and one, two, or three fetuses could continue gestating. They viewed the decision to withdraw treatment equivalent to fetal selection. They wanted the stronger twin to survive. The nurses were surprised by the parents' candor about wanting the strongest to survive. After the parents met with Dr. M. they did not come to Virgil's bedside, only to Matthew's. One nurse shared that she was uncomfortable with Virgil's DNR order since other infants in his condition have not had DNR orders. The social worker also commented that she was surprised about the DNR order.

The following day, Dr. M.'s rotation for the month ended and his associate, Dr. H., became the attending physician of the month. Both Dr. M. and Dr. H. met with the ethics consultant. Dr. M. explained that he believed that it was uncertain that continued treatment was in Virgil's best interest because he was likely to have significant disabilities if he survived. Because the parents wanted to discontinue treatment and he did not think he could withdraw treatment legally, he agreed to a DNR. Dr. H. stated that she did not believe a DNR was appropriate. She believed that because Virgil was only 4 days old, it was too early to tell what his outcome would be. The parents would not bond with him if they expected him to die, so she rescinded the DNR. Dr. H. met with the parents and informed them that in her opinion, the DNR order was inappropriate. It was difficult to prognosticate on the impact of neonatal events, but both Matthew and Virgil deserved further treatment. She suggested that the parents attend the parental support group meeting and talk to other parents. Over the next few days, Matthew continued to stabilize and improve, but Virgil's condition deteriorated. He required increased respiratory and hemodynamic support, and the IVH involved more brain parenchyma. Dr. H. advised the parents that she believed DNR was appropriate at that time. Despite maximal efforts, Virgil was dying. She wanted to maintain current efforts, but not resuscitate if he became bradycardic. The parents agreed. The father stated that he appreciated the efforts of the NICU staff and he was glad that the DNR was instituted when Virgil's outcome was more certain. The mother was angry. She believed that Virgil had to endure 3 more days of suffering.

Discussion. Dr. M. believed that he was mandated to treat Virgil, although he did not believe treatment was in Virgil's best interests. He justified his decision to withhold resuscitation on the basis that he believed that to be disabled is worse than being dead. Dr. M.'s position puts autonomy, parental autonomy, and nonmaleficence—preventing harm—as the priorities in treatment decisions. Dr. H. believed that Virgil's outcome could not be known with certainty. It was likely that he would have had some degree of motoric or mental impairment, but the degree of severity could not be known. She did not think it was fair to deny Virgil the opportunity to receive continued treatment, even if he survived with disability. She also prioritized autonomy, in terms of respect for persons, and viewed Virgil as a person worthy of respect, regardless of ability or disability. Continued treatment was viewed as a good and beneficent act.

Two ethical theories supported the physicians' positions and were in conflict. Dr. M. viewed the consequences of treatment, possible disability, as the reason to withhold treatment. Consequentialism was a form of utilitarianism. Dr. H. took a nonconsequentialist approach and examined the "act" of providing care. In her analysis, the consequences were not important, but the act of rendering treatment and not withholding treatment was obligatory.

The parents, as decision makers for the child, may have analyzed the situation differently. They may have believed that they had the option of withdrawing treatment because they were told they could selectively terminate unwanted fetuses. They may have attempted substituted judgment and tried to imagine what life would be like if disabled. Should the parents have made a decision based on what they believed was in Virgil's best interests or the family's best interests if those interests were not mutually compatible? Baby Doe regulations directed that the infant's best interests should have guided the decisions, but was this reasonable? Who would be responsible for the child after hospital discharge, and for the rest of the child's life? Was there a single, correct decision?

Disability advocates recognize that parents are placed in an untenable position of having to choose between their family's goals and one child's survival. Attitudes toward people with disabilities; services for people with disabilities, such as education, health care, employment, housing, leisure pursuits, and transportation; and assumptions about the quality of life of people with disabilities do not reflect a society that values people with disabilities. The interest and support for the Human Genome Project and for physician-assisted suicide reveal society's search for answers in eliminating disabilities and suffering. Eliminating disabilities and suffering could take the shape of eliminating people through the termination of the pregnancy of a fetus with a genetic anomaly or opting for assisted suicide. Physician-assisted suicide is only available to adults who qualify in Oregon, the same state that began rationing health care to the poor. The Netherlands, which has not prosecuted physicians for performing voluntary euthanasia, recently debated the merits of permitting adolescents to request voluntary euthanasia without parental consent. The proposal was not approved by Dutch Parliament, but the Dutch experience and its evolution into involuntary euthanasia of infants and the elderly bears watching (van der Heide et al., 1997). Assisted suicide may seem removed from the pediatric area in the United States, but the attitudes it engenders affect attitudes toward children with disabilities (Pellegrino, 1998).

Ethical Issues Involving Children

Other ethical issues surface after the newborn period. Those concerning children with disabilities, brain death, children with neurobehavioral disorders, children in the juvenile justice system, and research on children are discussed here.

Children with Disabilities

A number of conditions in children beyond the newborn period pose similar ethical questions. When, if ever, is it justifiable to withhold or withdraw life-sustaining treatment? Children who have disabilities such as cerebral palsy, mental retardation, or other significant developmental disabilities challenge society to question what is in these children's best interests. As stated above, much of the affective positions toward children with disabilities stem from the presumption that their quality of life is poor. Research has shown that both health-care providers (Saigal et al., 1999) and nondisabled laypeople underestimate the quality of life of people with disabilities (Albrecht & Devlieger, 1999). The question may be that the quality of the family life is profoundly affected, but not all families view the experience of having a child with significant disabilities as negative (Savage, 2000). Depending upon support for the family for round-the-clock care of the child with disabilities, families can be resilient. Singer et al. (1999) found that the resiliency of mothers of children with severe disabilities exacted a psychologic toll, mediated by feelings of mastery and satisfaction in parenting.

Since Baby Doe, there has been a growing ethical consensus toward treatment of imperiled newborns and children with disabilities (Shevell, 1998). Two major pieces of legislation support this movement—the Individuals with Disabilities Education Act and the Americans with Disabilities Act. Beyond the battles in the hospital, parents have had to fight for educational programs appropriate to their children's needs. In the 1970s, Public Law 94-142, the Education for All Handicapped Children's Act of 1975 was passed. It was renamed the Individuals with Disabilities Education Act (IDEA) in 1990 (Public Law 101-476) and has four main provisions:

- parental involvement in the educational plan,
- least restrictive environment,
- an individual education plan (IEP), and
- multidisciplinary assessment of needs.

Children with disabilities were to be included in classroom activities and other school activities and not segregated. One major advantage of this integration is the education of the nondisabled students about children with disabilities. Integration of children with disabilities into the community can have a favorable impact on their attitudes toward people with disabilities.

To facilitate the integration into the community, the Americans with Disabilities Act (ADA) was passed in 1990. ADA's intent was to protect people with disabilities against discrimination in the workplace and in public. Access to public transportation, public buildings, movie theaters, restaurants, and physicians' offices were examples of the intent of the law. A decade later it is still being tested in court as to the applicable disorders covered by the ADA and the extent to which people must comply. Recently when patrons in a wheelchair were not able to enter Clint Eastwood's restaurant in California, a lawsuit was filed. Mr. Eastwood testified before Congress that he perceived the ADA as a means for lawyers to line their pockets, and he chose to fight the lawsuit at an expense probably greater than the cost of remodeling the entrance to his restaurant (Johnson, 2000). Such a public example of resistance to accommodations indicates there is still a long way to go before people with disabilities have equity in society.

Children with Brain Death

With the ability to maintain cardiopulmonary function in the face of extensive brain damage, there was a need to define death. Speculation exists that the impetus for a brain-based definition of death was the increasing need for transplantable organs (Fox & Swazey, 1992), but the primary impetus was the desire to use resources appropriately. If there was no possibility of survival, use of technology to maintain cardiopulmonary function was inappropriate. The distinction between sustaining life and prolonging death needed to be made, and the diagnosis of brain death was useful to that end. The following Harvard Medical School criteria were proposed: unresponsiveness, lack of reflexes, lack of spontaneous breathing, and an isoelectric EEG (Ad Hoc Committee, 1968). If the examinations done 24 hours apart were essentially unchanged, the patient would be declared legally dead and treatment discontinued. For children, these criteria were inadequate. With technologic advances, the techniques to assess brain function changed, but health-care providers were warned to use caution in applying these assessment techniques to infants under 7 days of age (Task Force for the Determination of Brain Death in Children, 1987). The guidelines offer specific criteria for assessing brain death in children between 7 days and 2 months, 2 months to 1 year, and over 1 year of age. Dorr (1997) noted that while the guidelines may be considered the national standard, other authors have found that there is wide variability in the diagnosis of brain death across the country (Mejia & Pollack, 1995). Although the Uniform Determination of Death Act has been widely accepted as the applicable law to allow for discontinuation of treatment, many states have specific case law that is applied (Blank, 1999).

However, a number of controversies surround the issue of brain death. The first issue involves the accuracy of diagnosis, the rigor in which the criteria are applied, and the lack of distinction between permanent unconsciousness and brain death. Lock (2002) described a number of cases where children had been diagnosed brain dead by various tests. In one case a child was diagnosed brain dead via the apnea test, only to breathe spontaneously in the Operating Room when organs were about to be harvested. In other cases, the electroencephalogram (EEG) was relatively, but not completely, isoelectric, or all tests showed brain death but there was a little blood flow to the upper brain according to the nuclear scan. For children who may have sustained a traumatic brain injury, such as in a motor vehicle accident or fall, or an anoxic injury, such as with a near-drowning or accidental strangling, severe brain damage can occur, but the entire brain may not be affected. The brainstem may be damaged but still functioning, so that the child does not meet the brain death criteria. The case of Sammy Linares, a toddler who became asphyxiated when he inhaled part of a latex balloon that burst, exemplifies the tragedy faced by the family when a child is technology dependent and permanently unconscious, but not brain dead (Goldman, Stratton, & Brown, 1989). Sammy's father removed him from his ventilator while keeping the pediatric intensive care staff at bay with a .357 Magnum handgun.

Mejia and Pollack's study (1995) suggested that there may be instances where children will be removed from the ventilator under the auspices of brain death, but they may not technically meet the criteria. Some philosophers have argued that the whole-brain criteria for brain death are inappropriate and that the death of the higher brain, or cortical functioning of the brain, should be acceptable for brain death (Veatch, 1993). Under the higher-brain criteria, children who are permanently unconscious, infants with anencephaly, and adults with late-stage Alzheimer's disease may qualify for brain death. Truog (1997), while critical of the whole-brain criteria, does not believe the public will accept diagnosing brain death in patients who are breathing unassisted. He maintains that brain death is no longer needed to justify withdrawal of treatment.

The other ethical issue is that some cultures, as well as some religions, do not recognize brain death. Some Orthodox Jewish rabbis reject brain death and state that a Jew is obligated to accept life-sustaining treatment because "so long as it is possible for a Jew to live, he ought to want to live" (Bleich, 1998). Health-care providers who may wish to discontinue treatment after making a diagnosis of brain death in a child may encounter opposition from families whose religious or cultural values do not accept brain death. The health-care team may view continued treatment as futile and an inappropriate use of resources, while the family may view continued treatment as a religious mandate. Recognizing that the decision to discontinue treatment is not just a medical one is a beginning in the dialogue with the parents. Rubin (1998) suggested that the concept of futility should be a negotiated reality. The health-care team's reasoning should be "transparent" to the parent; that is, it should be clearly explained how the team arrived at its diagnosis and why discontinuation of treatment is recommended. Rubin also accepts moral suasion, the health-care provider's encouragement of the patient or family to accept the provider's recommendation, as legitimate because the health-care team has greater experience and expertise in cases of brain death than the public. She acknowledged that the disagreement may not be reconcilable, so that ethics committee consultation or even judicial intervention may be needed if the heath-care team believes that continued treatment is not in the child's best interests, yet the parents insist on continued treatment.

Children with Neurobehavioral Disorders

As smaller and smaller infants were surviving and their development was being evaluated, a condition originally called MBD, or minimal brain dysfunction, was identified. These children were noted to be very active, distractible, and impulsive, and had difficulty with school performance. One theory was that they had been overprotected because of their fragile beginning (vulnerable child syndrome) and lacked discipline and limit-setting abilities. Over time, a condition known as attention-deficit/hyperactivity disorder (ADHD) was described, and both children born prematurely and at those born at term were affected. The presentation was usually parental observation about the high activity level of the child and the inability of the child to attend to tasks, follow directions, or inhibit inappropriate responses.

The specialty of developmental pediatrics grew in the 1970s and children with attention or behavioral problems were evaluated by this new specialty. Merging neurology, psychiatry, and education, this specialty views learning and development as an interweaving of processes that affect and influence each other. Children who may have an organic predisposition for inattention or impulsivity engender certain responses from their environment. The environmental responses (e.g., difficult relationships with parents, siblings, and peers) further shape the child's behavior. Academic performance may be poor although the child may test in a normal or high range of intelligence. The interplay between a child's intelligence, motor performance, interpersonal relationships, and self-esteem is not easily understood; often the child is identified as a "behavior problem" or the child's abilities are thought to be limited. Through evaluation, usually including neuropsychologic testing and a neurologic examination, the child's strengths and weaknesses are discovered, and they may fall into a pattern characteristic of a neurobehavioral disorder. The rubric of "learning disabilities" captures a multitude of disorders from dyslexia, central processing disorder, or nonverbal learning disability to attention-deficit disorder with hyperactivity. The latter condition has created a furor over its alleged overdiagnosis.

The standard approach to diagnosing and managing ADHD requires information and cooperation from the child, the parents, and the school or other structured environment such as day care. The American Academy of Pediatrics has issued practice guidelines for the diagnosis and evaluation of the child with ADHD. In it they state that the prevalence rates of ADHD in a community of school-age children vary from 4% to 12% (AAP, Committee on Quality Improvement, 2000). There has been concern in the lay and professional literature that ADHD has been overdiagnosed. DeGrandpre (2000) asserted that the changing culture has created a generation of people "addicted" to sensory stimulation, creating inattentiveness and impulsiveness. The response, according to DeGrandpre, has been to prescribe stimulants such as methylphenidate (Ritalin). He believes Ritalin is overprescribed, at high risk for abuse as a recreational drug, and sends a mixed message regarding the United States' "war on drugs."

The National Institutes of Health (NIH Consensus Development Panel, 2000) issued a consensus development conference statement on the diagnosis and treatment of ADHD. In the statement, the panel acknowledged that there is evidence that the disorder of ADHD exists, but there is no definitive test to diagnose it, and its treatment, especially the use of stimulants, is controversial. The panel also urged further research into the long-term treatment of ADHD with stimulants, as well as investigation into the cause or causes.

In a review of the literature and analysis of two national surveys, Hoagwood, Kelleher, Feil, and Comer (2000) concluded that the diagnosis of ADHD has increased significantly. Many more children are seen in various settings (physician's office, psychiatric inpatient units, and special education settings) with some complaint related to the diagnosis. Hoagwood et al. found that use of stimulant and other psychotropic medications were increased but varied across geographic locations. Although two thirds of children with ADHD had medications prescribed at some point, a smaller percentage was offered special instructional help or counseling, and even fewer were referred for psychotherapy or given a follow-up appointment. The trend is likely influenced by the cost containment culture in health care (Dunn, 2002).

Lay media noted cases where parents were accused of "medical ne-glect" by school personnel when the parents discontinued their son's Ritalin (Thomas, 2000). Parents have resisted the use of medication, some voicing that they did not want their child "dependent" or "addicted to drugs." Some-times the child resists medication when parents and teachers are in favor. Through the use of a double-blind, placebo–Ritalin trial, the efficacy of the medication can be determined for a child in that child's specific situation. In the trial, a pharmacist prepares identical capsules—one with low-dose Ritalin, one with a higher dose of Ritalin, and one with inert ingredients. A sufficient number of each type of capsule is made so that a 3- or 6-week trial of med-ication can occur. For the first 1 or 2 weeks, the child takes capsules from Bottle 1; the next period of time, Bottle 2; and the last period, Bottle 3. At the end of each week, the parents, teachers, and other adults (e.g., babysitter, tu-tors, coaches) are asked to complete a checklist rating the frequency with which certain behaviors are observed. The child may also complete a check-list. At the end of the trial, the checklists are reviewed and the code for the medication is broken. If the child has a positive response to Ritalin, then the most improved week or weeks should correspond with one of the Ritalin dosages. If there is no difference between weeks, Ritalin may not be an effec-tive drug for this child. This approach provides an empirical assessment of the likelihood of a therapeutic response to Ritalin. However, it involves an increased cost for the medication, because the pharmacist's time in prepara-tion is increased. It involves more vigilance and time from teachers and others who complete the weekly checklists. It presupposes that the parents and child will consider medication as part of the treatment. A conflict in values can occur at this juncture. The physician, trained to diagnose and treat, and having empirical data that the child's performance improves on Ritalin, may value a management plan that includes medication. The parents may fear drug dependency, potential for abuse, or some parents may consider medica-tion a "crutch." They believe children should apply themselves, try harder, and learn via the mainstream teaching methods.

Drug use in the United States, for many conditions, is stigmatized. There is a "pick yourself up by your bootstrap" mentality surrounding certain con-ditions, such as depression, anxiety, obsessive–compulsive disorder, and ADHD. Some believe that if only the people with these disorders would get control of themselves, they could overcome these disorders. A class action suit was filed in three different states against the company that manufac-tures Ritalin, the American Psychological Association (APA), and CHADD (Children and Adults with Attention Deficit/Hyperactivity Disorder) for "conspiring, colluding and cooperating in promoting the diagnosis of at-tention-deficit disorder (ADD) and attention-deficit/hyperactivity disorder (ADHD)" (O'Meara, 2000). The author accused the drug industry, the APA, CHADD, and the National Alliance for the Mentally Ill (NAMI) of promot-ing the diagnoses of mental disorders for the purposes of selling prescription drugs. NAMI has accepted contributions from drug companies to conduct antistigmatizing campaigns.

The question remains: Is ADHD a disorder with an organic component amenable to psychopharmacologic intervention, or is it a symptom of inappropriate expectations of society on its children? Is there a resistance to acknowledging and treating mental disorders, or are these disorders contrived for the purposes of explaining or excusing poor performance and promoting medication to solve the problems? Accardo and Blondis (2001) unequivocally responded that ADHD exists as a neurodevelopmental syndrome and that stimulants are the "gold standard" for treatment and are safe and effective, along with other behavioral supports.

There is also the argument that performance enhancement should be acceptable. Although not everyone will respond to Ritalin in a double-blind, Ritalin–placebo trial, many people who take Ritalin will experience increased focus, increased wakefulness, and appetite suppression. Students who believe that these features will improve their performance on tests or assignments may want to occasionally use Ritalin for performance enhancement purposes. Is it ethically permissible to prescribe and use Ritalin for these purposes? Medication, such as propranolol, has been used for anxiety associated with stage fright. Is treating stage fright medically necessary? Does stage fright have to be pathologized for the medical treatment of it to be ethical? Should the cause of the symptoms be irrelevant if the symptoms can be dissipated through treatment? These questions bring the focus back to the concepts of "normal" and "different." Are the medications being used to permit children to behave, learn, and perform in a more "normal" fashion? Are the medications being used in addition to or in place of changing other aspects in the environment that would also improve children's behavior, ability to learn, and performance? These are questions that society must wrestle with—in homes, classrooms, school boards, professional associations, advocacy groups, and in corporations. Parens (1998) offered a stimulating discussion from "The Enhancement Project" conducted by the Hastings Center on the morality of enhancement that provides an exploration into the philosophical arguments for and against enhancement.

Children in the Juvenile Justice System

Nearly half of all the violent crimes in the United States are committed by male teens (Steiner & Stone, 1999). Cocozza (1997) found that 2.7 million children under the age of 18 years are arrested each year, with approximately one million having some formal contact with the juvenile justice system. In addition, 50% to 75% of children in the juvenile justice system have substance abuse problems. Public outcry has focused on increasing the severity of the punishment of young offenders, rather than addressing the cause of the criminal behavior. In the United Kingdom, there has even been discussion about use of the death penalty for children who commit heinous crimes. In the United States, a 16-year-old boy was convicted of killing a woman and her son in Las Vegas in 1993, and was sentenced to death. The Nevada

Supreme Court upheld the conviction and sentence, and the U.S. Supreme Court let the ruling stand. According to one source, the United States is one of seven countries that permits the executions of minors (*New York Times*, 2000). The American Civil Liberties Union opposes treating juvenile offenders as adults and supports alternative incarceration programs. Their fact sheet noted that juvenile crime increased by 55% from 1983 to 1992, despite a 10% decrease in the number of 16- and 17-year-olds in the population, and a 115% increase in the number of juveniles prosecuted as adults between 1989 and 1994 (American Civil Liberties Union, 1996). Their point is that treating juvenile offenders as adults does not decrease juvenile crime.

Kestenbaum (2000) estimated that 60% of the children in the criminal justice system have behavioral, mental, or emotional disorders. The presence of these disorders does not excuse criminal behavior; however, there is growing interest in the organic influence over deviant behavior. Blank (1999) cited research suggesting that hate crimes may be the result of fear so deeply ingrained into the perpetrator that it is not accessible to the consciousness nor under control of the will. In referring to children, though, it is incongruent to deny them the right to make their own health-care decisions based on the belief that they have not yet developed sufficient decision-making abilities, yet hold them responsible as adults for criminal behaviors. There is a reluctance to accept that children can do evil deeds; one wants to believe that there are reasons, such as abuse, cruelty, or abject poverty, that explain why children commit crimes.

The search for these reasons involves the health-care system. A psychiatric evaluation that includes ruling out an organic basis for aberrant behavior is useful, but not fully explanatory. The medicalization of criminal behavior in children shifts the focus from punishment to treatment through rehabilitation. Is the adult justice system appropriate for children? As children develop decision-making capabilities, one might conclude that they are then also capable of bearing responsibility for their decisions and actions, yet they lack the experience to fully appreciate the consequences of their actions. Interjecting the health-care system into the social phenomenon of juvenile crime reflects an attitude of hopefulness toward salvaging lost souls. A shift toward addressing the health-care needs of girls in the juvenile justice system should occur because the female population is rapidly increasing and the system has primarily focused on boys (Guthrie, Hoey, Ravoira, & Kintner, 2002).

Research on Children

Willowbrook State School was the setting for one of the more infamous instances of unethical research on children. In the 1970s, children with significant developmental disabilities were enrolled in a hepatitis vaccine study; their parents were told that the children would not gain admission into the residential facility unless parents would consent for the children to be in the study. The children were inoculated with the experimental vaccine, then

Table 11.1

483

Categories of Permissible Research on Children

Level of Risk	Prospect of Direct Benefit	Child Assent Needed	Parental Permission Needed
No greater than minimal	N/A	Yes	Yes
More than minimal	Yes[a]	Yes[b]	Yes
Minor increase over minimal	No	Yes	Yes[c]
Same as the previous 3 categories	No	Yes	Yes[c]

[a] The relation of the anticipated benefit to the risk is at least as favorable to the subjects as that presented by available alternative approaches (45 CFR § 46.405). [b] Assent may be waived if the child is likely to directly benefit from inclusion in the research. [c] Consent from both parents is required unless one of the parents is deceased, incompetent, whereabouts are unknown or is not reasonably available, or when one parent is the custodial parent.

Note. From *Summary of Basic Protections for Human Subjects,* by the Office for Protection From Research Risks, 1997, Rockville, MD: Author.

exposed to the rest of the institution's population in order to contract hepatitis, which was thought be to inevitable. The parents were placed in the position of either keeping their children at home or submitting their children to an experiment regardless of the potential risks or benefits. Children in institutions were especially vulnerable to exploitation by researchers (Weisstub, 1998).

The Belmont Report (National Commission for the Protection of Human Subjects in Biomedical and Behavioral Research, 1978) was a presidential commission's report on biomedical and behavioral research on human subjects. Seventeen federal agencies adopted the recommendations as the "Common Rule" for regulation of human subjects research. Institutional review boards (IRB) were charged with oversight of research, using the Common Rule as a guide. The guidelines pertaining to children recognized that children are a vulnerable group who needed special conditions to justify inclusion in research. Those conditions are divided into four categories (see Table 11.1). The American Academy of Pediatrics policy statement "Guidelines for the Ethical Conduct of Studies to Evaluate Drugs in Pediatric Populations" (AAP, Committee on Drugs, 1995) offers additional groups of children for which there should be special circumstances before they are included in research. These groups are children with disabilities, children who are institutionalized, children requiring emergency care, children who are dying, children with chronically progressive or potentially fatal diseases, and children who are newly dead by virtue of being diagnosed brain dead.

Today, research with children as research participants constitutes only a small portion of research efforts (Kanner, Langerman, & Grey, 2004). As with consent for children in treatment decisions, parents are expected to weigh the risks and benefits to their child when considering the child's participation in research. In some areas, such as oncology, many of the treatments for childhood cancers are available only through enrollment in clinical trials.

The newest drugs and drug combinations are presented as one arm of a study, the currently accepted standard drugs and drug combinations are the other arm. Many studies are very complex, involving varying drugs, varying dosages, and varying schedules of treatment. In the informed consent process, the oncologist explains the complex study to the parents and, depending on the age and developmental level of the child, may also include the child in these discussions, or may have a separate discussion with the child. The parents give or refuse consent for their child to participate in the research, and may withdraw the child from the study. The child's assent, or affirmative agreement, to be a research participant is also sought. If the study is likely to provide a direct benefit to the child, such as most oncology studies, the parents may override the dissent of the child. In those instances where assent is desirable but not necessary, the child should not be asked to assent if the dissent will not be honored. The older or more mature the child, the more weight should be given to the child's preferences. Parents usually know their children best and gauge how and when to discuss the study protocol with the child. One of the more difficult situations for the health-care team is when there is disagreement between the professionals and the parents about discussing the diagnosis and treatment options with the child. In these instances the parents often want continued treatment, while the child may be indicating a desire to stop treatment. Although parents retain the legal right to consent, the team may wish to explore the disagreement further to ensure effective communication between the child and parents. The medical center's institutional review board (IRB), when reviewing the research projects for research on children, may stipulate when a child's assent is required, when it can be waived, and whether both parents, if reasonably available, must give informed consent.

The issue of nontherapeutic research with children was raised when the Supreme Court of Maryland ruled in *Grimes v. Kennedy Krieger Institute*. The Institute was being sued for negligence because their researchers conducted a study on lead abatement in low-income housing. In this study, the researchers knew the lead abatement in some of the housing was only being partially done, one child had a dangerously elevated lead level and the parents were not informed of this in a timely fashion, and none of the parents were fully informed of the risks of the study. The court held that parents cannot consent to enroll a child in nontherapeutic research where there is the possibility of harm to the health of the child (Glantz, 2002). Subpart B of the Common Rule (45 CFR § 46.404; Office for Protection From Research Risks, 1997) permits children to be enrolled in research if there is no greater than minimal risk, but the Maryland court raised the standard for nontherapeutic research to "no" risk of harm.

For those conditions in which an adolescent can consent to treatment without parental permission, some authors believe that the adolescent should be able to consent to research (Leiken, 1993; Santelli et al., 1995). As discussed previously, state statutes specify conditions in which an adolescent may be treated without parental consent, and the statutes may address consent for research. However, the institution's IRB should ensure that their requirements for consent are consistent with state law.

Conclusion

This chapter has explored a myriad of ethical issues in children's health care. Many of these ethical problems occur within hospitals, but with the health-care settings moving beyond hospital walls, health-care professionals need a broader appreciation of issues affecting children. The answers can be elusive, but it is worthwhile for health-care professionals to contemplate these issues.

Each setting should identify the current policies and guidelines for informing ethical decision making relevant to that setting. For example, school personnel should examine policies on medication, including self-medication, use of psychotropic medications, and administration of medication in emergent situations. Additionally, school personnel should explore how they would respond to a request for withholding resuscitation on a student with a terminal illness who still is capable and willing to attend classes.

Not all settings may have access to an ethics committee for assistance in analyzing ethical issues. However, there may be ethics consultants with expertise in pediatrics who may serve as ad hoc consultants. These consultants can perform case consultation and inservice education, and may assist in the development of an ethics committee for the specific setting.

The Internet provides many ethics resources. E-mail provides almost instant access to colleagues and consultants who can provide information, support, and advice. One caveat is the issue of confidentiality when using electronic communication methods (e-mail, fax); communications must be HIPAA (Health Insurance Portability and Accountability Act of 1996) compliant (Centers for Medicare and Medicaid Services, n.d.). Another is that the information available on some sites should be evaluated carefully, as there is no assurance that the information is correct or current.

Ethical issues will always be present in health care of children, so professionals should be prepared through education, networking, and accessing resources to face and resolve those issues in their setting. They should also participate in their professional organizations or other groups to share their experiences and expertise in shaping an ethically responsible and child-friendly society.

Study Guide

1. Discuss various approaches to identifying and analyzing ethical issues in children's health care.

2. List and discuss current ethical, moral, and legal issues in children's health care.

3. To what degree can, and should, children make decisions about their health care?

4. Compare current perspectives and issues on children's participation and decision making with those of 25 years ago.

5. Describe psychosocial, economic, cultural, and medical changes related to current concerns on ethics, morals, and legal aspects of children's health care.

6. Discuss the implications for practice from "the best interests of the child."

7. In what situations are parents as decision makers for children appropriate? Inappropriate?

8. Describe children's abilities to make health-care decisions at various stages of development, and draw implications for practice.

9. Discuss emerging issues in children's health care, and hypothesize future ethical, moral, and legal issues.

10. Outline situations in which a child can make health-care decisions, those in which parents can make decisions, and those in which surrogates must make decisions.

References

Accardo, P., & Blondis, T. A. (2001). What's all the fuss about Ritalin? *Journal of Pediatrics, 138*(1), 6–9.

Ad Hoc Committee of the Harvard Medical School to Examine the Definition of Death. (1968). A definition of irreversible coma. *Journal of the American Medical Association, 205*, 337–340.

Albrecht, G. L., & Devlieger, P. L. (1999). The disability paradox: High quality of life against all odds. *Social Science & Medicine, 48*, 977–988.

American Academy of Pediatrics, Committee on Bioethics. (1995). Informed consent, parental permission, and assent in pediatric practice. *Pediatrics, 95*, 314–317.

American Academy of Pediatrics, Committee on Bioethics. (1998). Female genital mutilation. *Pediatrics, 102*(1), 153–156.

American Academy of Pediatrics, Committee on Bioethics. (2001). Ethical issues with genetic testing in pediatrics. *Pediatrics, 197*(6), 1451–1455.

American Academy of Pediatrics, Committee on Drugs. (1995). Guidelines for the ethical conduct of studies to evaluate drugs in pediatric populations. *Pediatrics, 95*(2), 286–294.

American Academy of Pediatrics, Committee on Quality Improvement, Subcommittee on Attention-Deficit/Hyperactivity Disorder. (2000). Diagnosis and evaluation of the child with attention-deficit/hyperactivity disorder. *Pediatrics, 105*(5), 1158–1170.

American Academy of Pediatrics, Task Force on Circumcision. (1999). Circumcision policy statement. *Pediatrics, 103*(3), 686–693.

American Academy of Pediatrics. (1984). Joint policy statement: Principles of treatment of disabled infants. *Pediatrics, 73*, 559–566.

American Academy of Pediatrics. (2002). Perinatal care at the threshold of viability. *Pediatrics, 110*(5), 1024–1027.

American Academy of Pediatrics. (2003). Consent for emergency medical services for children and adolescents. *Pediatrics, 111*(3), 703–706.

American Civil Liberties Union. (1996). *ACLU fact sheet on the juvenile justice system.* Retrieved July 22, 2004, from www.aclu.org

American Psychiatric Association. (1994). *Diagnostic and statistical manual of mental disorders* (4th ed.). Washington, DC: Author.

American Society of Clinical Oncology. (2003). American Society of Clinical Oncology policy statement update: Genetic testing for cancer susceptibility. *Journal of Clinical Oncology, 21*(12), 2397–2406.

American Society of Human Genetics and American College of Medical Genetics Report. (1995). Points to consider: Ethical, legal, and psychosocial implications of genetic testing in children and adolescents. *American Journal of Human Genetics, 57*, 1233–1241.

Annas, G. J. (1982). Mandatory PKU screening: The other side of the looking glass. *American Journal of Public Health, 72*, 1401–1403.

Asch, A. (1998). The "difference" of disability in the medical setting. *Cambridge Quarterly of Healthcare Ethics, 7*, 77–87.

Blank, R. H. (1999). *Brain policy: How the new neuroscience will change our lives and our politics.* Washington, DC: Georgetown University Press.

Bleich, J. D. (1998). *Bioethical dilemmas: A Jewish perspective.* Hoboken, NJ: KTAV.

Brennan, W. (1995). *Dehumanizing the vulnerable: When word games take lives.* Chicago: Loyola University Press.

Buchanan, A. E., & Brock, D. W. (1990). *Deciding for others: The ethics of surrogate decision making*. New York: Cambridge University Press.

Carter, B. S. (1993). Neonatologists and bioethics after Baby Doe. *Journal of Perinatology, 13*(2), 144–150.

Catlin, A. J. (1999). Physicians' neonatal resuscitation of extremely low-birth weight infants. *Image: Journal of Nursing Scholarship, 31*(3), 269–275.

Centers for Medicare and Medicaid Services. (n.d.). *Health Insurance Portability and Accountability Act (HIPAA): Administrative simplification*. Retrieved January 12, 2004, from http://www.cms.hhs.gov/hipaa/hipaa2/

Charlton, J. I. (1998). *Nothing about us without us: Disability, oppression, and empowerment*. Berkeley: University of California Press.

Clark, P. (2002). Medical futility in pediatrics: Is it time for a public policy? *Journal of Public Health Policy, 23*(1), 66–89.

Cocozza, J. (1997). Identifying the needs of juveniles with co-occurring disorders. *Corrections Today, 59*, 7.

Council on Scientific Affairs, American Medical Association. (1995). Female genital mutilation. *Journal of the American Medical Association, 274*, 1714–1716.

Dankert-Roelse, J., terMeerman, G., Martijin, A., tenKate, L., & Knol, K. (1989). Survival and clinical outcomes in patients with cystic fibrosis, with or without neonatal screening. *Journal of Pediatrics, 114*, 362–367.

DeGrandpre, R. (2000). *Ritalin nation: Rapid-fire culture and the transformation of human consciousness*. New York: Norton.

Dorr, P. (1997). Outcomes manager: Brain death criteria in the pediatric patient. *Critical Care Nursing Quarterly, 20*(1), 14–21.

Duff, R. S., & Campbell, A. G. M. (1973). Moral and ethical dilemmas in special care nurseries. *New England Journal of Medicine, 289*, 890–894.

Dunn, M. (2002). Is Ritalin the answer? Strong clinical skills can prevent misuse of the drug. *American Journal of Nursing, 102*(12), 22.

Flavell, J. (1985). *Cognitive development* (2nd ed.). Englewood Cliffs, NJ: Prentice Hall.

Fost, N. (1999). Decisions regarding treatment of seriously ill newborns. *Journal of the American Medical Association, 281*(21), 2041–2042.

Fox, R. C., & Swazey, J. P. (1992). *Spare parts: Organ replacement in American society*. New York: Oxford University Press.

Gallagher, H. G. (1995). "Slapping up spastics": The persistence of social attitudes toward people with disabilities. *Issues in Law & Medicine, 10*(4), 401–414.

Gibeau, A. (1998). Female genital mutilation: When a cultural practice generates clinical and ethical dilemmas. *Journal of Obstetric, Gynecologic, & Neonatal Nursing, 27*(1), 85–91.

Gilligan, C. (1982). *In a different voice: Psychological theory and women's development*. Cambridge, MA: Harvard University Press.

Glantz, L. (2002). Nontherapeutic research with children: Grimes v. Kennedy Krieger Institute. *American Journal of Public Health, 92*(7), 1070–1073.

Goldman, G. M., Stratton, K. M., & Brown, M. D. (1989). What actually happened: An informed review of the Linares incident. *Law, Medicine, & Health Care, 17*(40), 298–307.

Goldman, R. (1999). The psychological impact of circumcision. *BJU International, 83* (Suppl. 1), 93–102.

Grisso, T., & Appelbaum, P. S. (1998). *Assessing competence to consent to treatment: A guide for physicians and other health professionals*. New York: Oxford University Press.

Grisso, T., & Vierling, L. (1978). Minor's consent in treatment: A developmental perspective. *Professional Psychology, 9*(3), 412–427.

Hadorn, D. C. (1991). Setting health care priorities in Oregon: Cost effectiveness meets the rule of rescue. *Journal of the American Medical Association, 265*, 2218–2225.

Hiller, E. H., Landenburger, G., & Natowicz, M. R. (1997). Public participation in medical policy making and the status of consumer autonomy: The example of newborn screening programs in the United States. *American Journal of Public Health, 87*(8), 1280–1288.

Hoagwood, K., Kelleher, K. J., Feil, M. M., & Comer, D. M. (2000). Treatment services for children with ADHD: A national perspective. *Journal of the American Academy of Child & Adolescent Psychiatry, 39*(2), 198–206.

Johnson, M. (Ed.). (2000). Cover story: 10 years and 90 days. *Ragged Edge Online, 21*(4). Retrieved June 20, 2004, from www.raggededgemagazine.com/0700/0700cov.htm

Kanner, S., Langerman, S., & Grey, M. (2004). Ethical considerations for a child's participation in research. *Journal for Specialists in Pediatric Nursing, 9*(1), 15–23.

Kestenbaum, C. J. (2000). How shall we treat the children of the 21st century? *Journal of the American Academy of Child and Adolescent Psychiatry, 39,* 1–10.

Kopelman, L. M. (1997). The best-interests standard as threshold, ideal, and standard of reasonableness. *Journal of Medicine and Philosophy, 22,* 271–289.

Kopelman, L. M., Irons, T. G., & Kopelman, A. E. (1988). Neonatologists judge the "Baby Doe" regulations. *New England Journal of Medicine, 318*(11), 677–683.

Kunk, R. M. (1998). Expanding the newborn screen: Terrific or troubling? *The American Journal of Maternal/Child Nursing, 23*(5), 266–271.

Lashley, F. R. (1999). Genetic testing, screening, and counseling issues in cardiovascular disease. *Journal of Cardiovascular Nursing, 13*(4), 110–126.

Learman, L. A. (1999). Neonatal circumcision: A dispassionate analysis. *Clinical Obstetrics and Gynecology, 42*(4), 849.

Leiken, S. (1993). Minors' assent, consent, or dissent to medical research. *IRB: A Review of Human Subjects Research, 15*(2), 1–7.

Lock, M. (2002). *Twice dead: Organ transplants and the reinvention of death.* Berkeley: University of California Press.

Lorber, J. (1972). Spina bifida cystica: Results of treatment of 270 consecutive cases with criteria for selection for the future. *Archives of Disease in Childhood, 47,* 856–867.

Maxwell, L. G., & Yaster, M. (1999). Analgesia for neonatal circumcision: No more studies, just do it. *Archives of Pediatrics & Adolescent Medicine, 153*(5), 444–445.

Mejia, R. E., & Pollack, M. M. (1995). Variability in brain death determination practices in children. *Journal of the American Medical Association, 274*(7), 550–553.

Merell, M., Huisman, J., Alderden-van der Vecht, A., Taat, F., Bezemer, D., Griffioen, R., et al. (2003). Early versus late diagnosis: Psychological impact on parents of children with cystic fibrosis. *Pediatrics, 111*(2), 346–350.

National Commission for the Protection of Human Subjects in Biomedical and Behavioral Research. (1978). *The Belmont Report: Ethical principles and guidelines for the protection of human subjects of research* (DHEW). Publication No. OS 78-0012. Washington, DC: U.S. Government Printing Office.

New York Times. (2000, August 22). Ranks of youth on death row growing. *New York Times.*

NIH Consensus Development Panel. (2000). National Institutes of Health Consensus Development Conference Statement: Diagnosis and treatment of attention-deficit/hyperactivity disorder (ADHD). *Journal of the American Academy of Child & Adolescent Psychiatry, 39*(2), 182–193.

Oberman, M. (1996). Minor rights and wrongs. *Journal of Law, Medicine, and Ethics, 24,* 127–138.

Office for Protection from Research Risks. (1997). *Summary of basic protection of human subjects.* Rockville, MD: Author.

O'Meara, K. P. (2000, October 16). Writing may be on wall for Ritalin. *Insight Magazine.* Retrieved June 20, 2003, from www.insightmag.com/news/2000/10/16

O'Neill, K. (2002). Kids speak: Effective communication with the school-aged/adolescent patient. *Pediatric Emergency Care, 18*(2), 137–140.

Orfali, K. (2004). Parental role in medical decision-making: Fact or fiction? A comparative study of ethical dilemmas in French and American neonatal intensive care units. *Social Science & Medicine, 58*(10), 2009–2022.

Parens, E. (1998). Is better always good? The Enhancement Project. *Hastings Center Report, 28*(1), S1–S17.

Pass, K. A., Lane, P. A., Fernhoff, P. M., Hinton, C. F., Panny, S. R., Parks, J. S., Pelias, M. Z., Rhead, W. J., Ross, S. I., Wethers, D. L., & Elsas, L. J. (2000). U. S. Newborn Screening System Guidelines II: Follow-up of children, diagnosis, management, and evaluation. *Journal of Pediatrics, 137*(4), S1–S46.

Pellegrino, E. D. (1998). The false promise of beneficent killing. In L. L. Emmanuel (Ed.), *Regulating how we die: The ethical, medical, and legal issues surrounding physician-assisted suicide* (pp. 71–91). Cambridge, MA: Harvard University Press.

Ross, L. F. (1997). Health care decision making by children: Is it in their best interests? *Hasting Center Report, 27*(6), 41–45.

Rubin, S. B. (1998). *When doctors say no: The battleground of medical futility.* Bloomington: Indiana University Press.

Saigal, S., Stoskopf, B. L., Feeny, D., Furlong, W., Burrows, E., Rosenbaum, P., et al. (1999). Differences in preferences for neonatal outcomes among health care professionals, parents, and adolescents. *Journal of the American Medical Association, 281*(21), 1991–1997.

Santelli, J. S., Rosenfeld, W. D., DuRant, R. H., Dubler, N., Morreale, M., English, A., & Rogers, A. S. (1995). A special issue of the *Journal of Adolescent Health* on guidelines for adolescent health research. *Journal of Adolescent Health, 19*, 262–269.

Savage, T. A. (2000, July). Factors influencing parental decision-making regarding life-sustaining treatment for children with severe disabilities. *Paper presented at the 5th International Family Nursing Conference*, Chicago, Illinois.

Shapiro, J. P. (1994). *No pity: People with disabilities forging a new civil rights movement.* New York: Times-Books, Random House.

Shevell, M. I. (1998). Clinical ethics and developmental delay. *Seminars in Pediatric Neurology, 5*(1), 70–75.

Singer, L. T., Salvator, A., Guo, S., Collin, M., Lilien, L., & Baley, J. (1999). Maternal psychological distress and parenting stress after the birth of a very low-birth-weight infant. *Journal of the American Medical Association, 281*, 799–805.

Steiner, H., & Stone, L. A. (1999). Introduction: Violence and related psychopathology. *Journal of the American Academy of Child and Adolescent Psychiatry, 38*, 232–234.

Stinson, R., & Stinson, P. (1979). *The long dying of baby Andrew.* Boston: Little, Brown.

Strasburger, V. C., & Brown, R. T. (1991). *Adolescent medicine: A practical guide.* Boston: Little, Brown.

Task Force for the Determination of Brain Death in Children. (1987). Guidelines for the determination of brain death in children, *Neurology, 37*, 1077–1078.

Thomas, K. (2000, August 8). Parents pressured to put kids on Ritalin: NY court orders use of medicine. *USA Today.*

Toubia, N. (1994). Female genital mutilation and the responsibility of reproductive health professionals. *International Journal of Gynecology and Obstetrics, 46*, 127–135.

Truog, R. D. (1997). Is it time to abandon brain death? *Hastings Center Report, 27*(1), 29–37.

van der Heide, A., van der Maas, P. J., van der Wal, G., de Graff, C. L. M., Kester, J. G. C., Kollee, L. A. A., de Leeuw, R., & Holl, R. A. (1997). Medical end-of-life decisions made for neonates and infants in the Netherlands. *The Lancet, 340*, 251–255.

Veatch, R. M. (1993). The impending collapse of the whole-brain definition of death. *Hastings Center Report, 23*(4), 18–24.

Wang, S., O'Leary, L., Fitzsimmons, S., & Khoury, M. (2002). The impact of early cystic fibrosis diagnosis on pulmonary function in children. *Journal of Pediatrics, 141,* 804–810.

Weisstub, D. N. (1998). *Research on human subjects: Ethics, law and social policy.* Kidlington, Oxford, England: Pergamon Press.

Wilder, M. A. (2000). Ethical issues in the delivery room: Resuscitation of extremely low birth weight infants. *Journal of Perinatal & Neonatal Nursing, 14*(2), 44–57.

Williams, T. (2002). Patient empowerment and ethical decision making: The patient/partner and the right to act. *Dimensions of Critical Care Nursing, 21*(3), 100–104.

Wisconsin Association of Perinatal Care. (1997). *Guidelines for the responsible utilization of neonatal intensive care.* (WAPC-PSI: 10/97/2500).

Relationships in Children's Health-Care Settings

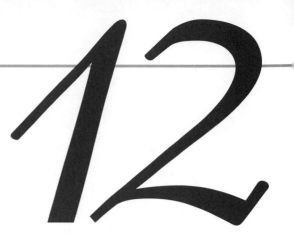

Judy A. Rollins

Objectives

At the conclusion of this chapter, the reader will be able to:

1. Discuss what relationships are, how they vary, and how and why they have changed in health-care settings over the past 25 years.

2. Determine the special issues of relationships in working with children in health-care settings and encounters, and draw implications for healthy relationships.

3. Outline relationships *among* professionals that are critical to optimal health care for children with special needs, and describe *optimal* relationships for today's health-care system and children's needs.

4. Determine the impact of *caring* and quality of relationships on children's psychosocial development as well as physical health. Summarize the major relationship factors that influence children's recovery.

*R*egardless of health-care setting, meeting the psychosocial needs of children and families occurs not in isolation but within the structure of relationships. Involvement, caring, and interpersonal connection form the basis from which care is delivered (Totka, 1996). Over the years, messages in the literature regarding professionalism and patient–provider relationships have changed in value from detachment and distancing to intimacy, commitment, and involvement (Williams, 2001). Discussions have addressed the issues of which types of relationships are most effective and which are most likely to result in harm, as well as the effects of under- or overinvolvement on children, families, and health-care professionals.

Before delving into the topic of relationships, it is important to acknowledge that fundamental differences exist between caring for children and caring for adults. For example, with children, physical boundaries are not the same. Health-care providers hold, kiss, and nurture children (see Figure 12.1). However, although physical boundaries of care are taken away, it is expected that emotional boundaries remain clear (Totka, 1996). Additionally, when children are ill, their parents are in crisis, making them vulnerable to the health-care provider's words and actions. Further, when parents are either physically or emotionally unavailable to their children, the struggle intensifies as the health-care provider tries to fill the gaps of care and advocacy. These issues add to the complexity of relationships in pediatric health-care settings.

We now know that there is no "one kind" of relationship that meets all needs and purposes of children, families, and health-care professionals in health-care settings. This chapter explores the types of relationships that develop between health-care professionals and the children and families they serve, as well as the relationships that develop among members of the health-care team.

Historical Perspective in Nursing

Nurses as a group typically have more contact with the child than any other members of the health-care team. Historically, the role of the nurse has been characterized by the provision of physical care under the control of the doctor, while at the same time remaining professionally detached from the patient (Pearson, Vaughan, & Fitzgerald, 1996). Within this biomedical model,

494

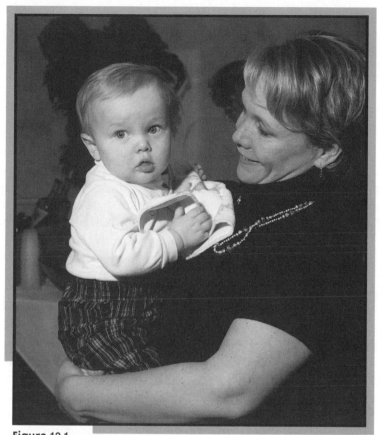

Figure 12.1.

In pediatrics, although the physical boundaries of care are taken away, it is expected that emotional boundaries remain clear.

the patient was perceived as a biologic body to be attended by the nurse, and emotional detachment and distancing were valued ideals (Williams, 2001). Gow (1982) offered the following account of a nurse that illustrates the confusing messages regarding professionalism that she experienced as a student:

> E. M. Jones tells us that when she was a student there seemed to be a motto, "Don't Become Involved with Your Patients." She felt that this was a protective device to spare the nurse from emotional breakdown as a result of "painful, disturbing, and depressing problems of their patients." I agree that this attitude was supposed to protect the nurses, but it seems to me that as a result, both the nurse and the patient ended up suffering. A nurse who felt distressed over a patient's predicament would use defense mechanisms (such as avoidance of the patient) to keep herself from getting emotionally involved. However, by the mere fact that

she was having these feelings she was already emotionally involved. Instead of admitting this, a process of denial went on, and the nurse never came to grips with her emotions; the patient suffered from loneliness and the feeling that the nurse was uncaring and coldhearted. The nurse was also useless in providing supportive care, since she required support herself, which she never received. (p. 12)

Nurses used distancing tactics to control interaction with patients, such as the use of closed questions, leading questions, a rapid succession of questions, and direct statements (Williams, 2001). Macloed Clark's (1982) comprehensive study of nurse–patient interaction in surgical settings found the average duration of contact to be 1.1 minute; further, this contact was superficial in nature and focused on the completion of physical tasks.

The introduction of the nursing process and later the focus on Primary Nursing challenged the notion of detachment (May, 1991). Both initiatives facilitate the provision of individualized care and focus on the nurses' personal relationships and commitment to patients. From this, a new definition of nurse–patient relationship emerges, one characterized by commitment, closeness, and involvement (Williams, 2001). These innovations, collectively referred to as "The New Nursing" (Savage, 1990), involve a clear redefinition of nursing care to include administering to the sick body and addressing wider, related psychological, emotional, social, and spiritual needs of the patient (May, 1991). Current perspectives lead to a broader interpretation of caring, which includes both "caring for" and "caring about" (Savage, 1995). Research findings indicate that "caring about" necessitates emotional involvement and commitment to the patient (Swanson, 1991).

Today, in place of distancing, the presence of the nurse has emerged as a key theme. Activities include giving time to and being with the patient and demonstrating an appreciation for the patient's experience. In exploring patients' and nurses' views on the beneficial effects of nursing care, Ersser (1991, 1998) found the potential for physical closeness and a psychological or existential closeness, which were considered valued and important. Further, communication that is patient-centered has been shown to facilitate a positive nurse–patient relationship (McCabe, 2004). It is clear that a fundamental change in perspective has taken place, whereby close, intimate nurse–patient relationships are increasingly prescribed rather than discouraged (Williams, 2001).

The Doctor–Patient Relationship

Dramatic changes have occurred in doctor–patient relationships during the past century. In the early 1900s, patients expected little from doctors and did not hold them in high esteem. The 1910 Flexner report revealed that diploma mills were churning out MD degrees, which served to further this attitude (Holoweiko, 1998). The flu epidemic and other infectious diseases were killing off entire families; doctors could do little to help. Family and friends provided most health care; asking a doctor to visit was a last resort.

Advances in medical science and technology changed the public's opinion of doctors. For example, pharmaceutical research post–World War II led to hundreds of potent compounds, dramatically expanding doctors' abilities to combat disease. Holoweiko (1998) also credited the media's portrayal of physicians—Ben Casey, Dr. Kildare, Marcus Welby—as almost god-like captains of the ship, not only curing patients' illnesses but resolving their emotional and relationship problems as well. Physicians were put on a pedestal, from which flowed a doctor-knows-best philosophy accepted with little question by patients.

With the movements for civil rights, peace in Vietnam, consumer rights, and women's equality during the 1960s and 1970s, most institutions were questioned. Paternalism was brought under fire, including the doctor–patient relationship (Holoweiko, 1998). Protestors of yesterday are now in their 50s or 60s and, better educated than previous generations, they are accustomed to challenging authority. Furthermore, the world of health information is available to anyone with Internet access.

Managed care also is changing the doctor–patient relationship, and with these changes, medical ethics. Most physicians were schooled in relationships that were convenantal, continuous, confidential, supportive, and personal. La Puma (1996) contrasted these relationships with the type more commonly seen today (see Table 12.1).

Forster (1998) offered examples of doctors who are unhappy with this depersonalization of doctors and patients and the language, such as "gatekeepers" and "clients," that accompanies it. He attributed this unhappiness with language as a symptom, masking depression over the loss of the traditional doctor–patient relationship, or, at the very least, a reflection of a fear that the idealized doctor–patient relationship is no longer attainable. However, Forster concluded that if doctors are competent and treat patients with compassion and concern, it matters little what someone chooses to call them.

Relationships Among Professionals

In recent years, under the constraints of cost-containment and with the rise of new technologies, shifts in division of labor have occurred among healthcare professions. For example, nurse technicians are performing certain tasks that in the past only registered nurses were permitted to do. Physician

Table 12.1

A Comparison of Characteristics of Doctor–Patient Relationships
of the Past and Today

The Past	Today
Covenant • Fidelity and altruism govern relationship. • Doctors put patients' interests before their own. • Relationship typically begins through recommendation from a trusted source.	Contract • Neither doctor nor patient truly has free choice. • Patients as a whole are increasingly wary of physicians as a group. • Relationship typically begins with selection from a list.
Continuous • Physician may care for several generations of the same family.	Episodic • Physicians couple and uncouple in group arrangements. • Physicians are selected and deselected by managed care plans. • Patients change doctors because of change in insurance.
Confidential • In 1976, approximately 70 physicians, nurses, managers, trainees, and students had access to a hospitalized patient's chart.	Wide Open • In 1996, approximately 210 physicians, nurses, managers, trainees, and students had access to a hospitalized patient's chart.
Collegial • Gaining the wisdom of another colleague or financial rewards provide incentives for referrals.	Solitary • Physicians face financial disincentives to refer patients or prescribe an off-formulary medication.
Personal • Focus is on the individual.	Population-based • Focus is on health of the public.

Note. Adapted from "Does the Doctor–Patient Relationship Mean More to Doctors than Patients?" by J. La Puma, 1996 [Electronic version], *Managed Care.* Retrieved from http://www.managedcaremag.com/archives/9601/MC9601.ethics.shtml

Assistants and Nurse Practitioners are prescribing medications and assuming other functions previously performed only by physicians.

Among physicians, questions are being raised about which tasks actually require the knowledge of a physician, much less a specialist physician, and which could be delegated to less skilled, but far more manageable, paraprofessionals. In fact, some experts argue that the best diagnostic and treatment knowledge and reasoning can be programmed into a computer, matching and surpassing the work of any physician or organization of physicians (Hughes, 1994).

Shifts in "who does what" can lead to confusion, turf issues, and tension. These factors must be considered alongside the normal conflicts that arise among professionals caring for children in health-care settings.

Types of Professional–Patient Relationships

"When a child is the patient, the patient is the family." This is one of the first lessons we learn when we enter the world of pediatrics. Thus, the discussion below may apply to relationships with individual children, with their parents or other family members, or both.

In researching and defining the nurse–patient relationship, Morse (1991) found that relationships can be either mutual or unilateral, according to the outcome of covert interactive negotiations or implicit interplay between the two persons. Mutual relationships fall into four broad types, and depend upon certain circumstances (e.g., length of time the nurse and patient have together), the needs and desires of the nurse and the patient, and personality factors. In a unilateral relationship, one person is unwilling or unable to develop the relationship to the level desired by the other. For example, a nurse who is "burned out" may not have the emotional energy to invest in the relationship when a patient clearly desires or needs a relationship with greater involvement.

The four broad types of mutual relationships, which are listed in order of involvement and intensity, are clinical, therapeutic, connected, and over-involved. The characteristics of each type are listed below (Morse, 1991; Stein-Parbury, 1993) and summarized in Table 12.2.

Clinical Relationship

Because of limited personal emotional involvement, the professional may not remember the patient, and the patient may not remember the professional. In a clinical relationship,

- professionals and families interact in a routine or standard manner;
- technical care is provided;
- the health situation involved typically is perceived by both parties as being minor and routine;
- the patient's vulnerability and dependence is almost nonexistent;
- little negotiation is involved;
- there is implicit agreement between both parties to keep the relationship at this level; and
- the relationship is short in duration. (Morse, 1991; Stein-Parbury, 1993)

Therapeutic Relationship

A therapeutic relationship is the most common type formed and is considered the "ideal" by most administrators and educators. At Rainbow Babies and Children's Hospital, for example, a therapeutic relationship is defined as

Table 12.2

Types and Characteristics of Nurse–Patient Relationships

Characteristics	Types of Relationships			
	Clinical	Therapeutic	Connected	Overinvolved
Time	Short/transitory	Short/average	Lengthy	Long-term
Interaction	Perfunctory/rote	Professional	Intensive/close	Intensive/ intimate
Patient's needs	Minor Treatment- oriented	Needs met Minor- moderate	Extensive/crisis "Goes the extra mile"	Enormous needs
Nurse's perspective of the patient; patient's perspective of own role	Only in patient role	First: in patient role Second: as a person	First: as a person Second: in patient role	Only as a person
Nursing commitment	Professional commitment	Professional commitment Patient's concerns secondary	Patient's concerns primary Treatment concerns secondary	Committed to patient only as a person Treatment goals discarded

Note. From "Negotiating Commitment and Involvement in the Nurse–Patient Relationship," by J. Morse, 1991, *Journal of Advanced Nursing, 16*, p. 457. Copyright 1991 by Blackwell. Reprinted with permission.

one that reflects the philosophy and values of the health-care institution, the department of nursing, and child life, and the individual nurse, while respecting patient–family values (McAliley, Lambert, Ashenberg, & Dull, 1996). In a therapeutic relationship,

- the patient typically is facing a situation that he or she perceives as neither life-threatening nor serious;
- care is given quickly and effectively;
- the patient's internal and external resources for meeting the demands of the situation are adequate and available;
- although the professional perceives the patient as a patient, there is also recognition and understanding of the patient as a person;
- the professional serves as support mobilizer and enhancer; and
- the relationship is usually of short or average duration. (Morse, 1991; Stein-Parbury, 1993)

Connected Relationship

A connected relationship may develop when the patient and professional have either been together long enough for the relationship to have evolved beyond a clinical and a therapeutic relationship, or the process is accelerated because of the patient's extreme need. Many children with cancer have identified this kind of relationship as being the single most important thing that has helped them to cope with the cancer experience (Rollins, 2003). Research findings indicate that developing reciprocal trust is the basic social process that enables professionals and children to reach the goal of becoming connected (Wilson, Morse, & Penrod, 1998). In connected relationships,

- the professional and patient perceive each other as people first and their roles as patient and professional become secondary;
- both the professional and patient choose to enter this level of relationship;
- trust and commitment are deep and complete;
- the professional will "bend and break the rules" and "go the extra mile" on the patient's behalf;
- the patient actively seeks the professional's advice and opinion;
- the professional functions as a source of support;
- self-disclosure is high; and
- both the professional and the patient experience change as a result of their relationship. (Morse, 1991; Stein-Parbury, 1993)

Overinvolved Relationship

This type of relationship usually develops when the patient has extraordinary needs and the professional chooses to meet them, or when the patient and the professional have spent an extensive length of time together and mutually respect, trust, and care for each other. In an overinvolved relationship,

- the professional is committed to the patient as a person, and this overrides the professional's commitment to the treatment regime, other professionals, the institution and its need, and the professional's responsibilities toward other patients;
- the professional is a complete confidant of the patient and is treated as a member of the patient's family;
- the relationship continues beyond the professional's work hours and the professional remains a key figure in the patient's life;
- the professional may become territorial and believe that he or she is the only one who can give proper and appropriate care to the patient; and
- the professional views the patient as a person, the patient relinquishes the patient role, and the professional relinquishes the impersonal professional relationship. (Morse, 1991; Stein-Parbury, 1993)

Special Considerations in Patient—Professional Relationships

Most researchers and clinicians agree that certain circumstances influence the type of relationship that is likely to develop between patients and professionals. The type of illness is a significant factor in the characteristics of the roles and resulting relationships. For example, patient passivity and professional assertiveness are the most common reactions to acute illness; patient cooperation and professional guidance are common characteristics in less acute illness; and professionals participating in a treatment plan where patients have the bulk of the responsibility to help themselves is common in chronic illness (Hughes, 1994).

Chronic Illness

With chronic illness, the opportunity exists for professionals and patients to come to know each other over a long period of time, and therefore for the possibility of a connected relationship to develop (Stein-Parbury, 1993). Both parties come to understand and appreciate each other as people, and often share on a personal level the pain of loss and the joy of successful adaptation that accompanies living with chronic illness.

Although the average length of hospital stay for children remain short, the increase in the number of children undergoing organ transplantation means very long stays for a growing number of children. Allenbach and Steinmiller (2004) found that inconsistent nursing practices created nurse–patient boundary issues on a cardiac step-down unit related to confidentiality, limit setting, and professionalism with children awaiting organ transplantation and their families. Nursing staff worked together to design and implement a plan to translate the principles of therapeutic relationships into daily practice. The plan outlined concrete solutions and resources available within the hospital to empower staff in the ongoing effort to manage relationships with children with chronic diseases and their families.

Life-Threatening Illness and Death

More involved and intense relationships tend to develop when a child has a life-threatening condition or is dying. Davies et al. (1996) conducted interviews with 25 nurses who had cared for at least one chronically ill child who had died. Findings indicated that nurses struggled with both grief distress and moral distress within the context of a mutually caring relationship between the nurse and child wherein both the patient and the nurse made a difference in each other's lives. These relationships evolved as nurses shared special times with children by sitting, listening, or being present during the child's vulnerable moments.

Totka (1996) also reported intense relationships between nurses and children who were dying. This theme represented some of the most significant stories in pediatric nurses' practices. She found that a child's death did more than affect the nurse emotionally; it actually transformed that nurse's practice. "Establishing a relationship with one who is dying is a privileged experience" (Stanley, 2000, p. 36). Talking about hopes and fears requires trust, and trust develops through getting to know each other. The connected relationship affords this important opportunity.

Home Care

Although a team of professionals are involved when a child receives home health-care services, families report that the single most important part of successful home care is the nursing staff (Creasser, 1996). Nurses come into the home as strangers and intrude into intimate family relationships that have been cultivated over years (Coffman, 1997; Petit de Mange, 1998). It is often difficult for the family and the nurse to set and maintain boundaries. In the words of a mother who has had home care services for her medically fragile child at home for over 10 years:

> Nurses can be in the home for long periods of time. This makes it difficult to remember they are not family or personal friends. They are professionals paid to take care of the child. It is not her role to baby sit with other children, clean the house, do laundry, pay bills, or criticize the family's lifestyle—unless that lifestyle affects the child's care. (Creasser, 1996, p. 42)

The home care nurse is exposed to private family conversations and interactions (Baptiste, 1996). Sometimes a nurse may be with the family for years. He or she may become the family's confidante or vice versa. The nurse may feel like both a "guest" and a "professional." Families, justifiably, may feel ambivalent about the nurse, for although they need the service the nurse provides, they also see the nurse as the cause of their loss of privacy.

Not only boundary but also authority issues can become a source of tension between parents and professionals. Wegener (1996) recommended that families establish "house rules" or guidelines with which they are comfortable: "These rules would then frame, from the beginning, the working relationship between the family, nurses, and nursing agency" (p. 21).

Negotiating Relationships

Morse (1991) described the process patients and nurses use to negotiate a relationship. The degree of intensity in the negotiation depends upon the patient's perception of the seriousness of the situation and his or her feeling of vulnerability and dependence. The patient first evaluates whether the nurse is a good person, asking questions such as "Are you from around here?" "Are you married?" and "Do you have children?" From there, he or she tries to determine if the nurse is a good nurse by asking, "Do you like nursing?" "Have you been a nurse long?" and asking other patients for references ("Is she good?"). When satisfied with the answers, the patient may then make some overtures toward the nurse (e.g., waving as the nurse passes; calling the nurse by name) so that he or she will willingly become involved.

While the patient is assessing the nurse, the nurse is assessing the patient, looking for a "personality click." Different from the nursing assessment, the nurse evaluates the patient's personal needs and support system, assesses the patient as a person, and consciously chooses whether to make an emotional investment in the patient or just do his or her job (Morse, 1991).

Power

Within the relationship, both the professional and the patient have power (see Table 12.3; Sully, 1996). The way in which professionals and patients interact depends in part on how they use their power. For example, professionals can assert their superior knowledge by using jargon, or they can attempt to use language patients can understand. Patients can be constantly demanding, or they can limit their requests to only the most urgent at busy times.

Professionals can examine their motives about their involvement with patients and families and determine whether these behaviors are empowering or paternalistic. Table 12.4 provides a guide. Once individuals have insight into their behavioral tendencies, they can be assisted in making changes in their interactions with children and families (Rushton, Armstrong, & McEnhill, 1996).

Power also can be asserted subtly (Ray, 1997). For example, *time* is a power issue. In any relationship, the person who controls the clock has more power. In a job interview, for instance, it is permissible for the employer to be late, but not the job applicant. Parents, not children, ultimately are the ones to decide how family time is spent (e.g., bedtimes, holidays, doctors' appointments). Bosses determine the time of the meeting, not the employees. Time has special meaning for people who are dying. One moment, time seemed more or less infinite; suddenly, this is no longer the case, which can result in intense feelings of powerlessness.

Table 12.3

505

Issues of Powerfulness and Powerlessness of Patients and Professionals

Variable	Patients	Professionals
Powerful	Are central figures and focus in health-care system Can be more or less cooperative Can have crises that demand immediate attention Have rights and can complain if rights are violated Can get worse and die, causing professionals to experience a sense of failure	Have specialist knowledge Speak a specialist jargon that patients may not understand Control access to tests and treatments Often require appointments Familiar with the health-care system Can close ranks to protect one another in the face of a patient's complaint
Powerless	Access to health-care professionals is often controlled May not understand the health-care system and have difficulty using it May be in a weakened state because of medical condition May fear serious illness or death	Must obey protocols and may feel they have little personal discretion Usually cannot choose whether to treat a particular patient Cannot relax vigilance because mistakes can have fatal consequences Constantly exposed to suffering and distress

Note. Adapted from "The Impact of Power in Therapeutic Relationships," by P. Sully, 1996, *Nursing Times, 92*(41), pp. 40–41.

Health-care professionals who demonstrate that they respect and value the child's and family's time can do much to equalize this balance of power and improve patient–family–professional relationships. Some methods include offering appointment times that are convenient for families, continually updating the family and offering apologies when there are unexpected delays, and providing pagers for families to allow them the freedom to move about while waiting for appointments, treatments, tests, or doctors to make hospital rounds. Health-care professionals can be flexible to changing plans. When a child is dying, the features of a connected relationship—breaking the rules, going the extra mile—can be put into play to accommodate the child's and family's wishes about how they wish to spend their time.

Touch also has power implications. The person with more power touches the other person more often (Ray, 1997). For example, teachers pat their students on the shoulder, yet a student returning this gesture likely would be considered disrespectful. A manager may congratulate an employee with a hearty pat on the back, but the employee patting the boss on the back likely

Table 12.4

Characteristics of Paternalistic and Empowering Behaviors

Paternalistic Behavior	Empowering Behavior
• Assumes needs of the patient and family without verification or mutual goal setting. • Replaces or subverts primary relationships. • Fosters dependency; projects own needs onto the patient and family. • Undermines confidence by conveying that parents are incapable of acting on their child's behalf. • Limits choices and opportunities for autonomous decision making. • Sabotages efforts of treatment team.	• Provides specific caregiving interventions based on a plan of care that is developed with the patient and family. • Supports and recognizes primary relationships. • Supports the autonomy of parents; assumes that parents have the capacity to act as their child's primary advocate. • Supports parents and patients to act on their own behalf; conveys support and affirms abilities. • Assists to reveal and explore the full range of options and choices pertinent to decisions. • Collaborates with the treatment team to achieve goals.

Note. Adapted from "Establishing Therapeutic Boundaries as Patient Advocates," by C. Rushton, L. Armstrong, and M. McEnhill, 1996, *Pediatric Nursing, 22*(3), p. 188. Copyright 1996 by Jannetti. Adapted with permission.

would be considered forward. In an effective parent–professional partnership, both partners are equals. The professional who overuses touch in this manner may be perceived as condescending and may threaten this balance.

Height, or looking down on someone, has power implications. Although much that professionals do in health-care settings must be done from above, there are still opportunities to get down on the child's level or sit by a parent with one's face looking up rather than down at the individual. The *chin* is the most powerful part of the body (Ray, 1997). When the chin is in the air, the person appears superior, condescending, or confrontational.

The use of *space* is another power consideration. Individuals who take up a lot of space are more powerful. Using big gestures, wide movements, arms akimbo or on the hips all send messages of power. Also, any sort of *pointer* or extension held in the hand, such as a pen or eyeglasses, operates as a symbol of authority. This reflects back to the days when parents or teachers shook their fingers at us (Ray, 1997).

Power shifts somewhat when the health-care setting is the home. In a study on negotiating layperson and professional roles in the care of children with complex health-care needs, Kirk (2001) found that being on home territory, and in possession of expertise in caregiving and in managing encounters with professionals, provided parents with a sense of control with which to enter negotiations with professionals. Kirk issued a caution regarding the importance of not letting changes in the balance of power lead to the development of parent–professional relationships that are characterized by conflict rather than partnership.

Boundaries

Within every relationship there are boundaries. Boundaries serve to help people to take care of themselves and prevent abuses (Rushton et al., 1996). The intense nature of relationships that professionals develop with children and their families may result in unclear boundaries. When professionals are either overinvolved or underinvolved, boundaries are ambiguous.

Boundary Violations

Professionals typically enter relationships with children and families with professional boundaries intact. However, in time, the relationship may begin to meet the professional's need for love, acceptance, meaningful relationships, affiliation, and regard by others (Pennington, Gatner, Schilit, & Bechtel, 1993). Because boundary violations often begin subtly, professionals frequently do not know that they have "crossed the line" until after the fact (Totka, 1996). The following behaviors can alert the professional to boundary problems (Willis-Brandon, 1990):

- Exaggerated feelings of shame, guilt, or inadequacy;
- Seeing oneself as a victim;
- An exaggerated sense of responsibility for things beyond one's control;
- Setting unrealistic expectations of oneself or others;
- Inability to tolerate differences in approach or human error;
- Avoiding conflict and confrontation;
- Giving help when it is not needed or requested; and
- Putting the needs of others above personal needs.

Rushton and colleagues (1996) recommended using mechanisms such as personal inventory questionnaires regarding professional boundaries, simulations of common clinical situations where boundary violations are possible, role-playings, and team strategy sessions.

Policy Statement for Pediatricians

In 1999, the American Academy of Pediatrics (AAP) issued a policy statement on appropriate boundaries in the pediatrician–family–patient relationship (AAP, 1999). Topics the document addresses include romantic and sexual relationships, inadvertent sexuality in the physician–patient relationship, and gifts or other expressions of affection or gratitude. Although intended for pediatricians, most of the issues discussed often are faced by other health-care professionals as well.

Reliable data on the prevalence of sexual contact between physicians and their patients or their patients' family members is difficult to find. The AAP (1999) pointed out that interpersonal entanglements raise at least two serious questions: (a) Can a patient or family member make clear and free choices to accept or reject affections, especially sexual, in the context of the unavoidably unequal physician–patient–family relationship? and (b) Once such intimacy develops, can the parties maintain a proper and effective therapeutic relationship?

Some professionals may feel sexually attracted to children, which may put children at risk of sexual abuse or exploitation. But the more likely situation to occur is a misunderstanding during routine discussions and examinations (Silber, 1994). For example, pediatricians, nurses, and other professionals may be misunderstood when they first discuss sexual maturation and sexuality with patients. Similarly, examining an adolescent's maturing genitals or breasts may be distressing or misunderstood, especially without the presence of a parent or other adult. Some kinds of touching may be confusing or offensive to children, depending on their stage of physical and emotional maturation. Words, body language, and other aspects of professional conduct may inadvertently offend or insult patients and family members, such as the use of endearments like "honey" or "dear" (AAP, 1999).

Conducting anticipatory discussions before a physical examination is performed can reduce fears and misunderstandings and lead to enhanced professional, child, and family comfort. Issues of concern can be clarified. For example, children may have a strong preference regarding whether a male or female performs their exam, and whether they would like someone else present.

Needless to say, romantic or sexual relationships with children and youth are always inappropriate. However, romantic or sexual relationships with adult family members of patients should also be avoided given the potential for adverse effects on professional judgment and family member behavior concerning the patient's health (AAP, 1999). Further, children should not have to be concerned about confidentiality or have anxiety over the potential for the professional to have a conflict of loyalty because of his or her involvement with a parent.

Gifts or other expressions of gratitude can be a concern. The AAP recommendations state that it may be appropriate to accept modest gifts from patients and their families. However, when the physician feels uncomfortable accepting a gift, he or she may want to suggest alternatives such as a charitable donation in the physician's name.

Models

Today, most institutions have rules and policies that establish clear boundaries in certain areas about what professionals can and cannot do. However, many boundary issues are not simply black and white, but fall into the grey zone. Perhaps what is more helpful is a process to help professionals sort out boundary issues. The Rainbow Babies and Children's Hospital in Cleveland,

Ohio, developed a therapeutic relations decision-making framework to (a) foster a proactive process of conscious deliberation regarding nurse–patient interactions, and (b) afford a nonthreatening mechanism for retrospective review of apparently nontherapeutic relationships (McAliley et al., 1996). The framework is based upon an "act utilitarian" approach to moral reasoning and promotes the clarification of personal philosophy and values.

The model encourages the nurse to contemplate the potential negative and positive outcomes of the interaction being examined within each of five contexts (McAliley et al., 1996):

- Philosophy and policy of the organization
- Impact upon desired patient–family outcomes
- Developmental stage of the relationship
- Potential impact on other patients, family, and staff
- The nurse's philosophy and values regarding role and the nature of a therapeutic relationship

The Rainbow Therapeutic Relations Decision-Making Model has been used successfully in a variety of situations, some fairly complex. See boxes for examples.

Establishing Relationships Between Professionals

When speaking of relationships between professionals in health-care settings, usually the first relationship to come to mind is the nurse–doctor relationship. Less common in clinical practice in recent years is the "doctor–nurse game," a stereotypical pattern of interactions, first described in the 1960s, in which (female) nurses showed initiative and offered advice while appearing to defer passively to the doctor's authority (Sweet & Norman, 1995). What remains, however, is each profession continuing to have ideal expectations of one another, which inevitably fall short as a result of differing views of qualities of doctors and nurses to be valued.

Changes in who performs certain health-care services and where these services are delivered quite naturally have doctors, nurses, and other professionals anxious about roles and turf issues. Regarding the advent of Primary Care Groups in England, Richards, Carley, Jenkins-Clarke, and Richards (2000) believe that the most successful approach to address these anxieties is to establish more equitable and less hierarchical models of multiprofessional teamwork.

The doctor–nurse relationship traditionally has been a man–woman relationship. The relationship often has been described as a dominant–subservient relationship with a clear understanding that the doctor is a man

Overinvolvement?

Co-primary nurses were contemplating becoming "Big Sisters" for a 10-year-old foster child who would continue to have periodic admissions to their unit. The Head Nurse Manager (HNM) and Clinical Nurse Specialist (CNS) had strong reservations about this. They were concerned that this interaction would interfere with the bonding process between the patient and her newly assigned (third) foster family. There was the potential that the nurses would not stick with the commitment very long (given their work and family/social lives were already very full), and that this already traumatized child would experience their withdrawal as yet another rejection. It was also likely that

and the nurse is a woman. However, in recent years the number of women studying medicine has increased. Gjerberg and Kjolsrod (2001) investigated what happens to the doctor–nurse relationship when both the doctor and the nurse are women. They reported that female doctors often find that they are met with less respect and confidence and are given less help than their male colleagues. The female doctors attribute this behavior in part to the nurse's desire to reduce status differences between the two groups. In response to this difference in treatment, female doctors in this study indicated that they do as much as possible themselves and attempt to make friends with the nurses.

English (1997) reported an increased emphasis for the team approach in which doctors, nurses, and other health workers adapt and develop new skills. Although the team approach to the delivery of health care has always been important, it has become more so as the boundaries between professional groups have become blurred:

> Doctors and nurses are becoming managers; nurses are taking on jobs previously done by doctors; support workers are taking over jobs done by nurses; and similarly, technicians, physiotherapists, and radiographers are all taking on tasks previously done by others ... unless there is dia-

Underinvolvement?

A generally sensitive and skilled nurse made the comment to the CNS that she really enjoyed working with the failure-to-thrive patients when their parents were not present (as was frequently the case). She viewed the parents as uninvested and antagonistic and felt they just complicated care. Although she was adept at implementing behavioral feeding plans and getting the children to grow while in the hospital, she had lost sight of the fact that failure-to-thrive is usually a family problem. Hospital gains would not be maintained if parents were not made partners in care and if nothing

other patients and families would hear about some of their adventures together. Although some might find the relationship laudable, others could view it as discriminatory. The nurses were not told that developing such a relationship was prohibited, but the Rainbow Framework was used to identify potential consequences and to help them examine their motives. The nurses chose to pursue the relationship. However, they reframed it for themselves and restructured it for the child involved, thus preventing most of the complications that had concerned the HNM and CNS.

Note. From "Therapeutic Relations Decision Making: The Rainbow Framework," by L. McAliley, S. Lambert, M. Ashenberg, and S. Dull, 1996, *Pediatric Nursing, 22*(3), p. 203. Copyright 1996 by Jannetti. Reprinted with permission.

logue and trust between the groups, one or more of them are likely to feel threatened as their roles are changed. (English, 1997)

The call throughout health care is the need for collaboration. Lockhart-Wood (2000) proposed that a number of characteristics are significant in influencing the collaborative process: (a) excellent communication skills, (b) respect for the value of colleagues' roles, (c) the ability to share points of view, and (d) trust.

Mutual respect for a profession's unique perspective and for an individual's unique strengths provide the basis for the trust needed for effective and rewarding working relationships between members of the child's health-care team. Finding ways to better understand each other is the path to mutual respect. One way in which doctors and nurses may come to understand each other is through receiving some of their training together and understanding more of each others' roles from the start of professional training.

Little can be achieved in isolation. To make a significant difference in improving the quality of health care for children, members of the health-care team and their representative organizations must learn to work together. Too much is at stake to do otherwise.

changed for them. The most helpful domains in the Rainbow Framework for discussion with this nurse were "patient–family outcome goals" and "philosophy and values of the nurse." She could be helped to see that the greater need and professional challenge lay with the family rather than the child. Engaging and empowering the family would result in long-term effects and reflect more positively on the nurse and institution.

Note. From "Therapeutic Relations Decision Making:The Rainbow Framework," by L. McAliley, S. Lambert, M. Ashenberg, and S. Dull, 1996, *Pediatric Nursing, 22*(3), p. 203. Copyright 1996 by Jannetti. Reprinted with permission.

Conclusion

Caring, in terms of health care, is something special. It is a process, a way of relating to someone; it needs to develop in the same way that a friendship only emerges over time (Castledine, 1998). Quality health care for children depends on caring individuals working well together. Establishing and maintaining effective relationships between professionals and the children and families they serve, as well as between the professionals themselves, is the key.

Study Guide

1. Discuss what relationships are, how they vary, and how and why they have changed in health-care settings.

2. How do relationships that nurses have with children in the health-care system differ from those of doctors, child life specialists, and other health-care providers? What factors have influenced changes in these relationships?

3. Compare and contrast the four types of mutual relationships.

4. How does nature of the illness or type of care required affect the type of relationship?

5. What are some of the sources of tension between parents and health-care providers, and how might they be addressed?

6. Describe power and empowerment in human relationships and their importance for children and their families in health care.

7. Boundaries exist in human relationships; explain boundaries and describe healthy boundaries in child health-care relationships.

8. Are there professional and institutional policies affecting professional relationships? Describe.

9. Relationships *among* professionals also are critical to optimal health care for children with special needs. Describe *optimal* relationships for today's health-care system and children's needs.

10. Caring has an impact on children's psychosocial development as well as physical health. Summarize the major relationship factors that influence children's recovery, maintenance, and quality of life.

References

Allenbach, A., & Steinmiller, E. (2004). Waiting together: Translating the principles of therapeutic relationships one step further. *Journal for Specialists in Pediatric Nursing, 9*(1), 24–31.

American Academy of Pediatrics (AAP). (1999). Appropriate boundaries in the pediatrician–family–patient relationship. *Pediatrics, 104*(2), 334–336.

Baptiste, G. (1996). A nursing perspective. In K. Gunter & R. Manago (Eds.), *Beyond discharge: Interdisciplinary perspectives for transitioning children with complex medical needs from hospital to home* (pp. 15–18). Bethesda, MD: Association for the Care of Children's Health.

Castledine, G. (1998). The relationship between caring and nursing. *British Journal of Nursing, 7*(14), 866.

Coffman, S. (1997). Home-care nurses as strangers in the family. *Western Journal of Nursing Research, 19*(1), 82–96.

Creasser, C. (1996). A family perspective. In K. Gunter & R. Manago (Eds.), *Beyond discharge: Interdisciplinary perspectives for transitioning children with complex medical needs from hospital to home* (pp. 39–44). Bethesda, MD: Association for the Care of Children's Health.

Davies, B., Clarke, D., Connaughty, S., Cook, K., MacKenzie, B., McCormick, J., O'Loane, M., & Stutzer, C. (1996). Caring for dying children: Nurses' experiences. *Pediatric Nursing, 22*(6), 500–507.

English, T. (1997). Personal paper: Medicine in the 1990s needs a team approach. *British Medical Journal, 314*(7081), 661–663.

Ersser, S. (1991). A search for the therapeutic dimensions of nurse–patient interaction. In R. McMahon & A. Pearson (Eds.), *Nursing as therapy* (pp. 43–84). London: Chapman & Hall.

Ersser, S. (1998). The presentation of the nurse: A neglected dimension of therapeutic nurse–patient interaction? In R. McMahon & A. Pearson (Eds.), *Nursing as therapy* (2nd ed., pp. 37–63). London: Thornes.

Forster, J. (1998). Remember when … doctors were doctors, not "providers"? *Medical Economics, 75*(13), 125–126. Retrieved July 31, 2001, from www.findarticles.com

Gjerberg, E., & Kjolsrod, L. (2001). The doctor–nurse relationship: How easy is it to be a female doctor cooperating with a female nurse? *Social Science Medicine, 52*(2), 189–202.

Gow, K. (1982). *How nurses' emotions affect patient care.* New York: Springer Publishing.

Holoweiko, M. (1998). Here's looking at: Doctor–patient relations. Good news—the pedestal is gone. *Medical Economics, 75*(20), 54–56, 63, 67.

Hughes, J. (1994). *Organization and information at the bed-side.* Unpublished doctoral dissertation, University of Chicago.

Kirk, S. (2001). Negotiating lay and professional roles in the care of children with complex health care needs. *Journal of Advanced Nursing, 34*(5), 593–602.

La Puma, J. (1996, January). Does the doctor–patient relationship mean more to doctors than patients? [Electronic version]. *Managed Care.* Retrieved March 2003, from www.managedcaremag.com/archives/9601/MC9601.ethics.shtml

Lockhart-Wood, K. (2000). Collaboration between nurses and doctors in clinical practice. *British Journal of Nursing, 9*(5), 276–280.

Macloed Clark, J. (1982). *Nurse–patient verbal interaction: An analysis of recorded conversations on selected surgical wards.* Unpublished PhD thesis, University of London.

May, C. (1991). Affective neutrality and involvement in nurse–patient relationship: Perceptions of appropriate behaviour among nurses in acute medical and surgical wards. *Journal of Advanced Nursing, 16*, 555–558.

McAliley, L., Lambert, S., Ashenberg, M., & Dull, S. (1996). Therapeutic relations decision making: The Rainbow framework. *Pediatric Nursing, 22*(3), 199–203, 210.

McCabe, C. (2004). Nurse–patient communication: An exploration of patients' experiences. *Journal of Clinical Nursing, 13*(1), 41–49.

Morse, J. M. (1991). Negotiating commitment and involvement in the nurse–patient relationship. *Journal of Advanced Nursing, 16*, 455–468.

Pearson, A., Vaughan, B., & Fitzgerald, M. (1996). *Nursing models for practice* (2nd ed.). Oxford, England: Butterworth Heinemann.

Pennington, S., Gafner, G., Schilit, R., & Bechtel, B. (1993). Addressing ethical boundaries among nurses. *Nursing Management, 24*(6), 36–39.

Petit de Mange, E. (1998). Pediatric considerations in homecare. *Critical Care Nursing Clinics of North America, 10*(3), 3339–3346.

Ray, M. (1997). *I'm here to help.* New York: Bantam Books.

Richards, A., Carley, J., Jenkins-Clarke, S., & Richards, D. (2000). Skill mix between nurses and doctors working in primary care—delegation or allocation: A review of the literature. *International Journal of Nursing Studies, 37*(3), 185–197.

Rollins, J. (2003). *A comparison of the nature of stress and coping for children with cancer in the United States and the United Kingdom.* Unpublished doctoral dissertation, DeMontfort University, Leicester, England.

Rushton, C., Armstrong, L., & McEnhill, M. (1996). Establishing therapeutic boundaries as patient advocates. *Pediatric Nursing, 22*(3), 185–189.

Savage, J. (1990). The theory and practice of the "New Nursing." *Nursing Times, 86*, 42–45.

Savage, J. (1995). *Nursing intimacy: An ethnographic approach to nurse patient interaction.* London: Scutari Press.

Silber, T. (1994). False allegations of sexual touching by physicians in the practice of pediatrics. *Pediatrics, 94*, 742–745.

Stanley, K. (2000). Silence is not golden: Conversations with the dying. *Clinical Journal of Oncology Nursing, 4*(1), 34–40.

Stein-Parbury, J. (1993). *Patient and person.* Melbourne, Australia: Churchill Livingstone.

Sully, P. (1996). The impact of power in therapeutic relationships. *Nursing Times, 92*(41), 40 41.

Swanson, K. (1991). Empirical development of a middle range theory of caring. *Nursing Research, 40*, 161–166.

Sweet, S., & Norman, I. (1995). The nurse–doctor relationship: A selective literature review. *Journal of Advanced Nursing, 22*(1), 165–170.

Totka, J. (1996). Exploring the boundaries of pediatric practice: Nurse stories related to relationships. *Pediatric Nursing, 22*(3), 191–196.

Wegener, D. (1996). A social work perspective. In K. Gunter & R. Manago (Eds.), *Beyond discharge: Interdisciplinary perspectives for transitioning children with complex medical needs from hospital to home* (pp. 19–24). Bethesda, MD: Association for the Care of Children's Health.

Williams, A. (2001). A literature review on the concept of intimacy in nursing. *Journal of Advanced Nursing, 33*(5), 660–667.

Willis-Brandon, C. (1990). *Learning to say no: Establishing healthy boundaries.* Deerfield Beach, FL: Health Communications.

Wilson, S., Morse, J., & Penrod, J. (1998). Developing reciprocal trust in the caregiving relationship. *Qualitative Health Research, 8*(4), 446–465.

Epilogue

Judy A. Rollins

As we imagine the future of children's health care and its psychosocial implications, those who advocate for children and their families will face ongoing as well as new challenges. We look at what some of these challenges might be, within the context of some of the more prominent trends of today.

Lack of Accessible and Affordable Health Care

As the last remaining industrialized nation without universal health-care coverage, the United States has never fully insured its population and the uninsured have never been guaranteed access to basic care. Conditions today, however, are worse because the gap between what the working poor could pay for out-of-pocket expenses years ago and what they can afford today is much wider. This is primarily because the cost of health care has risen faster than personal income, particularly for low-wage workers. Low-income workers further lose out because only 26% of those earning $25,000 or less have employers that offer health insurance benefits, compared to 83% of workers earning $75,000 or more (Nelson, 2003).

Managed care and other changes in the private health insurance system also have played a role by reducing surplus money that used to be available to cover free care for the poor. At the same time, government has moved to control taxpayer-financed health spending, leaving traditional safety-net services at public hospitals and clinics inadequate to meet the need. This has resulted in long waits for care and neglect of all but the most serious health problems of the poor. Today, even routine procedures are beyond the means of the uninsured.

Unfortunately, this trend is expected to continue. The number of uninsured individuals in the United States increased by 40% during the 1990s, from 31 million to 43.4 million in 1998 (Wielawski, 1998). Today, 12% of our nation's children are without health insurance (Annie E. Casey Foundation, 2004). In response to the millions of children with no health coverage, the federal government approved the State Children's Health Insurance Program (SCHIP) in 1998 (Web site: www.insurekidsnow.gov).

However, children can only benefit from this and other programs if they are identified and enrolled. Families often do not know these programs exist or do not realize that their children qualify, but even if they do, there are other reasons that children are not enrolled. For example, many working parents cannot afford the time required to complete complex and confusing application forms, and the application process itself can be demeaning. Even when parents do enroll their children, the lack of coordination among children's health coverage programs means children may not get referred to or enrolled in appropriate programs (The Robert Wood Johnson Foundation, 1998).

Lack of a consistent source of medical care can have severe psychosocial implications for children. Lacking health-care insurance or the financial resources to pay for doctor visits, families in such circumstances tend to use the hospital's emergency department as their child's health-care provider. In the hustle and bustle of such a setting, sensitive, age-appropriate preparation for examinations and procedures is less likely to take place and children may be left with painful memories and emotional scars that may last a lifetime.

All-important prevention issues may go unaddressed for children who lack a "medical home." For example, although some prevention efforts, such as childhood immunizations, may be enforced through requirements for school entry, will children receive the critical psychosocial-focused prevention information they need to avoid adolescent pregnancy, substance abuse, and sexually transmitted diseases? And even if these issues are addressed in other settings, such as the school, will the provision of information be as effective when delivered by an individual who is not the trusted pediatrician or other health-care provider with whom the child has an established long-standing relationship?

Hospitals

We continue to see the hospital being reinvented to conform with the forces that are replacing the acute, inpatient-oriented illness model of health care with a disease-prevention, health-promotion, primary care model. Hospitals are merging with others, forming regional health-care systems with names sounding more like businesses than health-care institutions. Growing numbers of religious hospitals are finding it difficult to survive.

What does the future hold for hospitals? Hospitals will no longer conduct the "core business" of U.S. health care; however, they can play a key role by empowering others and facilitating the integration of health services across the continuum of care. In 1995, Shortell and colleagues predicted the following challenges:

> New management and governance structures will be required, as will population-based health status needs assessments, new relations with physicians, re-engineering of the clinical processes, organization-wide

commitment to improving quality, information systems that link patients and providers, and creation of an overall community care management system. (Shortell, Gillies, & Devers, 1995, p. 131)

We already see some of these challenges being addressed. For example, with the overwhelming trend toward vertical integration of health-care organizations, hospital-based case management programs have taken the lead in considering how existing case management models can expand to meet patient and provider needs along a continuum of care. Parents, particularly parents of children with special health-care needs, need to have a voice in the creation of these management models to ensure that psychosocial care and other important elements of comprehensive family-centered care are included.

The Hospitalist

In an era of cost containment, only very sick children are hospitalized and as quickly as possible are sent home or to a less costly medical setting. Shorter hospital stays mean that inpatient conditions are more acute and require more of the attending physician's time and personal attention—time that many ambulatory physicians no longer have. Today's pediatricians and other primary care physicians spend at least 90% of their time in an office or clinic where the skills a physician needs and the illnesses seen are fundamentally different from the skills needed in the hospital setting (Boodman, 1999).

Inpatient and outpatient medicine have become so dissimilar in recent years that a new medical specialist has emerged called a hospitalist. Hospitalists, sometimes called inpatient specialists, are physicians who spend 25% or more of their time in the hospital setting working as the physician-on-record of hospitalized patients. Although variations exist, the basic concept is that the hospitalist accepts patients from community physicians and manages their in-hospital care, keeps the primary physicians up to date on their patients' progress, and transfers care back to those physicians upon a patient's discharge (McConaghy, 1998).

The goals of the hospitalist approach are to increase the efficiency of inpatient care while decreasing its costs. Proponents of this approach argue that inpatient specialists can give more personalized care to hospitalized patients because they spend most of their time in the hospital rather than in the office. Being "in-house" allows them to see patients several times a day, adjust therapies more efficiently, better coordinate care among consulting specialists, and quickly respond to patient problems or complications. They believe that this intensive care shortens hospital stays, decreases medical costs, and improves the quality of care (Wachter & Goldman, 1996). Others cite benefits such as patient satisfaction and physicians enjoying having more time to see patients in the office without the often-competing demands of hospital work (Brandner, 1995; Henry, 1997).

Opponents argue that decreased cost of inpatient care does not necessarily equal more cost-effective or high-value care. The hospitalist is likely to be unfamiliar with the patient's history and current psychosocial milieu, and might order more aggressive work-ups and intervention than would the patient's personal physician, thus increasing the cost of care in both the short and long term (Epstein, 1997). Further, with shorter hospital stays and more complex problems, some opponents of the hospitalist approach point out that the physician–patient relationship and continuity of care are more important than ever before. For children with special health-care needs and the variety and number of coordinated services they often require, the hospitalist approach may result in less favorable outcomes. Ryan (1997) noted the inconsistency of preaching continuity of care but "abandoning it at the hospital door as an unnecessary burden."

The arguments on both sides of the issue are based on anecdotal data and personal experience. Studies are under way, but at this time solid data to support either view do not exist. The answers to the many challenging questions will likely affect pediatricians, family physicians, and others that provide primary health-care services for children.

Hospitalist groups are becoming increasingly common in managed care organizations, larger hospitals, and some large physician practices. They are commonplace in urban areas, especially in states such as California where managed care market penetration is typically higher than in other parts of the country. Results of a 1997 California Medical Association (CMA) survey revealed that three out of four responding hospitals were using inpatient physicians to some degree, and half of those not yet using them were considering their use (Morasch, 1998).

The Physical Environment

The physical environment of the hospital will take on increased importance. Over the past decade, the health-care industry, looking at the guest-service industry, has recognized that the physical environment is a valuable resource that can and does affect all of its "customers" (Fottler, Ford, Roberts, & Ford, 2000). The health-care industry has learned two important principles from the guest-service industry model: (a) to provide the setting customers expect, and (b) to create an environment that meets or exceeds customer needs for safety, security, support, competence, physical comfort, and psychological comfort.

Patient and family resource centers will become the norm for hospitals that want to stay competitive in the future health-care environment. A commitment to family-centered care, the public's interest in health issues, as well as the acknowledgement that a better informed patient leads to improved health outcomes provides further incentive (Institute for Family-Centered Care, n.d.). Centers typically begin as a consumer-oriented health library, offering information on community resources and services. Later, the center may expand to include opportunities for peer support, recreational reading and videos, and a space for rest and reflection. Some centers add concierge services, family sleeping rooms, kitchen and laundry areas, learning labs, and family classrooms. Others may set up satellite centers outside the hospital and also participate in community health fairs and school outreach programs.

As noted in Chapter 8, the physical environment plays an important role in psychosocial support for children and their families. The trend for increased attention to environmental details of health-care environments can translate into more informal support as well as more comfortable and humane care for children, families, and caregivers.

Professionals

What is ahead for professionals? At this writing, perhaps the most crucial issue is the nursing shortage. Studies have shown that the higher the patient-to-nurse ratio in the hospital, the more likely there will be patient deaths or complications after surgeries that can lead to death (Aiken, Clarke, Sloane, Sochalski, & Silber, 2002). In a survey by Ludwick and Silva (2003), registered nurses attributed most of their clinical errors and untoward clinical incidents to the nursing shortage.

An aging workforce makes this shortage different from previous ones. Today, about one third of the nursing workforce is over 50 years of age and the average age of full-time nursing faculty is 49 years (Nevidjon & Erickson, 2001). Buerhaus (2000) predicts that 40% of nurses by 2010 will be 50 years old or older. Patient care delivery models may need to be redesigned to support an older workforce, using new technology and offering flexibility in scheduling, increased time off, and sabbaticals.

Will the nursing shortage and other changes affect psychosocial care for children in health-care settings? We already see that faced with less time for each patient, nurses often are forced to abbreviate, but hopefully never eliminate, preparation or other essential elements of psychosocial support. Nursing technicians already have assumed some tasks that were commonly performed by nurses (e.g., checking vital signs). Such tasks provide opportunities to conduct psychosocial assessments and deliver psychosocial support. As this trend is predicted to continue, how can we ensure that critical elements of psychosocial care will not be neglected? Perhaps future training for such personnel will place a greater emphasis on psychosocial content.

The shortage of pediatric subspecialists also will have an impact on children's psychosocial care. The proportion of pediatric residents choosing advanced training declined from 33% in 1986 to 21% in 2001 (National Association of Children's Hospitals and Related Institutions, 2002). This decline is mainly attributed to managed care's focus on primary care, which has guided reduced support for specialist fellowships and reduced reimbursement income for specialists. Within the next 15 years, specific subspecialties are predicted to "age out." Children may have to travel far from home to receive the services of a pediatric subspecialist, resulting in an increase in separation from family members and friends. Health care at a distance also can mean greater disruption for other family members, especially siblings.

In an effort to keep health-care costs down, many health-care services that were traditionally provided by physicians are increasingly being pushed down to less expensive providers (Malugani, 2001). For example, hospitals may use a certified registered nurse anesthetist rather than an anesthesiologist. Physician assistants and nurse practitioners are stepping into other areas in which physicians traditionally have had a monopoly. We must ensure that psychosocial knowledge and skills are essential elements of the education for all health-care professionals who assume these roles.

The increasing percentage of children from racial and ethnic minority groups will influence recruitment efforts for diversity among pediatricians, pediatric nurses, and others in the pediatric health-care workforce. It is projected that by the year 2025, the child population will comprise 15.8% Blacks, 23.6% Hispanics, 1.1% American Indian/Native Alaskans, 6.9% Asian/Pacific Islanders, and 52.6% Whites (*Statistical Abstract of the United States*, 1997). Gray and Stoddard (1997) found that patient and parent satisfaction with care may be higher when the physician is of the same racial or ethnic group as the patient. Does this "sameness" foster trust, which is essential in any caring relationship between children and professionals? More research is needed on the relationship between pediatric workforce diversity and satisfaction, access, quality, and outcomes of pediatric care (AAP, Committee on Pediatric Workforce, 2000).

We are hopeful that more hospitals and other pediatric settings will employ child life specialists. In 2000, the American Academy of Pediatrics (AAP) issued a formal position statement that concluded that child life services make a difference in pediatric care and made the following recommendations (AAP, Committee on Hospital Care, 2000, p. 1158):

1. Child life services are important for children and some of these services may be performed by different health-care professionals. The services could be offered in pediatric settings, including inpatient units, ambulatory units, and emergency departments.
2. Whenever child life services are provided, an adequate ratio of caregivers to patients needs to be developed. This ratio should be adjusted for the severity and acuity of illness of the patients served.
3. Child life services should not be withheld regardless of reimbursement.
4. Home health services may include child life services that help the child and family cope with the child's condition and treatment.

Children in all health-care settings will benefit if these recommendations are followed. However, because of cost implications, this expansion is only likely to occur if families as consumers understand the importance of psychosocial support for their children and the child life specialist's ability to provide such support. Greater efforts must be undertaken to educate families and health-care professionals about the role of the child life specialist as an essential member of the child's health-care team.

Continuum of Care

Parent–professional partnerships will become even more essential as more care shifts to families and from hospital to home. In many instances, this shift occurs without any increase in support. Because of their more frequent contact with the health-care system, families of children with special health-care needs find that partnerships are especially important. Families also need increased collaboration with professionals when accessing educational and other community services for their children. For example, pediatricians, nurses, and other professionals can take a more active role in helping families and educators to create more meaningful Individual Education Plans (IEPs) and Section 504 Plans for children.

Although some health-care professionals currently address the need for transition services as increasing numbers of children with special health-care needs live beyond childhood, much more collaboration and comprehensiveness are needed in this area. Again, health-care professionals can move beyond transition from child to adolescent to adult health-care services, and partner with families in sorting out education opportunities, independent living arrangements, and ongoing or new psychosocial issues related to the child's condition. A current focus on issues for survivors of childhood cancer reflects this trend.

Complementary and Alternative Medicine

Although complementary and alternative medicine (CAM) remedies vary greatly in safety and effectiveness, their use is increasing in the United States. Estimates of pediatric CAM use from children sampled at health-care facilities, with chronic conditions, or from countries other than the United States range from 10% to 15% (Davis & Darden, 2003).

As the use of CAM approaches in the United States increases, especially among children with chronic illness or disability, distinctions among unproven therapies, CAM, and biomedicine may become blurred (AAP,

Committee on Children with Disabilities, 2001). The AAP stresses the importance of providing balanced advice about therapeutic options, guarding against bias, and establishing and maintaining a trusting relationship with families.

Certain complementary therapies may hold special interest for children, especially school-age children who are curious about the world around them. Among all complementary therapies used by nurses in the Unite States, aromatherapy is the fastest growing (Buckle, 2001). Nurses throughout the world have been using aromatherapy during the last 2 decades; however, only recently the U.S. State Boards of Nursing recognized aromatherapy as a legitimate part of holistic nursing. Will children, often more eager to try new things than their adult counterparts, be more likely to use aromatherapy and other CAM methods?

A growing number of individuals consider the use of the arts to be a form of CAM, and, in fact, music was one of the therapies funded for research by the Office of Alternative Medicine (now the National Center for Complementary and Alternative Medicine) in the National Institutes of Health. Each year, more artists join children's health-care teams at hospitals, hospices, and in the home (Rollins & Riccio, 2002). Because of the "playful" nature of many art activities, health-care professionals may be more likely to introduce and integrate the arts into a child's plan of care than into that of an adult.

Research

Advances in medical research should continue at an accelerated rate, with an emphasis on genetic research. When the Human Genome Project formally began in 1990, its original goal was to map and sequence the complete set of human genes by the year 2005. This goal, quite remarkably, was achieved in early 2000. Genetic research holds promise for great strides in the diagnosis and treatment of many childhood diseases. However, emerging genetic technology often enables testing and screening before the development of definitive treatment or preventive measures, opening the door to ethical issues to ensure that the use of this technology promotes the best interests of the child (AAP, Committee on Bioethics, 2001). Chandler and Smith (1998) also pointed out that through striving to eradicate congenital disability, a community risks promoting a cult of perfectionism that may have discriminatory effects on people—whether children or adults—with disabilities.

We may see an increase in research with children in general due to federal funding requirements. In 1996, the National Institutes of Health (NIH) and the American Academy of Pediatrics held a joint workshop concerning the participation of children in clinical research. There was a valid concern that treatment modalities developed based on research conducted on adults, without adequate data from children, were being used to treat children for many diseases and disorders. From this workshop came the recommendation that the NIH develop a policy for including children in clinical research.

> The NIH concluded that when there is a sound scientific rationale for including children in research, investigators should be expected to do so unless there is a strong overriding reason that justifies their exclusion from the studies. Although this is the same scientific rationale that is the basis for the policy requiring the inclusion of women and minorities in clinical research, this policy does not mandate the inclusion of children in all clinical research. Because the issues and sensitivities surrounding children's participation in research are significantly different from those regarding women and minorities, such a mandate would be inappropriate. Nonetheless, even though the inclusion of children is not an absolute requirement, applicants for NIH funding will be expected to address this issue in their proposals. (NIH, 1997, p. 34)

With the likelihood of more children participating in research, researchers will have a greater obligation than ever before to help assure that children have adequate understanding of a research project before assenting or consenting to participation. Creative methods also will need to be devised to help children express their wishes and understanding in nontraditional ways. And, of course, attention to risk factors specific to children's developmental levels will remain a priority. For example, a developmental concern of school-age children is rule conformity. Thus, school-age children are vulnerable to coercion to participate due to respect for authority (Conrad & Horner, 1997). Researchers may need reminders to avoid using authority figures to recruit subjects, to approach a child with his or her parent present, and to reinforce the right to decline to participate.

Future decades likely will see an increase in African American and Latino children's participation in research. A dramatic increase in childhood obesity, especially among African American and Latino children, has stirred the research community. Additionally, ethnic and racial differences have surfaced in other areas. For example, researchers at the Children's Hospital of Pittsburgh in Pennsylvania have released findings that suggest that a significant number of children, mainly African American, may have "double diabetes," Type 1 and Type 2 (National Association of Children's Hospitals and Related Institutions [NACHRI], 2003).

Although race, or ethnicity, and gender often are viewed as variables that exert their effects through innate or genetically determined biologic mechanisms, there is a growing body of research that suggests that these variables have strong—and in may areas predominately—sociologic and psychologic dimensions (AAP, Committee on Pediatric Research, 2000). Studies that do not address the importance of social determinants as fundamental causes or contributors to disease and unfulfilled potential limit the scope and impact of research conclusions (Link & Phelan, 1995).

The American Academy of Pediatrics points out that community-based research with children raises ethical issues not normally encountered in research conducted in academic settings (AAP, Committee on Native American Child Health and Committee on Community Health Services, 2004). Conventional risk–benefits assessments often fail to recognize harms that can occur in socially identifiable populations as a result of research participation. Many such communities will require more stringent measures of beneficence that must be applied directly to the participating communities. In its recommendations, the AAP emphasizes the need for community involvement in the research process.

Outcomes research is of critical importance in exploring the efficacy of interventions. The move from episodic care to a continuum of care emphasizes the need for continued research across all organizational boundaries (Dunham-Taylor, Burton, & Leggett, 1996). The family—"as the constant in a child's life, while the service systems and support personnel within those systems fluctuate" (Shelton & Stepanek, 1994)—likely will be called upon to play a more collaborative role in outcomes research. Health status measures—functional outcome, well-being, or quality of life—are more likely to be used than reliance on medical information alone (Fleming et al., 1998). A multidimensional definition of health encompasses physical, psychological, and social aspects, as well as asking meaningful questions, such as "Can the child participate in normal school activities? Can the child play with friends? Can the child live a life free of painful symptoms?"

End-of-Life Care

The past decade brought an awareness of the need to look at end-of-life issues for everyone, including children. Families with children with life-threatening conditions face many challenges, such as

- lack of funding and limited access to the full scope of services the child and family need, including family support services and bereavement services;
- forced choices between potentially life-prolonging treatment and palliative care services due to funding requirements;
- fragmented care due to multiple providers in a variety of settings; and
- inadequate pain and symptom management. (Dull, 2001)

Several national initiatives, such as The Robert Wood Johnson Foundation's "Promoting Excellence in End-of-Life Care" and Children's Hospice International's Program for All-Inclusive Care for Children and Their Families (PACC) model of care for children with life-threatening conditions, set the stage for a continued focus on end-of-life issues for children in the years to come.

Technology

Technology has been and will continue to be increasingly visible across the health-care continuum. Some hospitals have become nearly paperless in this digital age (Fisher, Bands, Bowlen, & Holbrook-Preston, 2002). Nurses are using handheld computers—small personal computers weighing about 14 ounces—to facilitate real-time documentation. The device stores the majority of the patients' medical record information, including current orders, recent laboratory results, scheduled nursing interventions, and history, which all remain secure through individual security passwords (Fox & Lyon, 1999). The nurse downloads information to the hospital information system throughout the shift through connection ports located throughout the unit. This system is designed to give the nurse more time at the bedside by eliminating the need for one-time charting at the end of shift in the nurses' station. Ideally, for pediatric nurses, a portion of this "saved time" will be devoted to addressing psychosocial issues for children in their care.

Telemedicine—the use of electronic communication and information technologies to provide or support clinical care at a distance (Office for the Advancement of Telehealth, 2001)—is gaining popularity, especially in rural or remote settings. Creative strategies will be needed to meet challenges in some areas of practice, such as appropriate criteria for supervision of nonphysician clinicians, reimbursement for telemedicine services, privacy of patient information, universal standards for telemedicine technologies, professional and medical liability, regulatory and jurisdictional issues related to multistate licensure of clinicians, and high costs of transmission of medical information (AAP, Committee on Pediatric Workforce, 2003). To date, most telemedicine has addressed emergency or critical care. Health-care professionals that recognize the importance of psychosocial care for children must advocate for also addressing psychosocial issues as telemedicine networks are established and expanded.

As nearly half of the children in the United States have Internet access in their homes (Annie E. Casey Foundation, 2003), e-mail transactions between families and providers are becoming more common. E-mail, a hybrid between letter writing and the spoken word, is more spontaneous than letter writing and offers more permanence than oral conversations (Kane & Sands, 1998). Follow-up e-mail allows retention and clarification of advice provided in the health-care setting when parents and children under duress may forget to ask important questions. Educational handouts can be attached to e-mails. Further, e-mail messages are less likely to accidentally fall through the cracks of a busy practice. Several medical groups, including the American Medical Association, have developed guidelines for e-mail use that address topics such as when e-mail should and should not be used, expected response time, who else in the office will have access to messages, and so on. Although current guidelines are intended for adults, with the high level of comfort that even very young children often have with computers

Questions To Consider in Evaluating a Health-Related Web Site	1. Is it clear who has written the information on the Web site? Are his or her credentials listed? Is the author qualified to write on the given topic? 2. Is the site maintained by a credible, reputable, medical organization, government agency, or university? 3. What is the purpose of the Web site? To inform? To persuade? To sell? 4. Is there any potential conflict of interest involved? Does the site sell products? Have commercial advertising? Can you tell who sponsored or paid for this site? 5. What is the source of information on the Web site? Is the information based on clinical or scientific studies? Testimonials? Opinion? Are references provided for information cited on the Web site? 6. Does the Web site seem to provide a balanced, unbiased view? Is a range of reference sources identified? If treatment options are described, how much information and detail are offered regarding options? Are claims of benefits of specific treatments substantiated?

and other technology, can guidelines for the use of e-mail with child patients be far behind?

Families also are accessing the Internet for health-related research through Web sites, newsgroups, chat rooms, and listserves. Ahmann (2000) pointed out that although the use of the Internet can empower consumers, encourage both collaboration and a family-centered approach to care, and could contribute to improved outcomes and cost savings, at the same time, care and caution are needed regarding interpretation of health-related information from this source. The questions in the box can be used by both professionals and families for evaluating a health-related Web site.

Concern for patient privacy has developed as more private health-care information shifts to electronic medical records. To address these concerns, the Health Insurance Portability and Accountability Act (HIPAA) was passed in 1996 and became effective on April 14, 2001, with a 2-year implementation period built in before compliance with the regulation was required. (The Web site http://aspe.hhs.gov/adminsimp/pl104191.htm has a copy of the complete regulation.) Covered entities under HIPAA include health plans, health-care clearinghouses, and certain providers who use computers to transmit health claims information. Regulations cover only the use and disclosure of protected health information, which is any type of information that can be used to identify the subject. It also establishes the legal right for individuals to see and copy their own health information and request corrections. Children and families may need help in interpreting the regulation and health information. Will more meaningful child–parent–professional partnerships develop as an outcome of such interactions?

7. How current is the information? When was the site produced? Updated?
8. Does the Web site provide a means of contacting its webmaster?

Sources

DISCERN Instrument
www.discern.org.uk/
Click on "Discern"; click on "discern instrument."

HONCode Site-Checker
www.hon.ch/HONcode_check.html

Information Quality (IQ) Tool
www.hitiweb.mitretek.org/iq

Siwek, J. (April 25, 2000). One last piece of advice. *The Washington Post,* Health Section, p. 23.

The Quality Information Checklist (QUICK)
www.quick.org.uk/menu.htm

Note. From "Supporting Families' Savvy Use of the Internet for Health Research," by E. Ahmann, 2000, *Pediatric Nursing, 26*(4), p. 421. Copyright 2000 by Jannetti. Reprinted with permission.

Care for the Caregiver

A family-centered approach to care embraces caring for caregivers as well as the patient. Although progress has been made in addressing some of the many needs of family caregivers, initiatives for professional caregivers have not kept pace. Institutions must apply the principles of family-centered care to their own "family." Dissemination of information about successful programs, such as the Days of Renewal program for caregivers at Shands Hospital in Gainesville, Florida, can provide a starting point for others to develop model programs for caregivers in their institutions (Graham-Pole, Sonke, & Henderson, 2004).

2020

What will health care look like in the year 2020? In 1998, D'Amaro predicted that in 2020 technology will allow consumers to monitor their health just as easily as making a cup of coffee. CAM therapies, such as acupuncture, massage therapy, and aromatherapy will be taken for granted as a synergistic element of overall health. There will be more specialized facilities for conditions such as diabetes and arthritis. Organizational leaders will embrace consumerism and service will be king.

D'Amaro (1998) anticipated that with these changes, managed care organizations will change dramatically—from intermediaries that process claims, perform utilization management, and manage financial risk, to patient-friendly care facilitators. Instead of dictating what patients must do, managed care will focus on helping to integrate health management and patient care into daily life. Doctors will extend their practices to personal wellness and health management counseling. In place of an HMO panel of 2,000 patients, doctors will differentiate themselves from other practices by developing more involved and specialized relationships with fewer patients. We already see evidence of this happening in the concierge doctor movement, which at this time is only accessible to the financially privileged.

According to D'Amaro (1998),

> Though the road toward a fully consumer-sensitive system will have many unexpected twists and turns, momentum for such a system is increasing every day. Like many journeys, the arrival may not be readily perceived, but the progress along the way will surely be worth the trip. (p. 3)

How these predicted changes translate for children and their families remains to be seen. Considering the number of children without health insurance coverage in our nation today, a system such as that expected by D'Amaro seems far removed. However, without defining the elements of a sensitive, respectful, humane, and family-centered health-care system for all children that values psychosocial as well as physical care, how will we know what steps to take to get there, and how will we know when we have arrived?

References

Ahmann, E. (2000). Supporting families' savvy use of the Internet for health research. *Pediatric Nursing, 26*(4), 419–423.

Aiken, L., Clarke, S., Sloane, D., Sochalski, J., & Silber, J. (2002). Hospital nurse staffing and patient mortality, nurse burnout, and job dissatisfaction. *Journal of the American Medical Association, 288*(16), 1987–1993.

American Academy of Pediatrics, Committee on Bioethics. (2001). Ethical issues with genetic testing in pediatrics. *Pediatrics, 107*(6), 1451–1455.

American Academy of Pediatrics, Committee on Children with Disabilities. (2001). Counseling families who choose complementary and alternative medicine for their child with chronic illness or disability. *Pediatrics, 107*(3), 598–601.

American Academy of Pediatrics, Committee on Hospital Care. (2000). Child life services. *Pediatrics, 106*(5), 1156–1159.

American Academy of Pediatrics, Committee on Native American Child Health and Committee on Community Health Services. (2004). Ethical considerations in research with socially identifiable populations. *Pediatrics, 113*(1), 148–151.

American Academy of Pediatrics, Committee on Pediatric Research. (2000). Race/ethnicity, gender, socioeconomic status—Research exploring their effects on child health: A subject review. *Pediatrics, 105*(6), 1349–1351.

American Academy of Pediatrics, Committee on Pediatric Workforce. (2000). Enhancing the racial and ethnic diversity of the pediatric workforce. *Pediatrics, 105*(1), 129–131.

American Academy of Pediatrics, Committee on Pediatric Work. (2003). Scope of practice issues in the delivery of pediatric health care. *Pediatrics, 111*(2), 426–435.

Annie E. Casey Foundation. (2004). *KidsCount.* Baltimore: Author.

Boodman, S. (1999). The education of Dr. Kulick. *The Washington Post Health, 15*(5), 12–15, 17.

Brandner, J. (1995). Will hospital rounds go the way of the house call? *Managed Care, 4*(7), 25–28.

Buckle, J. (2001). The role of aromatherapy in nursing care. *Nursing Clinics of North America, 36*(1), 57–72.

Buerhaus, P. (2000). Implications of an aging registered nurse workforce. *Journal of the American Medical Association, 283*(22), 2948–2954.

Chandler, M., & Smith, A. (1998). Prenatal screening and women's perception of infant disability: A Sophie's choice for every mother. *Nursing Inquiry, 5,* 71–76.

Conrad, B., & Horner, S. (1997). Issue in pediatric research: Safeguarding the children. *Journal of the Society of Pediatric Nurses, 2*(4), 163–171.

D'Armaro, R. (1998). Checkup 2020. *Hospitals & Health Networks, 72*(17), 3, 18, 20.

Davis, M., & Darden, P. (2003). Use of complementary and alternative medicine by children in the United States. *Archives of Pediatric Adolescent Medicine, 157*(4), 393–396.

Dull, S. (2001, Fall). Enhancing the quality of life for dying children. *Children's Hospitals Today.* Retrieved on May 31, 2003, from www.childrenshospitals.net/content/contentGroups/Publications/Childrens_Hospitals_Today/Articles/20016/Enhancing_the_Quality_of_Life_for_Dying_Children.htm

Dunham-Taylor, J., Burton, J., & Leggett, V. (1996). Leading the research initiative: The role of the nurse manager. *Seminars in Nurse Management, 4*(4), 234–239.

Epstein, D. (1997). The role of "hospitalists" in the health care system. *New England Journal of Medicine, 336,* 444.

Fisher, J., Bands, J., Bowlen, N., & Holbrook-Preston, S. (2002). Straight talk: New approaches in healthcare. The digital hospital comes of age. *Modern Healthcare, 32*(43), 59–62.

Fleming, G., Olson, L., Asmussen, L., Risley, K., Couto, J., & Prassas, M. (1998). *Functional outcomes project.* Accessed September 7, 1998, from www.aap.org/research/outcome.htm

Fottler, M., Ford, R., Roberts, V., & Ford, E. (2000). Creating a healing environment: The importance of the service setting in the new consumer-oriented healthcare system. *Journal of Healthcare Management, 45*(2), 91–106.

Fox, L., & Lyon, K. (1999). Real-time documentation: Hand-held computers. *Nursing Spectrum, 9*(4), 4–5.

Graham-Pole, J., Sonke, J., & Henderson, J. (2004). The University of Florida Center for the Arts and Health Research and Education "Days of Renewal" program, a case study. In L. Kable (Ed.), *Caring for caregivers: A grassroots USA–Japan initiative* (pp. 21–28). Washington, DC: Society for the Arts in Healthcare.

Gray, B., & Stoddard, J. (1997). Patient-physician pairing: Does racial and ethnic congruity influence selection of a regular physician? *Journal of Community Health, 22,* 247–259.

Henry, L. (1997). Will hospitalists assume family physicians' inpatient care roles? *Family Practice Management, 4*(7), 54–60, 65–66, 69.

Institute for Family-Centered Care. (n.d.). *Patient & family resource centers.* Retrieved May 31, 2003, from www.familycenteredcare.org/special_topics/familyresource/main.html

Kane, B., & Sands, D. (1998). Guidelines for the clinical use of electronic mail with patients. *Journal of the American Medical Informatics Association, 5*(1), 104–111.

Link, B., & Phelan, J. (1995). Social conditions as fundamental causes of disease. *Journal of Health and Social Behavior, Spec No: 80–94.*

Ludwick, R., & Silva, M. (2003). Errors, the nursing shortage and ethics: Survey results. *Online Journal of Issues in Nursing.* Retrieved July 25 from www.nursingworld.org/ojin/ethicol/ethics_12.htm

Malugani, M. (2001). *Who's hot and who's not: Trends in healthcare recruiting.* Retrieved August 19, 2003, from http://www.jasneek.com/traveler/who_hot_who%27s_not.asp

McConaghy, J. (1998). The emerging role of hospitalists: Will family physicians continue to practice hospital medicine? *Journal of the American Board of Family Practice, 11*(4), 324–326.

Morasch, L. (1998). The hospitalist: A threat to the family physician? *Hospital Practice, 33*(7), 117–119.

National Association of Children's Hospitals and Related Institutions (NACHRI). (2002). The shortage of pediatric subspecialists: What can children's hospitals do? *Children's Hospitals Today.* Retrieved May 31, 2003, from www.childrenshospitals.net/nachri/aboutn/cht_subspecialistshortage.html

National Association of Children's Hospitals and Related Institutions (NACHRI). (2003). Children's hospitals on cutting-edge of pediatric research. *Child Health Trends Update, 2*(3). Retrieved July 25, 2004, from http://www.childrenshospitals.net/Content/Content Groups/Media_Center1/Child_Health_Trends_Update1/2003/Child_Health_Trends_ Update_-_Pediatric_Research_and _Obesity.htm

National Institutes of Health (NIH). (1997). Policy on the inclusion of children as subjects in clinical research. *NIH Guide, 26*(3), 34.

Nelson, D. (2003). The high cost of being poor. In *Kids count 2003* (pp. 11–33). Baltimore: Annie E. Casey Foundation.

Nevidjon, B., & Erickson, J. (2001). The nursing shortage: Solutions for the short and long term. *Online Journal of Issues in Nursing, 6*(1), Manuscript 4. Accessed August 20, 2003, from www.nursingworld.org/ojin/topic14/tpc14_4.htm

Office for the Advancement of Telehealth. (2001). *2001 Report to Congress on telemedicine.* Rockville, MD: Author.

Robert Wood Johnson Foundation. (1998). Covering Kids expands program and funding. *Advances, 4,* 9, 12.

Rollins, J., & Riccio, L. (2002). ART is the heART: A palette of possibilities for hospice care. *Pediatric Nursing, 28*(4), 355–362.

Ryan, C. (1997). Writer questions the inevitability of FPs' declining role in inpatient care. *Family Medicine, 29,* 382–383.

Shelton, T., & Stepanek, J. (1994). *Family-centered care for children needing specialized health and developmental services.* Bethesda, MD: Association for the Care of Children's Health.

Shortell, S., Gillies, R., & Devers, K. (1995). Reinventing the American hospital. *Milbank Quarterly, 73*(2), 131–160.

Statistical Abstract of the United States: 1997 (117th ed.). (1997). Washington, DC: U.S. Government Printing Office.

Wachter, R., & Goldman, L. (1996). The emerging role of "hospitalists" in the American healthcare system. *New England Journal of Medicine, 335,* 514–517.

Wielawski, I. (1998). Rationing medical care: The growing gulf between what's medically available and what's affordable. *Advances, 4*(Suppl.), 1–4.

Index

About the Authors and Contributors

Authors

Judy A. Rollins, PhD, RN, Rollins & Associates, Inc., Washington, DC, is a nurse with a fine arts degree in the visual arts, an MS in child development and family studies, and a PhD in health and community studies. She is an adjunct instructor in the Department of Family Medicine at Georgetown University School of Medicine in Washington, DC, and associate editor of *Pediatric Nursing*. Dr. Rollins consults, writes, and researches on children's issues, with a special interest in the use of the arts for children in health-care settings and a focus on children with cancer and their families.

Rosemary Bolig, PhD, is currently on the faculties of the University of the District of Columbia and Walden University as a professor of early childhood education. Formerly a faculty member at The Ohio State University and at Mount Vernon College, Dr. Bolig has published many articles on children in health care, children under stress, and child life programs. She has been an advocate for change in children's health care and a recipient of the Child Life Council's Outstanding Contributor award.

Carmel C. Mahan, MSEd, CCLS, is currently an early intervention specialist with the Baltimore County Public School System in Baltimore, Maryland. She has a BS in Human Development and Family Relations from the University of Connecticut and a MSEd in Special Education from Fordham University. She has over 20 years' experience as a child life specialist in a variety of acute-care settings. She has published articles and a chapter for a nursing textbook as well as co-authoring a book with Dr. Rollins on training for artist-in-residence programs. She and Dr. Rollins have collaborated on a number of projects to benefit children and families in health-care settings and to educate the professionals who care for them about their psychosocial needs. This is her first collaboration with Dr. Bolig.

549

Contributors

Elizabeth Ahmann, ScD, RN, has a background in nursing and public health. She has written numerous articles on family-centered care and families of children with illness and disability, and is section editor of the "Family Matters" column in *Pediatric Nursing*. She is a consultant in private practice in Cheverly, Maryland, and adjunct faculty at Columbia University School of Nursing, New York, New York.

Lynn B. Clutter, MSN, RN, BC, CNS, has over 25 years of experience in nursing of children and families. She is a nursing instructor at Langston University, Tulsa, and a certified doula and childbirth educator. She has worked in a variety of hospital and clinical settings, primarily in pediatrics, and has served as an instructor in the nursing schools of Oral Roberts University, the University of Tulsa, and Tulsa Community College. She has applied her clinical nurse specialist role toward parish nursing, adoption, and assisting adolescents with pregnancy, labor, and delivery. Her research and publications have focused on spiritual care, bonding and attachment, and children's pain.

Lacretia Johnson, MA, is the assistant director of student life for community service at the University of Vermont. She was the coordinator of service-learning of College Park Scholars Living and Learning Community at the University of Maryland, and a former artist-in-residence for the Studio G program at Georgetown University Medical Center and WVSA Arts Connections' ART is the heART, an arts-in-health-care program for children and families in home and hospice care.

David A. Julian, PhD, is a co–principal investigator for Partnerships for Success Academy at the Center for Learning Excellence, The John Glenn Institute for Public Service & Public Policy in Columbus, Ohio. He was educated at Miami University in Oxford, Ohio, The Ohio State University in Columbus, Ohio, and Michigan State University in East Lansing, Michigan. His teaching and research interests include community psychology and program evaluation.

Teresa W. Julian, PhD, RN, CFNP, is a research investigator at Columbus Children's Research Institute, Columbus Children's Hospital, Inc.; and a clinical assistant professor in the Department of Psychiatry at the College of Medicine at The Ohio State University in Columbus, Ohio. She received her education from Southeast Missouri State University, the University of Tennessee, and The Ohio State University. Her teaching and research interests include families and health, violence, and substance abuse.

Lois J. Pearson, MEd, CCLS, has been a child life specialist for more than 20 years, first starting a child life program in a community hospital. For the past 17 years, she has worked at Children's Hospital of Wisconsin in Milwaukee in the Intensive Care Unit. She also facilitates an ongoing support group for children who have experienced the death of a parent.

Mardelle McCuskey Shepley, DArch, is a registered architect and professor in the College of Architecture at Texas A&M University. She is also associate dean for student services and the associate director of the Center for Health Systems & Design. Dr. Shepley received her BA and MArch degrees from Columbia University and an MA (psychology) and DArch from the University of Michigan. Dr. Shepley currently serves on the research committees of the Coalition for Health Environments Research and the Center for Health Design. Co-author of *Healthcare Environments for Children and Their Families*, she has published more than 40 articles and book chapters.

Teresa A. Savage, PhD, RN, has over 30 years of experience in the nursing of children. Her interest in ethics grew from the issues encountered in neonatal care and follow-up, but expanded to include all aspects of bioethics. She served as an ethics consultant at a major academic medical center in the Midwest while a clinical nurse specialist in joint practice with a pediatric neurology service. She has taught pediatrics at four universities. Currently she is associate director of the Center for the Study of Disability Ethics at the Rehabilitation Institute of Chicago, and is an assistant professor, research, in Maternal–Child Nursing at the University of Illinois at Chicago College of Nursing. Her research interests include parental decision making regarding life-sustaining treatment for children with significant disabilities, and informed consent in adults with intellectual disabilities.